Elements of
RESEARCH IN NURSING

Elements of
RESEARCH IN NURSING

Eleanor Walters Treece, R.N., B.A., M.Ed., Ph.D.

James William Treece, Jr., B.R.E., B.A., M.A.

with 115 illustrations

FOURTH EDITION

The C. V. Mosby Company

ST. LOUIS • TORONTO • PRINCETON   1986

Editor: Nancy L. Mullins
Assistant editor: Maureen Slaten
Production coordination: Publication Services
Book design: Diane M. Beasley
Cover design: Christine Leonard Raquepaw

FOURTH EDITION

The C.V. Mosby Company
11830 Westline Industrial Drive
St. Louis, Missouri 63146

Library of Congress Cataloging-in-Publication Data

Treece, Eleanor Mae Walters.
  Elements of research in nursing.

  Includes bibliographies and index.
  1. Nursing—Research. I. Treece, James William.
II. Title. [DNLM: 1. Nursing. 2. Research.
WY 20.5 T786e]
RT81.5.T7 1986   610.73'072   85–25899
ISBN 0-8016-5105-0

PS/VH/VH 9 8 7 6 5 4 3 2 1   01/C/033

PREFACE

Keeping with nursing research has become a monumental task. When the first edition of this textbook was published, the number of articles and books written by nurses was considerably limited. Now there are so many references that it is impossible to complete a list without overlooking important names. In 1973, when the first edition of *Elements of Research in Nursing* was published, many nurses who were only beginning to develop research skills are now directing sophisticated nursing research projects and holding positions as directors in health care institutions worldwide.

In accordance with our original intentions, we have tried to keep the book readable, concise, and practical. We expect our readers to be able to conduct and critique research as well as apply findings in the appropriate situations.

Elements of Research in Nursing is a comprehensive textbook for students learning research methodology as part of their educational program and a guide for individuals who want to learn the principles of scientific investigation. We have found that the book is useful for undergraduate and graduate students on an international basis. The additions, deletions, and modifications contained in this edition are the results of several overseas teaching assignments to nurses and nonnurses.

Suggestons, recommendations, and personal experience have resulted in several chapter additions and rearrangements. Additional chapters, figures, and a glossary have been included. The rationale for some chapter and content rearrangement is to present a more coherent and useful order and to prevent the user from having to refer to future chapters to learn something that should have been covered earlier. Some chapters which covered the same general topic have been combined and new chapters and sections have been added or expanded based on reviewer suggestions or requests.

Guidelines are provided so that students can learn to write each step of their research project as it is planned and implemented. By the time students complete these research projects, they will have prepared the entire research report in rough draft form.

Some class activities and discussion questions have been rearranged or revised.

The fourth edition has been divided into six parts. Part One, The Research Process, deals with an introduction to research and includes a chapter on research and nursing.

Part Two, Preparation for Quantitative Research, reviews scientific method, critiquing, the research problem and question, and the relationship between theory and method.

Part Three, Preparation for Collecting Data, comprises Chapters 7 to 15. These chapters cover the library search, designing and conducting a study, proposals and grants, ethics, hypotheses, relationship between variables, approaches to research, the sample and sampling, the instrument, and reliability and validity.

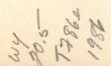

Part Four, Collecting Data, includes some discussion about questionnaires, interviews, records, observations, other techniques, the pilot study, and pretesting the instrument.

Part Five, Analyzing Data, contains three chapters which encompass the following topics: the analyzing process, descriptive and statistical data analysis, and the evaluation process.

Part Six, Presentation of Findings, is made up of three chapters concerning writing the research report, publishing, and the critical consumer.

The fourth edition came together during busy and exciting times. As professors at Liberty University, we have continued to pursue our usual administrative and teaching responsibilities while enrollment has doubled. Our private lives have been filled with exposure to several foreign cultures and professional meetings. These activities add yet another dimension to this edition.

We are especially grateful to Beverly Jean Kreider, our work-study student who typed most of the manuscript. Deborah Ann Cherry, another student, cheerfully sacrificed her time during the desperate race to the finish. Again, we hope that you will enjoy our product.

Eleanor Walters Treece
James William Treece

CONTENTS

PART ONE

THE RESEARCH PROCESS

Chapter 1 is an introduction to the subject of research and, more specifically, to nursing research. Other topics include definitions of nursing research, problems of research, and research and health.

Chapter 2 deals with nursing research in greater depth. We consider the reasons that research is needed in nursing, the nurse who enters the research field, the different kinds of studies that have been carried out in nursing, and those that are needed. Finally, there is a discussion concerning the trends in nursing research.

CHAPTER 1

INTRODUCTION

The importance of research in nursing continues to grow with each successive year. Nurses must be able to understand the accumulating quantities of research literature in order to apply the results to health care needs. For this reason, an appreciation for and skills in research should be developed early in undergraduate nursing programs.

Research takes time—it cannot be hurried. It also takes time to develop research skills through practice. For a beginning course in research methodology to be meaningful, it is important that a complete study be carried out so that the entire research process can be learned and understood. This means that the study should begin with a research proposal and conclude with the written research report. It is only through carrying out the complete process that a person can learn from experience and errors. One beginning researcher verbalized the feelings of many students, "I really learned more from my errors than from lectures and reading." We expect, therefore, that the steps of the research process will be practiced as they are discussed in the following chapters.

DEFINITIONS OF RESEARCH

Research in its broadest sense is an attempt to gain solutions to problems. More precisely, it is the collection of data in a rigorously controlled situation for the purpose of prediction or explanation. Every discipline relies heavily on research. Barnes says that "research is a way of dealing with ideas. It is nothing more than this, and it is nothing less. Most research deals with ideas."[1]

Sweeney and Oliveri point out that the goal of nursing research is to expand the theoretical foundation of nursing.[2] According to Best, "The terms *research* and *scientific method* are sometimes used synonymously...." in the educational field, although, some differences are recognized: "*research* is considered to be the more formal, systematic, and intensive process of carrying on a scientific method of analysis" for the purpose of "discovery and the development of an organized body of knowledge."[3] In problem

---

[1] Barnes, Fred P.: Research for the practitioner in education, Washington, D.C., © 1964, National Association of Elementary School Principals, NEA, p. 13. All rights reserved.
[2] Sweeney, M.A. and Olivieri, P.: An introduction to nursing research, Philadelphia, 1981, J.B. Lippincott Co., p. 28.
[3] Best, John W.: Research in education, ed. 4, Englewood Cliffs, N.J., © 1981, Prentice-Hall, Inc., p. 18.

solving, the *scientific method* "may be an informal application of problem identification, hypothesis formulation, observation, analysis, and conclusion."[4] Research projects range from major studies funded by grants to individual investigations conducted to meet the requirements of a course. Research may be implemented during working hours or carried out on personal time. Barnes suggests that projects may be as ambitious or as simple as the researcher desires:

> And if it is steeped in humility, so much the better. Far from being an inordinately complicated set of distant rituals dressed in a white gown, research is best when it becomes as personal and comfortable as a well-worn suit of clothes with baggy trousers.[5]

In a narrow sense, research is a manner or method of inquiry which is conducted in essentially the same manner in all disciplines. All professions utilize their own theoretical perspective, but the potential methods of investigation are similar.

Research also is a state or condition of the mind which attempts to be objective. It is a conscientious effort to find factual evidence of both the positive and the negative aspects of a phenomenon.

Nursing researchers must realize that all research questions cannot be answered by dealing with quantities; sometimes they must be studied with qualitative processes. Innovative techniques must be developed and the fresh insight of beginning researchers can prove fruitful.

Perhaps the term research has a frightening connotation because it is often accompanied by the stereotype of formality, advanced educational preparation, secluded rooms with specialized equipment, and limited socialization. Because of this stereotype, students tend to be apprehensive about their ability to carry out a project successfully. They often feel they are incapable of doing worthwhile research. And yet, if they are asked to do a small study, the request seems more reasonable. Is not research equivalent to a study?

PURPOSE OF RESEARCH

Research without purpose is meaningless. Students sometimes feel that an assignment to carry out a research project for a class is nothing more than that—an assignment. It is important to remember that the goal of research is finding answers to problems or questions. If beginning researchers will spend their time investigating a question or a hunch that will give a meaningful answer not only to themselves but to others who might be curious about the same question or problem, they will discover that research can be stimulating and exciting. Since research can be interesting, those who carry it out can expect to receive satisfaction and enjoyment as a concomitant result of their effort.

A course in research methodology and techniques sometimes becomes an end in itself; topics selected by students bear no relationship to one another and are not replicated by subsequent student researchers. If, within a given school of nursing or laboratory setting, the majority of students would carry out their research projects as replications or

---

[4]*Ibid.*, p. 8.
[5]Barnes, p. 10.

extensions of those already reported, not only would students have an opportunity to develop research skills, but with their findings could verify and add to the stockpile of existing research in nursing.

One nursing class pursued a single theme, "The image of the nurse." All students were instructed to design a study dealing with perceptions. The sample was to be selected from individuals on campus. Each student chose a different focus of the theme from a list generated during a brainstorming session. Then they developed their projects based on their particular topic. Some of the topics were:

How much education does a nurse have?

What courses do nurses take?

What socioemotional characteristics do nurses have?

What socioemotional characteristics should nurses have?

Students selected various segments of the campus population including other students, secretaries, and security guards. Their findings were used to plan strategies for advising, recruiting, and educating potential students and consumers about nursing.

The chief reason for conducting research is to find answers to queries by means of scientific methodology. To be answerable by research, questions must be conceived that will produce answers through some form of data collection either quantitative or qualitative. The scientific research question is precise, is based on prior knowledge, and allows the researcher to test conditions and influences as they affect each other. Obviously there are many different ways to discuss research; each discipline has its own particular methods and each researcher has some pet ways of approaching a problem.

Research points in a number of directions: nursing practice, nursing services, nursing service administration, nursing education, the practitioner, and consumer client.

Depending on their individual area of concern and interest, researchers eventually become experts within their sphere of investigation. They are expected to share information regarding their methods as well as findings in the form of oral presentations and publications for use by students, nurse-researchers, and interested persons representing other professions.

Nursing research as an academic process provides the same benefits as research in any other disciplines.

1. It can develop new techniques of nursing intervention.
2. It can be used to evaluate the utility of new nursing techniques and processes.
3. It can provide the tools for assessing and evaluating new nursing interventions.
4. It can provide answers to problems concerning health maintenance, health delivery, and health care.
5. It can help in determining areas of need relating to education, patient/client teaching, interpersonal relations, and employment.
6. It can provide the impetus for disseminating research findings related to nursing and health care.

In a more abstract and broad manner, Schlotfeldt declares that "the ultimate aim of research is the ordering of related, valid generalizations into systematized science."[6]

[6]Schlotfeldt, Rozella M.: Reflections on nursing research, Am. J. Nurs. **60**:493, April 1960. © American Journal of Nursing Co.

Page reminds us that the value of science is not that it is infallible but that it can correct itself when in error.[7]

Some argue that research is not needed for all decision making. Rarely do we use research for our personal, emergency, and emotion-laden decisions. We tend to base our judgments on experience, tradition, or professional opinions. Nevertheless, a need to undertake research is justified, but it is impractical to believe that all decision making will ever be based on research. Research, however, can benefit us personally and result in a contribution to others and to the nursing profession.

KINDS OF RESEARCH

Research is categorized according to different points of view. It is generally divided into two types: basic and applied. The goal of basic research is knowledge for its own sake, which differs from applied research in which practical application for the theoretical or abstract knowledge is sought. In other words, in basic research, the researcher is trying to find truth, and in applied research, the truth is adapted to the everyday situation.

Hayes believes that pure research is done for the intellectual pleasure of learning, whereas applied research results from present problems or from socially disorganized situations. The nurse-researcher should be involved in both types of research.[8]

Ackoff distinguishes between pure and applied research on the basis of answering a question or solving a problem. Pure and applied types of research have a reciprocal relationship since eventually most pure research filters down into real life situations and applied research frequently raises theoretical questions that must be answered by pure research. Pure research should be tested for errors by applying it in a measurable situation.[9]

Steward contends that basic research also endeavors to fill the gaps in current knowledge.[10] Nursing professionals are rapidly identifying such gaps as they gain research skills and more insight into their own discipline.

In order to conduct basic research, the investigator must have a breadth and depth of understanding about the components of a discipline as well as its relationship to other sciences. Ability to deal with the abstract, with ideas, and with mental images is important.

Researchers who conduct applied research specialize in the concrete; therefore, they have less need to deal with the abstract as they solve problems and investigate day-to-day phenomena. Both types of research are necessary and one type is not more important than the other.

Best refers to three types of research, based on the time element. Historical research, the first type, describes what *was*; descriptive research describes what *is*; and experimental

[7] Page, Ellis B.: Accentuate the negative, Educational Researcher **4**(4):4, April 1975. © American Educational Research Association.

[8] Hayes, Marjorie: Nursing research is *not* every nurse's business, Can. Nurse **70**(10):17, October 1974.

[9] Ackoff, Russell L., Gupta, Shiv K., and Minas, J. Sayer: Scientific method optimizing applied research decisions, New York, 1968, John Wiley & Sons, Inc. © 1962 by John Wiley & Sons, Inc., pp. 7–8, 24.

[10] Stewart, D.W.: Secondary research information sources and methods, Beverly Hills, 1984, Sage Publications, Inc., p. 16. Applied social research methods series Vol. 4.

research describes what *will be* when certain variables are carefully controlled and manipulated.[11]

Dickoff, James, and Semradek discuss eight-to-four research, sometimes called implementation or reality research. An attempt is made to integrate judgments concerning methodology, nursing care, and remaining factors.[12]

Weiss compares the analytic and holistic approaches to research. In the analytic approach the researcher attempts to identify and isolate the components of the research situation, whereas the holistic approach begins with the total situation, focusing attention on the system and its internal relationships.[13]

Altschul identifies another category of research, called action research. This type is consumer oriented and deals with health care procedures on the part of both the nurse and the patient.[14]

For the purpose of reporting nursing research abstracts, the journal *Nursing Research* has divided the subject into six categories: general, behavioral sciences, education, health care systems, health manpower, nursing practice, and related care. The major areas then have a variety of subdivisions.

Kosekoff and Fink point out that the term evaluation is used in at least three ways in research: evaluation research, evaluation survey, and evaluation process.[15]

Evaluation research developed and grew into a discipline as a result of the proliferation of human services programs that began during World War II. Because public money was used to create these programs, questions of worth and merit demanded answers. Evaluation practice and evaluation research were initially influenced by such researchers as Campbell, Stanley, Scriven, and Donabedian. The development of terminology, concepts, and perspectives enhanced the evaluation approach to research. Most federal agencies now require an evaluation component in human services programs.

Evaluation is the systematic appraisal of a phenomenon through the use of a set of procedures. Evaluation research is commonly conducted to rate the extent to which a program has attained its goals considering such factors as cost, impact, activities, and results. Evaluation of innovative programs is especially important because it adds to the knowledge base of a discipline. However, the measurement of changes in attitude, behavior, knowledge, and values resulting from public and educational programs is hindered by an inadequate number of valid and reliable tools and comparison-experimental groups.

The evaluation survey, which is discussed in Chapter 12, is one type of descriptive research in which data are collected to provide a critical inspection or a comprehensive view of the situation. The evaluation survey determines and reports the findings as they currently exist.

Chapter 24 focuses on the evaluation process as it is related to a research project. After the data have been collected, the raw data must be prepared for analysis. The researcher

[11] Best, p. 15.

[12] Dickoff, James, James, Patricia, and Semradek, Joyce: Eight-to-four research. Part I: A stance for nursing research—tenacity or inquiry, Nurs. Res. **24**(2):84, March–April 1975.

[13] Weiss, Robert S.: Alternative approaches in the study of complex situations. Human Organization **25**(3):199, Fall 1966. © 1967 by The Society of Applied Anthropology, University of Kentucky, Lexington, Ky.

[14] Altschul, Annie: Beginning and end, Nurs. Times **70**(19):718, May 9, 1974.

[15] Kosekoff, J. and Fink A.: Evaluation basics, Beverly Hills, 1982, Sage Publications, Inc., p. 21.

then interprets the meaning of the results as it is related to the phenomenon under study, to other individuals or groups, and to future research. Decisions concerning the phenomenon result from the arbitrary evaluation by the researcher.

CHARACTERISTICS OF RESEARCH

Certain characteristics have been attributed to research, and Best has cited such characteristics:

1. Research involves gathering new data or using existing data for a new purpose from primary or firsthand sources....
2. Research is directed toward the solution of a problem....
3. Although research activity may, at times, be somewhat unsystematic, it is more often characterized by carefully designed procedures, always applying rigorous analysis....
4. Research emphasizes the development of generalizations, principles, or theories that will be helpful in predicting future occurrences....
5. Research requires expertise....
6. Research demands accurate observation and description....
7. Research strives to be objective and logical, applying every possible test to validate the procedures employed, the data collected, and the conclusions reached....
8. Research is characterized by patient and unhurried activity....
9. Research sometimes requires courage....
10. Research is carefully recorded and reported....[16]

When we are told about the results of a research project or read a study for ourselves, certain factors must be considered as we think through what we have learned. Fox and Kelly have suggested five guidelines. First, identify the problem that was investigated, and second, consider who did the study. Third, give attention to the methodology that was used to answer the question. Fourth, notice which of the potential data sources were selected. Finally, consider the process of analysis, the conclusions, and the implications of the findings for people in general, for nursing, and for nurses.[17]

Other characteristics of research are concerned with the process of investigation. These characteristics are inherent within the actual procedure for conducting research. The following list describes the distinct characteristics that serve as the foundation of research.

1. Research is concerned with facts and their meaning and relationships.
2. Research is the result of a question that has intrigued the investigator.
3. The guiding principle of research is the development of tentative explanations.
4. In the process of thinking about the research project, the investigator develops a plan or strategy of approach.
5. Data (measures of quantity and quality) are collected for the purpose of testing the tentative explanation.
6. On the basis of the data, answers are found which lend insight into and knowledge about the question.

[16] Best, pp. 18–20.
[17] Fox, David J., and Kelly, Ruth Lundt: The research process in nursing, New York, 1967, Appleton-Century-Crofts, p. 17. © 1967 by David J. Fox and Ruth L. Kelly.

7. The new information stimulated additional insights and suggests new problems.
8. Research results in the discovery of new knowledge about the real world.

LIMITATIONS OF RESEARCH

The word *limitations* has two connotations in research. The first refers to the limitations or weaknesses that are the result of faulty planning and implementation of the project. These are recognized by the researcher and reported to the reader. The second connotation is the composite of situations that exists at the moment an investigation is begun. The research consumer and reader should be aware of the extent of their existence.

The limitations of the individual researcher may also be a factor. Does he or she have sufficient background and skills to study the subject area, to identify the problem, and to carry through the research process? If not, then the necessary skills must be developed.

The scope of knowledge or information available about the topic and the problem under study also must be considered. How much information is already available?

Finally, the tools of measurement may be inadequate or entirely lacking. The correct instruments must be used to assess and analyze data. What kind of tools are available or needed for obtaining and evaluating data?

In summary, the ability of the researcher and the availability of an adequate amount of knowledge and correct tools of measurement are major limitations of research.

DEFINITIONS OF NURSING RESEARCH

We have been looking at research from various points of view, and now we turn our attention to nursing research. In what way is this different from research in general? Nursing research is only one area of research, one piece of the whole pie, so to speak. Therefore, when we discuss nursing research we are talking about one type of research—that which is related to the whole of nursing.

Nursing research includes the breadth and depth of the discipline of nursing: the rehabilitative, therapeutic, and preventive aspects of nursing, as well as the preparation of practitioners and personnel involved in the total nursing sphere.

Nursing research may not actually be different from research in general, although it utilizes additional tools of measurement for those activities peculiar to nursing (for example, clinical nursing).

There is no need for nursing research to be carried out in isolation. Cooperation among disciplines leads to greater insight into a given problem or question. Nurses should profit by the knowledge available in other fields and the weaknesses cited by researchers in other disciplines. Assuming that nursing research is based on insight gained by others, nurse-researchers should not be guilty of repeating the same errors in research methodology and techniques that pioneers in research have made. It is important that tools perfected by other disciplines and deemed appropriate for nursing be utilized in nursing research. Fortunately, creative thinking is now being done by nurse-researchers so that new tools, unique to the profession, are being developed.

Since the nursing process takes place in a milieu of human behavior and personal relationships, it seems reasonable that nursing research relies heavily on the methods used in the behavioral science field. The behavioral sciences deal with people, as do nurses; both assess needs, observe, and evaluate. The difference lies in the fact that the behavioral sciences theoretically are not geared to making changes.

Nursing education can benefit from using, when appropriate, tools and techniques developed for educational research. Practice teaching bears some similarities to clinical laboratory experience, so that some types of research methodology from education may be considered for use.

Because nursing students and nurses will find many opportunities to apply some of the basic tools and skills of research from the fields of education and the social sciences, these techniques have been selected for description in this book rather than the techniques used in the physical sciences.

DISSEMINATING RESEARCH FINDINGS

One of the problems in disseminating information is the time lapse that occurs as a natural result of research from the time the researcher designs and carries out a project to general implementation of the findings, if considered useful, by the profession.

It may take 1 to 2 years to carry out even a modest research project and to write up the results for publication, and it may be an additional year before the results are published. Then the article or monograph must be read and studied by the curriculum committee of a school of nursing or a committee within a health care agency. If the results of the study are to be acted on and incorporated into the curriculum or affect the function of nurses, then other faculty members or those individuals who will be involved through implementation of changes will have to become familiar with them. Time must be planned for discussion; and if the change affects students, if may take from several weeks to the following year before modifications are made in the curriculum. Additional time is needed for evaluation following implementation, and refinement may or may not result (Fig. 1-1). It is evident that a long period of time elapses between the germination of an idea for a research study and final acceptance by a school of nursing, institution, or the profession.

A second problem is finding effective measurement tools and methods for studying clinical nursing practice. The development of useful tools and sound methodology is of prime importance if there is to be rapid progress in nursing research.

A third problem is the danger that questions and hypotheses will be phrased in terms meaningful to disciplines other than nursing. With nurses as co-investigators there should be less error in this regard.

The fourth problem is one of research omission. Too often, policy changes are made without systematic follow-up. A school may change its policies or make innovations simply because it is the popular thing to do, without regard for research findings. Institutions and agencies, likewise, may use the trial-and-error method rather than base changes on research results.

A fifth problem is the lack of trained personnel to carry out research in nursing because of insufficient funds. The need for research funds must always be recognized, but

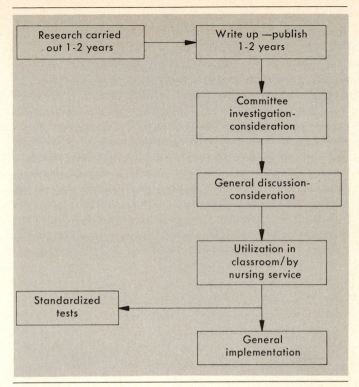

FIGURE 1-1   Time span from research to implementation.

it should not be an excuse for omitting research altogether. It is up to nurses to work with what is available at present and to be creative in designing and planning their studies.

The sixth problem is that research has yet to be carried out in many undetermined areas. Gaps are also evident in topics already studied. Even though many areas of nursing education have been investigated, more research is needed. The varieties of study include those involving the student, the instructor, the teaching-learning process, the curriculum, and relationships between students, students and teachers, and teachers and the learning process. Systematic comparisons must be made between nursing programs; the products of the various levels of nursing programs; students within a given program on various traits, characteristics, and abilities; and students in programs in different academic levels. Experimental programs must be developed, assessed, and evaluated. New teaching methods are still to be conceived and old methods reevaluated and sometimes refined. New knowledge, available to nurses from other disciplines, should be assessed and utilized in clinical nursing.

RESEARCH AND HEALTH

We sometimes repeat old wives' tales without realizing that our statements are not scientific facts. History records the acceptance of potions and remedies for illness along with seemingly justifiable reasons for not feeling well or lacking good health. On the other hand, many of the old prescriptions that have been ballyhooed contain ingredients that modern medicine has shown to be actually effective in curing illness.[18] But today, through health education, we no longer must rely on neighbors or relatives for explanations of illness, or for remedies brought by the medicine man, whose assistance was sought in the past. Health measured are now taught in schools, and certain procedures and programs are provided when needed. Free literature is available from many health-oriented agencies and companies for the education of the consumer.

Whereas many ancient civilizations thought demons to be the cause of illness, India, Greece, and Rome gave other reasons. As early as 300 years before Christ, India enjoyed a high level of health care through medicine, surgery, hygiene, and sanitation. A high standard in nursing care (which was probably given by men), in hospital construction, and in asepsis had been reached. These provisions for illness indicate that concern for health is not new.

The Greeks' desire for health was seen in their worship of such deities as Apollo, the sun god, who also was the deity of health and medicine. Hygeia was the goddess of health, and Panacea, the restorer of health. Health centers that provided hospital facilities were established, Epidauros being the most famous.

About the time Moses was born, the famous Papyrus Ebers, filled with prescriptions based on the medical knowledge of the day, was written in Egypt. These were different from the medical directions Moses later gave the Israelites and were the basis of codes of sanitation and personal hygiene for both the family and community. The impact of the positive suggestions of Moses on the prevention of infectious diseases is recorded in history. When people followed the procedures recorded in Leviticus 13:46, the major plagues of the Middle Ages were brought under control.

Throughout the ages, China has made extensive provision for remedies of illness in addition to acupuncture, which is practiced today to relieve pain. Chinese medicine is practiced in many countries outside China.

However, even in the twentieth century, on remote parts of the earth, there are tribes who have been untouched by modern culture and are illiterate or have no written language. These people are yet to be reached with appropriate health care and education.

Volunteers in the Peace Corps and the Agency for International Development (AID) and medical missionaries have contributed in many countries to the improved health of the people with whom they have worked. In addition to carrying out treatment and dispensing medicines, volunteers and other workers teach the people how to care for themselves and their families. Christian agencies and mission boards assist with the prevention of disease and care of the sick by establishing and maintaining clinics, health care centers, and hospitals, and by staffing them until there are sufficient numbers of trained nationals to take full responsibility. In some countries medical caravans are sent into the remote countryside not usually reached by professionally prepared personnel.

Because we hear so much today about poverty, famine, needs of the underprivileged, and needs of people living in the ghetto, the public is gaining more knowledge about the environment and its effect on health. This is not to say that people in past generations were not interested in the needs of their fellow human beings. For example, as fear of

[18]Bauer, W.W.: Potions, remedies, old wives' tales, Garden City, N.Y., 1969, Doubleday & Co., Inc.

epidemics increased, records were kept in Rome of the numbers of individuals contracting certain diseases. Religious and secular orders contributed to the care of the ill, with varying numbers of hospitals and monasteries providing nursing care through the centuries.

The standard of health that every individual is entitled to expect, according to the constitution of the World Health Organization (WHO), should be the highest attainable and "one of the fundamental rights of every human being without distinction of race, religion, political belief, economic, or social condition." As a means of attaining this standard, WHO provides for an exchange of ideas and experience among individuals from public health and medical professions of more than 100 countries in an endeavor to eradicate or control health problems common to several or all of them. This organization provides reports of the world health situation that gives us a greater understanding of trends in health care as well as a greater understanding of the primary problems to be solved.

Some of the major health needs have to do with famine, malnutrition, and urban squalor. In some instances people may be helpless to improve the environment in which they live. In other instances, if each family would make an effort to clean up its own living quarters, even in poverty there could be cleanliness. But both health education and a measure of feeling well are necessary for an individual to be concerned about the status of his/her health. Urbanization has brought with it certain problems, and so too has population growth. Pollution increase parallels population increase in intensity.

The WHO has identified four major areas where citizens are expected by their governments to take responsibility for health care and in which there are gaps of deficiencies: shortages in health service manpower, lack of training facilities, gaps in research in certain fields, and inadequate financial resources. It is encouraging, however, that so many countries have expressed a desire to coordinate health planning with economic and social development.

Before the WHO was established, the International Sanitary Bureau was founded in this hemisphere in 1902. The name of the bureau was changed several times until in 1958 it became known as the Pan American Health Organization. Since 1949, Washington, D.C., has been the location of the regional office of WHO for the Americas. The objectives of the organization are focused on the major health problem areas such as nutrition, mental health, radiation health, eradicating ancient diseases, and increasing the numbers of qualified nursing personnel. The ultimate goal of the Pan American Health Organization is to improve the health of all individuals living in the Americas.

SUMMARY

The research process is the attempt to gain new knowledge through the scientific method of systematic investigation. The purpose of research is to discover answers to questions through the collection of data. Nursing research uses the same scientific principles and procedures as other disciplines.

The approach of nursing research to nursing education is little different from that of educational research in general; nursing administration may borrow from administrative and managerial research, but clinical nursing is in a unique position and may demand a peculiar type of research that borrows from several disciplines, including medicine and the social and behavioral sciences.

Basic (pure) research strives to gain knowledge, whereas applied research adapts the finding to life situations. Unfortunately, many of the results of nursing research are never adopted. Some of the reasons that findings are not used are inconclusive results, noncommunication of findings, and failure to experiment with the findings. These weaknesses also are evident in many other disciplines. Research has several characteristics that serve as its foundation and are used in the investigative process.

Treatment of illness is not new but is evident throughout history and around the world. There is a growing concern about raising the health standards of all nations without distinction to race, religion, political belief, economical, or social conditions.

Research is needed not only to provide a satisfactory definition of nursing but to clarify the functions of nursing in the health field.

DISCUSSION QUESTIONS

1 What comes to mind when you hear the word research?
2 Why should practitioners do research?
3 In what ways is nursing research different from research conducted by medical doctors?
4 What is the relationship between nursing research and nursing education?
5 How does population growth affect health delivery? What is the effect of population increase on quality of health care?
6 How is a knowledge of research methodology valuable to nonscientists?
7 Why is there a relatively long time span between research and implementation of the findings?
8 Should nurses conduct only pure research? Why or why not?

CLASS ACTIVITIES

Tracks I and II

A pretest is given by the instructor to determine the students' knowledge of the research process.

SUGGESTED READINGS

Abdel-Al, H.: Ask a stupid question…, Int. Nurs. Rev. 29(4):112–117, July–August 1982.
Abu-Saad, J.: Nursing, a world view, St. Louis, 1979, The C.V. Mosby Co.
ANA center for research collects data on nursing, American Nurse 14(8):7–11, September 1983.
Bata, C.: Motivating nurses to do nursing research, Nursing Health Care 4(1):18–22, January 1983.
Bauer, W.W.: Potions, remedies, old wives' tales, Garden City, N.Y., 1969, Doubleday & Co., Inc.
Beckingham, A.C.: Identifying problems for nursing research, Int. Nurs. Rev. 21(2):49–50, March–April 1974.
Beckingham, C.R.: Science, the humanities, nursing research and nursing practice, Int. Nurs. Rev. 29:41–45, March–April 1982.
Bergman, R., Stockler, R.A., and Gilad, Z.: Opinion on nursing, Int. Nurs. Rev. 18(3):195, 1971.
Boone, J.: Focus on developments in British nursing: nursing research, nursing education, Journal of Advanced Nursing 9(1):93–95, January 1984.
Campbell, D.T., and Stanley, J.C.: Experimental and quasi-experimental designs for research, Chicago, 1963, Rand McNally & Co.

Church peace corps places nurses worldwide, Am. J. Nurs. **75**(12):2224, December 1975.

Cornelius, Dorothy: Report of the ICN President, 1973–1975, Int. Nurs. Rev. **22**(6):168–176, November–December 1975.

CNR adopts proposals on research, health workers, Int. Nurs. Rev. **28**(5):135, September–October 1981.

Crocker, L.M.: Linking research to practice, AJOT **31**(1):34–39, January 1977.

Cuban nurses society encourages research, contributes to practice and education progress, Int. Nurs. Rev. **18**(2):60, March–April 1981.

de Garine, I.: Tabu, food and society, World Health, February–March 1974, WHO, Geneva, pp. 44–48.

Diers, D.: Research for nursing, J. Nurs. Adm. **2**(3):7, 61, May–June 1972; **2**(5):8, 94, September–October 1972; **3**(1):8, 11, January–February 1973.

Donabedian, A.: A guide to medical care administration, Vol 2: Medical Care Appraisal. New York: American Public Health Association.

European researchers explore contribution of research to practice, Int. Nurs. Rev. **29**(2):35, March–April 1982.

Fawcett, J.: Integrating research into the faculty workload, Nurs. Outlook **27**(4):259–262, April 1979.

Fink, A., and Kosecoff, J.: An evaluation primer, Beverly Hills, 1978, Sage Publications, Inc.

Foster, S., Astei, J., and Sumner, S.: Cardiovascular research past, present, future, Heart & Lung **13**(2):111–116, March 1984.

Freebury, D.R.: The long arm of research, Can. Nurse **68**(10):40-45, October 1972.

Gortner, S.R.: Nursing science in transition, Nurs. Res. **29**(3):180–183, May–June 1980.

Greenwood, J.: Nursing research: a position paper, J. Adv. Nurs. **9**(1):77–82, January 1984.

Hanson, R.L.: Research: a necessity in nursing service, J. Nurs. Adm. **3**(3):61–62, May–June 1973.

Hayes, M.: Nursing research is not every nurse's business, Can. Nurse **70**(10):17–18, October 1974.

Hockey, L.: Bridge building...the importance of nursing research, Nursing Times **79**(22):64, June 1983.

Hollswander, C.H., Kinsey, D., and Paradowski, M.: Teacher-practitioner-researcher, Nursing & Health Care **5**(3):144–149, March 1984.

Horsley, J.A., and others: Research utilization as an organizational process, J. Nurs. Adm. **8**(7):4–6, July 1978.

Humphreys, D.: Recipe for research, Nurs. Times **68**(14):397–399, April 6, 1972.

ICN issues discussion guides on research and exploitation of public through marketing of drugs/ health products, Int. Nurs. Rev. **28**(4):99, July–August 1981.

ICN report, survey of nursing research units, Int. Nurs. Rev. **31**(4):116–121, July–August 1984.

India holds first national nursing research conference, Int. Nurs. Rev. **30**(2):61, March–April 1983.

Inman, U.: Nursing research—fact or fiction?, Nurs. Times **68**(2):46, January 13, 1972.

International guidelines for biomedical research proposed, Int. Nurs. Rev. **29**(2):36, March–April 1982.

Kelly, D.N.: What is research in nursing? (editorial), Superv. Nurs. **8**(4):9, April 1977.

King, D., Barnard, K.E., Hoehn, R.: Disseminating the results of nursing research, Nurs. Outlook **29**(3):164–169, March 1981.

Lambertsen, E.C.: Research in nursing—the task and the tools. In Focus on the future, Geneva, 1970, International Council of Nurses.

McMillan, S.I.: None of these diseases, Old Tappan, N.J., 1963, Fleming H. Revell Co.

Meeting explores present, future of nursing research, The American Nurse **15**(10):6, November–December 1983.

Meier, L.: Editorial: research on patients needed to dispel nursing myths, The American Nurse **15**(3):4, March 1983.

Mereness, D.A.: Graduate education, as one dean sees it, Nurs. Outlook **23**(10):638–641, October 1975.

Notter, L.E.: The case for nursing research, Nurs. Outlook **23**(12):760–763, December 1975.

Nursing's future outlined in New League Report, Nurs. Outlook **23**(10):604, October 1975.

Priorities for research in nursing, Kansas City, 1976, American Nurses' Association, ANA Pub. No. D-51.

Ramalingaswami, V.: Health professions tomorrow, World Health, April 1973, WHO, Geneva, pp. 30–33.

Report of European research conference available, Int. Nurs. Rev. **29**(4):104, July–August 1982.

Research Council sets August program, Am. Nurse **7**(7):6, July 1975.

Research in nursing: toward a science of health care, Kansas City, 1976, American Nurses' Association, ANA Publ. No. D-52.

Research is vital to nursing, British nurse tells conference, Int. Nurs. Rev. **21**(6):167, November–December 1974.

Researchers to develop field's future directions, Am. Nurse **6**(6):8, June 1974.

Schlotfeldt, R.M.: Planning for progress, Nurs. Outlook **21**(12):766–769, December 1973.

Schoor, T.M.: Building a firm foundation, AM. J. Nurs. **72**(8):1391, August 1972.

Simpson, M.: Research in nursing—the first step. Int. Nurs. Rev. **18**(3):231, 1971.

Steckel, S., and others: Implementing primary nursing within a research design, Nurs. Dimens. **7**(4):78–81, Winter 1980.

Stevenson, J.: Developing staff research potential: part one, J. Nurs. Adm. **8**(5):44–46, May 1978.

Stewart, D.W.: Secondary research, information sources, and methods, Applied social research methods series, Vol. 4, Beverly Hills, 1984, Sage Publications, Inc.

Sune, B.: WHO and research, World Health, WHO, Geneva, April 1980, WHO Monograph Series, 10-5.

Sweeney, M.A., and others: Driving nurses to research, Nurse Educ. **3**(4):7–13, July–August 1978.

Syphax, O.: Futuristic view of health occupations education, American Vocational Journal **50**(2):47–51, February 1975.

World health experts stress research in nursing, better defined role of psychiatric nursing, Am. J. Nurs. **75**(7):1097, July 1975.

World nursing research experts gather in Edinburgh, Int. Nurs. Rev. **29**(2):62, March–April 1982.

Young, B.: Research...whose responsibility is it?, Med. Rec. News **50**:23–24, June 1979.

Zyambo, B.: A tropical diseases research centre and the role nurses play, Int. Nurs. Rev. **30**(4):107–109, July–August 1983.

CHAPTER 2

RESEARCH AND NURSING

Greater emphasis is placed on research than on probably any other topic in nursing education. Not only are nurses involved in research, they are writing and publishing scholarly material about the latest methods and statistical techniques. Nurses seem to have moved toward research faster than any other discipline in the past 15 years.

There are three major areas, of concern in nursing research: (1) nursing education, (2) the practice of nursing and (3) nursing service. Increasing numbers of nurses are being prepared to do research and are gaining insight into their own problems. Nurses no longer stand back and wait for someone else to supply all the answers to nursing problems.

Florence Nightingale, product of the nineteenth century, is credited with being the first nurse-researcher, as well as the first modern nurse. According to Dolan, she lived at a time of growing dissatisfaction among women, who desired more education and the opportunity for a career. The climate was right for her spirit of determination and farsightedness to make waves in her chosen field, nursing. She clarified the role of the nurse, placed nursing firmly among the healing arts, and planned the education and continued professional growth of nurses. Since Miss Nightingale was aggressive and forceful, she went after those things that she believed necessary and appropriate for her profession. She founded the school at St. Thomas, laying down principles that have made it an example of an educational institution.[1] Her concern for systematic procedures, which classifies her as a modern researcher, was demonstrated by her careful recording and analysis of facts. Florence Nightingale led the way for nursing education, control of nursing by nurses, and nursing research by nurses.

Simmons and Henderson divide the history of professional nursing into three phases. First, the trained nurse of the late 1800s was a product of a hospital school of nursing. Second, from 1900 to 1930 there was expansion of hospital programs accompanied by the beginning of nursing education in institutions of higher education. Third, from 1930 to the present there has been a tendency to look inward for the purpose of improved quality of nursing care and nursing education.[2]

Other than Miss Nightingale's contributions, almost no published research by nurses was done during the first of these periods. The first significant study by a nurse in this

[1] Dolan, Josephine A.: History of nursing, ed. 12, Philadelphia, 1968, W.B. Saunders Co., p. 340.
[2] Simmons, Leo W., and Henderson, Virginia: Nursing research: a survey and assessment, New York, 1964, Appleton-Century-Crofts, pp. 7, 8.

country was perhaps that carried out by M. Adelaide Nutting: a survey of nursing education published in 1906 by the United States Commissioner of Education.[3]

REASONS FOR NURSING RESEARCH

One goal of research in nursing is to provide a basis for decision making at all levels of the profession. Schlotfeldt adds another dimension. "The primary task of nursing research is the development and refinement of nursing theories which serve as guides to nursing practice and which can be organized into a body of scientific nursing knowledge."[4] Thus, it has been suggested that the major reasons for doing research in nursing are providing the profession with a body of scientific knowledge and identifying and developing nursing theories. These reasons are similar to and as potent as those for any other profession.

Even though much of nursing research can be carried out in a manner similar to educational and social science research, new techniques will be needed as nursing and general knowledge grow, as findings are analyzed, as insight is gained into these findings, and as evaluation is carried out. It is necessary to develop new methods and techniques in patient care as nursing responsibilities change and expand. Nursing research should provide the foundation for these changes.

Christy claims that nursing research is needed because there are so many questions of vital importance to nursing that require a trained investigator. Nursing discussions can then be based on facts rather than on supposition.[5] We believe there is a need for nursing research because nursing has moved into an era of substantial independence. Nurses are questioning, creative, thinking analytically, and systematically solving some of their problems. The National Commission for Study has stated:

> It is regrettable that so little research has been conducted to determine the relative effectiveness of various forms of nursing intervention, and the impact of particular innovations in nursing practice.... We are confident that only through research can we begin to determine and fully exploit the capabilities of nurses to contribute to the health system.[6]

The National Commission cites research among the basic priorities in nursing: "(a) Increased research into both the practice of nursing and the education of nurses; (b) Enhanced educational systems and curricula based on the results of that research."[7]

The Panamerican Regional Group, which held its first meeting in Caracas, Venezuela, in November 1970, included the need for research as one of its recommendations: "There is a need to carry out research in every country to identify the needs of nursing and

[3] *Ibid.*, p. 17.

[4] Schlotfeldt, Rozella M.: Reflections on nursing research, Am. J. Nurs. **60**:494, April 1960. © American Journal of Nursing Co.

[5] Christy, Teresa E.: Portrait of a leader: M. Adelaide Nutting, Nurs. Outlook **17**:20, January 1969.

[6] Recommendations of the National Commission for the Study of Nursing and Nursing Education, Am. J. Nurs. **70**:285, February 1970. © American Journal of Nursing Co.

[7] *Ibid.*, p. 285.

available resources in order to increase the number of schools at basic and university level."[8]

The WHO Expert Committee on Nursing, in its fifth report, mentioned the need for research to identify community needs, since nursing care is good only when it is appropriate to the community that it serves. Nursing skills determined and taught without regard for the consumer are futile.

Beckingham quotes from the address of Dr. Quenum to the Directors of Nursing Schools in Africa, who cited the necessity for doing research in nursing administration, nursing education, and clinical nursing in order to develop critical thinking and to improve nursing procedures.[9]

Jacox stresses the need for nursing service administrators to know something about research so that some of them can carry out research in their own field (nursing service administration), support research done by clinical nursing service personnel, and read research literature intelligently.[10]

Schlotfeldt has suggested three reasons for pursuing empirical research: establishing the existence of order in human phenomena, finding inadequacies in explanations concerning human health, and developing theoretical systematized statements capable of improving future health practice.[11]

Nuckolls asks three questions that nursing research can answer. These involve recognition of need for change, of the most effective change, and of the effectiveness of change. She suggests that the answers to these questions may point the direction for future research.[12]

We believe that research is the most important process for instituting change in nursing and in other disciplines. A scientific investigation can answer the basic questions: Am I effective? How effective am I? How can I be more effective?

NEED FOR RESEARCH

Some questions we should consider: What is the need for doing research? What is the value of investigating a topic? What are the benefits to be gained from the results and conclusions of research? Let us answer these questions through an illustration.

A student was constantly asking her instructor, "Why must we do research? Why must we study people? What is the purpose? What is the reason?" And the answer given her was, "In order to predict and to explain." But this answer was not sufficient for her.

While doing a research project for a class in research methodology, she was employed in a clinic to which people came because of the relatively inexpensive and prompt medical attention provided there. There were no waiting lines, and the medical personnel tried to

[8] Panamerican Regional Group holds first meeting in Caracus, ICN Calling **3**:4, June 1971.
[9] Beckingham, Ann C.: Identifying problems for nursing research, Int. Nurs. Rev. **21**(2):52, March–April 1974.
[10] Jacox, Ada: The research component in the nursing service administration master's program, J. Nurs. Adm. **4**(2):37, March–April 1974.
[11] Schlotfeldt, Rozella M.: The significance of empirical research for nursing, Nurs. Res. **20**(2):141, March–April 1971.
[12] Nuckolls, Katherine B.: Nursing research—good for what? Nurs. Forum **11**(4):377, 1972.

avoid the appearance of being strictly professional types. For her project this student analyzed the clinic's records. She was amazed to find that people with certain types of problems came from certain sections of the city. For example, she found that women from one section of the city came frequently for abortion information, whereas from another section of the city, people came for flu and cold shots. She was able to relate these findings to her job, and the information proved to be valuable to her employer. The scheduling of specialists to give particular services to certain types of people became possible. She suddenly saw the value of research.

GROWTH OF NURSING RESEARCH

Research in nursing was slow to begin. But we must look at the milieu in which nursing existed. In a profession dominated by women, nursing research could begin and expand only as women were educated; as the nursing field grew and gained status; as increased numbers of individuals enrolled in the profession; as schools of nursing were established in institutions of higher education; as professional organizations clarified their roles, goals, and objectives; as science and technology contributed new knowledge; and as information was disseminated and applied to the medical and health care field. Only as women have gained their own identity have they had the opportunity and desire to continue their basic education, leading to an interest in research.

In the latter part of the nineteenth century, nurses used the results of medical research to determine procedures and nursing treatments and then turned to educational research to apply some of its methods and aims. Neither of these, however, was sufficient for guiding clinical nursing practice. As industrial research increased, nurses turned to industrial management, which provided limited findings that were helpful. These methods and techniques did offer help in the utilization of personnel.[13]

We do not believe that the application by nurses of research techniques used in other fields in the past should be entirely criticized. Nurses utilized what was available at the time and could not be expected to be as research oriented as some other professions because they were not prepared with the necessary skills. Perhaps they were wise in moving ahead steadily and adapting to the nursing profession the useful techniques of other disciplines.

More recently, the physical and social sciences have been of benefit to nursing and nurses. Social scientists, especially, have studied nursing because of their interest, and nursing has benefited from their research. Since the 1960s, researchers educated as nurses (nurse-researchers) have become available. Although their number is still inadequate, the number of nurses with research skills is increasing, the number of research reports in professional journals is growing, and workshops and seminars related to methodology are more frequently reported in the literature.

There are two major reasons why research methodology and techniques should be studied on the undergraduate level. First, as students become familiar with and gain the skills of scientific investigation, it is hoped that they will develop a positive attitude

13 Wald, Florence S., and Leonard, R.C.: Toward development of nursing practice theory, Nurs. Res. 13:309, Fall 1964.

toward nursing research and that many students will become interested to the extent that they will take the initiative to carry out fruitful studies of their own. Furthermore, by studying research methodology, students are alerted to the need for accuracy in any research project in which they might participate as registered nurses.

Nursing is now in a position where its own members are conducting research within the profession. A substantial number of nurse-researchers will certainly be needed in the future. In fact, nursing needs a substantial number of research-oriented nurses who can add to the store of knowledge that is beginning to accumulate as the result of increased numbers of studies. It is hoped that eventually there will be a wide base of prepared people contributing to nursing research.

Two reasons for the delay in the advance of nursing science, according to Schlotfeldt, are the lack of research concerning the ability to cope in the sphere of health and illness, and the uncritical acceptance and reliance on theoretical constructs of others.[14] Nevertheless, positive signs are evident that nursing research is gaining stature.

At present we are excited about the prospect of nursing students becoming familiar with the methodology and techniques of research. It is important that the findings from research studies, no matter how small, be disseminated, at least on a local basis. Students' findings should be reported to the class and to the institution where the research is carried out and, when appropriate, applied to the work situation.

WHERE TO DEVELOP RESEARCH SKILLS

A profession, in its entirety, should profit from all types of studies carried out by students and researchers. Replication of investigations, as well as original research, is called for if valid generalizations about nursing are to be the basic content of nursing science. Such replications should be reported and verified and any errors indicated. Published reports are necessary when facts that will add to nursing knowledge are found.

Small research projects can be carried out in any area in which a student (learner) has gained the understanding and skills necessary for execution of the study. This means that the student, enrolled in a course in methodology and techniques of research, but not yet familiar with clinical practice, may be limited to research topics dealing with familiar interests and situations.

If students have progressed in their nursing program to the point where they have some understanding of the patient, his/her family, and the environment, clinical nursing may then be the area for carrying out a research project. At least it is expected that most students will explore some topics of interest in the clinical setting. The student should be aware that we do not as yet have all the tools necessary to assess nurse-patient relationships, although instruments are being developed. The beginning student in research methodology can, nevertheless, utilize valid tools that have been made available to researchers in other disciplines, as well as in nursing.

Simon and Pitel report on the way in which an organization (hospital center) acquainted its professional nursing staff with the field of nursing research and its potential use by

[14]Schlotfeldt, p. 140.

potential use by means of a colloquium. Apparently, at least one third of the nurses had minimal or no previous formal introduction to nursing research.[15] In-service education is an avenue whereby research methodology can be conveniently taught to nurses who are employed in hospitals and agencies. The result is a staff who can understand research literature, appreciate their own contribution to ongoing research in their place of employment, become increasingly skillful in the art of critical thinking, and realize the possibilities that research holds for solving nursing problems.

Johnson and Okunade challenge community nurses to conduct their own research. Community nurses, they say, have assisted in the research of others and it is time that they do the initial planning by themselves or with consultative assistance of others.[16]

PREPARATION OF NURSE-RESEARCHERS

Researchers are not "born"; they learn the development of skills. Hochbaum points out the widespread idea that any intelligent nurse can go into research because nurses have been trained to be sharp observers.[17] But observation is not enough. Researchers also must be trained in designing studies, carrying out whatever technique is most appropriate, analyzing data, and reporting the findings. Judgments and decisions must be made by the investigator and later by those who are in a position to apply the findings in the work situation.

Nurses sometimes try to research certain topics or problem areas, but they are incapable of researching at present simply because they do not have the skills. Worthwhile research depends on the skills and the limitations of the researchers and whether or not they are aware of them. Nurses may expect too much from the research process—that it will solve all the problems of nursing and nurses, whereas it may only assist in solving some of the problems.

Until recently, the number of doctoral programs in nursing has been extremely limited, so nurses have tended to select majors in other disciplines. We do not believe that, with the growing number of graduate programs available in nursing, all nurses should continue their education entirely in nursing. Nurses who have gained knowledge and skills that can be brought into the field of nursing from other disciplines are still needed. Nurse educators may select the best that other disciplines have to offer and then apply what can be utilized by nurses and nursing.

Doctoral students have provided a sizable amount of research in the various disciplines, and nursing is no exception. Doctoral studies by nurses provide information as varied as the disciplines in which the nurses are enrolled and their areas of interest in nursing. It is expected that all research carried out by doctoral students will be published so their findings may be shared with others who could benefit from them.

However, nurses should not be required to continue their education to the doctoral level in order to become familiar with research methodology, and it is with just such a

[15]Simon, Helen M., and Pitel, Martha: Colloquium boosts practitioners' interest in clinical nursing research, Nurs. Res. Report 9(1):1–2, March 1974.
[16]Johnson, Margie N., and Okunade, Adebimpe O.: Roles that nurses in the community can play in nursing research, Int. Nurs. Rev. 22(5):148, September–October, 1975.
[17]The nurse in research as seen by behavioral scientist Godrey M. Hochbaum. In Fox, David J., and Kelly, Ruth Lundt, editors: The research process in nursing, New York, 1967, Appleton-Century-Crofts, p. 25.

conviction that this book has been written. A beginning student in nursing is academically prepared to learn the basic methodology and techniques of research.

Nurses who argue that research methodology should not be taught on the undergraduate level may not realize that research courses in the behavioral sciences are taught at the baccalaureate level. It is becoming increasingly important that students anticipating graduate school receive an introduction to research. An introduction to statistics and research methods at the bachelor of science level will provide the new graduate student with a degree of confidence and understanding that is absent in nonresearch-oriented students. The nurse who is well prepared to conduct research always has need of other individuals or groups with similar preparation for identification and feedback.

As nursing programs have moved into institutions of higher education and as nurses have become better educated, and have been granted degrees on the undergraduate and graduate levels, they have become better prepared to carry out responsibilities in education and administration. More recently, clinical nursing has moved into the graduate level. Nurses who have been exposed to research methodology and who have developed skills have begun to carry out research studies of their own. Others have begun to teach research methodology and techniques to increasing numbers of students as they themselves have gained insight and an understanding of the investigative process.

Schools of nursing vary in the year in which nursing research is taught and the requirements that are made for satisfactory completion of the course. As a result, graduates of baccalaureate nursing programs vary in their understanding of the research process and in the kinds of skills they have attained. Nurses who pursue graduate education may leave a master's program with an even greater variety in the amount of knowledge and skills they have attained because of their previous educational preparation and the amount of emphasis on nursing research included in their graduate work. The fact that a nurse has graduated from a baccalaureate or a master's level nursing program is no guarantee that a certain degree of competency in nursing research has been achieved. We believe that it is crucial that some minimum standards be established on both the baccalaureate and graduate levels of nursing education.

What should students be expected to know about the research process in order to become researchers? They should gain skill and knowledge in principles and methods of scientific investigation. Beginning students must realize that it is impossible to learn everything about research in one course. A good solid foundation can be laid for carrying out basic studies, but additional courses (such as statistics and computer use) will be required in order to add breadth and depth to a student's understanding of the research process. The nurse who is especially interested in research should become acquainted with the present tools available in the allied disciplines.

To be most effective and to make the greatest contribution to the nursing profession, the nurse-researcher must be knowledgeable about the content of nursing, the trends in the allied health fields, and any advances in research techniques. Nursing must be visualized in its proper perspective in the total health care system if a balance of function is to be maintained.

The educational preparation of the nurse-researcher is in a state of flux. It is expected that the nurse-researcher who directs a project or who is responsible for developing a major research design has gained skill and knowledge in areas necessary for carrying out the project. However, there is always the possibility that the person with limited research skill may use techniques in a way for which they were not intended, so the learner should read reports of studies in nursing as well as studies that have been done in other fields and are related to the area of investigation.

Conant has classified nurse-researchers into three categories: those prepared in another discipline who make little, if any, effort to apply their findings to the field of nursing; those who study nurses and nursing but do not participate in nursing itself; and those who continue to practice nursing while doing research. Encouragement is given for nurses to remain in clinical practice while carrying out research, since only nurses who continue in nursing as such are likely to study nursing practice problems and to develop theories of nursing practice.[18] Thus, nursing students, too, must be encouraged to carry out studies in the clinical area.

Not all nurses prepared at the doctoral level are interested in focusing all or part of their attention on research. The Ph.D. is a research-oriented degree with research skills built into the program. However, a nurse with academic preparation that includes a high level of performance in research may not want to become a researcher. Even when funds are available for research, the nurse prepared on the doctoral level may find more personal challenge in other professional avenues. This same situation may exist for those nurses granted other types of doctoral degrees.

Many institutions of higher learning require or offer programs that include a research experience on the master's degree level. Departments of nursing within these institutions may vary in their provisions for a nursing research experience.

Even though nurses may not have sufficient skills to do all their own research, they should be well enough acquainted with the principles of research to recognize areas for study and to be able to seek out others with the appropriate skills.

Not only must nurse-researchers have certain abilities, they also must overcome certain problems. First, nurses must learn to be independent in their thinking so that if they conduct research with someone of the opposite sex, their role as a man or a woman will not dominate the other. Second, nursing students are taught to make no mistakes; however, researchers expect errors to occur and accept the fact that they will. Third, nursing students are taught to deal with individuals, but researchers go a step beyond and generalize from the single case to the population of which they are a representative part. Fourth, researchers do not prove their hypothesis; they only test it. Fifth, nurses do not test or try out their solution to a situation before they apply it to the particular case.

PREVIOUS STUDIES IN NURSING RESEARCH

In this section we consider, first, the categorization of nursing research as compiled by Simmons and Henderson and then follow with examples of the types of nursing research that have been done. The description of these studies is purposely brief since in this book we are concerned with presenting methods of doing research rather than presenting a broad and lengthy discussion of what kinds of nursing research have been reported in recent years.

In the latter part of the 1950s, Simmons and Henderson categorized past nursing research; the following is a brief compilation of their major category headings:

[18]Conant, Lucy H.: On becoming a nurse-researcher, Nurs. Res. **17**:69, January–February 1968.

A. Historical, philosophical, and cultural studies
B. Occupational orientation and career dynamics (studies concerned primarily with supply and demand in nursing; job opportunities, satisfactions, and working conditions; economic and legal status; career appraisals and distributional characteristics)
C. Specialties in nursing (studies in this category focus on the nurse as she functions in a particular position, specialty, or place of employment)
D. Nursing organizations and organizations including nursing (studies of structure, policies, programs, operations, and relationships)
E. Administration of nursing services in hospitals, clinics, public health and other agencies
F. Nursing care (in homes, schools, industries, health agencies, or any institution)
G. Patients' reactions and adjustments to identifiable variables related to their illnesses
H. Interaction patterns between nurse, patient, patient's family, other nurses, physicians, and other members of the health team
I. Nursing education
J. Conducting research (facilities, personnel, support and method)[19]

One type of research survey report was that done by Dr. Faye Abdellah, in which an overview of 175 nursing research projects was published in a series of three articles. All these projects were supported in part by the Division of Nursing, National Institutes of Health, U.S. Department of Health, Education, and Welfare between 1955 and 1968. Such a survey report is an excellent source of ideas for further research.[20]

Much of nursing research in the past has focused on the nurse rather than on nursing. This is not to say that there should not be continued emphasis on the nurse or the student, but clinical nursing does need to be emphasized. Nursing service is concerned with the patient, the nurse's role, the process of nursing, and a multitude of topics classified as clinical nursing.

It has been traditional for nurses to repeat a procedure as taught without questioning its value or accuracy. One study, reported by Schmidt, demonstrates what can be done to investigate a single nursing procedure. A temperature-pulse-respiration (TPR) study was done before a new TPR procedure was developed. It might be wise for this same study to be repeated in other settings.[21] Likewise, research should precede changes in any nursing procedure. There should be a factual basis for change, not just a desire to do something differently.

An example of a study done by nonnurses, involving nursing care, was the one by Duff and Hollingshead and published in *Sickness and Society*.[22] The authors studied medical and social factors that influenced the care of patients in a general hospital. This assessment of care given each patient during the course of a single illness experience is an example of

[19]Simmons, Leo W., and Henderson, Virginia: Nursing research: a survey and assessment, New York, 1964, Appleton-Century-Crofts. By permission of Appleton-Century-Crofts, Educational Division, Meredith Corporation.
[20]Abdellah, Faye G.: Overview of nursing research 1955–1968, part I, Nurs. Res. **19**:6–17, January–February 1970; part II, **19**:151–162, March–April 1970; part III, **19**:239–252, May–June 1970.
[21]Schmidt, Alice: TPRs: an old "habit" or a significant routine? Minnesota Nursing Accent **43**:47–50, April 1971.
[22]Duff, Raymond S., and Hollingshead, August B.: Sickness and society, New York, 1968, Harper & Row Publishers.

studies that are done by nonnurses but that should be considered by nurses in their concern for better patient care. Students learning the research process would do well to become familiar with such investigations in their reading of research methodology.

Loomis found that 78.4% of doctoral dissertations in nursing for the years 1976–1982 were predominately in clinical nursing research. The topics of the dissertations were divided into three categories: actual potential health problems, human response problems, and clinical decision problems.[23]

The U.S. Public Health Service has provided grants for a number of research projects. Among these was a 5-year project by the Michigan Nurses' Association to help RNs utilize new nursing research knowledge[24] and an 18-month contract to the Western Interstate Commission for Higher Education "to develop new ways of analyzing manpower requirements...to aid manpower policy making at state, regional, and national levels.[25]

At the 1974 American Nurses' Association convention, reports were made on research topics ranging from management of selected nursing care procedures to studies about perceptions, attitudes, and leadership roles in nursing.[26]

Authors of many articles appearing in the various professional nursing journals are researchers as well as writers. Numerous other individuals are making contributions to research in nursing through books and monographs. Compilation of such a list runs the risk of omitting names of talented and dedicated researchers who are quietly pursuing truth and knowledge.

There is ample evidence that nurses around the world are aware of the need for nursing research. Nurses in most countries want research to be conducted on the same general topics and they express the same concerns.

CLINICAL RESEARCH

Traditionally, nursing research has centered around nursing education, nursing administration, and the nurse. Clinical nursing has been the primary focus of nurses throughout history, but it has been largely ignored by researchers until recently. Because of the increased emphasis on clinical research, we feel the need to include a special section dealing with patient-oriented research.

The subject area of clinical nursing is such that any of the research approaches described in this book can be implemented in clinical research. At the same time, because clinical nursing is a unique field of research, it requires appropriate instruments, techniques, and approaches. Clinical nursing lies somewhere on the continuum between behavioral-social science research and medical research. At the same time it clearly overlaps both. Social and behavioral research is concerned with the personality and interaction of

[23] Loomis, M.E.: Emerging content in nursing: an analysis of dissertation abstracts and titles: 1976–1982, Nursing Research **34**(2):113–118, 1985.

[24] Project on research use started in Michigan, Am. J. Nurs. **75**(9):1424, September 1975.

[25] Western nursing council to study manpower analysis and quality measurement, Am. J. Nurs. **75**(7):1105, July 1975.

[26] Implications of research to be topic, Am. Nurs. **6**(4):19, April 1974.

individuals and groups, whereas medicine is involved with organic, physiological, and biological relationships to disease and bodily function. The nurse comes in contact with the patient from times of health to death. This period allows the nurse to run the entire gamut of human relationships, social settings, and physiological situations. Generally, the concern of the medical profession is diagnosing and treating organic and psychiatric problems.

The positive reasons for doing clinical research include the following:
1. Problems and data are an everyday part of the work situation.
2. There is personal satisfaction gained from finding a better way to provide nursing care.
3. No one else has access to the patient to the same degree that the nurse does.
4. The very process of participating in clinical research may be a therapeutic and enjoyable activity for the patient.
5. Clinical nursing research is a practical way whereby the individual nurse can improve the health care of patients and benefit mankind in general.

Reasons for the lack of clinical research are the following:
1. Nurses tend to feel that they are "too busy taking care of the patients" to find time to conduct research.
2. Unless the nurse has had academic training geared toward theoretical conceptions, research may not seem important.
3. Unless the importance of research is learned, nurses may not be able to identify problems that are researchable.
4. Many nurses do not have the academic training necessary to feel confident in carrying out clinical research.
5. The ethics of research frighten some individuals. The requirement to obtain administrative-patient-relative approval for projects may deter some investigators. The fear of harming a patient is an obstacle for other researchers.
6. Unless the administrators of nursing service in health care institutions and agencies are research oriented, the nursing staff tends to feel that it is futile to expect support for nursing research; therefore, they have little or no motivation to pursue research.
7. Research takes time, time costs money, and money must be budgeted. That is, research may not be conducted because of lack of funds.

The need for clinical nursing research has been recognized for several years and from the literature it appears that inroads are being made. It is hoped that nurses will continue to concentrate on research related to the nurse-patient arena.

RESEARCH NEEDED

Some areas which are receiving limited attention in doctoral dissertations are: cultural/environmental; family, social, and cultural human response systems; stressors; and clinical decision making. Needs exist for research in such social issues as history, culture, economics, intervention studies, and politics.[27]

[27] From Loomis, *op. cit.*, p. 118.

Burgess believes that nursing research should be testing strategies and interventions which have come from nursing practice models especially relating to stress. She also emphasizes the need for qualitative research.[28]

From our experience the following are areas which need to be researched:

1. More replication studies of a basic nature which test some of the usual nursing care plan procedures.
2. A universal statistical procedure applicable to all forms of data, with a universally accepted meaning.
3. Greater reliance on case studies and other qualitative methods.
4. Multivariate research on the effects of several forms of simultaneous stressors—for example, the patient is worried about how to pay medical bills, how the spouse will get along, who will take care of the lawn, who will handle the job in the office, and if it will be possible to work in the future.
5. Why are some individuals always healthy while others seem to go from crisis to crisis? In other words, research that centers on wellness, not illness.
6. Research on grant productivity. Great discoveries are not so much the result of huge expenditures as they are enormous insight. For example, consider the heart recipient who was given a heart designed by a dentist from spare parts.
7. Priority research for priority problems. The more critical a problem, the greater the need for research. Apparently great numbers of people have cancer; therefore, why not place a priority on cancer and heart research?
8. International priorities. Nurses in the United States need to broaden their scope from purely domestic concerns to those of the world. Who has more knowledge, talent, funds, and resources? The people in many developing countries are suffering from parasites, worms, tuberculosis, yellow fever, malaria, cholera, typhoid, leprosy, schistosomiasis, venereal diseases, and hepatitis.
9. Nursing skills that are, versus those that should be, practiced in the community. Could nurses be utilized more effectively in the community?

As the role of the nurse expands and new areas of specialization arise nurse-researchers ought to be studying change and its effect on the student, the educator, the patient, the patient's family, the nurse, the nursing profession, and other professions as they relate to nursing. Most disciplines, including nursing, need a great deal of replication of research in order to refine, quantify, and verify original findings. The need for experimental research has been and is urgently needed if cause-effect relationships are to be established. If nurses who are already prepared to propose and assist in research projects would demonstrate initiative, much of the needed research could be undertaken immediately. It is the desire and commitment of nurses, not their ability, which will decide the fate of nursing research.

RESEARCH TRENDS

It is encouraging that research sessions were featured for the first time in the formal program of the International Council of Nursing (ICN) Congress in 1969 in Montreal.

---

[28] Burgess, A.: The American Nurse 17(3):18, March 1985.

The creation of the Commission on Nursing Research is another important step in the establishment of research as one part of the triad: education, service, and research. Just as these three are the functions of a university, they are the primary characteristics of a profession.

It appears from the literature that all major organizations whose membership is composed of nurses have added or are in the process of adding some phase of nursing research to their objectives. Many organizations, when reporting their goals, make suggestions for future research or offer grants for specific types of research. A synthesis of this information provides a glimpse into the future of nursing research.

We believe that in the future the gaps that have been recognized in research will slowly be closed through the process of original and repetitive studies. There will be increasing amounts of research carried on in all areas of nursing as research methods and techniques are taught in undergraduate nursing programs. Certainly many students will be stimulated to initiate their own studies or to suggest possible studies to others.

As for types of nursing research that will be done, nurses who are challenged by clinical nursing will pursue this field, increasing the amount of clinical nursing research done in the future. Experimentation with curriculum will increase as faculties attempt to provide the opportunity for mobility and more individualization of student learning. New patterns of personnel utilization in nursing service, studies of the relationship between nursing and allied health workers within the hospital, interdisciplinary health service problems, and new patterns of health care service are among the problems to be tackled.

It can be stated unequivocally that interest in research is growing. Further, the quality and quantity of research studies are improving.

Other trends in nursing research are:

1. The demand for doctoral degrees with research capabilities.
2. More educational institutions, hospitals, and organizations are creating special departments of research. Even the U.S. Department of Health and Human Services has established a Center for Nursing Research.
3. A greater emphasis on research in the undergraduate programs.
4. The proliferation of research texts, and series of articles on research methodology in nursing speciality journals.
5. Published and funded research studies as a basis for promotion in the academic area.

Following upon the increasing number of nurses who are knowledgeable about research methodology has come the rise of nursing research centers in colleges and universities. The centers are evidence of the acknowledged value of research to nursing.

There is an awareness on the part of nurses of the need to document their statements with facts. The expanded role of the nurse has reinforced vocal concerns with hard data from rigorous, methodologically sophisticated research findings.

In the 1980s some concerns of nursing researchers are the limited acknowledgment of nursing research findings within other health professions and the difficulty some segments of the public have in accepting a woman with advanced degrees as a researcher rather than solely as an "angel in white." Another concern is the myth that research methodology is only an academic subject appropriate for nurses in graduate school. Finally, nurse themselves must learn to view research as a tool for improvement, not as a threat to their lifestyle.

Again, trends in nursing research will depend somewhat on trends in nursing, higher education, economics, scientific breakthroughs, technological advances, the interests of individuals who enroll in nursing, and the identification of those students who are especially fitted for research. The nursing profession will be able to satisfy its third function, research, only to the degree that students in basic nursing programs learn research skills and become intrigued and challenged by systematic methodology.

SUMMARY

Nursing has arrived at the point where it must assume responsibility for its own research. The need for research has arisen sharply because of the changing world of nursing. There is a continuing need for educational, administrative, and managerial research.

We contend that research methodology should be studied at the undergraduate level. The expanding role of the nurse demands research to provide a wide philosophical base for health care, to stimulate interest in research, and to increase the pool of potential researchers.

Students are encouraged to conduct small research studies in replication, introductory clinical investigations, and nurse-patient relationships. The beginning nurse-researcher should not expect to become a professional investigator or to be able to solve all the problems of nursing after taking only a beginning course in research methodology. An introductory course is designed to stimulate the interest of the student and to provide a basic understanding of the research process. High-level research requires additional academic preparation.

Common criticisms of past nursing research are that it was focused on the nurse rather than on nursing and that it was done by nonnurses. Encouraging prospects for the future of nursing research are evident in international interest, in increasing numbers of schools offering courses in research methodology, and in nurses seeking graduate degrees involving research.

Organizations such as the ANA, ANF, WICHE, Sigma Theta Tau, WHO, ICN, Division of Nursing of the National Institutes of Health, and some universities are actively supporting research activities. Response to the needs and demands for clinical research is increasing.

DISCUSSION QUESTIONS

1 What are three of the major social forces that prompted nurses to undertake research?
2 What education or experience is necessary to conduct research?
3 How does the subject matter of clinical nursing research differ from medical research?
4 How does the United States rate with some developing countries in degree of interest and in nursing research?
5 Respond to the following statements: Clinical research *will* dominate the research arena in the next decade. Clinical research *will not* dominate the research arena in the next decade.
6 Comment on the following statement: Nurses have spent too much time researching nurses rather than nursing.
7 In your opinion, what aspect of the nursing profession should have priority in nursing research? Support your response.

CLASS ACTIVITIES

Tracks I and II

The students are to bring copies of research articles or reports that they have found interesting. Each student is to describe the study and tell why it is interesting.

SUGGESTED READINGS

ANA Center for research collects data on nursing, The American Nurse 15(8):7, September 1983.

ANA Commission outlines priorities for nursing research in the '80s, Am. J. Nurs. 80(5):846, May 1980.

Bauknecht, V.: Capital commentary: nursing groups testify on education research, The American Nurse 16(5):2, May 1984.

Bergman, R.: Omissions in nursing research, International Nursing Review 31(2):55–56, March–April 1984.

Boore, J.: Focus on developments in British nursing: nursing research—nursing education, J. Adv. Nurs. 9(1):93–95, January 1984.

Bowie, R. B.: Research responsibilities of the clinical nurse, AORN J. 31(2):238–241, February 1980.

Bowie, R. B.: The nurse researcher's role and responsibilities, AORN J. 31(3):609–611, March 1980.

Carnegie, M. Elizabeth: A serious omission, Nurs. Res. 24(2):83, March–April 1975.

Carnegie, M. Elizabeth: Nursing research centers on the rise (editorial), Nurs. Res. 27(4):211, July–August 1978.

Chenitz, W., and Swanson, J.M.: The postdoctoral research fellow in nursing: in between the cracks in the academic wall, Nursing Outlook 29(7):417–420, July 1981.

Conway, M.E.: Clinical research: instrument for change, J. Nurs. Adm. 8(12):27–32, December 1978.

Corbin, J., and others (eds): Cooperative research in nursing, monograph series 76, publication 1, May 1976, Sigma Theta Tau.

Currie, O.J., and others: Respiratory nursing research, Alberta Association of Registered Nurses Newsletter 35:1–2, December 1979.

deTornyay, R.: Nursing research—the road ahead, Nurs. Res. 26(6):404–407, November–December 1977.

Duffy, M.E.: When a woman heads the household, Nursing Outlook 30(8):468–473, September–October 1982.

Dumas, R.G., et al.: Should there be a National Institute for Nursing? Nurs. Outlook 32(1):16–22, January–February 1984.

Fagin, C.M.: The economic value of nursing research, The American Journal of Nursing 82(12):1844–1849, December 1982.

Feldman, H.R.: Nursing research in the 1980s: issues and implications, Adv. Nurs. Sci. 3(1):85–92, October 1980.

Francis, G.: Research comes out of academia, Virginia Nurs. 46:7–8, Spring 1978.

Francis, G.M.: Nursing research in Virginia, Virginia Nurse 49(2):31–33, Summer 1981.

Gortner, Susan, and Nahm, H.: An overview of nursing research in the United States, Nurs. Res. 26(1):10–33, January–February 1977.

Gottlieb, L.: Nursing research: where are we now, Canadian Nurse 77:26–28, November 1981.

Greenwood, J.: Nursing research: a position paper, Journal of Advanced Nursing 9(1):77–82, January 1984.

Gustaffsen, G.: The important part research plays in infection control, Nursing Times 77:15–16, September 1981.

Henderson, Virginia: Research in nursing practice—when? Nurs. Res. 4:99, February 1956.

Henderson, Virginia: We've come a long way, but what of the direction? Nurs. Res. 26(3):163–164, May–June 1977.

Hodgman, E.C.: Closing the gap between research and practice; changing the answers to the 'who', the 'where', and the 'how' of nursing research, Int. J. Nurs. Stud. 16(2):105–110, 1979.

Johnson, J.E.: Power: nursing's challenge for change. Translating research to practice, Kansas City, 1979, American Nurses' Association, ANA Pub. No. G-135, pp. 125–133.

Keighley, T.: Prologue for the future…in nursing research, Nurs. Mirror 158(1):22–23, 26, January 1984.

Kendrick, V.M., Sullivan, J.H.: Nursing research at the VNA, Home Health Care Nurse, p. 44–46, September–October 1984.

Ketefian, S.: The code for nurses: a research perspective, Perspectives on the code for nurses, Kansas City, 1978, American Nurses' Association Pub. No. G-132, pp. 27–34.

Kotthoff, M.E.: Current trends and issues in nursing in the United States: the primary health care nurse practitioner, Int. Nurs. Rev. 28(1):24–28, January–February 1981.

Krueger, J.C.: Utilization of nursing research: the planning process, J. Nurs. Adm. 8(1):6–9, January 1978.

Lancaster, J.: Bonding of nursing practice and education through research, Nursing & Health Care 5(7):379–382, September 1984.

Lang, N.M., and Clinton, J.F.: Assessment and assurance of the quality of nursing care, a selected overview, Evaluation and the Health Professions 6(2):211–231, June 1983.

Leininger, M.M.: Creativity and challenges for nurse researchers in the economic recession, Journal of Nursing Administration 13(3):21, March 1983.

Lindeman, C.A., and Krueger, J.C.: increasing the quality, quantity, and use of nursing research, Nurs. Outlook 25(7):450–454, July 1977.

MacPherson, K.I.: Feminist methods: a new paradigm for nursing research, Advances in Nursing Science 5(2):17–25, January 1983.

Maraldo, P.J.: Guest editorial—the nursing institute veto: a Monday morning quarterback session, Nursing & Health Care 5(9):459, November 1984.

McHugh, N.G., and Johnson, J.E.: Clinical nursing research: beyond the methods books, Nurs. Outlook, 28(6):352–356, June 1980.

Measuring quality of care is object of major research project, Int. Nurs. Rev. 28(6):187, November–December 1981.

Murphy, S.A.: Approaches to research in graduate education, J. of Nurs. Ed. Vol. 3:97, March 23, 1984.

Newman, M.A.: What differentiates clinical research, Image XIV(3):86–88, October 1982.

Noble, M.A.: Teaching clinical research: idealism versus realism, J. Nurs. Educ. 19(2):34–37, February 1980.

Nursing potential recognized in the Americas, Int. Nurs. Rev. 25(2):36–39, March–April 1978.

Nursing research options in PHS assessed, The American Nurse 17(1):2, January 1985.

Nursing research unit established at London University, Int. Nurs. Rev. 24(4):101–102, July–August 1977.

Nursing research—what is it and do we need it? The New Zealand Nursing Journal, 26–27, November 1983.

Pank, P., Rostron, W., and Stenhouse, M.: Using research in nursing, Nursing Times 80(11):44–45, March 14, 1984.

Parker, M.L., and Labadie, G.C.: Demystifying research mystique, Nursing & Health Care 4(7):383–386, September 1983.

Reeves, D., Underly, N., and Beckwith, B.: Establishing a research subcommittee in a service institution, Nursing & Health Care 3(4):189–191, April, 1982.

Research corner: registered nurses involved in research, Virginia Nurse 52(1):14, Spring 1984.

Research project produces 10 protocols on nursing care, The American Nurse 14(1):7, January 1982.

Richie D., and others: Nursing in clinical research: an extended role for the staff nurse, Canadian Nurse 79(2):40, February 1983.

Rubin, R., and Erickson, F.: Research in clinical nursing, J. Adv. Nurs. 3(2):131–144, March 1978.

See, E.M.: The ANA and research in nursing, Nurs. Res. 26(3):165–171, May–June 1977.

Shaver, J.P.: The productivity of educational research and the applied-basic research distinction, Educational Researcher, 8(1):3–9, January 1979.

Slavin, R.E.: Basic vs. applied research, a response, Educ. Res. 7(2):15–17, February 1978.

Steckel, S.B.: If you want to make a positive difference in nursing, become a nurse researcher, Nurs. '78, 8:78–80, July 1978.

Stinson, Shirley, M.: Staff nurse involvement in research—myth or reality? Can. Nurse 69(6):28–29, June 1973.

Wadle, K., and Munns, D.M.: A plea for research-based curriculum revision, Nursing & Health Care 4(5):261–264, May 1983.

Walker, M.: As I see it ... research with patients requires commitment, savvy, The American Nurse 15(7):5, July–August 19, 1983.

Werley, H.H.: Nursing research in perspective, Int. Nurs. Rev. 24(3):75–83, May–June 1977.

White, J.H.: The relationship of clinical practice and research, J. Adv. Nurs. 9(2):181–187, March 1984.

WHO goals could change nursing by year 2000, Am. J. Nurs. 79(9):1496, 1500, September 1979.

WHO session on European research, Am. J. Nurs. 80(1):36, January 1980.

Williams, C.A., editor: Image-making in nursing, papers of the 1982 Scientific Session, American Academy of Nursing, Kansas, 1983, ANA.

PART TWO

PREPARATION FOR QUANTITATIVE RESEARCH

Four chapters make up the second section of this book. Chapter 3 probes the broad area of scientific theory and methodology. The discussion focuses on the scientific method, its relationship to problem solving, the need for investigative tools, and nursing and the methods of science. Also included is an introduction to scientific terminology used extensively in the research process. Chapter 4 focuses on the steps of critiquing research projects and research reports. Chapter 5 introduces the beginning investigator to the process of developing a researchable problem and a research question. Chapter 6 discusses the relationship between research theory and methodology and explains theoretical perspectives, the kinds of theory, theory building, and the importance of theory to health science.

CHAPTER 3

SCIENTIFIC METHOD

Scientific method is a process of investigation. This process involves objectivity (viewing a situation on the basis of factual evidence without bias) and the use of empirical data (sensory material) in a systematic manner. The scientific method has not always been an acceptable means of investigation. It is not certain when the scientific method was adopted, but it probably started with some individual who was curious about nature and who began to make some systematic observations.

As early as 4700 B.C. the Babylonians had developed a calendar. The Greeks appeared to be the first people to make advances in science. Thales, in 580 B.C., Anaximander, in 550 B.C., and others made systematic observations. Plato, however, thought that experimentation was a base mechanical art and condemned it.

Gillespie states that Greek science was subjective, rational, and intellectual with its starting point in the human mind. If an explanation was satisfying to reason and curiosity, it was sufficient. In contrast, modern science, starting outside the mind, confirms reason with facts and collects hard realities to provide answers.[1]

It has always been people of leisure and wealth, along with craftsmen, who have turned to science. However, artists seem to have led the way. Although engineers and other inventors were often involved in inquiry, artists were not only working and inventing for improvements in painting and their arts, they were experimenting with new types of metal that would make weapons and tools. They found that in order to test, they had to experiment. One of the greatest experimenters the world has ever known was Leonardo da Vinci (1452–1519).

Galileo (1564–1642), the Italian physicist and astronomer, found that the earth and other planets rotate around the sun, not the other way around. Galileo may be called the father of modern science, for he was the first to use modern experimental methods.

However, Dr. Don Martindale[2] says that it was the Greeks who almost developed the scientific method. They were aware of the need for objectivity, especially in history. These early historians observed that they could not take one person's word for what happened in a battle. They found that if they listened to several versions of what happened in a specific battle incident, they could understand much more about the event. This objective method of history, if combined with the logic of philosophy, could have produced the scientific method. According to Martindale, the modern scientific method was waiting in

---

[1]Gillispie, Charles C.: The edge of objectivity, Princeton, N.J., 1960, Princeton University Press, p. 10.

the wings with the Greeks, but somehow it was lost and finally squelched in the Dark Ages. The following story furnishes us with insight into the attitudes toward inquiry that hampered the search for truth.

> In the year of our Lord, 1432, there arose a grievous quarrel among the brethren over the number of teeth in the mouth of a horse. For thirteen days the disputation raged without ceasing. All the ancient books and chronicles were fetched out, and wonderful and ponderous erudition was made manifest. At the beginning of the fourteenth day a youthful friar of goodly bearing asked his learned superiors for permission to add a word, and straightway, to the wonder of the disputants, whose deep wisdom he sorely vexed, he beseeched them in a manner coarse and unheard of, to look in the mouth of a horse and find answers to their questionings. At this, their dignity being grievously hurt, they waxed exceedingly wroth; and joining in a mighty uproar they flew upon him and smote him hip and thigh and cast him out forthwith. For, said they, "Surely Satan hath tempted this bold neophyte to declare unholy and unheard-of-ways of finding truth, contrary to all the teachings of the fathers." After many days of grievous strife the dove of peace sat on the assembly, and they, as one man, declaring the problem to be an everlasting mystery because of a dearth of historical and theological evidence thereof, so ordered the same writ down.[3]

The Renaissance brought with it a period of contrasts. Even though there were bitter wars and a revival of superstition, there were also great voyages of discovery, a study of nature firsthand, the Reformation, and the invention of printing. The search for truth had not been set aside.

In a general discussion with colleagues as to why social science research was so slow in developing, several ideas surfaced. Almost all the ideas seemed to be tied directly or indirectly to religion. For some individuals there has been a feeling that to pry into the lives of human beings is really not ethical, whereas others have the notion that we cannot really learn much about human beings.

The matter of authority has also slowed the development of social science research. People need to appeal to some higher authority, and when this higher authority disagrees with what they have observed, in spite of firsthand knowledge they tend to go along with the higher authority. A good example of this is seen in the following account:

> The story is told of a young student in the early days of universities who was dismissed because he argued with his instructor to the point of claiming that tigers had stripes. After all, who was this student to disagree with a famous Greek predecessor who had written that tigers did not have stripes. The student had only seen tigers, and one's observations could not be tolerated as a way of obtaining facts. The only truths were those stated by the authority.[4]

Many conflicts also have arisen over the possibility of using scientific procedure to study human behavior. Goode and Hatt cite four such problem areas: (1) over a period of time, changes in human behavior prevent exact predictions from being made; (2) individual behavior is too complex to place into quantitative analysis for investigation through the

[2]Classroom lecture, University of Minnesota, Minneapolis, Minnesota, 1965.
[3]From Francis Bacon as cited in Best, John W.: Research in education, ed. 3, Englewood Cliffs, N.J., © 1977, Prentice-Hall, Inc., p. 3.
[4]Helmstadter, G.C., editor: Research concepts in human behavior: education, psychology, sociology, New York, © 1970, Appleton-Century-Crofts, p. 9. By permission of Appleton-Century-Crofts, Education Division, Meredith Corporation.

instruments of science; (3) when individuals are studied by other individuals, the emotions of both the observed and the observer compound the problem; and (4) the free will of human beings allows them to deliberately upset predictions.[5] These four reasons are at least a partial explanation for the failure of scholars to adopt the scientific method for the study of human beings.

Stein has divided the progress of the scientific method, as related to medicine, health, and rehabilitation, into seven chronological stages.

1. Biological. An accurate description of the anatomy and physiology of the body was accomplished.
2. Methodological. The development of precise instruments enabled scientists to accurately measure internal body processes.
3. Etiology. An integration of the function of body systems and methodology was used to provide a diagnosis of disease.
4. Prevention. Sanitation, purification, and vaccination were used to prevent disease.
5. Treatment. Disease conditions were treated by use of chemicals, surgery, and hospital care.
6. Rehabilitation. Maximum rehabilitation of the mentally and physically disabled was achieved through the development of allied health techniques.
7. Habilitation. The use of special education and psychological technology was developed to identify and treat developmental and social disabilities.[6]

In summary, the process began with an accurate anatomical description of the body followed by the development of precise measuring devices such as microscopes, stethoscopes, and thermometers. The germ theory led to the understanding of the cause-effect relationship between germs and disease. The prevention of disease was the next logical step; this was improved by the use of new methods in the field of public health. Advances in technology and in theory improved the treatment of disease. As cure is not always sufficient, steps were taken to restore the disabled to maximum physical and mental function.

Specialties in the health professions arose as a result of expanding knowledge and technology. Finally, attention was given to individuals who had social demands that were not being met by the medical and public health professions.[7]

Conservatism has been cited as a major reason for the slow acceptance of new approaches to health care.

> We should not fail to remember that the great anatomist Vesalius was ridiculed mercilessly by his colleagues when he attempted to describe the human body as it is actually constructed. William Harvey was professionally berated after he asserted that the blood really circulates through the body. Bodington, when he suggested that tubercular patients be exposed to fresh air, was laughed down as a faddist. Semmelweiss, whose work with puerperal fever is now world acclaimed, was held up to scorn when he recommended that careful hygienic measured be employed at childbirth; his persecution was so brutal that he went insane. The

[5]Goode, William J., and Hatt, Paul K.: Methods in social research, New York, 1952, McGraw-Hill, Inc., p. 2.
[6]Stein, F.: Anatomy of research in allied health, Cambridge, Mass, 1976, Schenkman Publishing Co., Inc., pp. 3–40.
[7]Ibid., pp. 3–40.

Royal Society of Physicians of London rejected the discovery of Marshall Hall of the reflex function of the spinal cord and the brain. Andrew Still was ostracized from the medical profession after he voiced his osteopathic concepts. Daniel David Palmer was persecuted when he initiated modern chiropractic to the world. And even most recently, the Australian nurse Sister Kenny was assailed for her different, yet more successful, approach to the handling of polio in the 1930s–50s.[8]

Any society that does not constantly seek new answers to old problems is destined to become stagnant if not ineffective. It has been the natural history of medical orthodoxy to resist change, often to the point of obstinancy. While such a conservatism offers stability to the status quo and a safety factor against faddism and competition, it must not be allowed to prevent objective analysis of the new theories developed beyond the medical pale.[9]

STEPS OF THE SCIENTIFIC METHOD

The number of steps listed in the scientific method tends to vary depending on whether some steps are grouped or stated separately. Here they are considered as five in number:
1. The problem is stated (purpose of the project is determined).
2. An hypothesis is formulated for testing.
3. Facts are gathered from observations or experimentation.
4. Data are compiled and interpreted.
5. Conclusions are drawn.

Seven steps are often identified as necessary in the research process. However, different authors may name different steps. For instance, Barnes, in describing the steps in educational research lists them as formulation of the problem, collection of background information, incubation period, formulation of the hypothesis, development of methodology, analysis of data, and conclusions concerning the hypothesis.[10]

French, on the other hand, suggests a more precise first step, that of identifying, limiting, and defining the problem. Next, French identifies basic assumptions prior to accumulating the relevant facts and principles. Before beginning a plan of action, the researcher arranges assumptions, premises, and conclusions. Then a plan of action is selected and carried out. Finally, the researcher evaluates the outcome.[11]

Notice that there is no reference to the hypothesis formation or the design for testing the hypothesis in French's approach. This may be a matter of semantics, and both writers may actually be advocating the same steps but emphasizing aspects of them differently.

Stein considers the scientific method to have eight steps including problem identification, library searching, hypothesizing, method application, examining results, and discussion of findings. In additions, he includes titling and writing an abstract.[12]

---

[8] From Chiropractic health care by R.C. Schafer, Published by the Foundation for Chiropractic Education and Research © 1977, Des Moines, Iowa.
[9] *Ibid.*, p. 27.
[10] Barnes, Fred P.: Research for the practitioner in education, Washington, D.C., 1964, Department of Elementary School Principals, National Education Association, pp. 24–25.
[11] French, Ruth M.: The dynamics of health care, New York, 1968, McGraw-Hill, Inc., p. 112.
[12] Stein, pp. 50–51.

Abdellah and Levine include 12 steps. Defining variables, quantifying variables, delineating target population, and formulating method to analyze data are additional steps not included in some of the other writers' guidelines.[13]

Polit and Hungler have fifteen steps that include doing a pilot study and revising. Most authors agree on the method, but vary in the number of substeps in each step.[14]

THE RESEARCH PROCESS: AN EXPANDED VERSION

The steps of the research process are an elaboration of the steps of the scientific method. They are described here briefly as an aid to gaining an overview of research as it is discussed in the following chapters.

1. General problem or question. Research may begin with the question, "*What* am I going to study?" or "*What* is the problem?" The general topic may be hazy at first, but careful thought and study eventually shed light on the true problem. Productive research is often the result of observing a familiar phenomenon from a different perspective.

2. Specific problem or question. Since the general problem or question tends to be too complex or too broad for a single investigation, focus is made on a particular area of concern, and the research project deals with the most pertinent aspect of that problem or question. Unless there is a target, it is difficult to know when a mark has been hit.

3. Purpose of this research. For the benefit of informing others about the project and clarifying the reason for this particular investigation, the researcher determines and states the specific purpose or goal of this inquiry. Within the boundary of the phenomenon under study, the researcher selects one aspect for investigation at this time. Later, other aspects of the phenomenon can be studied. The statement of purpose is concise and leaves no doubt in the reader's mind as to the focus of the project.

4. Library search. Searching for appropriate background literature and nonverbal materials may begin during step 1 and continue to the point of data collection. However, the researcher must return to the library periodically to keep abreast of the latest information concerning the topic under investigation. Literature searching can and should occur when looking for instruments and when investigating how data were collected in other research projects, how the data were analyzed, how statistical techniques were used, and how the results were written up.

5. Hypothesis. An hypothesis(es) is (are) a statement(s) to be tested. By the time the library search is completed, the researcher is ready to predict the findings of his/her research. It is important that the hypothesis or the question to be answered is determined relationships, and on the basis of the findings the hypothesis is accepted as true or rejected as false.

6. Research design. The researcher begins by developing a framework based on theory or concepts (theoretical framework or conceptual framework) before plunging into the project. Once the overview of the research is determined, the investigator is able to fit the research plan together. Consideration must be given to each of the following steps:

---

[13] Abdellah, F., and Levine, E.: Better patient care through nursing research, ed. 2, New York, 1979, Macmillan, Inc., pp. 97–98.
[14] Polit, D., and Hungler, B.: Nursing research: principles and methods, New York, 1978, J.B. Lippincott Co., pp. 41–53.

a. Approach to be taken. The researcher decides which approach will best answer the research question or meet the objective: a survey, a case study, an experiment, or an historical investigation. Considerations must include permissions that might be required, ethical dilemmas that could occur, the timing of each step of the project, and defining of terminology.

b. Instrument. Should one or more tools be used to collect the data? Should the researcher develop a new tool or use one that has already been tested? What instrument would yield the most significant information? The library is the best source of ideas and information concerning the instrument. The researcher must constantly ask himself/herself if the instrument tests what it proposes to test. If there is any doubt, then a new or revised instrument is needed.

c. The researcher must determine the criteria to be used in the selection of the sample, the proportion of the population to be used in the study, and the method of contact. When selecting a sample of the population (all the possible subjects), the more the researcher knows about the sample, the easier it is to determine the sampling procedure.

d. Data collection process. The researcher identifies alternative procedures for collecting the information sought. The advantages and disadvantages of each data-collecting technique are evaluated, and the most appropriate one is chosen. Necessity of travel, time allotted for collecting the data, and cost are concerns.

e. Tables. Since tables are used to present a systematic arrangement of data in tabular form, the format of the tables must be well planned. The format must provide for all data pertinent to the study. By planning the format and titles of each table as part of the research design, the instrument will be easier to develop.

7. Pilot study. During the planning stage for the investigation, the researcher decides on the location, the subjects, and the permission that must be obtained to carry out the ministudy. During this stage, the instruments may be pretested, and proposed techniques are evaluated to ascertain weaknesses in the study design. Revisions may be necessary. The pilot study is actually a ministudy so it includes all the steps of data collection and analysis except the number of subjects are on a smaller scale.

8. Data collection. Actual information (data) desired by the investigator is gathered, using the instrument that has been developed and tested in the pilot study. Worthwhile research demands that each piece of data collected has a reason and purpose relating to the goal of the project.

9. Analysis of data. Research data are categorized, scrutinized, and cross-checked. Tables and other visual aids organize the findings. Included in the analysis is the quantification of data and application of statistics, where appropriate. The process of analysis is determined by the research approach that is taken; a survey and an historical investigation will produce different types and amounts of data.

10. Evaluation process. After analyzing the data, the researcher ponders the true meaning of the results. What do they imply? Is it likely that the population from which the sample was drawn is so similar that generalizations can be made from the sample to the larger group?

11. Conclusions. Concise summary statements of the findings are formulated from the analysis. The researcher ponders the question "What did I actually learn from my data?" The answers are then listed as the conclusions of the study.

12. Implications. The question to be answered is, "What do the findings mean for others (for example, the profession, the administration, and the faculty)?" What is the value of the study for them? Should it result in changes in some of their policies? In their curriculum? In their assumptions?

13. Recommendations for further research. Based on the conclusions, the investigator makes suggestions for further research that will provide more insight into the topic. Included are suggestions to future researchers on how to improve any part of the research methodology (such as hypotheses), how to collect additional or different data, pilot studies, analysis of data, and so on.

14. If the research project is sponsored by an organization or agency, it may request a report of the researcher's recommendation for action. An oral report may be given at the time the written report is submitted.

PROBLEM SOLVING

The concept of problem solving and the scientific method are often considered synonymous; both are ways of finding answers to problems. However, research is more rigorous and broader in scope than problem solving. One basic difference between the two seems to be that in the problem-solving method there is a problem that needs a solution; whereas in the scientific method, we may not have a problem, we may be merely interested in the answer to a question.

An analysis of differences between research and problem solving reveals that nursing theory is developed and tested through research, whereas problem solving has as its goal finding solutions. It is narrower in purpose; its aim is to solve a well-defined problem.

An interesting example of defining the problem was given by Mrs. Pansy Torrence during a classroom presentation.[15] In a speech on creativity she told of a family who was in very poor circumstances. The family had an old broken baby crib, but not enough money for another one. The baby had jumped up and down in the crib and had broken the bottom out, so the crib needed to be replaced. The question arose, "Was replacing the crib the important thing?" Was this the problem to be solved? No, the class finally decided that the problem to be solved was "Where is the baby to sleep?" The baby did not necessarily have to continue sleeping in the crib. Recognizing the problem is not always easy. In the problem-solving technique, part of the process is recognizing the problem.

Diers advocates that nursing research should give first priority to solving nursing practice problems.[16]

In the problem-solving technique one must identify the problem, collect and analyze the data, make a decision, and evaluate the decision. The conclusion is that if the problem is solved, lessened, or eliminated, the solution has passed some kind of test of validity, simply because it has worked.

The main purpose of any kind of research, whether it is problem solving in the health field, an experiment in physical science, or an investigation in the social sciences, is to describe, predict, control, or explain.

[15]Classroom lecture, University of Minnesota, Minneapolis, Minnesota.
[16]Diers, Donna: This I believe—about nursing research, Nurs. Outlook **18**:54, November 1970.

According to Folta and Deck, problem solving does not always involve research. They believe that the aim of research is to make a contribution to general knowledge, whereas problem solving is concerned with a single situation rather than broad problems.[17]

Problem solving is accomplished in five steps: (1) an obstacle is perceived; (2) the difficulty is identified and put into behavioral terms (specific overt actions that can be identified); (3) an investigation is made (all the steps of the scientific method and the appropriate tools are used to collect and analyze the problem); (4) possible solutions are suggested and evaluated, one or more of the solutions are accepted, and the most plausible one is tried out; and (5) the decision is evaluated on the basis of consequences. Problem solving and the scientific method follow in a logical sequence. In other words, the investigator does not propose a solution before identifying the problem; data must be gathered before the results can be analyzed. Most research texts do not discuss problem solving because it is not considered to be true scientific research.

Differences between the scientific method and problem solving are presented in Table 3-1. Four major factors must be noted. First, it is not necessary to have a problem when utilizing the scientific method. For instance, an organization that sponsors a radio or television series of programs on health care may be interested in learning the composition of their listening-viewing audience because it would be helpful for future programming. There may not be a problem involved, only the desire to produce programming that is suitable for the majority of the audience. For example, an interesting series of first aid demonstrations was presented on the local TV station by several students enrolled at the University of Panama School of Nursing in 1974. It was a means of teaching the public how to meet the emergency needs of the family.

Second, the scientific method usually tests an hypothesis, unless the researcher is conducting an exploratory survey. In the latter case a descriptive study provides factual information on such factors as respondents' perceptions, their attitudes, and their socioeconomic status.

Third, the scientific method goes beyond problem solving. After conclusions are drawn, implications for specific groups are determined, and recommendations for further research are reported, based on the present findings.

Fourth, statistics are frequently omitted in the problem-solving method because they may not be needed in dealing with a single case.

TABLE 3-1 Comparison Between Scientific Method and Problem Solving

Scientific Method	Problem Solving
1. May not have a problem; may have a question or an hypothesis	1. Identify the problem
2. Study design developed	2. Usually the same as scientific method
3. Data collected	3. Usually the same as scientific method
4. Analyze and report results	4. Analyze and decide which solution to attempt
5. Conclusions, implications, recommendations determined	5. Evaluate decision on basis of consequences

[17]Folta, Jeannette R., and Deck, Edith S.: A sociological framework for patient care, New York, © 1966, John Wiley & Sons, Inc. By permission of John Wiley & Sons, Inc.

ABILITIES NEEDED FOR RESEARCH

In order that the steps of the scientific method be carried out accurately, there are certain skills that the researcher must develop. Dressel has suggested that these are eight in number.

1. Ability to recognize the existence of a problem
2. Ability to define the problem
3. Ability to select information pertinent to the solution of the problem
4. Ability to recognize assumptions bearing on the problem
5. Ability to make relevant hypotheses
6. Ability to draw conclusions validly from assumptions, hypotheses, and pertinent information
7. Ability to judge the validity of the processes leading to the conclusion
8. Ability to evaluate a conclusion in terms of its application.[18]

Practice is the mechanism by which these skills are attained. The learner is expected to accept the rigorous standards of the research process and to work unhurriedly and painstakingly in each step. Accuracy is a must in a systematic investigation as all data are carefully recorded and reported. These data, gathered from firsthand or primary sources, are organized into quantitative terms, with the learner using logic and objectivity in place of presumptions and biased opinions. A scientific attitude enables the individual to seek rationality as the basis of verification, rather than to depend on intuition or emotion.

NURSING RESEARCH AND THE SCIENTIFIC METHOD

The principles of the scientific method such as rigid control, objectivity, careful measurement, systematic organization, and rigorous standards are as necessary in health research as they are in any other discipline. These principles, however, are applied in a manner unique to nursing. Medicine has a whole series of ethical and methodological problems related to research on human beings. A new type of drug for humans cannot be used in experiments until it has been tested in a laboratory using animals. In some instances, the animal may be destroyed. Social and behavioral sciences stress the study of human interaction through verbal and nonverbal means (observation, opinions of subjects, and historical records). Since nursing research is primarily concerned with human subjects, it tends to utilize techniques, methods, and ethics similar to those employed by social and behavioral scientists.

Research involves the implementation of the scientific method to answer questions and study problems. It is more than quoting, paraphrasing, and writing a paper. The student who limits inquiry to the use of the library in order to learn about the effects of malnutrition, for instance, is not doing true scientific research. If malnutrition is compared with the consumption of a certain food, this could be studied as a scientific inquiry. Use of the library to report on a condition or situation is a single step of the scientific method.

[18] Dressel, Paul: Evaluation in higher education, Boston © 1961, Houston Mifflin Co., pp. 72, 73.

It can no longer be said that there is a dearth of nursing theory. Graduate education has provided nurses with the skills and opportunity to conduct research in their own discipline. This has led to a major interest in the development of theory and a modest increase in theory development. Discussions, books, and articles now refer to nursing theory as they once did to research. This situation is an influencing factor in how and what nurses are investigating. Lack of theory in the past probably influenced nurses to be problem-solving oriented and more motivated to find answers than to apply rigorous scientific methodology to the development of theory.

SCIENTIFIC TERMINOLOGY

Before the initial stage of a scientific investigation, it is necessary to consider certain preliminary steps. Definitions are an important part of the communication process, and in research, clear, precise defining of terms takes on special emphasis. The student researcher needs only to look up the definition of a single term to find that no two writers seem to agree on exactly the same meaning for a word. It is important that the definition of the following words be understood.

A *concept* is a generalized idea of some group of objects, or an abstract idea generalized from several specific instances. A workable definition of the term concept is that it is an image or mental picture of some phenomenon. The phenomenon or concept may require several words to describe it adequately. To save time here we give these words a name. This name now substitutes for the description of the phenomenon. When the name of a concept is used, it gives the idea of the long verbal definition. Examples of concepts are "health," "nursing intervention," "nursing process," "holistic," "society," "status," and "happiness."

Conceptualization is the process of forming ideas, designs, and plans. The term need not be limited exclusively to research; it is an important process in the formulation of plans for problem solving. Conceptualization may result from attaining a great deal of background information, or it may come as a flash of inspiration. If creativity is 90% perspiration and 10% inspiration, the same is probably true of conceptualization. There is no substitute for gaining knowledge, experience, and background information in order to produce fruitful conceptualization of a good research plan. During the conceptualization stage, strategies are planned, operational definitions are identified, methods of approach are selected, and types of instruments are given a mental examination. Problems of confusing or obscured language and clarity of wording may force us to reconceptualize the research plan.

Conceptualization is the process of moving from an abstract idea to a concrete proposal. Suppose a nurse researcher is interested in self-care as related to diabetics. Suppose, further, that she has observed that diabetic patients are often grouchy and irritable on some occasions but pleasant and agreeable at other times. The conceptualization process will be used by the researcher to answer the following questions:

How do the swings in mood relate to diabetes?

Do all diabetics have shifts in mood?

Are changes in mood always extreme and noticeable?

Are diabetics aware of their changes in mood?

Why do diabetics allow unpleasant moods to harm their interpersonal relationship?

What safeguards can be used to counterbalance mood changes?

While some of these questions may not have instant answers, they nevertheless come to mind during the process of conceptualization. If the diabetic recognizes his or her own mood changes and relatives and friends report that they observe them too, this must be a clue. The researcher begins to develop a plan at this point in the conceptualization process.

Suppose a number of diabetics self-rate their mood changes and then family and friends rate the diabetic subjects on mood changes. Both groups could use the same rating scale. If selected characteristics could be ranked from high to low, the data would lend itself to a statistical analysis by rank-order correlation. Suppose there was a positive correlation between relatives and the diabetic (they agreed on mood changes)? What would it mean?

We will not carry this example of conceptualization further, but it is evident that conceptualization is analogous to a maze puzzle. In his or her mind, the researcher explores the pros and cons of various schemes, plans, and courses of action. In turn, each plan is analyzed for strengths and weaknesses. Some plans are rejected or combined. Hypotheses are changed, concepts developed, terms defined, and instruments considered. Conceptualization is "the look before you leap"; it considers alternatives and maps out a useful strategy for the researcher's blueprint of action. Even though conceptualization is the most difficult aspect of research and often requires considerable time, the effort can make the difference in the quality of the results.

A *fact* is the most basic term in research. It is the irreducible object. For example, it is a fact that there are 12 chairs in a given room. We can say that a fact is something that has actual existence, that can be verified. It is a statement of actuality. The more facts we have at our disposal or are able to obtain, the more completely we are able to do research. We analyze the facts to interpret the meaning of their relationships. Therefore, if we do not have sufficient facts, our research results will not have reasonable assurance of acceptable value. Facts are the building stones for hypotheses, propositions, and theories (Fig. 3-1).

A *hypothesis* is one kind of statement or declaration—usually one that can be tested. Quite often several propositions make up a hypothesis. However, a proposition, unlike an hypothesis, is more closely allied to the level of a fact. A hypothesis can be an assumed or proposed possibility that is used for testing. Normally, a hypothesis has some logical or empirical possibilities for its testing, so that we can determine exactly how true, how relevant, or how correct it is. It is a type of guiding idea, a tentative explanation, or a probability. A hypothesis is often used to initiate or guide some type of observation. A hypothesis can quite possibly be true but usually it is now known to be true. If it is found to be true, it is advanced to a higher order, perhaps that of a scientific theory. Sometimes a hypothesis is assumed or conceded merely for the purpose of testing or merely for the purpose of an argument.

A *theory* is a kind of general principle or explanation of some phenomenon. Usually a theory is much broader and more complex than a fact. A specific theory has probably been based on facts or propositions that have been found to be true. Therefore, a theory is likely to be a rather detailed technical explanation of how phenomena have happened. However, a theory does not always provide an overall general explanation. A theory may

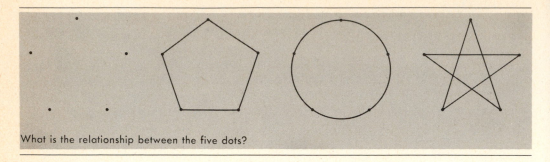

What is the relationship between the five dots?

FIGURE 3-1 Relationship between facts. Additional information may result in a more complete or different picture.
From Dr. Donald K. Smith, Daystar Communications, Nairobi, Kenya.

express the relationship of facts, and the analysis of facts and explanations; or it may explain the relationship of facts to other facts, or of propositions to other propositions. Quite often a theory generates one or more hypotheses to be tested. Theories serve as spotlights in the dark that are hopefully pointing us toward finding relevant knowledge. A theory can be a hypothesis that has been tested and found to be acceptable in certain cases under certain conditions.

Dr. Donald K. Smith believes that theory is correctly understood to be a grouping of facts that shows the relationships between them. From the grouping we can see new relationships and develop new applications from old knowledge. Since facts can be put together in different ways, it is necessary to find enough facts to develop one complete picture. Figure 3-1 illustrates what happens when there are lines drawn instead of just five dots; a more complete picture is represented. Dr. Smith suggests that theory is much like the five dots; further research provides information that leads to a more and more complete picture, until finally, the relationships can be stated with certainty and serve as a guide in practical work.[19]

Laws, on the other hand, are certain. We have called some ideas laws, such as the law of gravity, but we have never called evolution anything beyond a theory. In the field of mathematics, we might call a law a general principle to which all things respond or to which everything is applicable in every case. A law always implies regularity, a constant thing that continues to happen.

The process of searching for scientific truth begins with facts that can be developed into propositions. The relationship of fact to fact or proposition to proposition may suggest a hypothesis. After sufficient testing, a hypothesis may become a theory. Orem's and Roy's theories are examples of nursing theories that are receiving considerable application and evaluation. A theory may suggest other hypotheses that can be tested.

[19]Smith, D.K.: Paper given at the All India Christian Communications Conference, Nagpur, India, November 1978, and classes at Daystar International Institute, Nairobi, Kenya.

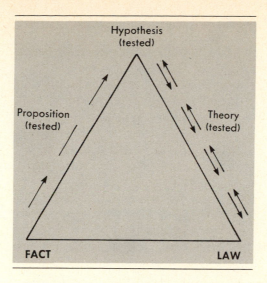

FIGURE 3-2   Relationship of scientific terminology.

When a theory has been subjected to much testing, the theory may attain the status of a law. The relationship between these steps is illustrated in Figure 3-2. The development of each step is further presented in Figures 3-3 to 3-5.

Facts and laws are two basic constants of knowledge that serve as the foundation of science. Between facts and laws is the working arena of doubt: propositions, hypotheses, and theories (Figure 3-5).

Sometimes research begins with a hypothesis that eventually leads to a scientific fact. However, even then, the hypothesis is based on some prior factual knowledge.

A *model* is a copy or an imitation of something that actually exists. It is a conceptual idea, formulated in the mind or on paper, that diagrams or explains a situation in real life. We may be able to make changes on a model to see the results and then infer that these same results will happen in real life. A model is a pattern, a standard, or an example that can be used as a form of comparison. Several types of models are referred to in research literature: analog models are analogies that show comparisons between theoretical concepts and real life; iconic models are scale representations of actuality; symbolic models are figurative representations of concepts and phenomena; mathematical models employ symbols that represent quantities and are frequently used to express laws and theories.

Models are often used in both research and theory. The basic format for models is a mathematical form and line drawings, referred to as schematic drawings or schematic models. A mathematical model shows the relationship of numbers through symbols, whereas the schematic model presents the relationship of variables through lines.

[20]Williamson, J.B., and others: The research craft, Boston, 1977, Little, Brown & Co., p. 332.

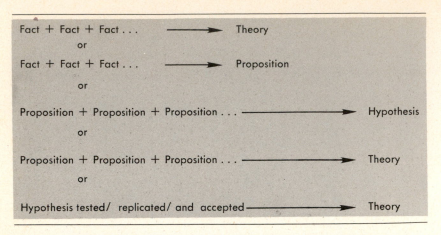

FIGURE 3-3   Examples of development of new knowledge.

Williamson and associates state that models have two major characteristics: (1) they are composed of the most influential factors that describe or explain an event, and (2) they clearly specify the causal relationships among variables.[20] Figure 3-2 is a schematic model that shows the relationships among five concepts.

The Roy adaptation model grew out of Sister Roy's experience as a nurse and is defined as a deductive model. Roy has done some theory construction from the model as well as developed some propositions deduced from axioms to be tested empirically.[21]

A *paradigm* is somewhat akin to a model, as both are a type of representation. Usually a paradigm is a picture of parts that are interrelated to each other. Some writers may call a conceptual diagram a paradigm; other writers may call it a model.

A paradigm also is used to visually represent a grammatical structure and as an anthropological device for analyzing cultural contrasts. Figure 3-1 may be considered a paradigm.

SUMMARY

The scientific method refers to the way techniques are selected for the acquisition of systematic knowledge. Although the scientific method is only about 400 years old, men were observing and collecting facts as early as 4700 B.C. Galileo was the father of modern

---

[21]Roy, Sister Callista: The Roy adaptation model comment, *Nurs. Outlook* 24(11):690–691, November 1976.

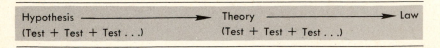

FIGURE 3-4   Process of theory and law building.

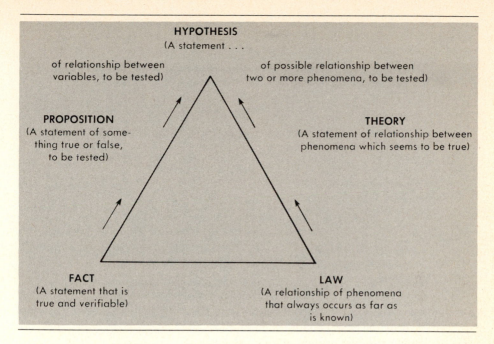

HYPOTHESIS
(A statement . . .

of relationship between
variables, to be tested)

of possible relationship between
two or more phenomena, to be tested)

PROPOSITION
(A statement of some-
thing true or false,
to be tested)

THEORY
(A statement of relationship between
phenomena which seems to be true)

FACT
(A statement that is
true and verifiable)

LAW
(A relationship of phenomena
that always occurs as far as
is known)

FIGURE 3-5 Development of scientific knowledge.

science. The basis of the scientific method in sociobehavioral research is a little more than 100 years old.

The steps of the scientific method are as follows: problem is stated, hypothesis is formulated, facts are gathered, data are compiled and interpreted, and conclusions are drawn. Implications of the study for nursing, for the community, or for the general public, and recommendations for further research are given.

An expanded version of the research method includes the following steps:

1. General problem or question
2. Specific problem or question
3. Purpose for this research project
4. Library search
5. Hypothesis
6. Research design
   a. Approach to be taken
   b. Instrument
   c. Sample
   d. Data collection process
   e. Tables
7. Pilot study
8. Data collection
9. Analysis of data
10. Conclusions

TABLE 3-2   Examples of Scientific Terminology

Scientific Terminology	Definition	Example
CONCEPT	A term or construct which is present but not readily visible	**Wellness**—implies a state of mental and physical health in which no pain is present
		Altruistic—a self-sacrificing love or concern for another. Animals and humans often sacrifice their own lives to save the life of their child or a friend.
HYPOTHESIS	A statement concerning two variables which is believed to be true and which is capable of being tested:	The more educated the nurse the less time he or she spends with the client.
		The more responsibility nurses have, the more time they spend on paper work.
		Nurses can better perceive patients' needs (as evaluated by the patient) than the physician.
FACTS	A statement which can be verified by objective measures:	There are four registered nurses assigned to surgery on Wednesday.
		The American Nurses' Association headquarters is located in Kansas City, Missouri.
THEORY	An explanation or principle which has been tested and accepted.	Orlando's theory of nursing is: nursing is the process of interacting with the patient.
		Roger's theory of nursing is: nursing is the science of humanity.
LAW	A statement of some phenomenon which is always true.	A straight line is the shortest distance between two points.
		Mercury expants when heat is applied (there are no laws in nursing identified as such).
MODEL	Models are conceptual analogies which explain reality. Theories are testable assertions while models are untestable.	Stress is the final cause of all disease.
		The world is being overpopulated in direct proportion to the number of illegitimate births.
PARADIGM	An explanatory framework which is often the result of considerable research or theorizing by a particular group.	The purpose of meditation is to prevent pain.
		As long as pain is present, the cause is undetermined, therefore pain is necessary to determine the cause.

11. Implications
12. Recommendations for further research
13. Recommendations for action, if sponsored; may include oral report

Problem solving, through similar to the scientific method, is narrower in scope and less rigorous. It is usually relegated to answering some question that needs a solution and is a type of methodology rather than a tool.

The researcher must develop an objective attitude that includes following rigorous standards and logical sequence and methods.

In a given research project, there is a variety of ways of collecting data, and it is seldom possible to say that any one method is better than another for collecting information. Training is often necessary if someone other than the researcher is going to be using the research tools.

The principles of the scientific method are utilized in nursing research just as they are in other disciplines; however, the uniqueness of nursing makes its own particular demand on how and what is studied.

The research process is related to the ideas of concepts, conceptualization, facts, propositions, hypotheses, models, paradigms, theories, and laws. A *concept* is a mental picture of a phenomenon. *Conceptualization* is the process used in clarifying wording and formulating a plan of attack in the research process. A *fact* is a common, verifiable truth and the basic unit for research. *Propositions*, which may be either true or false, are expressions of possible relationships between facts. A *hypothesis* states a relationship between variables. A *model* is an imitation of something that actually exists and is used for comparison in the research setting. *Paradigms* are conceptual diagrams that show the interrelationship of parts to one another. A *theory* is a general explanation of a phenomenon. A *law* implies regularity and complete dependability. It is considered to be at a higher level than a theory.

DISCUSSION QUESTIONS

1 What is the relationship between research and the scientific method?
2 Why is it important to follow the steps of the scientific method in chronological order?
3 Comment on the use of concepts as a means of advancing the field of knowledge.
4 Defend the following statement: The scientific method would have been a mockery to the reasoning power of man, a dead weight to the natural progress of the ages, and a useless plaything of academia had it been discovered and utilized before the Renaissance.
5 What are the possibilities that the scientific method will be superseded by a new breakthrough in knowledge acquisition?
6 How can the methods of science be used by an individual in the process of daily living?
7 In what ways does the scientific method differ from problem solving?
8 Describe an incident in which you would use the problem-solving process in preference to the scientific method?
9 Comment on the following statement: It is necessary to know the scientific method to do problem solving.
10 Is the scientific method more useful than problem solving? Support your response.
11 What is the relationship between the scientific method, problem solving, and pure and applied research?

CLASS ACTIVITIES

Tracks I and II

1 The class is divided into groups of two or three individuals. Each groups lists in detail the steps of the scientific method that should be followed when designing a project that could be conducted before the course is completed.
2 Each person is to select and describe a common health problem. The individual then outlines the steps that should be taken in order to study the problem scientifically.

SUGGESTED READINGS

Abdellah, F.G., and Levine, E.: Better patient care through nursing research, ed. 2, New York, 1979, Macmillan, Inc.

American Nurse, research project produces ten protocols on nursing care, Am. Nurse **14**:7, January 1982.

Batey, M.V.: Conceptualizing the research process, Nurs. Res. **20**(40):296–297, July–August 1971.

Brown, J.S., Tanner, C.A., and Padrick, K.P.: Nursing's search for scientific knowledge, Nurs. Res. **33**(1):26–32, January–February 1984.

Conant, James B.: Science and common sense, New Haven, 1951, Yale University Press.

Cotgrove, Stephen: The sociology of science and technology, The British Journal of Sociology **1**:1–15, March 1970.

Deets, C.A.: Methodological concerns in the testing of nursing interventions, Adv. Nurs. Sci. **2**(2):1–11, January 1980.

Dempsey, P.A., and Dempsey, A.D.: The research process in nursing, New York, 1981, D. Van Nostrand Company.

Elmes, D.G., Kantowitz, B.H. and Roediger, H.L., III: Research methods in psychology, ed. 2, St. Paul, 1985, West Publishing Company.

Gortner, Susan R.: Scientific accountability in nursing, Nurs. Outlook **22**(12):767, December 1974.

Hemple, Carl G.: Philosophy of natural science, Foundations of Philosophy Series, Englewood Cliffs, N.J., 1966, Prentice-Hall, Inc., p. 8.

Henderson, Virginia: Research in nursing practice—when? Nurse Res. **4**:99, February 1956.

Keresey, Elinor P.: Reaction to Ada Jacox, the research component in the Nursing Service Administration Master's Program, J. Nurs. Adm. **5**(1):6–8, January 1975.

Kratz, C.R.: Research—how can we challenge nursing practice? Nursing Times **78**(32):128, November 3–9, 1982. Occasional papers.

McManus, R. Louise: Today and tomorrow in nursing research, Am. J. Nurs. **61**(5):68–71, May 1961.

Manuel, B.J.: Research, a logical problem-solving method, AORN J. **27**(1):56–61, January 1978.

Morse, J.M., and others: Putting research into practice, Can. Nurse **79**(8):40, September 1983.

Orr, J.A.: Nursing and the process of scientific inquiry, J. Adv. Nurs. **4**:603–610, November 1979.

Padilla, G.V.: Incorporating research in a service setting, J. Nurs. Admin. **9**(1):44–49, January 1979.

Polit, D.F., and Hungler, B.P.: Nursing research: principles and methods, New York, 1978, J.B. Lippincott Co.

Rinehart, J.M.: One way to learn the research process, Nurs. Outlook **24**(1):38–40, January 1976.

Rotenberg, A.: Local studies—the way to solve local problems, Int. Nurs. Rev. **25**(2):53–54, March–April 1978.

Scriven, M.: Self-referent research, Educ. Res. **9**(6):11–18, 30, June 1980.

Silva, M.C.: Philosophy, science, theory: interrelationships and implications for nursing research, Image **9**(3):59–63, October 1977.

Stein, F.: Anatomy of research in allied health, New York, 1976, Schenkman Publishing Co., Inc.

Stember, M.L., and others: Job satisfaction research—an aid in decision making, Nurs. Adm. Q. **2**(4):95–105, Summer 1978.

Tinkel, M.B., and Beaton, J.L.: Toward a new view of science: implications for nursing research, Adv. Nurs. Res. **5**(2):27–36, January 1983.

Williams, P.D.: The scientific method, research, and nursing, Philipp. J. Nursing **46**:135–141, April–May 1977.

CHAPTER 4

CRITIQUING AN ARTICLE AND CRITIQUING SKILLS

CRITIQUING A STUDY

A critique is a critical evaluation of the strengths and weaknesses of any work—in this case, research. The word critique carries the connotation of being a negative reaction. Actually, the term refers to a process rather than an attitude.

Frequently, when teaching research methodologies, the learner is given an assignment to critique an article in a professional journal. Obviously, the beginning student has no previous experience, and little understanding of terminology, and is poorly equipped academically to evaluate the components of the research that was conducted.

We reject the notion that the research study was "poor" if the hypothesis was not accepted. All research has value and any subjective statements of worth must be regarded. Although the hypothesis was rejected, something was learned from the data. That is, to learn what is *not* true is as important as to learn what *is* true.

Often, both students and researchers critique research projects. The critiquing process is a critical estimate of the research report. It includes comments on the information provided as well as comments about omissions that should not have been made. A critique could include most of the topics covered in this book. However, such a critique would be too lengthy. The major points that should be included in a critique are provided in this section. The length of a critique is limited by its purpose and by the amount of time available for the task. Instructors and publishers may provide guidelines for a review, including its suggested length. In that case the guidelines should be followed.

After the initial perusal of the research report, the reviewer gains a general impression of the quality and the organization of the material. Following a second thorough reading, this impression may change. The reviewer should be sure to give consideration to each of the following topics.

Problem

Was the general problem stated clearly? Preferably the opening sentence will be definitive: "The problem of this study was…"
Does the author differentiate between the general problem and the specific problem?
General problem refers to national or universal while specific is local or personal.

Is the problem a practical one that needs a solution or one of a theoretical nature? If the problem is practical, it will relate to some specific or personal need. Theoretical problems should involve explanations, definitions, or the name of an individual associated with the theory.

What was the background of the problem? How did the author learn about the problem? What incident stimulated the problem?

What is the significance of the problem for future research? For the discipline? For the welfare of mankind? The value of the research and the beneficiary should be named. If the study is of a broad nature, the value should be implied. A new nursing intervention technique implies better health for all.

Purpose

The reviewer should note that there are two purposes for the study: (1) what the researcher hoped to achieve, and (2) why the researcher did the study.

The author will make a definite statement of purpose: "The purpose of this research is to evaluate the effectiveness of..."

Who will benefit from the research? A general group should be identified. Often research is done purely out of curiosity on the part of the investigator in which case it should be mentioned.

Was the study done for an organization? For a course requirement? For the personal interest of the investigator? It is especially important to identify the organization or course associated with the project. Also important is how the research will be used.

Conceptualization

Are the concepts of the author well defined? To understand research, it is important that concepts be adequately defined. Too often, concepts receive cursory, inadequate definitions. The author may be very familiar with the concepts, but readers also must be considered.

Are the concepts clearly understandable? The minimum treatment for an understanding of a concept is a definition and an illustration.

Are the concepts relevant? A relevant concept is one that is adequate and appropriate for the situation. It should be natural and not forced.

Is there a logical route from theory to research problem? Research based on theory is desirable since theory rests on a firm foundation. It is necessary that the path from theory to problem be defined. Such knowledge is valuable and provides an important learning tool for beginning researchers.

Does the total research plan indicate a creative conceptual framework? A clever conceptual framework is preferable to a laborious plan that is poorly or inadequately explained.

Do the steps of the conceptual framework have a logical, natural flow? The conceptual framework should move logically step-by-step from problem to data analysis. This movement should be evident in the flow of the research report.

Review of the Literature

Was the literature review specific to the purpose of the study? Did it include general background material? Or both? Literature reviews often take one of two extremes.

They either refer to two or more authors per sentence or one author for several sentences. The reader needs to know how much of the information is related to a given author and what is supplied by the researcher.

Was the literature review ample? Do the authors provide adequate information for the reader to gain an understanding of the topic? Some references should be made to classics as well as to current literature. Many scholarly journals include 30 to 50 references in the bibliography. Probably 20 to 30 is ample.

Did the material include professional journals, books, and general literature? A mix of references is valuable and all three sources should be included. Journals are more scholarly than the popular press. Professional journal material is often older than that found in popular magazines because it has taken so long to go through the process of manuscript review and printing. Books, as opposed to professional journals and magazines, seem to be more interesting and readable as resource material.

Are the authors authorities in their field? The reputation of the author(s) is important but not absolutely essential. Literature should be evaluated on its own merit.

Did the study include both current and noncurrent information? It is important that the literature review include historical and contemporary material.

Hypothesis or Question

Was the hypothesis stated clearly or was it hidden within the context of the report? The hypothesis should be stated very early in the report: "The hypothesis is...."

Was the hypothesis based on theory: If so, what theory? The name of the theorist and the theory should be identified. Theoretically-based research stands on tested ground and is preferable to nontheoretical research.

Did the hypothesis state a relationship between variables? An hypothesis should indicate the direction and relationship between two variables. If several hypotheses are used, each should be included.

Were the variables identified? Variables which have an effect on the hypothesis should be reported. The possible effect should be included.

Was the hypothesis defined in operational terms? Are the words in the hypothesis explained so that they could be tested? Replication studies are more difficult to conduct if operational terms are not reported.

If a question was researched, was the question clearly stated? Clarity and conciseness are necessary. The most frequent complaint about professional journals from students is that they are redundant, too wordy, difficult to understand, and concepts are not clearly defined.

Is the question worthy of study? The term worthy has a subjective connotation. Yet, a success-predicting scale appears to have more worth for more persons than a study of dating habits.

Design of the Study

Did the study show evidence of thorough planning from beginning to end? The study design is often a weak link in research projects; too often, the researcher completes one step before planning the next step.

Was this an original study or a replication of another study? It is important to give other authors credit when borrowing their ideas. The researcher should state if the study is a replication and/or how it deviated from the original.

Were all the steps of the scientific method included so that another researcher can replicate it? Research becomes useful and valuable as details are reported. Unfortunately, it is easier to critique a thoroughly reported study than an incomplete one.

Was a pilot study reported? If so, did it result in any changes in the major study? Pilot study results and changes should be described. The revision of instruments adds valuable insight to readers who may be considering similar research.

Was the instrument pretested for reliability and validity? Many research studies neglect to mention validity and reliability, which suggests that probably no effort was made to pretest the instrument.

What measures were taken to protect the rights of the subjects? Ethical dilemmas are becoming a legal issue. Many journals and funding organizations require that ethical standards be met before results are published or funds granted. If ethical safeguards are not mentioned, readers will be suspicious that ethics were not considered.

Were organizations or individuals identified in the report? Organizations, individuals, and groups should not be named or in any manner be identified in the research article unless permission is given.

Methodology

Was the sample appropriate for the hypothesis or question? Sample size can be affected by time and money. It is important to inform the reader what criteria were used to select the sample.

Was the sample representative of the population? Representativeness is a factor about which the researcher is most aware. It is the researcher who must inform the reader if the sample is representative.

What percent of the population was sampled? Was this adequate? Sample size is controlled by many variables. It is easy to criticize the researcher for the size of the sample, but the investigator may have reasons for including a particular size—personal preference or inability to gain access to additional subjects, for example.

Was the population specifically defined? In reporting sample size, it is important to inform the reader what group of subjects composed the population.

Were the descriptive measures or statistical tests appropriate? The beginning researcher may need assistance in interpreting the appropriateness of the statistical measures used to test the hypothesis. Regardless, the researcher should have explained how statistics were applied.

Were the researcher's biases reported? Every human being has some preferences and beliefs that are unrelated to factual evidence. Researchers must be aware of personal biases and warn the reader. Bias may appear in the selection of the sample or in the interpretation of the findings.

Did the researcher use a valid and reliable instrument? Investigators are obligated, in the interest of good research, to explain efforts to test for validity and reliability. It is desirable to perform two tests of validity and one of reliability. If the instrument does not test what it proposes to test, the research is of limited value.

Was an effort made to control the variables? The researchers should report the extent to which an attempt was made to control the variables.

How were the intervening variables controlled? The writer should indicate the methods used to prevent the influence of intervening variables. A conscientious researcher should identify all the steps in the study so the reader is aware of control factors.

If the study was an experiment, was manipulation of the variables well controlled? In experimental research, the controlling of variables is necessary and especially important to the critic. Any effort to improve the quality of the research must be reported, otherwise it is assumed that no measures were taken to control variables.

If the study was conducted by observation, was the researcher a participant? Observational research can be conducted with permission, by participant observation, lurking, without permission, and so on. The writer should indicate the kind of observation used and any ethical safeguards taken.

Was it necessary for the researcher to have assistants? If so, were they trained? When research requires the director to hire assistants, training must take place to ensure that all investigators give the same directions and collect the same type of data. Every part of the project must be conducted in an identical manner; the number of assistants and the training program should be described.

Analysis of Data

Were the results of the statistical test or the descriptive measure reported correctly? The usual complaint is not the correctness of results but how the statistics were used and interpreted.

Were the findings and data interpreted correctly? The writer must use concise but thorough descriptions if the reader is to make judgments concerning correctness. The reader should be able to understand the intent of the researcher and decide on the matter of correct interpretation.

Was the level of significance reported? Probably the second most important aspect of the research report is the statement of the level of significance. It is not sufficient to show the level of significance by a symbol at the bottom of a table. There should be a statement in the text of the report as well as in the abstract (brief summary).

Was the hypothesis accepted or rejected? The most important fact contained in the report is whether the hypothesis was accepted or rejected. It should be stated in the published report.

Were the tables set up correctly? The table format should be easy to understand and the data placed correctly in columns and rows.

Can the tables stand alone or is it necessary to read the authors descriptions to understand what they mean? Tables should be self-explanatory. If it is necessary to read the narrative for understanding, the tables are inadequate.

Was there consistency between the content of the tables and their descriptions? The reader's interpretation of the tables and the explanation provided by the researcher will be in agreement if the writer has set up the tables and explained them correctly.

Were there sufficient visual aids to make the findings easily understood? Some facts are more readily comprehended if provided by means of visual aids rather than in tables.

Conclusions

Were the conclusions supported by the data? Certainly, conclusions and data should agree. Conclusions should reflect the information that has been provided by the subjects.

Were the conclusions supported by the tables? The conclusions can be compared with the tables and the report text to determine if they agree. The tables should provide a visual presentation of the findings so that it is possible to determine if the two are in agreement.

Do the conclusions follow from the stated purpose of the study and the hypothesis? The conclusions should provide evidence that they are based on the purpose of the study and the hypothesis(es). The reader must be informed of all the important facts from the analysis of data.

Were the conclusions stated clearly and concisely? Each conclusion should be stated concisely and clearly so that the reader knows exactly what the researcher's final judgments are.

Implications

Were implications included in the research report? Implications entail extracting further meaning from the data. Implications have an "if, then" component. *If* this is true, *then* we can expect that...

Were implications suggested for practical use? It is hoped that the writer will suggest some practical points that will assist other groups in applying the findings. The report should be detailed enough for identified groups to make application of the findings.

What are the implications for the profession? The general public? The client? The discipline? The writer should inform the reader of those groups for whom the study holds special importance. Actual uses of some research findings may be restricted to additional research; application by the profession, client, public, or discipline may not be stated. Other groups, unknown to the researcher, may understand the value of a particular set of data from their own point of view.

Recommendations for Further Study

Were further studies suggested by the researcher? It is essential that the writer suggest further studies to be conducted. One of the major reasons for conducting a literature search is to become aware of suggested research.

Were recommendations realistic and meaningful? Future research suggestions should include broad (macro) studies which need grant support as well as smaller (micro) studies suitable for beginning researchers. Students should glean enough information from the report to develop additional ideas for research.

Were other hypotheses suggested by the investigator? An insightful researcher will suggest other hypotheses that might or should be tested in the future.

Miscellaneous

What were the strengths and weaknesses of the study? Strengths and weaknesses should be discussed by the writer. There have been few, if any, perfect studies. If the investigator does not mention weaknesses, the critics will. It is better if the researcher reports the flaws than for the critics to assume that he/she did not notice them.

Were the limitations and delimitations presented? Limitations are weaknesses or problems in the research such as a small sample or uncontrolled variable. Delimitations are restrictions imposed on the study by the researcher. For example, "only full-time nursing students should be included in the sample."

How extensive was the bibliography? Was it current? The bibliography should contain a good sampling of classics, current books and periodicals, and popular literature (if relevant).

Did the report provide suggested readings? Suggested readings are useful, but an adequate bibliography may be sufficient.

Did the author use a consistent style for the footnotes and bibliography? Consistency in footnoting also should include complete documentation. Month, year, and number are often ommitted from the bibliographies of professional journals and many authors do not include the page number for the books they cite. Any or all of these deletions may add difficulty when the reader wants to locate the literature for further investigation.

Were the grammar and writing style conducive to making the report interesting and understandable? Unfortunately, many writers use the jargon of their discipline instead of words that can be easily understood. This is one reason why research reports go unread by potential consumers.

Was an abstract included? If so, does it state the purpose, hypothesis, and results? An abstract including answers to the basic who, what, where, when, how, and why questions is very useful to the busy reader. An abstract should always be provided.

These major topics have been suggested for evaluation of the research report. Obviously, additional elements could be evaluated and criticized. However, if the suggested topics are thoroughly discussed, the resulting critique could conceivably be as long as the original research report. An evaluation of such details as footnoting, titles, grammar, spelling, questionnaire length, time of interviewing, details of the abstract, and so on could become mere nit-picking and might discount the value of the research.

Critiquing is a valuable exercise for beginning researchers. It can help them to gain an understanding of the investigative process. It should not become a critical game of faultfinding, but an evaluation that teaches beginners new research techniques.

SUMMARY

The critique of a research report should contain comments about the general impression the study makes. Background about the problem should include the value that can be expected from the results. The purpose should be in the form of a definitive statement.

Conceptual frameworks should reveal a logical route from theory to problem. Concepts should be clear and well defined.

Attention should be given to the literature review relating to topics such as relevancy, the number of appropriate journals, current literature, and classics consulted and evidence of depth of review.

Hypotheses should be operationally defined, understandable, and stated in definite terms so as to be testable.

The study design should show evidence of thorough planning in such areas as instruments, ethics, pilot studies, validity, and reliability. The section on methodology should evaluate sampling techniques, control of variables, and a consideration of various approaches. The analysis of data should contain a critical review of the uses of appropriate statistics, descriptive measures including self-explanatory tables, and reporting of statistical results. An evaluation of the conclusions should consider the purpose of the study, the findings as compared with tables, and the amount of support given the conclusions by the data.

The implications section should suggest uses for the findings as related to the profession, public good, and field of knowledge. A thorough study should suggest additional research, alternative methods and hypotheses, and advice on better methodology. The final, general evaluation should include summary statements of strengths and weaknesses and broad evaluations of the research study.

DISCUSSION QUESTIONS

1 Why is it desirable to critique a research study?
2 Comment on the following statement, "If you can critique research studies, you will most likely be able to conduct good research." Defend your position.
3 Why do you suppose some educational programs require a critique of a research study in place of actually conducting a research project?
4 Comment on the following statement: Novice researchers have a few skills or experiences which qualify them to critique research.
5 Comment on the following statement: If critics do not find as many positive as negative features in their evaluation, they are overly critical.
6 Why is criticism of research studies often the result of reader misunderstanding? Is it? Defend on point of view.

CLASS ACTIVITIES

Track I

1 The instructor distributes research articles or reports to each group of three to five students. The groups are to critique the handouts.
2 The instructor distributes two research articles to each group of three or four students. Each group reads research articles A and B and then compares the quality of the articles as to their clarity, their completeness, and the quality of their research designs.

SUGGESTED READINGS

Aamodt, A.M.: Problems in doing nursing research: developing a criteria for evaluating qualitative research, West J. Nurs. Res. 5(4):398–401, Fall 1983.
Diers, Donna: Research for nursing, JONA 3(1):11, January–February, 1973.
Fleming, J.W., and Hayter, J.: Reading research reports critically, Nurs. Outlook 22(3):174–175, March 1974.

Gulick, E.E.: Evaluating research requests: a model for the nursing director, J. Nurs. Admin. **11**(1):26–30, January 1981.

Issues in evaluation research, An invitational conference, Dec. 10–12, 1975. American Nurses' Association, ANA Publication Code No. G-124.

Knafl, K.A., and Howard, M.J.: Interpreting and reporting qualitative research, Research in Nursing and Health **7**:17–24, 1984.

Rescher, N.: Scientific explanation, New York, 1970, The Free Press, p. 152.

Schantz, D.: Reading a research article, Journal of Nurs. Admin. **12**:30, March 1982.

Snow, R.E.: Representative and quasi-representative designs for research on teaching, Review of Educational Research **44**(3):270, Summer 1974.

Some common-sense suggestions for nurses new at the research game, Can. Nurs. **77**:32–33, November 1981.

Stetler, C.B., and Marram, G.: Evaluating research findings for applicability in practice, Nurs. Outlook **24**(9):559–563, September 1976.

Ward, M.J., and Fetler, M.E.: What guidelines should be followed in critically evaluating research reports? Nurs. Res. **28**(2):120–126, March–April 1979.

CHAPTER 5

THE RESEARCH PROBLEM AND RESEARCH QUESTION

Research is motivated by several factors. Among these, is the necessity to always have goals or reasons for conducting an investigation. These goals or reasons are usually identified as problems and questions.

A problem is a condition requiring a solution. A question is an inquiry concerning a situation about which something is not known. When investigating a problem, the researcher is aware that a situation exists that needs an answer, whereas in the investigation of a question, curiosity or interest may lead the researcher into pioneer work in an area about which little or nothing is known. It is possible to develop hypotheses when conducting research on the basis of a question, but it is more likely that the study will be done without hypotheses. In this chapter, we will limit the discussion first to the research problem and then to the research question.

DEVELOPING A RESEARCHABLE PROBLEM

Wilson says, "Many scientists owe their greatness not to their skill in solving problems but to their wisdom in choosing them."[1] We might ask why one choice is better than another. Wilson has suggested that the problem should strongly interest the investigator. We agree with him because if one is not interested in the problem under investigation, it is difficult to become involved and keep going with the research.

Scientific research is not a routine process; it requires originality and creative thought. Therefore, the researcher must be in an environment that permits freedom of inquiry as well as nonconformity. The value of research is sometimes questioned, and the fear of what research will reveal may be threatening to the subjects being studied.

A research problem is based on any situation that needs answering. Developing a researchable project implies that not just any problem is researchable, and that it must be developed. "How many beds are there in Hospital X?" is not an appropriate topic for research. Anyone can simply count the beds in the institution. "What is the

[1]Wilson, E. Bright, Jr.: An introduction to scientific research, New York, ©1952, McGraw-Hill, Inc., p. 1. Used with permission of McGraw-Hill, Inc.

relationship between the number of beds and the quality of patient care?" can become a researchable inquiry.

On an abstract level, problems can be suggested by theories or other research. Suppose it is observed that residents in a particular high-rise apartment building are not availing themselves of a nurse's services. To the nurse this seems to be a problem because a much higher percentage of the residents in similar buildings are availing themselves of such services. On reflection, the nurse decides that there may be several reasons why the residents have not been coming to the high-rise clinic office. Do people need such services? Do they receive follow-up care somewhere else? Are "personalities" responsible for the seemingly negative situation? If the nurse already knows the answer, the situation is not a problem. If health care of the residents is inadequate, then there is a problem for investigation.

Problems needing research are to be found in every area of life—personal, professional, social, and institutional. Rarely is a problem so specific that refining is not necessary. In almost any research situation there is a general problem that can be redefined into a specific problem. For the nurse, the general problem is concern that all people in high-rise apartment buildings have adequate health care. The specific problem is that residents of a certain high-rise apartment seem to be receiving less nursing care than in similar buildings.

In an attempt to narrow the scope of the problem further, the nurse must ponder several questions. What evidence is there to indicate that a lower percentage of referrals is being made in this case? What evidence indicates that the health care of residents is less adequate than in similar high-rise apartment buildings? Is the problem relevant? Can it be that the nurse's real concern stems from a feeling of pressure from the sponsoring agency? Are people in the high-rise complaining about the services they are offered? It is possible that the residents in this case have good health, are receiving health care from other sources, cannot afford health care, are not aware of the services available, have racial prejudices, or are affected by personality conflicts.

Selecting a problem seems to be particularly difficult for the beginning researcher. The investigator who lacks insight into potential problem topics ought to read broadly in areas of personal interest and concern, talk with people knowledgeable in the discipline, and reflect on meaningful personal experiences.

Problems are problems only when they are perceived as such. This suggests that identifying the problem may be at the very heart of the research process. Superficial covering of the selected problem must be stripped away before the study can be initiated. After considerable thought, what at first seems to be the major problem may be recognized as only obscuring the real problem.

Many methodological approaches can be used to provide a solution. Some of the factors instrumental in deciding the approach to take include extent of institutional or administrative cooperation, finances, time, and level of skill attained by the researcher.

Frequently, a selected research problem is too extensive and must be limited to one aspect. The original problem may be so broad that only one segment at a time can reasonably be investigated. Remaining segments may be worthy projects for future study. Inexperienced researchers often try to solve the problems of the disciplines with one study and end up frustrated and discouraged because of inconclusive results. In other words, one should select a topic of concern, define the "real" problem, refine it to a single segment for study, and finally decide the purpose of the investigation.

A problem and a purpose are different. Problems are the *what* of research, and purposes are the *why*. It is customary to state the problem as the topic of the study; the purpose indicates the reason that the research is being conducted. Both the purpose and the problem should be closely related in a tight methodological research plan.

An illustration of developing a researchable problem is presented from the field of education. The researcher hears the complaint, "Children living in Northeast Neighborhood are receiving a poor education," from a parent. The complaint is based on the following statements:

1. The children are seen sitting on the front steps and curbs at all hours of the day.
2. Teachers report that their students are frequently absent from school.
3. The children can't read.
4. The kids can't get jobs after they leave school.

The researcher must verify the statements through such procedures as observation, checking school records, and interviewing teachers. If the parent's statements are valid, the question becomes, "Is this situation typical of all schools in the area?" A comparison of Northeast Neighborhood school records with records from other schools in the district and the state will confirm or refute the parent's contention.

The problem is then narrowed to, "What causes the children in Northeast Neighborhood schools to receive lower scores on the standardized achievement test?" For the purpose of research, the question could remain, "What causes children in Northeast Neighborhood schools to receive lower scores on the standardized achievement test than students in other district schools?" The research could be conducted by testing an hypothesis such as, "The cause of low achievement scores by students in Northeast Neighborhood school is lack of parental involvement in their children's education." Such terms as low achievement scores and parental involvement would need to be operationally defined.

For this particular study, the investigator could state that the purpose of the research is to learn more about parental involvement in their children's education in Northeast Neighborhood schools.

Suppose it is hypothesized that absenteeism decreases as motivation increases. Absenteeism might be defined as three or more days per year away from work, exclusive of vacation, paid holidays, and agency business. Motivation could be defined as a positive attitude which is manifested by offers to do extra work, arriving and/or beginning work early, and working to or slightly beyond quitting time. The topic could be studied as applied research if there is an absentee problem in Agency Y and the researcher wants to provide information for decision making, for instance. The approach could be that of qualitative research if the investigator studies the topic of absenteeism in general as it relates to motivation.

LeCompte and Goetz believe that developing a research problem requires the researcher to select a content area as well as choose the design of the study which includes methodology. The two authors differentiate between qualitative and ethnographic research as opposed to quantitative and positivistic research.[2] These will be discussed in greater detail in Chapter 20.

An initial step in problem selection is identifying variables and giving them abstract and concrete definitions. It is also necessary to distinguish between irrelevant and relevant ideas, material, or concepts.[3] After considering both the general and specific aspects of the problem, the researcher is prepared to develop the purpose of the study and move on into the library search.

DEVELOPING A RESEARCHABLE QUESTION

A researchable question is not as tangible as a researchable problem. Problems irritate people causing hardships and unpleasant situations; thus they are easier to identify than questions. Questions ask why; they are the result of observation or other research. Questions imply that the researcher is aware of some problem and is interested in why it occurs. The evidence that smoking causes cancer is well known. But the question is, "Why do people continue to smoke when they know it causes cancer?"

It cannot be stressed too strongly that good questions require background knowledge either from experience or from review of the literature. Even then it is necessary to narrow the topic to something more specific. "Nursing" is not a researchable question. "Why are nurses interested in politics?" is a much more specific question.

Fig. 5-1 illustrates an approach for generating researchable questions. A productive starting place is the experience of the researcher. Each person has experienced a particular set of events which provide opportunities for researchable questions. Researchers searching for a question could ask themselves the question listed on the left. On the right are some hypothetical answers. As the researcher moves down the list of questions, it becomes evident that it is possible to generate both problems and questions. Both the complaints and improvements listed yield problems, but finally, in the last section, the research question is formulated. This is not the only possible way of arriving at questions but it illustrates a principle.

GENERATING HYPOTHESES FROM QUESTIONS

The use of questions to generate hypotheses is provided here not only as an example but as a reminder that the researcher can begin a study with a problem or a question.

The researcher could begin by asking the question: What are some variables associated with the topic of special interest? The nurse who is interested in the care of infants might proceed along the thought process as follows:

> *Why do small babies have different personalities?* Some reasons I can think of are sex, race, parent's education, and stress during pregnancy. Some of these seem reasonable. However, others might include the amount of attention that is given the child by the mother, its weight at birth, or the cultural practices of the family.

[2]LeCompte, M.D. and Goetz, J.P.: Problems of reliability and validity in ethnographic research, Rev. of Educational Research **52**(1):31−60, Spring 1982.
[3]Cooper, H.M.: The integrative research review, a systematic approach, Applied Social Research Methods Series, Vol. 2, Beverly Hills, 1984, SAGE Publications, Inc.

Developing Researchable Questions	
	Hypothetical Answer
1. What is my nursing specialty interest?	—Pediatric nursing —Surgical nursing —Gerontological nursing
2. What is my area of expertise within my specialty?	—Premature infants —Orthopedic surgery —Rehabilitation of the aged
3. What complaints do I have either in my specialty or my area of expertise?	—Too busy or nothing to do —Pressure to start next patient before the last is completed —Patients often are taking one or more medications for each of several problems
4. What improvements would I like to see?	—More general staff nurses working in the evening —Schedule surgery patients on all shifts —More research on the substitution of nursing interventions for selected medications
5. What topics do I find especially interesting in my specialty?	—Behavior of infants and cultural practices of new mothers
6. *What is the relationship between birth weight and diet of the pregnant woman in _____? country	

*The last sentence could be the question to be researched.

FIGURE 5-1   Approach for generating researchable questions.

The second question might be, *How do children differ in personality?* Answers could include the amount of smiling and crying, ability to follow objects with their eyes, amount of movement of their arms and legs, amount of sleep required, amount of time used in rolling over, and so on.

The researcher would add other questions and responses to this list and then relate two of the variables into an hypothesis (a statement of the relationship between two variables). A few of the possible hypotheses are:

Male babies smile more (or less) than female babies.

Babies born to unmarried parents cry more (or less) than babies born to married parents.

Babies born to mothers who experienced stress during pregnancy will cry more than babies born to mothers who did not experience stress during pregnancy.

Numerous other hypotheses can be generated with no more than the variables listed here.

SUMMARY

Identification of a researchable problem is basic to research. The purpose and the problem (topic) for study should be closely related in the research plan. The steps of the scientific method are followed in solving or exploring the problem. Various approaches may be implemented to obtain data for testing and analysis.

DISCUSSION QUESTIONS

1 What is the relationship between the problem and the hypothesis?
2 How would you evaluate whether or not a problem is suitable for a research project?
3 Differentiate between a research problem and a research question.
4 Suggest three problems from your experience in nursing that would make good research studies.
5 Give an example of developing a research problem. Use an experience in which the original problem as first perceived was only an artificial coating for another problem.
6 Why are you well qualified to develop a researchable question from your own nursing experience?

CLASS ACTIVITIES

Track I (Activities Related to the Chapter, Not to a Single Project)

1 Divide the class into groups of two or three persons. Each group is to select two problems relating to nursing or health care and then determine what is the evidence that a problem exists.
2 Each student is to write a problem of interest and then list the assumptions that are inherent in it.

Track II (a Continuous Activity That Leads to the Completion of a Scientific Investigation)

1 Each beginning researcher writes a description of a problem of personal interest suitable for study during the course and lists assumptions.
2 The class is divided randomly into groups of two or three persons. Each individual reads his or her description to the other members of the group. Each group or individual student then selects the problem to be researched during the remainder of the course.

SUGGESTED READINGS

Adebo, A.O.: Identifying problems for nursing research, Int. Nurs. Rev. **21**(2):53–54, 59, March–April, 1974.
Artinian, Barbara M., and Anderson, N.: Guidelines for the identification of researchable problems, J. Nurs. Educ. **19**(4):54–58, April 1980.
Frazer, G.H., *et al*: Research questions in health education: a professional evaluation, J. Sch. Health **54**(5):188–192, May 1984.
Lindeman, C.A.: The research question, Journal of Nursing Administration, **12**:6–10, January 1982.

Lindsey, A.M.: Research questions and answers. Research: the problem and the purpose, Oncol. Nurs. Forum **10**(3):97–98, Summer 1983.

Thomas, B.: Using nominal group techniques to identify researchable problems...research preparation in nursing, Journal of Nursing Education **22**(8):335, October 1983.

Watson, J.: How does a nurse interested in research identify a researchable question?, J. Nurs. Res. **25**(6):439, November–December 1976.

Watson, P.G.: Formulating a research question, J. Enterostom Ther. **11**(3):125–126, May–June 1984.

Wechsler, H.: Choosing a research design and a study sample, in Wechsler, H., and Kibrick, A., editors: Explorations in Nursing Research, New York, 1979, Human Sciences Press Inc., pp. 89–95.

CHAPTER 6

THE RELATIONSHIP BETWEEN THEORY AND METHOD

At first glance, it would seem that an appropriate title for this chapter should be theory and research, but since methodology is the theme of the book, we find it more utilitarian to consider the relationship between theory and method. Thus, method refers to the use of theory in research.

Advocates of theory and research continue to proclaim their point of view as the source of new knowledge. Theorists usually claim that theory should guide research, whereas researchers claim that new theory is developed through research. Some scholars see a happy marriage between the two...theory and method complementing each other.

It may come as a surprise to the beginning researcher that it is difficult to separate method and theory because the two are closely related. It has often been stated that the physical sciences have laws, but the social sciences have only methods. This need not be the case in nursing, because nursing can draw from both areas while developing nursing science. The nurse-researcher should be aware that *how* information is found is as important as *what* is found. Unless the process or method of obtaining information is well conceptualized, the findings cannot be trusted.

The importance of methodology is also apparent in a health care institution. Suppose, when studying the quality of nursing care in a clinical unit, nursing students ask just the patients to whom they are assigned, "Were you given good nursing care this morning?" and all patients answer. "Yes, I was given good care." Can the students who asked the question assume that they gave good nursing care to their patients just because the patients said, "Yes"? No, they must criticize the method used to obtain their information. Obviously, there are at least two factors influencing the responses. First, the patients may not want to respond negatively, and therefore formulate an answer that will be sure to please the student. Second, the students and the patients may not be defining the word *good* in the same frame of reference. Again, it is not the findings but the method used that is the important factor. When we present or publish results, readers, after scrutinizing how we studied the problem, will criticize the results of such a study because of the methods used.

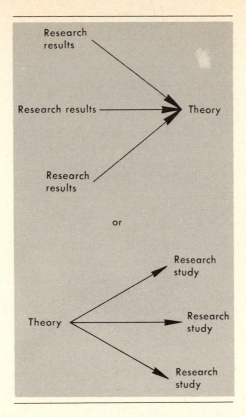

FIGURE 6-1   Which comes first—research or theory?

WHICH COMES FIRST—RESEARCH OR THEORY?

The question that seems to present itself immediately is, "Which comes first—research or theory?" It is possible to begin with either. We may need to do research in order to arrive at a theory, or we can select a theory on which to base our research (Fig. 6-1). It has been our experience when talking to young students that they will say, "I don't know what to research." In this case, our advice is, "Go out and look into the area in which you are going to do research. If you take a long, close look, you will notice some unusual circumstances or events that suggest research possibilities. You cannot sit home in your armchair and expect good theories to come floating to your mind. It is imperative that first you observe what is out in the real world, then go back and develop a theory. Unless you know what to look for, you may just have to observe broadly until you find something that interests you."

Two students recorded the number and types of individuals who came to the outpatient department at 9:00 AM. The findings gave them an idea for an hypothesis. Another student went to a restaurant located next door to a downtown hotel from 8:30 to 9:02 AM to observe the breakfast habits of the local residents. From her observations she developed an hypothesis concerning the importance of eating breakfast.

It seems that many researchers in various disciplines gather facts and figures for the pure enjoyment of collecting data. Instead, data need to be put in a larger context. There should be an overriding theme into which information can be categorized for the development of theory. Additional studies may be needed to clarify and amplify some neglected aspect of the theory. Some studies also should be repeated to learn whether or not the results are consistent.

Some researchers argue that research must begin with a theory; otherwise they are not sure what to research. Talcott Parsons suggests that numerical data must be placed in a broad analytical category—if we are to produce facts that can be utilized in a generalized theoretical perspective.[1]

THEORY

Theory is derived from the Greek word theoros given to the holy representative of the public festivities of Greek cities. The representative was an impersonal observer (theoria) of sacred events. Philosophically, theoria has taken on the connotation of contemplation of the cosmos.[2]

Although to many people theory is synonymous with speculation, to the scientist it goes further. Empirical evidence provides facts, and the relationship between these facts is the theory regarding the phenomena. An important, even primary, use of theory is to lead the researcher along the empirical route in order to accept or reject the nature of the theory. The results can be reinvested in the theory to modify or change some of its dimensions. The process can be repeated for further enrichment of both theory and practice.

It is interesting and important to find out how theory develops. Many scholars develop theories from being shrewd observers of their surroundings or from reading literature. New theories are often the result of riding "piggy-back" on the ideas of others. It is often mentioned that anything of value has been said before. Some people take delight in pointing out previous discoveries that are the forerunners of many ideas the innovator considered original.

Is creativity stimulated or suppressed by studying the history and development of certain theories? Is new theory developed in the armchair or in the laboratory? What process is used to generate theory? Do we use history as the springboard, since, as we have shown, there is nothing new; or do we attempt original discovery and ignore others who have discovered the idea years before?

For the purpose of increasing knowledge, knowing the name of a theorist does little to benefit mankind; but knowing the steps of a theorist's thought process provides insight into how theories can be formulated.

In showing the difference between the orientation of the sciences and the humanities toward classic works, Merton finds some disturbing features.[3] The pure sciences, such as

[1] Parsons, Talcott: The role of theory in social research, American Sociology Review 3:19, 1938.
[2] Habermas, Jurgen: Knowledge and interest. In Emmet, Dorothy, and MacIntyre, Alasdaire, editors: Sociological theory and philosophical analysis, New York, 1970, Macmillan, Inc., p. 37.
[3] Merton, Robert K.: Social theory and social structure. New York, 1968, The Free Press. Copyright © 1968 and 1967 by Robert Merton.

mathematics, physics, and chemistry, are cumulative, whereas the social sciences stop with the old classics. The average undergraduate student in many of the pure sciences is solving problems that early giants did not even comprehend. Theory and findings of the past are incorporated in the cumulative present knowledge. The actual discovery and discoverer are treated merely as history and have no other value.

In the physical sciences students traditionally repeat some of the old experiments, whereas in the social sciences retesting is rarely done. Strangely, contemporary scholars of the abstract disciplines rarely retest the theories or concepts of the founding fathers.

In the humanities, the classic works are treated with greater relevancy than present writings. Firsthand acquaintance with the founding fathers of the discipline tends to be all important for the social scientist, but meaningless for the physical scientist.

Duffey and Muhlenkamp have suggested four questions to serve as a framework for examining nursing theories: (1) What is the origin of the problems with which the theory is concerned? (2) What are the methods used? (3) What is the character of the subject matter dealt with by the theory? and (4) What are the results of testing propositions generated by this theory that you would expect to get?[4]

METHOD

Research method can generally be assumed to be the technique used by the scientist to collect and order data, to use statistical manipulation, and to arrive at a logical conclusion. After the process of collecting, refining, and analyzing data from the information gathered, we can develop a theory—an explanation of what is occurring. The explanation concerns the relationship between two or more variables or phenomena. We do not find isolated events, but correlations that are part of a much broader context of the relationship that exists between facts or events or both.

Methodological and theoretical considerations are dependent on each other for direction. Certain methods may be more appropriate for testing theory A than for testing theory B. It is generally accepted that most scientists use "pet" methods of research with which they are more familiar or feel most compatible. Questionnaires happen to be the most frequently used method for gathering data. Chapter 16 shows that questionnaires are often nothing more than opinionnaires.

THEORETICAL PERSPECTIVES

A theoretical perspective involves an entirely different viewpoint toward a situation than does a problem-solving approach. To the individual on the firing line in a face-to-face confrontation with reality, theories are of little value. It is generally conceded that everyday situations call for practical, everyday solutions.

Theories are general explanations of reality; they seldom attain the status of laws. The theoretical perspective is the broad look; it is the view from the highest point in the land.

[4]Duffey, M., and Muhlenkamp, A.F.: A framework for theory analysis, Nurs. Outlook **22**(9):571, September 1974.

The theoretical perspective is the "germ theory of medicine," not a treatment for a simple headache. The theoretical perspective tries to explain the cause of all illness and the "why" for every case.

Research is often conducted for the purpose of contributing to the body of theory. Haphazard selection of projects without theoretical bases ignores one of the primary purposes of research, namely, theory building.

Theorists usually explain reality with a theory specifically related to a rather limited situation. The nutrition expert, for example, might theorize that excessive use of preservative Y contributes to malady X. Such a theory, more on the order of an hypothesis, is valuable and commendable but does not qualify as a theoretical perspective approach because of its limited scope. If the researcher were to expand the project to include other health factors such as exercise, medication, and stress as they are related to malady X and preservative Y, he/she would be demonstrating a use of the theoretical perspective that might eventually lead to a more inclusive theory of health care in general. Such a perspective might explore such questions as, Can this particular theory be woven into a broader network of theories? If this theory is valid, what is the effect on other theories of health? If research fails to confirm the theory, is the theory valid or is the research inadequate?

USE OF THEORY TO GAIN KNOWLEDGE

Historically, many new discoveries were made by accident. Only in the last few hundred years has scientific experimentation been the basis for gaining knowledge that is raising safety standards, increasing efficiency, and improving health.

Early attempts at improving crop production probably did not involve deliberate experimentation. For example, it was found that dead fish made good fertilizer for increasing corn production. Probably the discovery of the relationship between using dead fish for fertilizer and the increase in crop yield was accidental.

Presently, theories are used by scientists in almost the same manner as fishermen use nets. Scientists cast their theoretical nets into the world in hopes of capturing knowledge that will predict and explain phenomena. Neither the fisherman nor the scientist casts his net just anywhere.

Scholars realize that even if the evidence indicates that a theory is unacceptable, some knowledge is still gained . . . they know what is false. The theory provides a point of focus for attacking the unknown in a specific area. If a relationship is found between two or more variables, a theory should be formulated to explain why the relationship exists.

When a theory is able to suggest research, encounters resistance to its acceptance, or encourages scientists to attempt to find evidence to reject it, this capacity is known as heuristic influence.[5] Note that theories are either accepted or rejected, never proven true or false. Hall and Lindzey say that a theory is accepted or rejected on the basis of *utility*. If a theory is verifiable (evidence to substantiate it) and comprehensive (complete, covering

[5]Snow, R.E.: Theory construction for research on teaching. In Travers, R.M., editor: Second handbook of research on teaching, Chicago, 1973, Rand McNally & Co., p. 82.

a wide range), it is said to have utility.[6] Such a theory should predict and explain results where the components of the theory are involved.

The necessity to "know" has pushed scientists and scholars to develop theories. It is not our purpose to proclaim that theory is the most productive vehicle for acquiring knowledge, but it is an effective one. Perhaps the future will reveal other successful ways to learn more about reality.

An engineer remarked that electrical engineering is all theory. A friend of his responded, "But the light above your desk works. You know exactly how to perform all the functions necessary to make the bulb light. How can you call it theory?" The engineer replied, "We have a theory of why it works but it is only a theory. Each year new, more conclusive theories are being developed, but we can never know all truth."

KINDS OF THEORY

Theories do not easily fall into convenient categories, but writers often classify theories according to use. Many disciplines specify categories for theories according to subareas in their field. Business administration has management theories; sociology has game theories; and social psychology has group theories. More than one discipline may have the same subarea. For example, psychology and education are both interested in learning theories.

Some scholars distinguish between theories and scientific theories, hinting that a scientific theory is on a higher level. Scientific theories as conceived by chemists and physicists are usually empirically testable, whereas social and psychological theories have numerous variables that do not always allow for empirical testing.

Explanatory theories are often proposed that seem plausible, but are too general to be verified. Theories have been developed to explain the appearance of unidentified flying objects. Yet these explanatory theories are difficult to test because the data are always in question. Few theories have caused more controversy than Darwin's theory of evolution. A search of the literature from various disciplines reveals that many authors accept his theory as law, though it is only speculation.

THEORY BUILDING

There are numerous routes for developing theories. Some of the following methods of theory building can be combined or refined. Imagination and creativity are desirable companions on a theory-building excursion.

Inductive theory construction.   In inductive theory construction the theorist moves from the specific to the general. One or more hypotheses or propositions are used as a springboard to launching a more general or a more inclusive theory. For example, an investigator believes that the laying on of hands has a positive affect on pain. By projecting this belief one step further using induction, the theory might be formulated that laying on of hands regularly prevents illness.

---

[6]Hall, C.S., and Lindzey, B.: Theories of personality, ed. 2, New York, 1957, John Wiley & Sons, Inc., p. 12.

Combining two or more hypotheses.   Combining two or more hypotheses may be used to develop a new theory. For example, research found that the staff employed at Agency H had a higher rate of absenteeism than the staffs employed by similar agencies in the region. It also was discovered that the employees at Agency H were allowed more days of paid sick leave than employees at other agencies. It was further noticed that the employees felt that Agency H owed them the extra time because they were not given bonuses or allowed overtime pay. One hypothesis could be that work incentive programs are effective for reducing absenteeism. If this hypothesis was tested repeatedly and found to be true in each instance, it would move up to the level of theory.

Theory reworking.   A new theory may be developed by revising an existing theory. If our hypothesis concerning work incentive programs had reached the stage of being a theory, we might want to rework it as follows. We could theorize that work incentive programs are effective for reducing absenteeism when employees perceive the monetary return as high enough to offset the loss of personal time.

Theory borrowing.   If a theory is developed, tested, and accepted into the teaching experience of teacher education students, the faculties in other disciplines might want to apply the theory in the health care field. The theory could be used in the clinical experiences of nursing, medical, and dental students. Later it might be applied to the paramedical fields.

Theory extension.   Results of a reworked theory can be refined again. Reworking a theory is advantageous, because the researcher is already involved with a theory that has been tested and accepted. Since it has served as an established foundation in the past, the credibility of the theory can be extended for additional study.

Theory integration.   At first glance, theory integration might be mistaken for combining theories. When the researcher combines theories, they are used together but may retain their own identity. The integration of theories proposes not only to combine other theories, but to use the combination to produce an entirely new idea. Theories are not sacred; theories are tools and can be modified much as a chemist may alter the chemicals in a formula. Burr has developed a taxonomy of theory-building strategies, which extend from grounded strategy to theory reworking as the ultimate level.[7]

Building with metaphors.   Snow proposes that metaphors can be used to develop theories.[8] Metaphorical comparisons help to shift patterns of thought from one medium to another. They illustrate ideas and compare one thought with another. The relationship between A and B might suggest the possible relationship between X and Y.

Schematic drawing.   Schematic drawings are visual aids that diagram the relationships between elements or units. Schematic visualizations and line drawings can be produced to predict relationships between variables. These drawings can be converted to theories or hypotheses by substituting variables for the elements or units (Fig. 6-2).

Miniaturizing.   Miniaturizing is a process whereby a partial theory or subtheory suggests a path that might be developed to produce a larger, more complete, or conclusive theory. In miniaturizing, it is assumed that it is easier to develop theories covering subsystems or subunits than to develop theories for a complete system.

[7]Burr, W.R.: Theory construction and the sociology of the family, New York, 1973, John Wiley & Sons, Inc., p. 281.
[8]Snow, p. 87.

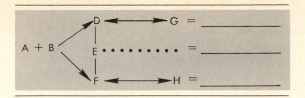

FIGURE 6-2   Example of a schematic drawing.

Taxonomy.   Taxonomy is the science of classification through scientific ordering or arranging. Taxonomy is a theory-building device that exploits possible relationships among categories. One well-known example is Bloom's taxonomy of educational objectives.[9]

Models.   Jacox says that models representing conceptual relationships can aid the development of theories.[10] A theory from one area of study may provide a model with which to develop theory in another field. Burr, in following Gibson's idea of factor strategy, contends that new theoretical insights can be gained by learning how independent variables influence dependent variables.[11] In recent years several models have gained prominence in nursing such as the model in Orem's self-care theory.[12]

Cross-disciplinary library searching.   This technique will often provide stimulation and new insights which will furnish ideas for hypotheses in other disciplines.

WHY THEORY IS IMPORTANT TO THE HEALTH SCIENCES

A theory is of no more importance to the health sciences than to science in general, except that the health sciences deal more directly with the well-being of mankind than any other discipline.

Elderly individuals, the wealthy sick, and all sick individuals declare that they would give anything if they "could just be well again." Good health is universally desired. It involves physical, spiritual, mental, and social states. Only a small percentage of the world's population has good health according to these four conditions.

Medicine, one of the oldest of the sciences, has abounded with theories of causes or cures for various health problems. Probably no other discipline has accumulated as large a body of written knowledge as medicine nor has any other science had more control over the application of its knowledge. Because of the great pool of knowledge, which is well organized in the *Index Medicus* and revised daily by computer printout, the health sciences have at their disposal an excellent opportunity to develop and utilize theory.

There are a number of reasons why theory is so important to the health professions.
1. The life and death seriousness of health care demands high-level thought processes.

[9]Bloom, B.S., and others: Taxonomy of educational objectives. Handbook I. Cognitive domain, New York, 1956, David MacKay Co., Inc.

[10]Jacox, A.: Theory construction in nursing, Nurs. Res. **23**(1):9, January 1974. © American Journal of Nursing Co.

[11]Burr, W.R., p. 281.

[12]Dorothea Orem's theory of self-care, Amer. J. Nurs. **80**(2):248, February 1980. Also, Orem, Dorothea: Nursing: concepts of practice, ed. 2, New York, 1980, McGraw-Hill, Inc.

2. A theory focuses special attention on a specific illness or cure. The goal is to develop theories that will wipe out diseases, prevent illness, and assist the individual to attain an optimum standard of health.
3. Theories hasten the process of obtaining answers to specific causes of pathological conditions.
4. A theory is able to predict when certain health conditions will occur or recur, thus making it possible to alleviate or prevent poor health.
5. Theory provides an important means for improving the health professions' service to the community and society as a whole. Adequate distribution of services is as important as a new discovery in a discipline.
6. Theories have added to the knowledge of health care in the past, so it is logical to assume that they will add to it in the future.

RELATIONSHIP BETWEEN THEORY AND METHOD

Why is there a relationship between two events? By observing a certain group of people or a situation, perhaps we can formulate an explanatory theory of why this event or situation occurred.

Suppose we start with an explanatory theory of why a situation exists. We must then test for the truth of the theory. By testing the theory, we hope to be able to identify the one variable that appears to be the causal factor. After testing the theory, we may find that it has not been supported by the evidence. Even though the hypothesis may require revision, we have still learned one bit of truth—there is no relationship between the variables. We also may have found another hypothesis to test.

In this chapter, theory and hypothesis have been used almost synonymously, although theory is actually of a much higher intellectual level than hypothesis. Nevertheless, there is a reciprocal relationship between the two. As we test our hypothesis, we learn new knowledge, reformulate our idea, and test it again, hoping to develop a theory. Such a theory, in turn, may suggest new hypotheses.

Theory has as its subject matter certain aspects and results of the interaction of human beings. Methodology transcends the theories of any one discipline and deals with those common to groups of disciplines, or those common to all scientific inquiry. A method is not just a way of dealing with a nursing problem, but a way of researching and gathering data in all disciplines. Method is concerned with the way in which inference is used in investigation.

In general, the problem is circular. Should we devise a theory and then attempt to verify this theory by collecting data? Or should we collect some kind of data and then devise a theory? Before we continue the discussion, the concept of theory should be clarified. Hardy defines theories as "sets of interrelated hypotheses which are subject to reformulation and refinement. The development of adequate theories to describe, explain, predict, and control phenomena is a slow process and requires the cooperative effort of many persons."[13]

[13]Hardy, Margaret E.: Theories: components, development, evaluation, Nurs. Res. 23(2):105, 1974. © American Journal of Nursing Co., 1974.

Theories and research are partners in that theories provide an explanation of relationships which are then tested and verified by research.

Wallace suggests that the power of a theory is based on the strength of the method of gathering data. Theory has two roles in generating information contained within it: first, it specifies the factors we should be able to measure before we start the research, such as formulating hypotheses and collecting data, and second, it serves at the end of the study as a common language into which the generalizations may be translated to compare and integrate the results with other research.[14] Thus, theory comes both before and after the research is carried out.

The debate between theory and facts is a continuing discussion today. A further point of debate that is of concern in this selection is related to the appropriate time for fact gathering. Should facts—empirical data—be collected before or after a theory is formed? Should a theory be based on facts or should facts be gathered to test theories?

Glaser and Strauss, in discussing grounded theory (theory obtained from data systematically obtained for research) say that generating theory goes hand in hand with verifying it.[15] Theory based on data usually cannot be completely refuted by more data or replaced by another theory. In contrast, logically deduced theories based on ungrounded assumptions can lead their followers far astray in trying to advance a discipline. Grounded theory can help to limit the use of theory to the data at hand rather than to serve as an afterthought from an empirical study. Glaser and Strauss believe that explaining data from one source with a different theory results from a lack of training.

The armchair researcher often finds examples of other research that support his theory. In such cases the theory "receives the image of a proof where there is none, and the theory obtains a richness of detail that it did not earn."[16]

Theory may suggest a method, but the method also may control the type of theory that we get. Selecting the best method to fit a theory is the concern of all disciplines.

Merton believes that research plays an active role and performs at least four major functions that shape the development of theory. It initiates, it reformulates, it deflects, and it clarifies theory.[17] Theory is often found by the serendipity pattern, which means finding the unanticipated or the unexpected. We might be looking for silver, and we find a gold mine. Suppose we are testing a hypothesis concerning nurses and patients, and we discover some new understanding of the nurse-physician relationship, possibly suggesting a new hypothesis for testing. Serendipity happens more frequently in experimental research and in broad general surveys than in problem-solving situations. A 100-item questionnaire covering patients' backgrounds is more likely to reveal unexpected insight (serendipity) into the subjects' needs than a 10-item questionnaire.

Research done by Phyllis Tyzenhouse is an ideal example of serendipity. The purpose of her study was "to describe the response of family members of men who had been hospitalized with manifestations of coronary artery disease to a risk factor intervention program." Although the focus of the study was on the response of the family members,

---

[14]Wallace, Walter L., editor: Sociological theory, Chicago, 1969, Aldine Publishing Co., p. x.

[15]Glaser, Barney S., and Strauss, Anselm: The discovery of grounded theory, Chicago, 1967, Aldine Publishing Co., p. 2.

[16]*Ibid.*, p. 5.

[17]Merton, p. 157.

she found that almost 76% of the patients' wives had one or more risk factors that attribute to atherosclerosis: overweight and cigarette smoking. The second serendipity finding was that 83% of the siblings also had risk factors, the most serious factor being overweight.[18]

Merton has suggested that theory does not precede research. The theorist cannot be considered as leading the way to new knowledge. It is only through the interrelationship of theory and research that a discipline is able to advance. Theory and research are the alternating steps up the ladder of science.[19] Roy G. Francis concludes:

> The relation between data and theory is not simple and direct. Techniques of measurement are also techniques of assembling and reporting data, and techniques make theoretical commitments and, hence, can alter data. Moreover, data are not allowed to speak for themselves; they are joined together in ways such as to force a certain conclusion. Data and form are thus intrinsic issues in theory building. The logical sequence is from theory to data—not from data to theory; for there is no way to verify inferences drawn from the latter formulation.
>
> Deductive logic permits a testing of inferences from theory to data. To those trained in logic, the reason should be clear: data are immediately available and data statements can be falsified. Theory is not immediately present to the scientist; hence, theory statements themselves cannot be directly falsified. If, however, a data statement deduced from a theory is falsified, the theory statement itself is falsified. This being so, the theory must be regarded as being logically prior to the data it encompasses.[20]

NURSING THEORY AND METHODOLOGY

Williamson differentiates between a theory of nursing and a theory for nursing. A theory of nursing seems very broad and would attempt to describe the field of nursing through its concepts. A theory for nursing seems to indicate that there are several theories which might explain some aspect of nursing. This is an insightful look at a dilemma relating to nursing theory. Not too many years ago it was claimed that nursing did not have any theories. Now, many theories exist which explain the purpose of nursing, and within which nursing can, should, or does operate.[21]

According to Meleis, the purpose of theory is to formulate a minimum of statements that explain a maximum number of questions or relationships.[22]

Some authors believe that nursing has borrowed theories from sociology, education, and psychology, which is true. However, in defense of nursing theorists, it should be noted that great strides are being made in the development of theories which are strictly nursing and have much to offer sociology, education, and psychology. The discipline which has the most to gain from nursing theory is medicine.

[18]Tyzenhouse, P.: An intervention program for risk factor reduction in first degree relatives of men with premature coronary disease, (abstract), March 1980. By permission of the author.
[19]*Ibid.*, p. 171.
[20]Francis, Roy G.: The relation of data to theory, Rural Soc. **22**:266, 1957.
[21]Williamson, U.M.: Research methodology and its application to nursing, New York, 1981, John Wiley & Sons, Inc.
[22]Meleis, A.I.: Theoretical nursing: development and progress, Philadelphia, 1985, J.B. Lippincott Company.

Nurses are struggling with their role, education, history, clinical practice, accreditation, licensure requirements, career mobility, health issues, and relationship to the medical profession. The nursing profession seems to be more concerned with developing theory than with testing it. Scholars of most other disciplines are developing and testing theories relating to the subject matter of their discipline.

Methodology is usually not an issue with nurses since they have few nursing theories. Rather, they are concerned with problem solving, problem stating, historical research, and evaluation of research. This is not a criticism of nurses and nursing, but simply an observation that the profession as such is not interested in methodology.

A few individuals are making an effort to assist other nurses in developing skills in theory building and theory evaluation. Benoliel believes that theory can interpret and explain reality, as well as health and illness. She concludes that nursing knowledge will be more the result of the nurse investigator's creativity and imagination than of theories, philosophies, and methods.[23]

A new kind of replication study, called successive research, has been used to investigate different aspects of an original project. This approach appears to offer a satisfying answer to the need for replicating research studies. It is only when theories are repeatedly tested, refined, and retested that the worth of a theory can be evaluated. In this instance, an intensive care unit environment was investigated by Noble, and then several masters and doctoral students replicated the original study or conducted a secondary study. The result was to establish the reliability and validity of the data-collecting instrument (an interview guide), to produce new hypotheses, and to provide beginning researchers with a learning experience. This also is an excellent example of doing research based on theory and then using the results of the project to refine and retest a theory.[24]

FRAMEWORKS: THEORETICAL AND CONCEPTUAL

Krueger, et al envision a conceptual framework as a paradigm or a representation of predictive relationships between theoretical and operational concepts as indicated by the theory. The conceptual framework is a structure in which to gather and analyze data. The actual results as found by analysis of the data can be compared with the predictive relationship in the conceptual framework.[25]

When designing a scientific investigation, the researcher envisions the framework through which the crucial objective of the study can be attained. The systematic schema shapes the extent of the relationships within the frame and provides the imagination with a means of understanding the structure. By developing a framework within which ideas are organized, the researcher is able to show that the proposed study is a logical extension of current knowledge. When building a framework, the researcher is not dealing with the steps of the scientific process but with a search for knowledge. There may be more than

[23]Benoliel, J.Q.: The interaction between theory and research, Nurs. Outlook **25**:108–113, February 1977.

[24]Noble, M.A.: Successive research; a strategy for building on previous research, Nurs. Outlook **27**(9):600–603, September 1979.

[25]Krueger, J.C., Nelson, A.H., and Wolanin, M.O.: Nursing research, development, collaboration, and utilization, Germantown, MD, 1978, Aspen Systems Corporation.

one path to a new discovery, and the framework is a means of finding the shortest path. Treatment X may result in learning the cause of condition Y, but treatment Z also may lead to discovering the cause and require fewer steps in the process. It is imperative that the researcher be acquainted with the treatments, technology, and methodology already available. A new perspective may be all that is needed to discover a law.

Frameworks are developed out of a review of the existing literature. They organize current knowledge around a scheme of concepts or proposed theory and hypotheses that are to be tested. A conceptual framework consists of concepts that are placed within a logical, sequential design, whereas a theoretical framework consists of theories that seem to be interrelated. If a single theory is involved, generalizations and propositions will be key components. If the planned study is exploratory in nature, questions rather than hypotheses are appropriate. Such questions may be specific and directed toward possible options.

To design a research project loosely, without developing a conceptual or theoretical framework, may result in some interesting information but will not provide good, solid evidence that results in theory or theory building. Conceptual frameworks are effective tools in developing and refining nursing practice, nursing education, and nursing administration.[26]

In summary, both conceptual and theoretical frameworks are important. The researcher determines the objective(s) to be achieved by the research project, and the developed framework is the strategy for achieving those objectives. Methods and tools are the tactics selected to use in each circumstance.

FROM SCIENTIFIC THEORY TO RESEARCH PROCESS

Theories are useful in nursing and other disciplines in several ways.
1. Theories increase the body of knowledge since they are constantly being tested, verified, and rejected. The mere process of testing allows the researcher new insight into the theory and into nursing.
2. The consistency between parallel theories and conflicts between rival hypotheses, all contribute to understanding nursing.
3. Theories can clarify concepts or relate concepts through cross-disciplinary testing.
4. Hypotheses can be deduced from theories for testing. Theories from other disciplines can provide insight for hypotheses in nursing.
5. Nursing can apply theories directly to practice. For instance, Nightingale, Hall, Henderson, Peplau, Orem, Abdellah, Orlando, Weidenbach, Levine, Rogers, King, Roy, and others have theories which can be utilized (see the nursing theories conference group).
6. Most nurses are already practicing some aspects of a theory but are not aware of the theorists. An understanding of the theory will enable the nurse to better understand patient care.

In order to facilitate the transition from theory to hypothesis, the following procedure offers one possibility:

[26]Munjas, B.: Conceptual framework, Virginia Nurse, **48**(2):25, Summer 1980.

Theory:

Nightingale believed that providing an environment that was friendly to the patient contributed to wellness. Warmth not cold, good ventilation not poor, quiet atmosphere not noise, sunlight not darkness, pleasant clean air not foul odors, she believed, are the elements which contribute to being well or ill. It is quite simple to move from Nightingale's theory to an hypothesis.

Hypothesis:

Patients with an outside window as opposed to artificial light will: (a) rate the room higher, on a five-point scale, (b) express feeling more alert, (c) spend less time in the hospital, (d) express more desire to go home, (e) require less medication.

This illustration demonstrates that only one part of Nightingale's theory can produce five hypotheses. Each of the other environmental variables could be tested using the same or additional hypotheses.

Theory:

Sister Callista Roy has developed the adaptation model. Briefly, this model views people as caught between two forces: environmental change and their ability to adapt to change. Environmental changes could include diseases, viruses, illness, death in the family, loss of job, fires, accidents, and so on. Adaptation involves physiological needs, self-concept, role function, and interdependence. The term role function refers to interaction and communication with other individuals in society. Every person has a role or function in society and he/she interacts with others who also have role functions and positions. Failure to adapt to this interactional environment leads to maladaptation and nursing implementation becomes necessary.

Hypotheses:

1. More persons in hospitals have role function problems than the public in general.
2. Nursing implementation is more effective in treating role function problems than physician's orders. Without nursing intervention, role function problems will continue to increase.

Theory:

A different approach to Roy's adaptation model is her health continuum scale from death on one extreme, extremely poor health, poor health, normal health, good health, high-level wellness to peak wellness on the other extreme.

Hypotheses:

1. Nursing intervention can move a client from the low extreme to the normal position but nursing intervention cannot move a client from normal to peak wellness.
2. Nursing intervention cannot (or can) move a patient higher on the continuum. (In other words, the nurse has to be at high-level wellness in order to help the patient to high-level wellness.)

The procedure of generating hypotheses from theories consists of selecting a theory and reducing it to two variables, a cause and an effect. Often, a complex theory such as Roy's adaptation model is so comprehensive that it is easier to select one aspect. Notice that Roy's model includes physiological needs, self-concept, role function, and interdependence.

The following are some possible ways of developing hypotheses:

1. Determine whether one of the four proponents of Roy's is more important or influential to health than another.
2. Compare each of the four variables with the same nursing intervention.

3. Compare a single proponent with two or more nursing interventions to learn which intervention is most effective.
4. Try to break some components of the model—say physiological needs—into specific items, such as relationship of exercise to self-concept.

If the beginning researcher believes that a certain hypothesis is not worth testing, then some critiquing skill has already been developed. There is probably no best way to develop hypotheses from theories, but, hopefully, these examples have helped the new researcher to move more readily from a theory to the hypothesis.

SUMMARY

The behavioral and social sciences and even nursing (whichever claim it) are more interested in how information is obtained than what information is found. The findings are always at the mercy of the methods and techniques used to obtain them.

Method and theory are the two links of the circle of the scientific approach. It is necessary to have theories to guide research, but it is also necessary to do research to produce theories.

Nursing theory, though decidedly lacking, must depend on the interplay of data and the theories of human interaction.

Theoretical perspective is the basing of one's research on a theory. Knowledge has increased to the extent that the scientific method has been applied. The routes to theory building include inductive theory construction, combining hypotheses, theory reworking, theory borrowing, extension and integration of theories, building metaphors, schematic drawing, miniaturizing, taxonomy, models, and cross-disciplinary library searching.

The weakness of the social sciences is noticeably evident in its lack of testing and retesting. On the other hand, the concrete disciplines of the physical sciences are not concerned with historical perspectives, but spend their energy building on the solid rock of empirical replications. The abstract disciplines of the social sciences read the historical fathers with almost the same reverence as Holy Scripture and avoid replication like a scourge of the plague.

Methodological and theoretical considerations are mutually dependent for direction. One theory may be tested more appropriately by questionnaires than by observation (methods). The results will suggest other theories and hypotheses for further testing.

A theory is only as strong as the test of its accuracy. An untested theory is useless; the more rigorous the testing, the more valuable the theory. As theories of human interaction are strengthened and developed, nursing theory should and must also develop. The nursing profession is struggling with the development of theory but has not yet reached the point of giving priority to the testing of theory.

DISCUSSION QUESTIONS

1 Do you believe that research comes before theory or vice versa? Defend your position.
2 If theory and research are locked together, what is the purpose of an hypothesis?
3 Why are health researchers interested in the methods of social and behavioral research?
4 Is there any overlap between medical and nursing research? Support your response.
5 What are the differences between medical and nursing research?

6 In what ways do theories suggest research methods?

7 Why do the physical science majors repeat experiments year after year, while the social and behavioral science students talk about the histories and theories of their disciplines?

8 What is meant by the statement that a theory is only as strong as its test?

9 Why is it better to know how a theory was developed rather than who developed it?

10 How does theory building contribute to new knowledge?

CLASS ACTIVITIES

Track I

1 Divide the class into two groups. One group debates why theory should precede research, and the other group debates why research should precede theory.

2 Divide the class into groups of three or four. Each group lists the types of theory that may be tested in nursing research.

Track II (Steps in Research Project)

1 Each research group or student is to determine the theory being tested in its selected project, or the question that it desires to study.

2 Each group or student is to list the concepts involved in its investigation.

SUGGESTED READINGS

Archer, S.E.: Community nurse practitioners: another assessment, Nurs. Outlook 24(8):499–503, August 1976.

Bohny, B.J.: Theory development for a nursing science, Nurs. Forum 19(1):50–67, 1980.

Brodt, D.E.: A re-examination of the synergistic theory of nursing, Nurs. Forum 19(1):85–93, 1980.

Bromley, B.: Applying Orem's self-care theory in enterostomal therapy, Am. J. Nurs. 80(2):245–249, February 1980.

Bush, H.A.: Models for nursing, part 2(2), Adv. Nurs. Sci. 1:13–21, January 1979.

Camooso, C., and others: Students' adaptation according to Roy, Nurs. Outlook 29(2):108–109, February 1981.

Chinn, P.L.: Practice oriented theory: a model for theory developed in nursing, Part 1, Adv. Nurs. Sci. 1(1):1–11, October 1978.

Crow, F.A.: Research and the standard of nursing care: what is the relationship? Journal of Advanced Nursing 6:491, November 1981.

Davis, T.M.: The kinetics of nursing: a conceptual framework for nursing practice, Virginia Nurse 48(2):31–32, Summer 1980.

Downs, F.S., and Newman, M.A.: A sourcebook of nursing research, ed. 2, Philadelphia, 1977, F.A. Davis Co., p. 4.

Ellis, L., and others: Implementing a conceptual framework, Nurs. Outlook 27(2):127–130, February 1979.

Engstrom, J.L.: Problems in the development, use and testing of nursing theory, Journal of Nursing Education 23(6):245, June 1984.

Farrell, A.M.: Conceptual framework for psychiatric nursing practice: the use of communication and nursing processes. Virginia Nurse 48(2):28–30, Summer 1980.

Fawcett, J.: A declaration of nursing independence: the relation of theory and research to nursing practice, J. Nurs. Adm. 10(6):36–39, June 1980.

Fawcett, J.: The relationship between theory and research: a double helix, part 1, Adv. Nurs. Sci. 1(1):49–62, October 1978.

Fenner, K.: Developing a conceptual framework. Nurs. Outlook 27(2):122–126, February 1979.

Flynn, B.C.: An action research framework for primary health care, Nursing Outlook 32(16):316–318, November–December 1984.

Foley, Joan: Wanted: a theory of nursing, Int. Nurs. Rev. 18(2):138–148, 1971.

Folta, Jeannette R.: Obfuscation of clarification: a reaction to Walker's concept of nursing theory, Nurs. Res. 20(6):496–499, November–December, 1971.

Fox, S.: The vitality of theory in Schwab's conception of the practical, in Curriculum Inquiry by the Ontario Institute for Studies in Education, 15(1), New York, Spring 1985, John Wiley & Sons, Inc.

Gudmundsen, A.M.: The conduct of inquiry into nursing, Nurs. Forum 18:52–59.

Hamilton, G.A.: Miller's living systems: a theory critique, part 2, Adv. Nurs. Sci. 1:41–52, January 1979.

Hanlon, J.H.: Theory and the practice of nursing, J. Contin. Educ. Nurs. 5(6):12–18, November– December 1974.

Hardy, M.E.: Perspectives on nursing theory, part 1(4), Adv. Nurs. Sci. 1(1):37–48, October 1978.

Henderson, B.: Nursing diagnosis: theory and practice. Adv. Nurs. Sci. 1(1):75–83, October 1978.

Johnson, Dorothy E.: Development of theory: a requisite for nursing as a primary health profession, Nurs. Res. 23(5):372–376, 1974.

Johnson, J.: The effects of preparatory information on the recovery of surgical patients, A tripartite research conference, part 2, monograph series No. 76, Burlingame, CA, 1976, Sigma Theta Tau, p. 6–19.

Johnson, J.L.: Some aspects of the relation between theory and research in nursing, Journal of Advanced Nursing 8(1):21, January 1983.

LaRocco, S.: An introduction to role theory for nurses, Superv. Nurse 9(12):41–45, December 1978.

Leedy, S., and Pepper, J.M.: Conceptual bases of professional nursing, Philadelphia, 1985, J.B. Lippincott Company.

Mastal, M.F., and Hammond, H.: Analysis and expansion of the Roy adaptation model: a contribution to holistic nursing. Adv. Nurs. Sci 2(4):71–81, 1980.

McFarlane, E.A.: Nursing theory, the comparison of four theoretical proposals, J. Adv. Nurs. 5(1):3–19, January 1980.

McMurrey, P.H.: Toward a unique knowledge base in nursing, Image Vol. XIV(1):12–15, February–March 1982.

Meleis, A.I.: Theoretical nursing: development and progress, Philadelphia, 1985, J.B. Lippincott Company.

Mooney, M.M.: The ethical components of nursing theory: an analysis of ethical components in four nursing theories, Image 12:7–9, February 1980.

Ohashi, J.P.: The contributions of Dickoff and James to theory development in nursing, Image Vol. XVII(1):17–20, Winter 1985.

Ostrow, C.: The care and feeding of theories, AJOT 34:272–273, April 1980.

Roy, Sister C.: Relating nursing theory to education: a new era, Nurse Educ. 4:16–21, March–April 1979.

Sellitz, C., Wrightsman, L.S., and Cook, S.W.: Research methods in social research, ed. 3, New York, 1976, Holt, Rinehart & Winston.

Silva, M.C. and Rothbart, D.: An analysis of changing trends in philosophies of science on nursing theory development and testing, Advances in Nursing Science 8(2):1–13, January 1984.

Stern, P.N.: Grounded theory methodology: its use and processes, Image 12:2023, February 1980.

Stevens, B.J.: Nursing theory: analysis, application, evaluation, Waltham, Mass, 1979, Little, Brown & Co.

Weatherston, L.: Theory in nursing: creating effective care, J. Adv. Nurs. 4(4):365–375, July 1979.

Wensch, P.C.: Conceptual framework of nursing practice, Virginia Nurse 48(2):25–27, Summer 1980.

PART THREE

PREPARATION FOR COLLECTING DATA

Part Three is divided into nine chapters, each dealing with some aspect of preparation for data collection. Since nursing research must include a firm base of literature review, Chapter 7 emphasizes the importance and techniques of an effective library search. The focus is on general procedures, practical application, and computer databases.

Chapter 8 deals with the design and conduct of a research project, logic, research proposals, and grants. A discussion of the ethical aspects of nursing research is presented in Chapter 9. The legality of research, informed consent, human rights, and dignity as related to biomedic and behavioral research are addressed. The function, sources, and testing of hypotheses are explained in Chapter 10. Operational definitions are discussed as well as research that explores a question. Chapter 11 includes a discussion of the relationship between the variables being studied. Cause-effect relationships and correlations also are considered.

Chapter 12 presents information concerning the major approaches to research. These include the survey, the experiment, the case study, and historical research. Evaluation research and policy research are presented as increasingly important new methods of investigation. Chapter 13 presents an extensive consideration of the sample and sampling techniques and Chapter 14 centers around a discussion of the instrument and data to be collected. Chapter 15 considers the importance of reliability and validity as they relate to instruments and research.

CHAPTER 7

THE LIBRARY AND COMPUTER-BASED LITERATURE SEARCHES

Beginning researchers often assume that using the library is a simple procedure. However, a literature search involves more than looking in the library card catalog. It seems that as computers become more common, students know less about libraries. Unfortunately, because the computer can conduct the search for some kinds of material, the beginning researcher frequently does not bother to conduct a personal search. Libraries prove to be interesting even exciting sources of knowledge when their services are fully utilized. A-nother assumption is that libraries are easy to use; consequently, people tend not to listen to lectures on library usage. One of the results of this attitude is that research papers frequently demonstrate weakness because of a poor library search. When questioned, beginning researchers often reply, "There was nothing written on my topic." Our response to this statement is, "Do you mean to say you are so original that you chose a topic no one else has written about?" There is almost no topic so unique that some phase of it has not been investigated. It is our intent in this chapter to help the beginning researcher overcome some of the obstacles that hinder progress in the library search.

Literature review is fun, but it is also demanding. There are times when it can be quite boring until suddenly there is a lead on the topic. Retrieval of pertinent information, therefore, need not be a painful process, but much depends on the researcher's attitude.

Another point of difficulty is getting new researchers to search broadly. They often select a very narrow approach to their topic and then say that there is nothing written about it. We have found that even though we stress the necessity of looking broadly, beginners still want to narrow their investigation of literature to a specific type of study exactly like the one they propose. Although an identical study may not have been done, there are many studies of the same general nature. A broad background search of a topic is superior to a narrow one. For example, let us use the subject of cross-cultural relationships. Suppose someone is conducting a study of dating patterns between males and females from different cultures. It may be difficult to find material on the specific topic, but any knowledge of cultural relationships, perhaps concerning medical care, income, or education, would be valuable. Any information about differences between the cultures pertaining to their lifestyles, beliefs, and customs would render further insight into the subject. If the beginning researcher will search broadly into the general background of the topic, results will be an overall view rather than a specific, limited point of view.

The library search is like a big puzzle. The investigators may not find the specific piece they want, but by searching and getting the basic outline of the puzzle, they will have a much better understanding of the project than if they have only one particular piece. Of course, we are not suggesting an either-or proposition. It is hoped that it will be possible for the investigators to find some specific studies during the library search, but if not, they should then try to locate similar studies along with general background material.

Researchers should not be satisfied to limit themselves to one or two libraries, but should do their investigation in as many appropriate local or regional libraries as possible. Most areas of the United States are within driving range of a university library, college library, or large public library. Many cities and towns have specialized private libraries as well. Hospitals, seminaries, and health care centers have large collections of professional journals, books, and abstracts for use by students, staff, and personnel.

PURPOSE

Nursing research may be considered a continuing process in which knowledge gained from earlier studies is an integral part of research in general. Before any research can be started, whether it is a single study or an extended project, a literature search of previous studies and experience related to the proposed investigation should be done. There are valid reasons why the search must be made, and there are guidelines and systematic procedures that will facilitate the search.

One of the most satisfying aspects of the literature search is the contribution it makes to the new knowledge, insight, and general scholarship of the researcher. There are also five pragmatic purposes for the search:

1. The researcher may find methods for research used by others that may be useful for the project.
2. The researcher may locate pertinent data or ideas useful for the present study or for a new project design.
3. The researcher may discover that certain aspects must be included in the study to confirm or refute earlier findings.
4. The researcher may find comparative data that will be valuable in interpreting the conclusions of the study.
5. The researcher can ascertain if some work has already been done on the question; thus, duplication can be avoided unless desired for retesting purposes.
6. The researcher may find information that will help in the development of the conceptual or theoretical framework of the project.

GENERAL PROCEDURE

Before entering a library, the researcher should have a general plan for conducting the search. There is no best or right way of searching, and certainly, experienced researchers will have developed methods that work for them. At the outset of the first literature search, beginning investigators will benefit from an established method and will soon learn to adapt it to their individual preferences.

Time and the Library Search

The first question is, "How much time should be spent on a review of literature?" Abdellah and Levine suggest that if a study is expected to last for 2 years, then 2 months should be sufficient for the literature search.[1] It is important that the investigator project the amount of time it will take for each phase of the research project and plan accordingly.

The second question is, "When should the hypothesis be determined, before or after the library search?" There is no rule. The topic may be identified prior to the beginning of the research process. On the other hand, it may be necessary to go to the library first and do some investigating before a subject of interest is found. Even with a topic in mind, researchers may change their opinions about the subject after reading a portion of the literature. This may simply involve a change in point of view or attitude toward the topic. In some instances, the investigator may start with knowledge gained from others, ride "piggy-back" on their findings, and use this added information to assist in the anticipated project.

Above all, it is important that the library search be done as an early phase of a study, not after the study is well underway. Furthermore, ample time must be set aside to read available pertinent information before launching the research design.

What and Where to Search

Two other important questions must answered when doing a library search: what and where. What is the topic called? Where can we look for it? Initially, the first question is more important: What do we call the topic we are searching for in the library? Will other authors and researchers use the same title we do?

A valuable source of ideas for topics is the reference source *Library of Congress Subjects.* This is a subject index to the Library of Congress classifications and has numerous cross-listings of subject titles. It opens doors to subject headings that people might not have been able to articulate or that are unfamiliar to the researcher. After looking through the two volumes, the next step is to look for the headings in the card catalog.

Abstracts are a valuable source of research. Other scholarly works can be found by title and topic. Many beginning investigators do not realize that there is an abstract for almost every discipline (an abstract is a brief summary of a scholarly writing or a research report). Frequently, new researchers who know of the existence of abstracts fail to understand their value and use in spite of library tours, discussions, and lectures explaining the library services.

Several problems interfere with ready access to library materials. First, articles written in professional journals in the last few months of the current year have not been listed in the abstracts. Since it takes time for an article to be published, read, abstracted, and

[1] Abdellah, Faye G., and Levine, Eugene: Better patient care through nursing research, ed. 2, New York, 1979, Macmillan, Inc., p. 121.

distributed, current material is not to be found in the abstracts. Current journals may be consulted individually, or *Current Contents* can be scanned.[2]

Second, after journals have become a year or more old, they are frequently bound together. So, while the current material has not as yet been abstracted, literature that is a year old may be at the bindery.

Third, books and periodicals are often in use around the library, have been checked out, or are lost, misplaced, or otherwise not available for use. The library may not subscribe to little known, foreign, and even some popular professional journals.

Some librarians specialize in the literature of specific disciplines and are prepared to assist the researcher with the techniques of librarianship. For those reasons it is important to utilize the expertise of the librarian.

BEGINNING THE SEARCH

After the researcher has clearly delineated the topic, the research proposal should be stated again; but now the emphasis should be on both specific and general terms applicable to the topic. Additions to synonymous terminology may be identified by consulting dictionaries, encyclopedias, and textbooks. These terms or subject headings will be the key to the primary and secondary source material needed to fulfill the purpose of the search. Because all reference tools do not use the same subject headings, a variety of headings will lead the researcher to a more thorough literature search. It is convenient to list all possible headings on a 3 × 5 card that can be checked during the searching procedure. New headings may be added as they are discovered.

If the researcher plans to use an unfamiliar library, it will be helpful to begin with a general exploration of the facilities. By determining the general arrangement of reference materials, books, and journals, and the availability of audiovisual materials, the policies for borrowing, the access to photocopy service, and the rules for interlibrary loans, the researcher will have some foreknowledge of the amount of materials and services available. This information may be obtained from the reference librarian, who will offer explanations and perhaps provide printed material about the library and its use. On occasion the librarian may not know as much about a specific topic as the researcher does but will know general sources of information.

An example of librarian assistance was a study in which the researcher needed to know the number of female college students enrolled in the United States. The figure was not readily available, so when the librarian was approached for assistance, she reached under her desk and said, "A new book came in just this morning, and it has that information in it."

During the general exploration of the library the researcher will undoubtedly have noted the card catalog and various reference tools. At this point some beginning researchers begin a trial-and-error search of the many indexes and other tools. To find material by this method is time consuming, and important sources may be overlooked. A more productive approach is to study several guidebooks to appropriate reference words that are applicable to the research topic. One of the better guidebooks is *Medical*

[2]Current Contents; Life Sciences, Philadelphia, January 1967, Institute for Scientific Information. Weekly.

Reference Works.[3] We suggest that a 3 × 5 card be used to record a list of the various library resources that are judged useful for the search.

After preparing the preliminary list of library resources, the researcher should consult with the librarian. When given a description of the subject matter, the librarian can check the list of reference works and subject headings and advise the researcher on the choices made, as well as suggest other topics and headings. The librarian also may be helpful in defining the extent of the search. Sometimes a comprehensive search of all the material on the subject is needed, but other times a more selective number of review articles, standard texts, and definitive research reports is adequate. For example, nurses should be familiar with *Nursing Research*[4] as an important source for research information and for abstracts of research in nursing.

Before beginning the actual literature search, the investigator should decide on how to record findings. Because the citations found during the search will compose the working bibliography, convenience and accuracy are important in recording what is found. A separate 3 × 5 card for each book and journal citation is most convenient. These cards are preferable to a sheet of paper because they make possible rearrangements, deletions, or additions as necessary in the working bibliography. As each appropriate title is found, a complete citation should be recorded. For books, this includes the author, title, year and place of publication, and name of the publisher. For journal articles, the complete citation includes journal title, volume and page numbers, date, and author and title of the article. If a uniform style for recording the citations is used, preparation of the final bibliography and footnotes will be simplified (Chapter 25). The few extra minutes needed to carefully record the complete citation can save hours of searching later, if it becomes necessary to verify the citation for the final bibliography. It is also wise to record the source of the citation. This can be an abbreviated notation, such as INI, p. 60, 1981. If it becomes necessary to recheck the citation or to obtain an interlibrary loan, the source of the citation will be immediately available.

The 3 × 5 card has ample space for the complete citation and source as well as any specific notes or reminders the researcher may wish to make (Fig. 7-1). When it is time to type the bibliography in alphabetical order, the cards may easily be placed in the desired order.

CONDUCTING THE LITERATURE SEARCH

The researcher may now begin a systematic search for book and monograph materials, journal articles, and special sources of information.

Books

The card catalog is the basic key to the book and monograph collection of the library. The approach to the card catalog is by subject, starting with a specific term and, if

[3]Blake, John B., and Roos, Charles, editors: Medical reference words, a selected bibliography, Publication No. 3, Chicago, 1967, Medical Library Association.
[4]Nursing Research, New York, June 1952, American Journal of Nursing Co. Six issues per year; not cumulated.

WY 3

A

Anderson, Betty. **Theories of Health**
Care. Midwest: Jackson Publishers,
1984, pp. 35-40.

FIGURE 7-1   Sample bibliography card for book.

necessary, moving to a more general term. The various topic headings on the previously prepared list should be checked, and as appropriate book titles are found, they should be copied on the 3 × 5 card. The complete citation should be copied, as well as the classification number, in the upper lefthand corner of the catalog card. This classification number is the locating device that will aid the researcher in finding the desired books. A sample catalog card for a book is shown in Fig. 7-2. Note the placement of information as well as the content.

Not all books on the topic will be available in the library; thus, the researcher may wish to examine the *National Library of Medicine Current Catalog*[5] for book titles available elsewhere. These titles should be recorded on the 3 × 5 cards as they are located, so the librarian may be asked to acquire these books through an interlibrary loan.

Journals

Most research is first reported in journal articles; therefore, these will be a primary source for other investigative work done on a particular topic.

Just as the card catalog is the key to the book collection, the many indexes and abstracting tools are the keys to journal literature. Selection of the best indexes and abstracting tools will depend on the topic being researched. In preparing for the literature search, the researcher should compile a list of possible sources and confer with the librarian as to its completeness. For the most part, the nurse-researcher will find that the following works have been selected from the guidebooks to medical nursing literature:

[5]U.S. National Library of Medicine, National Library of Medicine current catalog, Washington, D.C., 1966, U.S. Government Printing Office.

Mowry, Lillian.
    Mowry's Basic nutrition and diet therapy.

    Bibliography: p.
    Includes index.
    1. Diet therapy. 2. Nutrition. I. Williams, Sue
Rodwell, 1922-   II. Title. III. Title: Basic
nutrition and diet therapy.
RM216.M64   1980   615'.854   79-26165
ISBN 0-8016-5556-0

FIGURE 7-2   Sample catalog card for book.

International Nursing Index,[6] *Cumulative Index to Nursing and Allied Health Literature*,[7] *Nursing Studies Index*,[8] Index Medicus,[9] *Excerpta Medica*,[10] *Hospital Literature Index*,[11] and *Medical Socioeconomic Research Sources.*[12]

Some general guidelines for the use of indexes that facilitate the search for journal articles are as follows:

1. Learn how indexes can be used. Review the introduction and explanation for proper use and understanding of the index. Time spent becoming familiar with the special features of the index will save needless searching.
2. Explore various topic headings. This exploration will lead to a more comprehensive search. The previously prepared list of topic headings will now be most important. Many indexes include journal citations under several headings; therefore, there will be duplications, but these can be deleted when the working bibliography cards are arranged alphabetically. Some indexes have special subject heading lists. Two good examples of subject heading lists are MeSH (Medical Subject Headings) for *Index Medicus*, and *Nursing Thesaurus for International Nursing Index*. Any heading found in these lists should be added to the 3 × 5 topic heading list card.
3. Be alert for transposed subject headings, such as "cysts, ovarian" rather than "ovarian cysts."
4. Start with the most specific topic heading available and then use more general headings.

[6]International nursing index, I, New York, 1966, American Journal of Nursing Company in cooperation with the National Library of Medicine. Quarterly; cumulated annually.

[7]Cumulative index to nursing and allied health literature, I, Glendale, Calif., 1956, Seventh-Day Adventist Hospital Association. Quarterly; cumulated annually; 5-year cumulation, 1956 to 1960; 3-year cumulation, 1961 to 1963. Indexes more than 3,000 sources; updated every 2 months.

[8]Henderson, Virginia: Nursing studies index: an annotated guide to reported studies, research in progress, research methods and historical materials in periodicals, books and pamphlets in English, Philadelphia, 1963, J.B. Lippincott Co. Prepared by Yale University School of Nursing Index Staff.

[9]Index medicus, I, Washington, D.C., 1960, U.S. National Library of Medicine. Monthly; cumulated annually as reference 6.

[10]Excerpta medica, Amsterdam, 1947, Excerpta Medica Foundation. Currently in 24 sections.

[11]Hospital literature index, I, Chicago, 1945, American Hospital Association. Quarterly; cumulated annually under the same title and quinquennially as Cumulative Index of Hospital Literature. Covers all aspects of the literature.

[12]Medical socioeconomic research sources, vol. I, Chicago, 1973, American Medical Association. Four times yearly; cumulated.

5. Begin the search with the most recent cumulated index volumes and then use the monthly volumes and the older cumulated volumes.
6. Work systematically through one index at a time, recording each pertinent citation on the 3 × 5 cards.

A book is a valuable resource, but considering the date of the material in a book versus that in a periodical, it is our opinion that the periodical is somewhat preferred to a book. One point is that periodicals, especially current periodicals, are more up to date in their information simply because the content tends to reach the reader more quickly. Of course, this may not always be the case, but it is likely to be so. Professional articles for any discipline represent the highest and most sophisticated level of academic quality; exposure to this scholarship is not only stimulating, but helpful in preparing the beginning researcher for writing up the study results.

Other Sources

Although books and journals are often the prime source for information, there are other forms of material equally valuable. If audiovisual materials are available in the library, these should be checked. A search in *Dissertation Abstracts*,[13] *Research Grants Index*,[14] *Nursing Research, Journal of Advanced Nursing*,[15] *Advances in Nursing Science*,[16] and the *Western Journal of Nursing Research*,[17] often yields new research and acquaints the researcher with others working in the field.

Government publications are listed in the *Monthly Catalog*.[18] The government, of course, is the largest publisher of printed material, with a surprising number of articles and bulletins published on almost every subject. If such material is not on file in the library, the librarian will be able to order it.

A technique designed for easy storage and retrieval is microfilming. Most libraries now have on microfilm local newspapers as well as the *New York Times*. Each page is reduced to less than 1-inch square. The microfilm reader, used to view the microfilm, enlarges each page back to approximately original size and allows the viewer to stop or move rapidly through several pages in quick succession. Microfiche is a series of even smaller slides mounted on a card about the size of a postcard and is also viewed in a reader.

Since it is important to research broadly when doing a library search, materials other than those found on the shelves of a medical or nursing library or both will also provide background for a study. Professional journals and scholarly books are preferred to material in popular magazines or newspapers. Popular magazines are oriented to the lay reader and will not have the depth of content found in professional literature.

If a surplus of information on a subject is found, researchers may proceed in several ways.

[13] Dissertation abstracts, Ann Arbor, Michigan, University Microfilms..
[14] Research grants index, Public Health Service. Publication No. 925, Bethesda, Md., 1961, U.S. National Institutes of Health, Division of Research Grants. Annually.
[15] Journal of Advanced Nursing, England, 1976, Blackwell Scientific Publications, Ltd. Bimonthly.
[16] Advances in Nursing Science, Germantown, Md, 1978, Aspen Systems Corp. Bimonthly.
[17] Western Journal of Nursing Research, Anaheim, Calif., 1979, UCLA School of Nursing. Quarterly.
[18] U.S. Superintendent of Documents, monthly catalog of U.S. government publications, Washington, D.C., 1895, U.S. Government Printing Office. Monthly; title varies.

1. Select only the most current material.
2. Select literature from a more narrow focus on the topic.
3. Select only those references whose titles seem to be the most appropriate for the topic under study.
4. Select only those authors who have written several articles or whose names appear in several bibliographies since they are likely to be authorities.
5. Select articles from refereed journals or well-known publishers.

These suggestions are, of course, to be taken with caution. The very best reference may not fit any of these suggestions. An unknown journal may contain an excellent article, a previously unpublished author may have written an excellent book, or a very old article may still be recognized as a classic in the field so none of these should be overlooked.

Cooper discusses three types of literature reviews which summarize material relevant to research. Methodological reviews, found in many journals, synthesize various aspects of research methods. They may concentrate on such themes as the most popular methods, the least productive, and the latest methods. Integrative research reviews cumulative findings from several years of publishing on one specific type of research. The reviewer may reach conclusions on current trends or most productive techniques. Theoretical reviews propose to summarize theories, compare theories, assess trends, and so on.[19]

Other techniques for finding research studies include informal channels such as the researcher's own research studies, similar research by colleagues in other institutions, and attendance at professional conventions and conferences. Primary channels are the personal books the researcher owns or the professional journals to which he/she subscribes. Cooper believes that this source can often lead to a bias toward the point of view of the library sources. Since researchers read their own personal collection of journals within a specific area, they often get a narrow, restricted perspective. A final technique, called secondary channels, is less restricted than the other channels and more convenient because it includes compiled information such as listings of books and articles found in bibliographies of other researchers. The familiar indexing and abstracting services of any large library is included in secondary channels.[20]

THE COMPUTER-BASED LITERATURE SEARCH

Although it is essential that beginning researchers become experienced both in the use of the library and in techniques for manual literature searching, they also should be aware of the benefits of the mechanized literature search. Searching with the aid of the computer has been shown to save considerable time and cost.[21] Although new computer-based bibliographic services are constantly added, the one most generally available to health professionals is MEDLARS, the National Library of Medicine's *Index Medicus* database.

[19]Cooper, H.M.: The integrative research review, a systematic approach, Applied social research methods series, Vol. 2, Beverly Hills, 1984, SAGE Publications, Inc. p. 19.
[20]*Ibid.*, p. 11.
[21]Elman, Stanley A.: Cost comparison of manual and online computerized literature searching. Special Libraries **66**(1):12–18, January 1975.

MEDLARS is a computer-based system of literature retrieval located in the National Library of Medicine (NLM) in Bethesda, Maryland. More than 1,000 regional network centers located in universities, medical schools, and commercial networks provide access to the system. MEDLARS provides access to 4,500,000 references in books and articles published since 1965 dealing with the health sciences. Terminals located in the regional institutions are connected to commercial networks or telephone lines of the Library's IBM 370/158 computers. Reference retrieval is accomplished by a typewritten dialogue on a terminal keyboard. Continued dialog with the computer, called an "online" search, clarifies the topics of inquiry until the desired references are found and printed out on the terminal. There are 14,000 Medical Subject Headings (MeSH) used to index and catalog material. The 10 or 15 minutes necessary for an online search will yield an individualized bibliography that would usually require many hours of manual searching. the printout may include subject headings, abstracts, authors, titles, and publication sources. Any literature not available in the local library may be requested through one of the 11 regional libraries or through the NLM as a final recourse. Copies or originals of the requested material will be provided to health practitioners, researchers, educators, and students. Online centers will help those making requests by giving instructions or by performing the search. Charges vary from free to a modest fee, depending on the depth of the search, the length of online time, and the extent of the bibliography. An offline printout from the terminal is less expensive than online printouts and is sent by mail the following morning.[22]

The NLM in October, 1971 initiated the MEDLINE (MEDLARS On-Line), based on the MEDLARS (Medical Literature Analysis and Retrieval System) and the AIM-TWX (Abridged Index Medicus via Teletypewriter) experiences, the NLM initiated the MED-LINE (MEDLARS On-Line) in October, 1971. This decentralized online system serves more than 2,000 institutions; thus it is readily available in many institutions, including hospital, university, and research libraries. The MEDLINE data base contains *Index Medicus* citations from 1966 to the present. More than 200 nursing journals worldwide are indexed and listed in *International Nursing Index*. As shown by the following example, the MEDLINE bibliography provides full journal citations including authors, article title, journal, volume, issue number, pages, date, and often index terms (asterisks).

AU   Bryan NE
TI   Every nurse a teacher
LA   Eng
MH Attitude of health personnel
MH Ethnopsychology
MH *Health education
MH *Nursing
MH Patients/*education
MH Special list nursing
MH *Teaching

[22]MEDLARS, the computerized literature retrieval services of the National Library of Medicine. NIH Publication No. 80-1286, revised January 1980, Department of Health, Education, and Welfare, Public Health Service, National Institutes of Health.

CI D9GG-0000 4:31 74
SO Aust nurses J 4(1):31-3, JUL 74

Database

MEDLINE. Back files from 2,500,000 references can be obtained, including a search formulation that will automatically select any new references and mail them from the NLM.

TOXLINE (Toxicology Information Online). This system has a collection covering references on human and animal toxicity studies, chemical and pollutant effects, and negative drug reactions.

CHEMLINE (Chemical Dictionary Online). This computerized dictionary contains the names of chemical substances and compounds. In collaboration with the Chemical Abstracts Service (CAS), it contains CAS Registry numbers, molecular formulas, generic names, and other pieces of information.

RTECS (Registry of Toxic Effects of Chemical Substances). RTECS is a compilation of acute toxicity substances.

TDB (Toxicology Data Bank). This database contains chemical, pharmacological and toxicological references that have been extracted from books and reviewed by a group of subject specialists.

CATLINE (Catalog Online). This service provides users with access to cataloging information. With the CATLINE, libraries can save cataloging time and use the base for ordering, for reference, and for an interlibrary loan service.

SERLINE (Serials Online). Bibliographic information on serial titles is available, including all journals ordered or cataloged for the NLM collection.

AVLINE (Audiovisuals Online). There are 11,000 references to teaching packages for health sciences college courses in this system. Entries are screened for quality and can be retrieved by subject heading, name, title, and playing time.

HEALTH PLANNING & ADMIN (Health Planning and Administration). This database has 200,000 references on health planning, management, manpower, organization, financing, and other subjects. Eventually the base will refer to books and technical reports.

HISTLINE (History of Medicine Online). This base contains approximately 40,000 references to material relating to the history of medicine, and nursing, and related sciences, professions, individuals, institutions, drugs, and diseases.

CANCERLIT (Cancer Literature). This service of the National Cancer Institute contains more than 300,000 references to the various aspects of cancer. It includes abstracts from foreign and U.S. journals plus selected reports, meeting papers, and dissertations.

CANCERPROJ (Cancer Research Projects). This base is sponsored by the National Cancer Institute and has references from the present and past. Ongoing cancer research projects are described.

CLINPROT (Clinical Cancer Protocols). This base contains summaries of new anticancer agents and cancer treatment techniques. Although a reference tool for clinical oncologists, it is useful to others also.

BIOETHICSLINE. This file contains references from several disciplines dealing with such bioethical topics as euthanasia, abortion, and human experimentation.

EPILEPSYLINE.   This reference base contains sources sponsored by the National Institute of Neurological and Communicative Disorders and Stroke.

POPLINE (Population Information Online).   This base is a source of citations concerning reproduction, family planning, and demography. It is produced in cooperation with the Office of Population, U.S. Agency for International Development.[23]

PDQ (Protocol Data Query).   This database contains active, NCl-sponsored protocols from the CLINPROT file, a list of institutions where the protocol is being used, and the name of an oncologist to contact about the protocol.

Other data bases include Psychological Abstracts; ERIC, an education file; and CAIN, an agriculture database.

As an example of what can be accomplished with a computer-based search, Silva reported using two MEDLARS literature searches that generated nearly 700 citations related to informed consent in addition to online and offline computer searches, using MEDLINE, BIOETHICS LINE, and LEXIS (Law), which generated nearly 550 citations on the ethical and legal aspects of human experimentation.[24]

Making a Request

Before submitting a request for a computer-based bibliographic search, the researcher should be prepared to state the information needed completely and accurately. In an interview with the librarian, search terms and strategy can be discussed and the proper database selected. The researcher may elect to work with the librarian during the online search. During the online interactive session, different approaches to the topic can be explored until the search satisfies the researcher's need.

COMPLETING THE SEARCH

When the major indexes and the card catalog have been searched for relevant citations, the researcher is then ready to accumulate materials for the purposes of evaluation and use. The researcher will be familiar with the collection arrangement by now and should seek help from the librarian in locating materials.

As each book is located on the shelf, the table of contents, chapter headings, preface, and index should be scanned to determine possible relevancy. Journal articles, as well as books, can be evaluated by reading the introductory paragraphs and scanning topic sentences and conclusions. The author and date of publication are also indications of the usefulness of a work. Some books and journals will be chosen for immediate use, whereas others will be considered as possible choices. If the researcher makes a note concerning the possibility for use on the bibliography card, it will be a reminder to check these possible sources if adequate material is not found.

Many books and journal articles have quite complete bibliographies. These should be scanned and any pertinent citations copied on the 3×5 cards. After checking a number of these bibliographies, the researcher will notice that certain authors and titles begin to

---

[23]MEDLARS brochure.
[24]Silva, M.C.: Informed consent in human experimentation; the scientist's responsibility—the subject's right, Trial **16**(12):37–41, 62–63, December 1980.

stand out as key sources. The researcher also will gain some insight into the amount of material necessary to cover the subject. Certain works will be considered essential for the research project, and special efforts may need to be made to obtain them.

The researcher should not discard any of the working bibliography cards unless they are duplicates. These cards are the record of what has been checked, what has possible use, and what is essential for complete coverage of the subject. Although a work may appear inappropriate on first evaluation, as the search progresses the researcher may decide that some application could be made.

If a particular citation cannot be easily found or is not available in the library, the librarian will often be able to borrow the material or to obtain a photocopy.

When the investigator has reached this point in the literature search, it is time to explore further in those directions indicated by the materials already located. This is one of the more pleasurable parts of the search. Following upon clues that lead to some new source of information or to some unexpected knowledge that is just right for the research project is gratifying. Although systematic searching is necessary, a spontaneous break from the routine to follow some especially interesting facet has a definite place in the search process.

Since it is important to research broadly when doing a library search, materials other than those found in a health professions library also will provide background for a study. *Readers' Guide to Periodical Literature* should not be overlooked. Journals and literature from fields related directly or indirectly to the health sciences (such as psychology, home economics, music, religion, philosophy, speech and drama, sociology, education, special education, anthropology, economics, history, and literature) should be investigated. The reference librarian will suggest specific indexes or abstracting tools, such as *Sociological Abstracts*,[25] *Public Affairs Information Service*,[26] and *Education Index*.[27]

If such material is not on file in a small library, the librarian will be able to order it. Sometimes there is a nominal charge involved. Journal articles and books are usually available on an interlibrary loan basis, and for minimal cost microfilmed material may be obtained. If there is a great need for a specific book, it may be expedient for the library to purchase the book or have it put on microfilm. If the book was valuable enough to be microfilmed the library should have it in the reference file.

Library Networks

Obtaining materials or requesting computer-based bibliographic services not available in the local library is expedited by the medical library network. This network is hierarchical in design, with local hospital libraries serving as primary resources, followed by resource libraries such as large university medical libraries, the Regional Medical Library centers and finally, the NLM. An awareness of the network is essential, especially to researchers who lack local access to a good library. In such cases inquiries should be addressed to a resource library within the state or to the Regional Medical Library, which will provide material or refer the researcher to the appropriate resource library. The purpose of the Regional Medical Library is to extend library services throughout the region, thus

[25]Sociological abstracts, New York, 1952. Six times per year; cumulated every 10 years.
[26]Public affairs information service, New York, 1915, Bulletin of the Public Affairs Information Service. Forty-four issues per year; cumulated five times per year.
[27]Education index, New York, 1932, Wilson. Published monthly from September to June; cumulated annually.

making biomedical information more readily available to all health professionals. The Regional Medical Libraries are listed in Table 7-1.

TABLE 7-1   Regional Medical Libraries

Regions	States	Regional Medical Library
1	Connecticut Delaware Maine Massachusetts New Hampshire New Jersey New York Pennsylvania Puerto Rico Rhode Island Vermont	Greater Northeastern Regional Medical Library Program New York Academy of Medicine 2 East 103rd Street New York, New York 10029 (212) 876-8763 TWX: 710-581-6131
2	Alabama District of Columbia Florida Georgia Maryland Mississippi North Carolina Puerto Rico South Carolina Tennessee Virginia West Virginia	Southeastern Atlantic Regional Medical Library Services University of Maryland Health Services Library 111 South Greene Street Baltimore, MD 21201 (301) 528-2855 (800) 638-6093 TWX: 710-234-1610
3	Illinois Indiana Iowa Kentucky Michigan Minnesota North Dakota Ohio South Dakota Wisconsin	Greater Midwest Regional Library Library of the Health Sciences University of Illinois at Chicago Chicago, IL 60680 (312) 996-2464 Telex: 206243
4	Colorado Kansas Missouri Nebraska Utah Wyoming	Mid-continental Regional Medical Library Program Library of Medicine University of Nebraska Medical Center Library Omaha, NE 68105 (402) 559-4326 Interlibrary: (402) 559-6221 TWX: 910-622-8353
5	Arkansas Louisiana New Mexico Oklahoma Texas	South Central Regional Medical Library Program University of Texas Health Science Center at Dallas 5323 Harry Hines Boulevard Dallas, TX 75235 (214) 688-2085 TWX: 910-861-4946

TABLE 7-1—cont'd

Regions	States	Regional Medical Library
6	Alaska Idaho Montana Oregon Washington	Pacific Northwest Regional Health Sciences Library Service Health Science Library University of Washington Health Sciences Library Seattle, WA 98q95 (206) 543-8262 TWX: 910-444-1385
7	Arizona California Hawaii Nevada	Pacific Southwest Regional Medical Library Service UCLA Biomedical Library Center for the Health Sciences Los Angeles, CA 90024 (213) 825-1200 ILL: 213-825-5639

QUALIFICATIONS FOR RESOURCES

The researcher should be aware of the qualifications for good sources of information. A primary requirement is that they demonstrate high-level scholarship by being well written, factual, and current. If the research study requires a search into historical aspects of the topic, the literature utilized should have been pertinent and relevant at the time it was published. Generally, however, it is important that the material included in a review of the literature be as recent as possible because of social and technological change. Two or three hundred years ago a 10-year-old book would not have been a problem. Today, it is very important that references be up to date. For example, statistics that are more than 5 years old are of little value for current research projects.

References should be unbiased. The *Christian Science Monitor* and the *New York Times* are considered relatively unbiased newspapers. Some periodicals are extremely one sided, or politically biased, or their material is not as relevant as that of some other sources. For a library search, in addition to the literature cited in the card catalog, indexes, and bibliographical listings, the researcher should not forget dictionaries, encyclopedias, and abstracts, all of which provide factual information.

Special materials include periodicals from other professions and from international organizations (such as the World Health Organization and the International Council of Nurses), and government documents, state and local documents, directories, almanacs, and fact books among other sources of significant data. Researchers should become acquainted with the official organs and publications of professional organizations in other countries. More and more of these are becoming available in medical, nursing, and hospital libraries, and are written in English.

It has been our experience that rather than read lists of potential journals, most individuals, after learning the library search procedure, prefer going to the library to look over the card catalog or list of journals available in the library. Therefore, we are not including names of potential sources in this book but are recommending that a methodical investigation of possible literature references be made on a firsthand basis.

CATALOGING AND CLASSIFICATION

We present brief examples of the Dewey Decimal Classification system, the Library of Congress, and the National Library of Medicine Classification.

Dewey decimal classification

610	Medical sciences
611	Anatomy
612	Human physiology
613	Personal hygiene
614	Public health and preventive medicine
615	Therapeutics
616	Internal and clinical medicine
617	Surgery
618	Gynecology and obstetrics
618.9	Pediatrics
618.97	Gerontology

Library of Congress classification
(Class R—medicine)

R	Medicine (general)
RA	Public aspects of medicine: medicine and the state; public health, and so on
RB	Pathology
RC	Internal medicine; practice of medicine
RD	Surgery
RE	Ophthalmology
RF	Otorhinolaryngology
RG	Gynecology and obstetrics
RJ	Pediatrics
RK	Dentistry
RL	Dermatology
RM	Therapeutics; pharmacology
RS	Pharmacy and materia medica
RT	Nursing
RV	Botanic, Thomsonian and eclectic medicine
RX	Homeopathy
RZ	Other systems of medicine

National Library of Medicine classification
(Preclinical sciences)

QS	Human anatomy
QT	Physiology
QU	Biochemistry
QV	Pharmacology
QW	Bacteriology and immunology

QX　　　Parasitology
QY　　　Clinical pathology
QZ　　　Pathology

Medicine and related subjects

W　　　General and miscellaneous material relating to the medical profession
WA　　　Public health
WB　　　Practice of medicine
WC　　　Infectious diseases
WD　　　Deficiency diseases
WE　　　Musculoskeletal system
WF　　　Respiratory system
WG　　　Cardiovascular system
WH　　　Hemic and lymphatic systems
WI　　　Gastrointestinal system
WJ　　　Urogenital system
WK　　　Endocrine system
WL　　　Nervous system
WM　　　Psychiatry
WN　　　Radiology
WO　　　Surgery
WP　　　Gynecology
WQ　　　Obstetrics
WR　　　Dermatology
WS　　　Pediatrics
WT　　　Geriatrics
WU　　　Dentistry, oral surgery
WV　　　Otorhinolaryngology
WW　　　Ophthalmology
WX　　　Hospitals
WY　　　Nursing
WZ　　　History of medicine

PRACTICAL APPLICATION

Now that we have presented the process to be undertaken when doing a library search, we offer a number of suggestions that should be beneficial and time-saving for the beginning researcher.

1. Libraries usually have a number of files. Some of the larger libraries have departmental card files as well. Take time to become acquainted with these files. They may contain just the material you need.

2. Each library has its own idiosyncracies and its own location of books and journals, depending on space available and the classification system. Oversized books may be found in a different section of the library from the regular size books.

3. Certain types of research periodicals and small pamphlets may be stored in a special section of the library.

4. Find the classification number for the type of books needed. Then ask permission to go into the stacks and browse through the books. This does not mean that all books concerning a given topic are located in one section of the stacks. For instance, a book on nursing theory could be found under two categories, either nursing or theory. Just because a book is not listed in the card catalog under a certain category does not mean that such a book is not available.

5. Current periodicals are located in a special section of the library and are not yet included in the cumulative index. Only unbound current issues are displayed; older issues of the current year are stored nearby. Journals from previous years are usually bound and shelved by title and by year.

6. While perusing periodicals, notes may be taken, and sections of articles or entire articles may be photocopied for future reference, or duplicate copies may be checked out.

7. After searching through the literature of your discipline, repeat the process, using indexes and abstracts from related fields. Frequently they offer helpful information.

8. Never overlook the materials on reserve. Some books and periodicals are placed on the reserve shelf with limited or no checkout time. Occasionally the book you need has been taken from the stacks and is on reserve.

9. Every library has a variety of services, and no two libraries seem to function alike. Services such as book discounts, photocopying, and computer services for specific topics can be found in individual departments. Interlibrary loans, telephone references, and computer searches also may be provided.

10. Abstracts list not only professional journals but also books. Most disciplines are broken down by sections or classifications. Once the section or classification of the topic is located, it is easy to run through the various years of the publication, looking in that specific section.

11. Some journals concentrate on a specific topic. Rather than rely on an abstractor to categorize the subject matter, simply thumb through these journals yourself. Most journals have their own cumulative index, which can be checked for titles. Quite often the title may include words that are in the topic being studied. On the other hand, do not discard an article or a book on the basis of the title alone.

12. Because many authors specialize in certain areas of study or research, some material may be located by author as easily as by topic.

13. Generally, if a good reference source is found on the topic of interest, the author's bibliography will furnish other sources.

14. While searching for a topic such as theory in nursing, look in the index for the word *nursing* and then for the word *theory*. If theory and nursing are both listed as being on the same page in a work, then the author must be discussing nursing theory on that page.

Again, when looking for information dealing with the effect of music therapy on the rate of recovery from a certain illness, look up the term *music therapy* to see on what page it is listed and on what page the illness or disease is listed. If both topics are listed on the same page of the article, this must be where music therapy and the illness are being discussed. It is also possible to cross-reference music therapy and the name of an expert known to be associated with that form of treatment. Various combinations of cross-referencing may be used. This is a valuable technique for abstracts, books, and journals.

It has been our experience that when looking for current information, the more up to date the information is, the less likely it can be found without assistance. The reason for this is the length of time between publication and published abstract, plus the fact that the abstractor may use different terms. Abstracting publishers abstract month by month or quarter by quarter; therefore, they are always some months in arrears. Most of these publishers have a yearly cumulative abstract, and some are in 5-year periods. This means that the cumulative abstracts must be searched to date, then the annual abstracts to date, and finally, the monthly abstracts to date. The most current months have not been abstracted at all. Sometimes it is almost as wise to flip systematically through each issue of current professional journals on a month-by-month basis as to search by trial and error.

15. Locate and check out all the books that can be found on a topic when the sources are known to be valuable.

16. Photocopy any page that cannot be checked out if time becomes a factor. This may be fairly costly, but in the long run a few dollars will probably be sufficient for the amount of duplication that will be necessary. It is convenient to have all reference material at one location at home, in the office, or in a study area.

17. Be sure to note complete bibliographical citations on 3×5 cards.

Writing the Review of the Literature

Experienced researchers will have gone to the library often to review the literature. They will have searched for similar problems studied by other researchers. Investigators also will consider their particular problem in the study of nursing as it relates to the developing school of thought and the topic of nursing in general. The suggested order places the review of literature after the statement of the problem, although this is not necessarily a rule. One of my saddest moments as a teacher was when a student asked permission to have an additional day to work on a research project so that she could do library research before handing in her research paper!

A question frequently asked concerning the review of the literature is, "How is it written up?" It should be noted here that documentation style is not as important as consistency and thoroughness. Some authors have a very brief summary of the review of literature, stating other research findings in a few words. At other times investigators may combine the findings of two authors into a single sentence. Suppose we illustrate the point using fictitious names. "Dr. Meredith (1980) found that highly educated people usually have higher incomes; however, Dr. Smith (1985) found that the world's wealthiest people have not completed college." Reviewing literature in this manner provides a brief summation of findings.

Certain items should be included in the review of the literature. These are (1) the similarities and differences between the present study and studies done by other researchers, (2) the weaknesses and shortcomings of other studies, and (3) anticipation of how the present study will fill in the gap. The section on the review of literature should serve as a broad overview of the whole general area being researched. As an illustration, consider a possible study on the need for a well-baby clinic in a specific community. Review of the literature might focus on well-baby clinics in general. However, in the event that very little has been written about the specific topic, the researcher can broaden the search to include medical clinics and pediatrics. Furthermore, a review of the literature could include findings in overseas settings where well-baby clinics have been set up by the governments and medical missions. Of course, it is hoped that throughout the library aspect of the research process, the researcher will have help in developing the instrument, in formulating the problem, and in selecting the hypothesis.

For another illustration of how to find literature relevant to a topic under study, suppose a researcher is interested in interracial dating within the health professions. Possibly such a topic is difficult to locate or research findings have not been published; but interracial dating has been studied, and there has been a flood of information on interracial relationships in general. If the researchers are unable to find information on the specific topic, they should go to the broader, more general idea. Suggested sources are the health professions' literature, and then literature in the fields of psychology, sociology, and anthropology. Indexes, abstracts, and the card file are among the major sources of categorized listings.

After the literature has been searched and screened and valuable references have been determined, the researcher summarizes the findings in a brief presentation. This section in the report presents the rationale for the investigation.

SUMMARY

Contrary to student opinion that the card file lists all library references, making the procedure easy, a library search is both difficult and time consuming. Most student researchers limit their search to an extremely narrow topic and then complain about lack of reference material.

Two questions, what and where, continue to plague the person engaged in searching the library for information concerning similar studies: (1) "What do other people call my subject heading?" and (2) "Where do I find the material I need?"

Reasons for the library search include finding methods, ideas, and similar studies. Frequently, other researcher's findings are used for comparison with the proposed study.

Before beginning the literature search, develop an organized plan that suggests the proportion of the total time to be spent in the library, the topics to cover, the use of interlibrary loans, and the location of various resources. It cannot be stressed often enough that the librarian is one of the researcher's best friends.

Every reference or resource should be listed on a 3 × 5 card with a complete bibliographical citation.

Journals are generally more scholarly in their approach and contain more current information than books. Most disciplines have abstracts prepared of other publications. These are brief summaries of articles by title, author, and category.

Just a few of the valuable sources in the library are the card file, abstracts, government publications, microfilms, microfiches, cumulative indexes, and interlibrary loans.

Computer-based bibliographic services, such as MEDLINE, can provide comprehensive literature searches for researchers. Various databases are available in different subject areas.

It is suggested that you familiarize yourself with the library, find the topic classification number, and then browse the stacks for general and specialized literature; use abstracts and indexes from several disciplines, and make use of the library services.

In conclusion, the researcher is encouraged to utilize the library as one of the most valuable sources of help available.

DISCUSSION QUESTIONS

1 Distinguish between using the library for a term paper and using the library search for a scientific research project.
2 What is the purpose of an abstracting service?
3 In what ways is a library card catalog inadequate?
4 Why is it so difficult to locate books and periodicals in a library even though the particular literature is in the library collection?
5 Justify your belief that either the physical or the health sciences have better defined concepts, making it easier to locate its research results.
6 What are the merits of browsing through the shelves looking for source material in a specific section of the library rather than using the card catalog?
7 What are the advantages of using a learning resource center over a library? What are the disadvantages?
8 Why is the library search done during the preliminary part of the research process?
9 When is the library search completed?
10 What could be gained by eliminating the library search?

CLASS ACTIVITIES

Track I

1 The students are to search a particular topic in the library. When the students return to the classroom, several of them are to report what and where they found information. Suggestions and questions about future searches are discussed.
2 Copies of research abstracts are distributed to the students, who then list the words and topics that should be searched in the library.

Track II

1 The entire class goes on a tour to a library that is unfamiliar to the group.
2 Each student is to list specific sources in the library that will supply titles and authors of nursing research studies by topic (exact word or words). The students then look for them in a library search.
3 Students begin the library search for their project. As soon as the search is complete, the student is to submit a draft of the literature review plus bibliography to the instructor for evaluation and/or advising.

SUGGESTED READINGS

Armour, R.: How to find it: basics of research, The Christian Science Monitor, education page, July 2–August 20, 1979.
Ash, L.: Subject collections, ed. 5, New York, 1978, R.R. Bowker Co.

Aydelotte, Myrtle K.: Nurse staffing methodology: a review and critique of selected literature, Washington, D.C., 1973, U.S. Department of Health, Education, and Welfare, DHEW Pub. No. (NIH) 73–433, U.S. Government Printing Office.

Cooper, H.M.: The integrative research review, a systematic approach, Applied Social Research Methods Series, Vol. 2, Beverly Hills, 1984, Sage Publications, Inc.

Culkin, Patricia B.: Creative approaches to library service, American Libraries 3(6):643–645, June 1972.

Henderson, Virginia: Implications for nursing in the library activites of the regional medical programs, Bull. Med. Libr. Assoc. 59:53, January 1971.

Henderson, Virginia: Library resources in nursing: their development and use, I, Int. Nurs. Rev. 15:164, April 1968.

Henderson, Virginia: Library resources in nursing: their development and use, II, Int. Nurs. Rev. 15:236, July 1968.

Henderson, Virginia: Library resources in nursing: their development and use, III, Int. Nurs. Rev. 15:348, October 1968.

Lehmkuhl, D.: Techniques for locating, filing, and retrieving scientific information, Phys. Ther. 58(5):579–584, May 1978.

Library of Congress subject headings, 2 vols., ed., Washington D.C., 1984, Library of Congress.

Notter, Lucille E.: The significance of the literature search in the research process, ANA Pub. No. G-125:25–30, 1977.

Parkin, Margaret L.: Information resources for nursing research, Can. Nurse 68(3):40–43, March 1972.

Rajecki, A.A., and Muntz, M.L.: An introduction to medical/nursing libraries and available resource tools, Nurs. Forum 17(1):103–112, 1978.

Sheehy, E., and others: Guide to reference books, ed. 9, Chicago, 1976, American Library Association.

Sparks, S.M.: AVLINE for nursing education and research, Nurs. Outok ST37(11):733–737, November 1979.

Sparks, S.M.: The National Library of Medicine's bibliographic databases: tools for nursing research, Image XVI (1):24–27, Winter 1984.

Sparks, S.M., and Kudrick, L.W.: AVLINE: an audiovisual information retrieval system, J. Nurs. Educ. 18(7):47–55, September 1979.

Taine, Seymour I.: Health literature—a new world service, World Health, May 1974, p. 28.

Toward a national program for library and information services: goals for action. Washington, D.C., U.S. Government Printing Office, No. 052-003-00086-5.

CHAPTER 8

DESIGN AND CONDUCT OF THE STUDY: PROPOSALS AND GRANTS

The design and conduct of the study is the heart of the research report. It contains all the important information related to strategy and methodology and describes the instrument.

A research design is a scheme of action (framework) for answering the research question or questions. After formulating the specific problem and thoroughly reviewing relevant literature, the researcher thinks through the steps to produce a workable strategy.

The design includes such factors as the research setting, operational definitions, assumptions, relationships between variables, delimitations, sample, sampling procedure, instrument, approach to be used, and the method for analyzing data. Ethical questions concerning subjects' rights, use of data, debriefing, and permission must be resolved. To clarify the process of designing a research study, we will use a hypothetical situation for illustration.

Various members of the health team notice that many children in the community show evidence of poor nutrition, including underdevelopment, susceptibility to upper respiratory infection, and pallor, even with such factors as income and education are average or above. Using this information as a background, we present four possible research designs.

From the evidence, the researcher concludes that problem is "malnutrition in children in the community." The researcher proceeds by going to the library and checking the topic of nutrition in abstracts drawn from journals and books in such fields as home economics, dietetics, nursing, dentistry, and medicine. After a complete review of the relevant literature, the investigator can draw on the information relating to the problem of malnutrition. Eventually the decision is made that one hypothesis should be that poor nutrition in children is related to peer food preferences.

Developing the research design is the next step. The theories and concepts used to develop the hypothesis are the basis for the theoretical or the conceptual framework. Poor nutrition in children and peer food preferences are concepts that must be operationally defined in their relationship to the framework. One of the assumptions is that there are several factors related to poor nutrition in children, but for this particular study, only peer food preferences are being investigated.

In continuing the designing process, the four basic research approaches are considered. Within each of the approaches there are various data-gathering methods that can be applied. The investigator must evaluate the alternatives and select those that will provide the most suitable data for testing the hypothesis.

Historical Approach

The historical approach is the least likely to be used since it deals with the past and this is a current problem. If the researcher wanted to study past trends in nutrition in children, then the historical approach would be appropriate.

Survey Approach

Because this is an exploratory or descriptive study, and because new facts need to be gained in the actual setting, the survey approach is a likely possibility. Using the survey approach, the researcher must decide which instrument to use. If a questionnaire is selected, further decisions must be made regarding type, length, and other specifications. An interview guide or interview schedule requires similar decisions. What format would an observation tool require? What other tools are possible? Other important questions include "Where can the instrument be tested," and "Who will be used in testing the instrument?"

Questions that must be resolved when considering the sample are "What age group should be included." "How large should the sample be?," and "How should I go about obtaining permission from the parents to include their children in the study?" Of equal importance is the sampling procedure. "Should I take a random sample, a matching sample, a convenient sample, or some other sample?" The data-collection process poses many questions as to what methods and techniques should be used.

Case Study Approach

The case study is probably not an appropriate approach because it leads to an in-depth study of only one case or one unit, and a general picture is needed in this instance. If for some reason the case study approach was chosen, decisions for selection of the case would be crucial. An interview schedule or an interview guide is the usual instrument and yields probing information. Many of the alternatives to be decided when using the survey approach are not relevant in the case study. Such factors as sampling, data collecting, statistics, and tables are not vital because only one subject is involved.

Experimental Approach

The experimental approach can be applied by comparing a group of children who have received nutritious food with a group of children who have not. The samples and sampling procedure would involve some of the same questions as in the survey. However, since two or more sample groups are necessary in the experiment, the groups must be as nearly identical as possible in the variables being studied. Decisions concerning data collecting also would be similar to those in a survey. It would be wise to discuss which statistical tests should be selected with a statistician.

Tables may be more complex than in a survey, and a number of questions need to be asked. Is a table presenting a comparison of children who ate nutritious food versus those whose diet was inadequate sufficient information for the reader? Should tables show a comparison between such variables as socioeconomic background and prior medical history? What other comparisons should be made? Which variables should be held constant? What method will be used to manipulate the independent variables?

This brief introduction to research design is meant to answer basic questions that beginning researchers often ask. Detailed descriptions of the various aspects of the plan are the focus of this book.

PHILOSOPHY OF LOGIC

A discussion of logic is necessary because research is based on reasoning, the foundation of logic.

If A is larger than B, and B is larger than C, then A is also larger than C. Here we are using reason based on known facts. The fact is that A is larger than B, and B is larger than C; so then it is logical that A is larger than C. Logic is a form of convincing proofs that show beyond doubt that something is true. Logic is the core of physical sciences such as mathematics, physics, and chemistry. It serves the same purpose in all research.

Logic, scattered through the entire research process, is the necessary ingredient that welds together a systematic investigation from the time of conceptualization through the research design, data collection, and writing of conclusions and implications. Ideally, a research problem should be based on a theoretical perspective. Utilizing a tested and acceptable idea (theoretical perspective) as the basis for a research question is superior to proceeding without a theoretical foundation. It is logical that we use findings that have been tested rather than those that have not been tested. It is logical to proceed from the known to the unknown. A combination of two or more known facts should produce additional logically deduced truths.

All sciences except mathematics are empirical. That is, they are based on observations and experiments derived through the senses, and they can be verified. Logic is a method of reaching conclusions that satisfies the need for proof on the basis of other inferences considered true. That which is known to be true, valid, and reliable is used as the basis on which to advance to other truths. Logic is the process of moving from one statement known to be true to another that is true. This can be accomplished through inductive and deductive reasoning.

Inductive reasoning results in a generalization based on a number of individually observed phenomena, all of which are in the same class. It is an instance of reasoning from a part to the whole, from one to many, from particular to general, from singular to universal.

Deductive reasoning works in the opposite direction. It goes from general to particular, from the whole to a part, from many to one. For instance, we may by inductive reasoning sample a few students from a group and reach a conclusion about the whole student population. Using deductive reasoning, if we knew that student nurses in general tended to demonstrate a particular characteristic, we might deduce that those enrolled in a given school of nursing also might tend to demonstrate the same characteristic.

In regard to people, inductive logic and deductive logic are only probable, never certain. In true logic, a single instance of contradiction disproves the conclusion of previous reasoning. We assume on the basis of observations of people that human beings have two eyes. A single observation of a three-eyed person might therefore make us question the validity of our previous observation. In the observation of personality or other characteristics of people, it is only possible to make statements that are "usually" true or that may happen "60% or more of the time."

The Greek philosophers were well aware of the need for a rational interpretation of factual data, which could be supplied by logic. An example of Aristotle's distinction between knowledge of fact and knowledge of the reasoned fact by use of a syllogism is reported by Brody.[1]

E. (1) All planets do not twinkle.
   (2) All objects that do not twinkle are near the earth.
   _____
   (3) Therefore, the planets are near the earth.
F. (1) The planets are near the earth.
   (2) All objects that are near the earth do not twinkle.
   _____
   (3) Therefore, the planets do not twinkle.

E is knowledge of the fact; F is knowledge of the reasoned fact, correctly stating the cause. Nearness is the cause of nontwinkling; nontwinkling is not the cause of nearness. This illustration of the Greek application of logic to a problem shows the necessity of a penetrating analysis of facts.

Sometimes a conclusion is reached that seems reasonable but is criticized by others as illogical. An invited speaker—an inmate in a penal institution who was on parole for the day—was criticizing prisons. His contention was that prisons should be torn down. A young man in the class disagreed, "The prison census of the local penitentiary is down, but the newspapers say that crime is on the increase." He reasoned that crime was on the increase because the "bad" people were out committing crimes instead of being confined in jail. This may or may not be true. The point is that the student's reasoning was not logical; he simply associated two events that were occurring at the same time as being cause and effect, without considering other alternatives.

John Stuart Mill formulated two fundamental principles of causality. Rather than go into a detailed explanation of his principles, we shall make general statements about them.

Researchers may take phenomenon X and attempt to find its cause. Suppose they find that no other known variable occurs with X in every case. Sometimes Y is found; sometimes A, sometimes B, or sometimes several variables occur at the same time as X. There are, therefore, no instances of "Y always occurs with X," so it is not known what causes X.

Suppose on the other hand, that in every instance in which X is found, Y is always present; it might be concluded that there is some relationship between X and Y, but it cannot be concluded that Y causes X. Further research may reveal heretofore unknown variables that may be the cause of both X and Y. It is through this process of experimental addition and subtraction of variables that researchers arrive at conclusions.

The use of logic can be illustrated with a homey example. A garage mechanic noticed an unusual noise in the transmission of an automobile. He disassembled the transmission

[1]Brody, B.A.: Towards an Aristotelean theory of scientific explanation, Philosophy of Science 39(1):22. March 1972, Used with permission of the author and publisher.

and installed a new part, reassembled the transmission, and listened for the noise. The noise persisted, indicating that the trouble still remained. He then systematically disassembled the transmission, removed the new part, and replaced it with the old. Obviously, only one part could be interchanged at a time if the fault was to be located. Interchanging two parts at a time would confuse the issue. In the scientific process, we can manipulate only one variable at a time. The introduction of logic into research methodology has been immensely important to the development of research. Through it, scientists reach conclusions.

Further, the purpose of logic is the same as research—to interpret events of the past and present in order to predict and explain. Logical reasoning is the process of understanding events for predicting and explaining. It is therefore important that the researcher knows if some point of reference (an hypothesis, for example) is true or false.

In research, a body of knowledge (an accumulation of observations) is used as the basis of truth or error. The usual procedure of building a body of knowledge is to compare the new with the old. The new should confirm and verify the old. In the field of research, hypotheses based on theory should confirm the theory. If the theory has been verified (accepted) many times and the hypothesis does not support the theory then the hypothesis is quite possibly false. Probably the hypothesis is wrong because the methodology for testing the hypothesis is inappropriate.

A body of knowledge develops through testing (research) and the thought processes (logic). Knowledge is significant and useful when it is consistent. New knowledge when combined with the old, through thought processes in a logical fashion, is the creation of an entirely new body of knowledge. This process is known as inference. Inferences draw from the old body of knowledge to produce new ideas. This process of drawing and predicting is known as deduction and induction. Deductive inferences move from the general to the specific, from the universal to the particular, whereas inductive inference is just the reverse, from the particular to the universal. Inferences are the manner or process through which knowledge or judgment is revealed. A syllogism is an example of an inference which uses deductive reasoning. Women who wear white caps are nurses. Linda wears a white cap, therefore, Linda is a nurse. Syllogisms have a middle term upon which the logic of the inference depends.

Hypotheses in the field of logic are suppositions which explain the cause and effect relationship between two phenomena. The hypothesis provides a bridge between and upon which inductive and deductive inferences can be made. Induction results are used as a basis for deductive inferences concerning possible things which exist. Through this process the scientific method has verified inferences. Inductive and deductive reasoning through the application of logic has been the process by which science has developed new fields of knowledge.

THE RESEARCH PROPOSAL

A research proposal is a brief description of the projected investigation to be submitted for acceptance by governing bodies, funding organizations, or persons in authority. It may be written in the words of the researcher or as answers following the guidelines provided by the sponsoring organization. A review of the proposal submitted by the investigator helps both the investigator and the reviewers to better understand the purpose and procedures of the study. Reviewers, regardless of whether they represent an organization or teach a research course, will almost always give helpful criticism and suggestions for the proposal.

Proposals are comparable to blueprints and serve the same function. Just as the architect gives the contractor a blueprint of his building ideas, the researcher presents a proposal for evaluation.

Proposals are essential and are required for all research that must be funded or approved. They become a descriptive part of the contract for services that will be offered in exchange for funds or permission. Proposals are beneficial because they force researchers to make a complete analysis of the research process they intend to use as they contemplate and plan each aspect of the study.

Writing the Proposal

One of the major advantages of the well-written proposal is that it serves as a guide for writing the research report. Kielsmeier and Crawford suggest that changing the tense, adding the data, and discussing the findings are all that is needed for the research report. They go on to point out that a proposal deals with three general questions; *Why* should the study be done? *How* will it be conducted? and *What* will be the benefits after completion.[2]

During the development of the proposal, it is sometimes feasible to complete one step before moving on to the next. Other times it may seem more natural to move back and forth between steps.

If there is a dearth of information about the topic in the literature, the researcher must decide how this lack should be interpreted. Is it because the idea is innovative, because it does not have sufficient potential value, or because it is untestable with present technology? The latest research that has been done should be cited along with a statement as to the way in which it falls short of the proposed study.

Proposal Contents

The reviewer to whom the proposal is submitted is a specialist in evaluation. A proposal must be convincing and speak for the writer. It should have a neat physical appearance and be organized so that the reader can easily follow along from point to point by clear, summarizing statements. The well-written proposal is a demonstration of the scholarly capabilities of the researcher and, indirectly, an indication of the quality of the research. It should include the following general information:

1. Title of research proposal
2. Name of investigator and qualifications of researcher and staff involved in the project
3. Date submitted
4. Statement of problem
    a. Specific enough to be solved, yet can be generalized beyond the immediate study
    b. Manageable in size
    c. Stated in the form of a declarative statement or question, especially in exploratory research

[2]Crawford, J., and Keilsmeier, C.: Proposal writing. In Crawford, Jack, editor: CORD, national research training manual, ed. 2, Monmouth, Oregon, 1969, Oregon State System of Higher Education, p. ix–3.

5. Importance of problem
    a. Theoretical base, if any
    b. Need for such research
    c. Beneficiaries of the research
    d. Implications for special groups and further research
    e. Value of research, regardless of whether or not investigator's idea is effective
    f. Contribution to previous or new theory
    g. Contribution to public at large
    h. Uniqueness of project
6. Objectives of study
    a. Are achievable
    b. Are specific
    c. Are measurable
7. Résumé of relevant literature
    a. Provides overview of topic
    b. Review of past studies using selected references that are documented
    c. Strengths and weaknesses of previous studies
    d. Recommendations suggested by other researchers
    e. Emphasis on current research
    f. Synthesizes results of research cited
8. Research design
    a. Statement of approach to be used: survey, experiment, case study, historical, or other
    b. Statement of hypothesis(es) or questions to be investigated
        (1) Should be in logical order
        (2) Preferably, use operational or scientific form
        (3) Should be stated in a form that is testable
        (4) Wording should be clear and concise
        (5) Theoretical base is identified, if any
    c. Assumptions, definitions, delimitations, and limitations of study
        (1) Assumptions made by investigator
        (2) Operational definitions of terms and concepts as will be used
        (3) Delimitations set by investigator
    d. Outline of research procedure in complete detail
        (1) Description of the population and the sample, including size and use of a control group
        (2) Description of sampling procedure along with reasons for use if complex sampling plan is anticipated
        (3) Description of tool(s) to be used. Statement as to whether goal is to develop new tool or to develop one before data are collected
        (4) Description of how descriptive measures or statistics are to be used. Include statement concerning their appropriateness for type of data collected
        (5) Kinds of tables to be included
        (6) Description of data analysis methods and consistency with study design
        (7) Method of coping with procedural problems associated with data collection and ethics

    (8) Description of anticipated by-products and procedure for dissemination of findings and materials

    (9) Procedure for evaluating study should be clear and exact

9. Budget of projected expenses

    a. Names of director and other personnel. Backgrounds are included to show their competence for conducting research

    b. Evidence of approval, cooperation, or necessary contractual agreements

    c. Cost of research materials

    d. Salaries of director, assistants, consultants, and secretarial assistance

    e. Cost of office space, supplies, and services

    f. Cost of rental or purchase of computers and equipment

    g. Travel expenses, local and out of town

    h. Communications: phone, Telex, or other

    i. Cost of final report production and distribution

The research proposal must speak for itself. Therefore, one draft is not sufficient, and revision is necessary. By laying the proposal aside for a few days, the writer will be more alert to its degree of persuasiveness and to any grammatical weaknesses in it. The proposal forecasts the study results and is meant to convince the reader that the researcher understands precisely what he/she intends to study and that the researcher is using a logical, systematic approach.

In the classroom it is not likely that the student will be requested to prepare a proposal if the entire project is to be completed (including a written report) within one quarter or one semester. However, one the graduate level and in the professional setting, a proposal is expected to be developed and submitted to the appropriate committee before permission is granted to proceed with the project. When requesting funds from an organization for financial support, a proposal giving detailed information is mandatory.

Why Proposals Fail

Because proposals are not always accepted, the researcher must be alert to the reasons for rejection. According to Krathwohl, major reasons for the failure of government-sought proposals are that (1) they seem to have limited significance, (2) the procedures were not adequately described or there were flaws in the design, (3) the researcher was inadequately prepared to undertake the project, and (4) the budget was too high in relation to the anticipated results, or it included inappropriate costs.[3]

Taub adds to this list such factors as unsound hypotheses, nonspecific objectives, and invalid proposed methods.[4]

The proposal becomes ineffective when the researcher does not follow the guidelines, fails to complete the application form, does not meet the deadline, or does not match the study problem with the correct funding agency, according to area of interest.

If a proposal is not accepted, it should be resubmitted according to the suggestions of the reviewers or submitted to another appropriate funding agency. The researcher can expect a proposal to be eventually funded if it addresses an important problem in a creative manner.

[3]Krathwohl, D.R.: How to prepare a research proposal, ed. 2, Syracuse, NY, 1977, Syracuse University Press, p. 59.
[4]Taub, A.: Grantsmanship: getting school health funded, Health Educ, 9(5):2–4, September–October 1978.

GRANTS

Financial support, through grants, is frequently necessary for research projects to be conducted. Beginning investigators, however, normally do not initiate a project of such magnitude that funding is required. Even so, it is important to understand grantsmanship and the process of grant funding. Proposal preparation is closely linked to funding, since the grantor of financial support will want to know exactly what the researcher's idea is, the design of the project, and the proposed budget.

Prior to seeking a grant, the project must be completely conceptualized, and it should have the support of the institution that the researcher represents. The project is then matched with the most likely sponsor, and any written guidelines furnished by the possible grantor should be followed precisely. The proposal must be submitted prior to the published deadline date required by the funding agency. There is a great deal of hard work and preparation involved, but researchers do receive grant money.

The purpose of obtaining grants is to obtain the funds that will ensure continuance of the project. Grants cover the salaries of professional and clerical personnel (full-time and part-time), the cost of necessary equipment, and operating expenses, including travel expenses, and the rest of the budget. The last covers such items as heat, light, library services, rental of space, accounting, and other details.

The timing for getting a project funded must be considered as soon as the purpose of the research project has been identified. But first, the need for a grant must be determined by asking the following questions: Is it possible to conduct a preliminary study in the course of one's work routine and then seek funding if the findings warrant further investigation? Has preliminary research already been conducted, and is now crucial that funds be obtained for a full-scale project to be undertaken? Is there a need for additional funding to continue ongoing research?

The writer of the research proposal is acquainted with the situation and is the appropriate person to apply for a grant. The primary fact is that the project must be based on an extremely good idea—one that is above and beyond the relative face value of a good idea.

Proposals may be submitted on a form provided by the grantor or may be typewritten in prose. In either case, they should include information essential to understanding the worth of the proposed project.

Grantsmanship has been described as an art. The researcher matches the amount of funds needed with the sources who usually give grants of that amount and are interested in the area of the proposed research. For instance, a foundation that funds health-related projects is more likely to finance preventive health care projects than those aimed at the concerns of education. Locating possible sources of grants involves time and effort; however, the librarian can be of value in acquainting the researcher with the indexes, directories, books, and foundations that are on file.

Among the best sources of information on federal funding are the *Catalogue of Federal Domestic Assistance, The Federal Register*, and the *Commerce Business Daily*, which are available from the Superintendent of Documents, Government Printing Office, Washington, D.C. 20202. The official handbook used by the federal government that describes the programs and activities of most of its agencies is the *United States Government Manual*, published by the Office of the Federal Register, National Archives and Records Service, General Services Administration. It, too, is obtained from the Superintendent of Documents, Government Printing Office.

Private foundations on the national, state, and local levels may be asked for financial support. Because foundations invest in people, they are interested in the person behind an idea. Of course, each source of funds is geared to its own interests, and it is important that the proposed research fall within the scope of the foundation's program. The *Foundation Grants Index*, published by the Foundation Center as an insertion *Foundation News* magazine, is a major tool in locating possible funding. As a nonprofit organization, the center disseminates information on grants from philanthropic organizations. *The Foundation Directory*, published by The Foundation Center and distributed by Columbia University Press, reports data on the largest foundations. State directories may include a variety of funding sources with lesser annual grants. Nursing is one of the areas of research funding available in Comsearch printouts, which are generated from the Foundation Center's database.

A search through recent issues of *Foundation News* for current information on grants is a good way to determine which foundations are likely to be interested in the proposed research. New names of possible grantors may be found, and other names may be deleted because of funding guideline limitations.

Periodicals that provide space for news of grants awarded from federal and nonfederal sources include *The Chronicle of Higher Education* and *Foundation News: The Journal of Philanthropy*; the latter is published by the Council on Foundations, Inc., New York, N.Y. 10019. *The Register*, which is updated annually and covers both federal agencies and foundations, and the reference guide, *Grantsmanship: Money and How to Get It*, ed. 2, are published by Marquis Academic Media, Marquis Who's Who, Inc., 200 E. Ohio St., Chicago, Ill. 60611.

Selling the proposal is the second aspect of grantsmanship. It is one thing to match the project with appropriate sources of grants, but it is another thing to sell the source on the value of the proposal and on the investigator's ability to conduct the research. Often a cover letter, which provides a brief overview of the proposal, is sent to the funding agency. The aim is to convince the grantor that there is a problem, but there is also a solution. Who, what, when, where, and why are topics the cover letter should attack. Foundations are interested in funding worthwhile projects and have mixed portfolios of risky and not-so-risky projects.

Beginning researchers may use their first projects to gain skills and knowledge about the research process and in so doing become aware that further research on the same topic calls for "seed" money. Such funds may be available from a local or regional source.

SUMMARY

The approaches used in conducting research are classified differently, depending on the authors; survey research (sometimes called descriptive research) is nonexperimental in nature; a case study investigates a single subject in depth (in some instances this is an aggregate situation such as a town); experimental research is based on manipulation of the subjects, and historical research is an integrative account of the relationship of people, places, and events studied in historical perspective.

Definitions are welded together through the use of logic to provide the research setting. The philosophy of logic is related to inductive (going from specific to general) or deductive (going from general to specific) reasoning and the finding of cause-effect relationships through manipulation of variables.

Identification of a researchable problem is basic to research. The purpose and the problem (topic) for study should be closely related in the research plan. The steps of the scientific method are followed in solving or exploring the problem. Various approaches may be implemented to obtain data for testing and analysis.

A *research proposal*, submitted for acceptance by appropriate persons or groups, is a brief description of the problem to be solved or explored. Such factors as significance of the problem, hypotheses to be tested, assumptions, definitions, delimitations, limitations, pertinent literature, and the budget are included.

Grants cover the cost of research. Grantsmanship is the art of trying to match funding needs with a funding source.

DISCUSSION QUESTIONS

1 Evaluate this statement: The research proposal is the blueprint of science.
2 Develop your own breakdown of research categories based on your knowledge of nursing.
3 How is logic related to reasoning? To common sense?
4 Summarize the major points of a grant proposal.
5 Why would researchers want to base their investigations on theory?
6 How is the approach related to the topic to be studied? Why is a particular approach often right or wrong for a specific project?
7 What is the purpose of obtaining a research grant?

CLASS ACTIVITIES

Track I (Activities Related to the Chapter, Not to a Single Project)

1 Divide the class into groups of two or three, to draft a research proposal for a problem of interest or one that is presented by the instructor.
2 Divide the class into two groups and debate the pros and cons of obtaining grants for research.

Track II (a Continuous Activity That Leads to the Completion of a Scientific Investigation)

1 Each student begins to design a study based on the problem that has been developed. The student should write out the beneficiaries of such research, the uniqueness of the project, the achievability and measurability of the project, and the prevalence of previous studies.

SUGGESTED READINGS

Abarbanel, J.: Planning a do-it-yourself funding search, Health Educ. 9(5):8–12, September–October 1978.

Ackerman, W.B., and Lohnes, P.R.: Research methods for nurses, New York, 1981, McGraw-Hill Book Company.

Adebo, A.O.: Identifying problems for nursing research, Int. Nurs. Rev. 21(2):53–54, 59, March–April, 1974.

Adesso, N.A., and Brannon, J.H.: Writing for funding, Health Educ. 9(5):20–21, September–October 1978.

Andrew, B.J.: Can professional competence be measured? In Loveland, E.H., guest editor: New directions for program evaluation, measuring the hard-to-measure, No. 6, 1980.

Artinian, Barbara M., and Anderson, N.: Guidelines for the identification of researchable problems, J. Nurs. Educ. **19**(4):54–58, April 1980.

Bailey, A.L.: So you want to get a grant, Change **17**(1):40–43, January–February 1985.

Baker, F.: Data sources for health care quality evaluation, Evaluation and the Health Professions **6**(3):263–281, September 1983.

Barnard, R.: Writing grant proposals, Reflections **6**:8, May–June 1980.

Berkbuegler, J.: Proposal writing: essential first step to research, Med. Rec. News **51**:68–70, February 1980.

Brink, P.J., and Wood, M.J.: Basic steps in planning nursing research, North Scituate, Mass., 1978, Duxbury Press.

Campos, R.G.: Acquiring foundation funds, J. Nurs. Adm. **10**(6):16–23, June 1980.

Canadian nurse researchers discuss methodology, Int. Nurs. Rev. **25**(2):59, March–April 1978.

Claypoole, R.L.: The U.S. government manual, Health Educ. **9**(5):12, September–October 1978.

Crawford, J., and Kielsmeier, C.: Proposal writing. In Crawford, Jack, editor: CORD, national research training manual, ed. 2, Monmouth, Oregon, 1969, Oregon State System of Higher Education.

Cruise, R.J., and Cruise, P.D.: Research for practicing nurses...an introduction for all nurses who can and should be doing nursing research, Superv. Nurse **10**:52, October 1979.

Davitz, J.R., and Davitz, L.L.: Evaluating research proposals in the behavioral sciences: a guide, ed. 2, New York, 1977, Teachers College Press.

Debakey, L.: The persuasive proposal, Foundation News, pp 19–24, July–August, 1977.

Golden, A.: The grantsmanship center news, Health Educ. **9**(5):13–14, September–October 1978.

Gray, G.: Nursing research: is it justified? Aust. Nurses J. **9**:41–43, September 1979.

Harty, H.: What administrative help in preparing research proposals do professors find useful? Educ. Res. **6**(10):16–17, November 1977.

Hoult, B.: Oiling the wheels, Nurs. Mirror, pp. 25–26, May 4, 1978.

Jacobson, S.: An insider's guide to field research, Nurs. Outlook **26**(6):371–374, June 1978.

Kazdin, A.E.: Research design in clinical psychology, New York, 1980, Harper & Row Publishers.

Kim, H.S.: Critical contents of research process for an undergraduate nursing curriculum, J. Nurs. Ed. **23**(2):70–72, February 1984.

Krathwohl, D.R.: How to prepare a research proposal, ed. 2, Syracuse, N.Y., 1977, Syracuse University Press.

Krueger, J.C., Nelson, A.J., and Wolanin, M.O.: Nursing research, development, collaboration, and utilization, Germantown, Md, 1978, Aspen Systems Corp.

Lee, J.M.: Methods of funding, Physiotherapy **68**(11):365, November 1982.

Locke, L.F., and Spirduso, W.W.: Proposals that work, a guide for planning research, New York, 1976. Teachers College Poress.

Macilwaine, H.: How to get started, Nurs. Mirror, pp. 23–25, May 4, 1978.

Malia, K.: Students views of nursing, discussion of method—insights into social science research, Nursing Times **79**(20):24, May 18–22.

Marriner, A.: The research process in quality assurance, Am. J. Nurs. **79**(12):2158–2161, December 1979.

Mastal, M.F., and Hammond, H.: Analysis and expansion of the Roy adaptation model: a contribution to holistic nursing. Adv. Nurs. Sci. **2**(4):71–81, 1980.

Miller, J.R., and others: Obstacles to applying nursing research findings, Am. J. Nurs. **78**:632–634, April 1978.

Partridge, C.J.: The research process, Physiotherapy **68**(11):354–355, November 1982.

Reinharz, S.: On becoming a social scientist, San Francisco, 1979, Jossey-Bass Inc., Publishers.

Riehl, J.P., and Sister Roy, C.: Conceptual models for nursing practice, ed. 2, New York, 1980, Appleton-Century-Crofts.

Roy, Sister C.: The Roy adaptation model comment, Nurs. Outlook **24**(11):690–691, November 1976.

Schantz, D.: The research design, Journal of Nursing Administration **12**:35, February 1982.

Schmidt, M.H., and Chapman, M.K.: Alumni involvement in nursing research development, Nurs. Outlook **28**(9):572–574, September 1980.

Sexton, D.L.: Some methodological issues in chronic illness research, Nursing Research, **32**(6):378, November–December 1983.

Singleton, E.K.: An experience in collaborative research, Nursing Outlook **30**:395, July–August, 1982.

Slavin, R.E.: Basic vs. applied research: a response, Educ. Res. **7**(2):15–17, February 1978.

Sliepcevich, E., and Vitello, E.M.: A selective bibliography—proposal writing and grant sources, Health Educ. **9**(5):5–7, September–October 1978.

Sliepcevich, E., and others: Grantsmanship: Getting school health funded, Health Educ. **9**(5):2–30, September–October 1978.

Smith, J.P.: Is the nursing profession really research-based? J. Adv. Nurs. **4**:319–325, May 1979.

Spector, P.E.: Research designs, Series: quantitative applications in the social sciences, No. 07-023, Beverly Hills, 1981, SAGE Publications, Inc.

Spitzer, W.O.: Ten tips on preparing research proposals, Can. Nurse **69**(3):30–33, March 1973.

Sylvester, D.C.: Nursing research essential to professional practice, AORN J. **30**(6):1078–1082, December 1979.

Taub, A.: Grantsmanship: getting school health funded, Health Educ. **9**(5):2–4, September–October 1978.

Teaching and learning research grants announcement: Fiscal years 1981, 1982, 1983, 1984, Washington, D.C., August 1980, United States Department of Education, National Institute of Education.

Tyler, J.: The art of grantsmanship, Health Care Educ. **6**(2):14, 33–34, 40, April 1977.

Wagner, P.: Testing the adaptation model in practice, Nurs. Outlook **24**(11):682–685, November 1976.

Warren, M.P.: Preparing a research proposal, Physiotherapy **68**(11)(:357–358, November 1982.

Watson, J.: How does a nurse interested in research identify a researchable question? J. Nurs. Res. **25**(6):439, November–December 1976.

Wechsler, H.: Choosing a research design and a study sample. In Wechsler, H., and Kibrick, A., editors: Explorations in nursing research, New York, 1979, Human Sciences Press Inc., pp. 89–95.

White, V.P.: Grants: how to find out about them and what to do next, New York, 1975, Plenum Publishing Corp.

CHAPTER 9

ETHICS IN RESEARCH

Many disciplines, groups, and organizations are concerned with ethical matters regarding human subjects.

In research, the question usually raised concerns the ethical and moral issue involved in gathering data on individuals. Our society, indeed, has some strange codes of conduct. The mass media have freedom to publish all manner of scandal about the general public. Divorces, arrests, trials, and frauds are given exposure to the world. It is certain that publishing these proceedings causes a great deal of anguish to the persons and families involved.

Psychological tests are sometimes criticized as being too probing and too personal by prying into the lives of respondents. What then can be said to justify our researching the behavior and activities of people involved in the fields of medicine, health, and nursing? The issue is even more critical when it involves the manipulation of human beings as they are placed in a laboratory experiment—either knowingly or unknowingly.

Wolfe has suggested that the field of medicine does not provide a complete model for experimenting with human subjects. However, researchers should not overlook the fact that experience and knowledge gained through the medical process have made a valuable contribution to understanding human behavior. Such experimentation includes surgical techniques, medications, nursing care procedures, and types of health care delivery.

Ethical considerations were heightened some years ago when Laud Humphries published his study "Impersonal Sex in Public Places." Humphries collected research by observing homosexuals who participated in sexual behavior in isolated, public men's rooms. He was able to trace the subjects whom he had observed in homosexual acts through their license plate numbers. Some months later, after disguising his appearance and posing as a social researcher, he visited their homes and was able to gather specific socioeconomic data. A flood of complaints from researchers, reporters, writers, and moralists denounced his tactics as unethical. Van Hoffman[1], one of the critics of Humphries' study, raised three issues concerning such research. First, information was collected that could be used for blackmail and extortion. Second, the motives for such a study may be questionable. Third, such an invasion of privacy is not proper.

On the reverse side of the issue, the news media and other journalistic endeavors use opinions, attitudes, and interviews as sources of information in the same manner as some

[1]Von Hoffman, Nicholas, Horowitz, Irving Louis, and Rainwater, Lee: Sociological snoopers and journalistic moralizers, Transactions 7:4, May 1970. Used with permission of *Society* magazine and Mr. Horowitz.

other researchers. Scientific data gatherers are not supposed to identify individual subjects or manipulate the lives of the particular people researched. Horowitz and Rainwater say that the issues raised by Von Hoffman will replace the good, tight methodology of the 1960s. However, they agree that certain sociological findings can become political statements.[2]

Social scientists sometimes do research for prestige and status. Such research is often aimed at receiving recognition for the writer by having the author's name appear under his article when it is published in a prestigious professional journal. However, researchers in the pure sciences are able to produce results that save lives and improve health, while gaining status for themselves.

It may be that the crucial issue concerns the investigator's freedom to present to a wide variety of readers material gathered on unsuspecting or even informed respondents. Some types of professional and technological research from the pure sciences (for example, chemistry and physics) can be published in their entirety since the results are as beneficial as the technique used in arriving at the findings.

The health field, in general, has been and continues to be very open to publication of all types of research findings. Apparently people feel that revealing their personal health deficiencies and illnesses is not really harmful to them personally and is advantageous in the long run to the medical profession and the public at large. Obviously this freedom should not be abused.

In the beginning some nursing research was under the direction of the sociologist. Any definition of sociology includes the idea that the sociologist studies the interaction or behavior of people as they respond to their environment. Gathering data on human interaction, from the standpoint of the social scientist and the nurse, can only come about by some sleuthing, otherwise, the subjects may not react naturally. The question that this chapter tries to answer is what is ethically and morally acceptable in gathering and reporting information about human subjects?

CONSEQUENCES OF CONTROLLING BEHAVIOR

The debate over use of research findings is neither new nor old but a continuing dialogue. Leonardo da Vinci said of his design for a submarine:

> This I do not...divulge on account of the evil nature of men, who would practice assassinations at the bottom of the seas, by breaking the ships in their lowest parts and sinking them together with the crews who are in them....[3]

But in response to Leonardo it can be said that any findings are amoral. What is *done* with them becomes the moral issue.

To continue the example, nursing research also can be used for good or evil. If we find that patients recover more rapidly under expressive nursing care (concern for the patient

[2]*Ibid.*, pp. 4–8.
[3]Gjessing, Gutorm: The social responsibility of the social scientist, Current Anthropology, December 1968, p. 402. © 1968, The University of Chicago Press.

as a person) than under nonexpressive nursing care (concern with tasks and the disease), it would be immoral not to publish the findings simply because we are afraid that someone would resort to nonexpressive nursing care in a concentration camp.

Medical practice has not always been allowed freedom in studying the human body.- Reynolds criticizes the attitude toward human subjects in research. Between 332 B.C. and 280 B.C. Herophilus dissected between 200 and 600 human cadavers. But dissection of human beings did not become legal again until 1280 A.D., when Fredrick II, Emperor of Germany, allowed it. Even then some countries permitted only a single dissection every 5 years.

Reynolds has classified research procedures into five categories, presented in the order of increasing severity.[4]

1. No effect. In this category there is neither positive nor negative effect on the subject participating in the research. Most students' surveys done as a course requirement fall into this category.

2. Temporary discomfort. The participant experiences temporary anxiety, tension, or physical pain. Such discomfort is terminated at the end of the study and is no greater than that encountered in day-to-day living. An experiment in which a very quiet student is required to stand in front of the class and relate a brief account of his history may fall into this category.

3. Unusual levels of temporary discomfort. This condition may last beyond the research study but usually returns to a normal state at a later time. In some instances, a postexperimental treatment or a debriefing may be required. For example, a group encounter may later require the assistance of a psychiatrist if it is not conducted by well-qualified personnel.

4. Risk of permanent damage. Risk implies that some subjects may experience or suffer permanent damage. This is possible in medical research, but examples are rare in social research.

5. Certainty of permanent damage. Permanent damage is expected to occur as a result of the research procedure. This level of damage is rare in any type of research.

Best questions the ethics of experimenting on human subject who participate in it for reasons of money, coercion, or lack of competence.[5]

We have never heard of a single case of social science or nursing research that has resulted in permanent damage to an individual. But we have often wondered about the level of damage that the mass media inflict on individuals in high office through the use of cartoons. Nursing research, to our knowledge, has never ridiculed any individual by name.

ETHICS IN DATA GATHERING

Although clinical investigation must use any and all means available, certain limitations exist in human investigation. Some experiments in nursing care are completely impossible,

[4]Reynolds, Paul D.: On the protection of human subjects and social science, International Social Science Journal **24**(4):694–695, 1972.
[5]Best, John W.: Research in Education, ed. 4, Englewood Cliffs, 1981, Prentice-Hall, Inc.

and others would create grave anxiety. The questions discussed in the following paragraphs deal with data gathering in nursing research.

1. "What is the risk involved for the patient or subject in any study of subjective responses?" Will exposure of his concerns, attitudes, feelings, and emotional state be detrimental to the patient, his/her family, or friends?

The degree of risk is a factor to be dealt with in ethical research. Asking age in an interview seems less harmful than asking subjects if they had ever stolen thermometers, syringes, drugs, or other hospital supplies. Administering placebos to patients who are psychologically dependent on a drug seems less harmful than administering placebos to patients physically dependent for comparison with a control group that receives the real medication.

Even though subjects give their permission to be used in an investigative study, it does not mean that the researcher is free to ignore their welfare. For example, a film was produced of the worship ceremony of a minority subculture. The photographers were given permission to record the service, and the film received extensive use in the academic world. Numerous comments were made by the students such as, "Look at those weirdos," "Do they actually do that?" and "They must be crazy." Quite possibly, friends, relatives, or participants in the worship service might be embarrassed or insulted by such comments. Although the religious ceremony was open to the public, permission was allowed for filming, and the photographers were permitted to use the film as educational material, harm could be done to the subjects by the ridicule of the viewers.

Areas of harmful effects include deception (makes the subjects look like fools), physically painful treatment (receive an electric shock), embarrassing questions (subjects have low incomes for particular jobs), or psychological stress (are asked to administer what they believe is an electric shock to another person). Some individuals might consider all four of these situations unethical, while another might not object to one or more.

It is difficult for a researcher to know when a specific project, experiment, or question will be harmful to subjects. Just because one researcher or one subject does not consider a project harmful is no indication that other subjects will approve.

2. "Does the subject have a right to know the purpose of the research being done?" Many arguments exist both for and against getting the subject's permission to participate in a research study. For example, in the medical profession, any new drug must be more than 30% effective because even placebos are 30% effective. Therefore, if nearly one third of the patients get well because they think that they are receiving a certain treatment, do we have an ethical responsibility toward them?

It seems that blanket permission (permission without limits) from the respondent to use data would meet ethical demands. After the research is completed, a detailed description of the use of the information could be given to the subject. Normally a researcher should never divulge the question being tested until all the basic information is obtained. To reveal the question or hunch being tested would obviously influence the respondent to react differently in order to impress, fool, please, or in other ways respond to the researcher.

Captive audiences (such as college sophomores in a psychology class) may not be the same as subjects out in the real world, but they should not be ignored. Captive audiences can always be informed later as to the purpose of the experiment and then be given an opportunity to refuse to have their responses used for publication. For the television show Candid Camera, the subject's permission is obtained after the recording of a humorous situation. There is no reason why the health researcher cannot do the same.

3. "To what extent should the subject know the nature of the research instrument and of the study situation?" A standard procedure that we have used with nursing students anticipating an experiment in social psychology is to inform the class of the forthcoming experiment. Any student who objects to the experiment may skip the class session, observe the experiment rather than participate, or assist the instructor. In one or two instances students have asked to help the instructor, but none has ever refused to participate. After all information is gathered, the motive and purpose are revealed, and the students are allowed to discuss and criticize the process. The research process thus becomes an interesting and educational experience for both subjects and researcher. Most people enjoy being part of an experimental research group. In addition, they seem to learn a great deal about experimental research by participating in such groups.

4. "What secondary effect will the research have on subjects (such as patients in the hospital) and those immediately around the subject (nurses and other personnel) during or subsequent to the research process?" The Hawthorne effect can occur in many strange and mysterious ways, even extending to persons interacting with the subjects (Chapter 19). It is in this secondary aspect that subjects may need to be warned about the results of participation. For example, in a hospital setting, a researcher might collect data on some form of nursing care. In the process patients may become aware of yet unrevealed information about their physical condition, or have a false perception about some aspect of their care that would influence their relationship with hospital personnel, physicians, friends, or family.

5. "Must the investigator respect the confidence of the subject?" It has been said that the person who asks the questions must bear the burden of the answer. If we ask a question, the person we wish to study is under no obligation to answer; however, the respondent is always doing the researcher a favor by answering the question. Therefore the researcher is always obligated to guard the confidence of the subject.

People usually do not object if their responses are included in a larger collection of data. But in some situations, negative findings on even a group might be detrimental in the eyes of the group; then their identification must remain anonymous. To guarantee anonymity involves careful thought. How do we know who responds and who does not respond to a questionnaire if we do not keep track of who has returned it? How can we collect further data on a subject if the subject is not known and there is no way to match future responses with the original? Will respondents answer honestly if they know their names can be matched with their answers? The whole issue must be a matter of trust. Certainly researchers should ask questions only if they want to bear the responsibility of the answer given.

What do the researchers do if they become aware of some serious acts committed by the respondent that could and should be corrected? Do the investigators report the subject's behavior? No, the researchers cannot reveal what is told in confidence.

One investigator obtained permission from an organization to investigate the incidence of pilfering among its employees. The question of ethics arose when the researcher was asked by the administration for the names of persons who had been pilfering supplies. The investigator was reminded by his advisor that primary responsibility is toward the subjects. The administration would probably have used the information to dismiss the guilty employees.

On another occasion a student proposed a study involving a penal institution. Permission was granted by the administrators for the study to be carried out; however, all the subjects, guards, inmates, and medical personnel refused. The study design included using prison records from the medical department as a means of checking the number of beatings there were by inmates and by guards. The guards did not want it known that they beat the prisoners; the prisoners did not want it known that they had their own system of justice; and the medical personnel were afraid of both the guards and the prisoners. Of course the study was never attempted.

6. "What is the nature of the relationship between the subject and the investigator?" Should researchers pillage the land behind them? No, it is necessary to treat respondents with respect and concern. If we take unfair advantage of our subjects, they may not cooperate with the next researcher. If obtaining the information is really important but there is danger of hurting the subject, it may be necessary to try a different approach. In nursing research, names of people, of institutions, and of nursing programs may not be revealed if to do so would be detrimental to the individual or the reputation of the institution.

7. "Should the subject be allowed to see the research results if he/she is interested?" Not all participants are interested, but it is extremely important to send results to any respondents who request them. Usually a one- or two-page summary of the study findings is sufficient.

It is also ethical to inform subjects exactly what will be done with the results of the study. Subjects must be told why we want their opinions or help. If, for example, we want to make some improvement from which the subject will benefit, or if we want simply to add to the store of knowledge, to publish the results in a book or journal, or to evaluate a procedure or process, then we must inform the subject of our purpose for gathering data. A golden rule of ethics is to treat respondents as we would like to be treated if we were the subjects.

8. Does the research design require invasion of privacy? Some individuals feel that reporting income, age, marital status, dating habits, and so on is an invasion of privacy. Of course, if subjects object, their feelings should be respected. Some of the activities that may or may not be considered invasion of privacy are one-way mirrors, lurking tactics, "bugging," joining a group for the sole purpose of studying the members, and masquerading. When dealing with primitive people, anthropologists assume that there is legal consent if they are not run out of the village. Photographers usually follow the same guidelines, assuming that it is acceptable to take pictures unless they are stopped by someone. Conversations and interactions that occur in public are just that—public—and are not considered an invasion of privacy.

9. Does the researcher have the right to ask subjects to perform a task that is contrary to their profession's code of ethics? A few years ago a health-related journal reported research in which medical personnel were asked to administer a nonlethal overdose of a drug to patients. The purpose of the study was to see if the persons administering drugs would challenge the order. We question the ethics of such an experiment not only involving subjects but also the persons administering the drug. It seems unethical to place medical personnel in a position where they must make painful choices: disobey the

physician's order, administer an overdose, or delay administering what may be a needed medication.

10. Is it ethical to conduct genetic research? Recombinant DNA is a case in point. Genes from lower organisms such as bacteria are combined with those of higher organisms. It is then possible to technically create new cells, and to learn more about DNA and genes that control heredity. Critics of this form of research are fearful that the new organism might produce unforeseen and dangerous results in densely populated areas... a laboratory horror story, so to speak.

Not only is some genetic research under fire, but various forms of chemical and physical research are questioned on the basis of health and safety. The atomic, hydrogen, and neutron bombs have received long and continued attack. It has been recommended that biological studies such as the DNA project be carefully monitored by the National Institutes of Health and that this board should apply stringent guidelines to such projects.[6]

DEBRIEFING

The term *debriefing* as used by Aronson and Carlsmith refers to the process of explaining the complete experimental design to the subjects.[7]

Debriefing is often necessary in experimental research and it may be mandatory in other situations. The debriefing process is conducted to include the following:

1. Explain the purpose of the research.
   —who will benefit
   —how the subject will benefit
2. Inform the subjects.
   —why it was necessary to keep some aspect of the project secret
   —why the subject was not informed
   —why the method was concealed
   —why the purpose was concealed
   —what might have happened if the subject had known the real purpose
   —how the results are more valid or reliable or beneficial by having naive subjects
3. Assure the subjects that no harm was intended to any participant. Assure them that the researcher had the participants' safety and psychological well-being in mind before and during the research. Discuss any negative feelings, attitudes, or beliefs that are expressed.
4. Tell subjects the intended use of the results. Explain that the findings and results will be available to read or to retain, if desired. Assure the subjects that their names will not be revealed, nor will they be identified in any manner.
5. Inform subjects that trickery was not intentional on a personal basis; the use of any techniques to assure naive subjects was in the interest of valid results, not to make fun of participants.

[6]Chronicle of Higher Education **13**(20):1, January 31, 1977.
[7]Aronson, Elliot, and Carlsmith, J. Merrill: Experimentation in social psychology. In Lindzey, Gardner, and Aronson, Elliot, editors: The handbook of social psychology, ed. 2, Reading, Mass., 1968, Addison-Wesley Publishing Co., Inc., p. 31.

6. Ask the subjects their feeling about the research and how they felt when informed of the true nature of the study. Subjects should be encouraged to discuss and talk about their involvement in the project. Subjects should again be encouraged to talk about any negative aspects.
7. Ask subjects to suggest improved procedures to prevent any negative feelings and improve conditions for research participants.
8. Consider subjects as co-researchers by asking how the experiment or study could be improved, how the validity of results could be increased, how a specific variable could have been controlled, and what insights would be beneficial for the researcher.
9. Express gratitude for the participation of the subjects.

Reynolds reports a study by Milgram related to debriefing. Participants who were debriefed after an experiment were less likely to regret taking part in the research than those who were not debriefed.

When conducting small classroom experiments in which students have agreed to participate it is assumed that they will try to trick the professor. Personal evaluations have revealed that students enjoy class experiments greatly. They delight in trying to guess what the researcher is testing and the purpose of the research, and in discovering ways to invalidate the results. The classroom atmosphere develops into one of anticipation of an experiment, interest in the results, and suggestions for improving future research. Some students are more compliant than others, some more naive, some very difficult to deceive. Once subjects develop a basic trust in the researcher, debriefing is a pleasant, fun experience eagerly anticipated. It is concluded that the better an experimental design is developed, the more skeptical the subjects, and the more sophisticated the researcher, the more valid the results.

ETHICS IN HEALTH RESEARCH

Reynolds has proposed several procedures used to control ethics in research. Journal editors should and do have some responsibility for rejecting articles that include unethical procedures. Professional activity can be controlled through a code of ethics and a complaint procedure against violators. Professional assistance is sometimes warranted in order to protect the welfare of subjects. Each discipline should regularly upgrade its professional code of ethics and revoke licenses when there is evidence that the client or patient is in danger. There should be a review panel to examine and approve all research to be conducted on human beings before the research is begun.[8]

Florence Downs editorialized some of the concerns of nursing research. Protection of the rights of patients, informed consent, freedom to withdraw or refrain from participation, and full explanation of the risks are some of the major points. Editor Downs says that manuscripts for publication will not be considered without a statement of the methods used to protect subjects. This attitude is typical of the concern expressed by various organizations toward research.[9]

The nursing profession on the national and international levels has been aware of the need for such procedures and has taken steps to ensure the rights of subjects. The

[8]Reynolds, pp. 713–714.
[9]Downs, Florence: "Whose responsibility? Whose rights? (editorial), Nurs. Res. 20(3):131, May–June 1979.

Commission on Nursing Research voiced its concern about ethics in the resolution adopted at the ANA convention in 1974. It was recommended that (1) all nursing education programs provide organized content regarding the responsibilities of the participant in research in protecting the rights and safety of human subjects, and (2) organized nursing services develop and enforce written guidelines and policies to protect the rights of individuals. Such action assumes that ethics can be learned. On the state level the association is to provide a grievance procedure whereby nurses who are aware of violation of human rights can report such violations for redress.[10]

Guidelines for the ethics of nursing research have been set forth by Canadian nurses. These, too, stress the need for free and informed consent of subjects, and every effort must be made so that the subject understands the nature and purpose of the research. Confidentiality is to be maintained and priority given to the rights and concerns of the subject. Researchers must meet certain standards in order to be assured that they have the knowledge and skill necessary to conduct the research, are aware of personal limitations, use appropriate designs and procedures, and are honest in purpose and use of the research. Expected research results should be worthwhile financially, and the project reviewed by a group of professional peers.[11]

On the international level, the ICN Code for Nurses does not mention ethics in nursing research per se but it does place responsibility for proper conduct on the individual nurse: "The nurse, in providing care, promotes an environment in which the values, customs, and spiritual beliefs of the individual are respected.[12]

Federal guidelines for research on human subjects are applicable to all research subjects who may receive physical, psychological, or social injury. Subjects must be free to accept or decline participation in a research study. Grantee institutions are to follow prescribed review procedures when submitting proposals and conducting the research.[13] The National Institutes of Health have prepared their own policies to protect subjects involved in its research.[14]

The Steering Committee of the Nursing Research Special Interest Section prepared a statement which was accepted by the National Executive of the New Zealand's Nurses' Association. The following points were considered: respect for rights of the subjects to life, esteem, self-determination, privacy, and protection from injury; informed consent; confidentiality; qualified nurse-researchers; clear lines of responsibility in conducting research ethically; and funding agencies.[15]

The ANA has established a six-member group known as the Institutional Review Board to protect the rights of human research subjects. This board is required by the U.S. government's Office for Protection of Research Risks for ANA to receive federal research funds.[16]

[10]Resolutions, Am. Nurse **6**(8):5, August 1974.
[11]Ethics of nursing research, Can. Nurse **68**(9):24, September 1972.
[12]Code of Ethics, Int. Nurs. Rev. **20**(6):116, 1973.
[13]Protection of the subjects of social research, Footnotes **2**(7):7, October 1974.
[14]Boffey, Philip M.: Research on human subjects, The Chronicle of Higher Education **9**(8):4, November 11, 1974.
[15]Int. Nurs. Rev. **24**(2):61, March–April 1977.
[16]Group safeguards rights of human research subjects, Am. Nurse **12**(6). 7, June 1980.

With regard to ethics, the American Nurses' Association has developed a set of ethical standards titled *Human Rights Guidelines For Nurses in Clinical and Other Research.* The national commission for the Protection of Human Subjects of Biomedical and Behavioral Research produced the *Belmont Report: Ethical Principles and Guidelines for the Protection of Human Subjects in Research.* In educational research two pieces of legislation called the Buckley Amendment are concerned with the rights of human subjects in research.

Fry draws attention to the Belmont Report and three issues: respecting individual rights for protection, defining the benefits for subjects, and some just means of selecting research subjects that would result in maximum benefit for all.[17]

Recently, issues have been raised concerning subjects in various suppressed conditions. Young children of an undetermined age may not be capable of making decisions regarding their involvement in research. Critically ill patients, the mentally handicapped, and poorly educated individuals are examples of questionable research subjects. Such persons may not be capable of acting autonomously. Justification for research as it relates to subjects' health in general, or contributing to the field of knowledge may or may not be considered an adequate reason for involving them in research. The American Nurses' Association *Human Rights Guidelines* admits that collective rights can supercede individual rights.[18]

Some aspects of ethical consideration in nursing as proposed in 1973 by the American Nurses' Association are as follows:

1. Subjects must be assured that their rights will not be violated without their informed consent. Subjects also must know the advantages and benefits of participation.
2. Researchers must guarantee that the subject will not experience harm, invasion of privacy, or loss of dignity.
3. Subjects must not be coerced into participation or harassed because they do not participate.
4. Health personnel must be aware of any participation in research. If they are to administer medication, partake in double-blind experiments, or record data, informed consent must be obtained.
5. The rights of patients too ill to make decisions, small children, and others must be protected from risk of injury.
6. Privacy for subjects includes consideration of anonymity, confidentiality, and unanticipated physical, social, and psychological disadvantages from participation. Since loss of dignity may occur at a future time, the subject may encounter long-range implications.
7. Captive subjects' rights must be considered. Such subjects include organ donors, prisoners, the mentally retarded, and military personnel.
8. The public in general has the right to the knowledge which research has or can develop. It is assumed that qualified nurse researchers should be encouraged to pursue improved methods of health delivery.

[17]Fry, S.T.: Ethics and nursing research, Virginia Nurse **L**(2):16–21, Summer 1982.
[18]*Ibid.*, 17–21.

9. Institutions and agencies are responsible for ensuring that the rights of clients and patients are protected in research. It is suggested that research be approved and monitored by a review committee or board appointed by the institution.
10. It is the duty of the nursing profession to ensure that the rights of research subjects are protected. Nurses are encouraged to become active in developing guidelines, serve on review committees, and be alert to human rights violations.

Reynolds finds that covert research tactics on unwary subjects has produced little evidence of negative effects.[19] Most review boards demand that subjects be informed of the risks, the purpose, and the procedure of research, and that subjects know how to withdraw and are free to do so. Most research requires written consent of the subjects.

Reynolds cites the fact that some legal aspects dealing with subjects' rights came out of the Nuremberg trials of Nazi war criminals. The four areas of legal rights considered were whether subjects had legal capacity to consent, were not coerced or forced to consent, were aware of the consequences, and understood the extent of the consequences.[20]

The American Psychological Association cites the psychologist's concern for research subjects. The psychologist assumes obligations for the welfare of his/her research subjects, both animal and human.

a. Only when a problem is of scientific significance and it is not practicable to investigate it in any other way is the psychologist justified in exposing research subjects, whether children or adults, to physical or emotional stress as part of an investigation.
b. When a reasonable possibility of injurious aftereffects exists, research is conducted only when the subjects or their responsible agents are fully informed of this possibility and agree to participate nevertheless.
c. The psychologist seriously considers the possibility of harmful aftereffects and avoids them, or removes them as soon as permitted by the design of the experiment.
d. A psychologist using animals in research adheres to the provisions of the Rules Regarding Animals, drawn up by the Committee on Precautions and Standards in Animal Experimentation and adopted by the American Psychological Association.
e. Investigations of human subjects using experimental drugs (for example: hallucinogenic, psychotomimetic, psychedelic, or similar substances) should be conducted only in such settings as clinics, hospitals, or research facilities maintaining appropriate safeguards for the subjects.[21]

Parts b and c mention harmful aftereffects. It may be very difficult to decide what is harmful to the subject before the experiment begins. It is never known exactly what the result will be. The experiment may be routine, and yet something may happen that will psychologically upset some subjects. For this reason, it is necessary to exercise extreme caution. The researcher should not ask embarrassing questions or probe sensitive areas (sex, death, income, illegal activities, moral behavior), and the subject should not be asked to do anything illegal, immoral, or offensive to his/her sense of dignity.

It seems that most guidelines for conducting research on human subjects are too vague. What is physical harm? Psychological harm? Emotional harm? What is invasion of privacy? Certain topics are taboo depending on the issues of the day—for example,

[19]Reynolds, P.D.: Ethical dilemmas and social science research, San Francisco, 1979, Jossey-Bass Inc., Publishers, p. 225.
[20]Ibid., p. 334.
[21]Research precautions of ethical standards, Washington, D.C., Copyrighted 1963, American Psychological Association, principle no. 16. Reprinted by permission.

race relations, sex, abortion, birth control, and population control. Doing research on some topics is considered unacceptable by some organizations. For example, experimental research in the area of religion has been rejected by some people as being naive, immoral, and foolish. Euthanasia is considered murder by most individuals and is not acceptable for experimentation. Research that supports a position contrary to our value system is most likely to come under attack. Some scientists studying foreign cultures are finding their research restricted until it has been approved by the government of the proposed subjects. Developing countries often want research to be done that will benefit them as well as the researcher, and grant permission accordingly.

It is interesting to speculate on some recent advances in health care. When a new nursing intervention or medical procedure is conducted on a patient in a critical state, is this considered research? What about the accident victim who arrives unconscious without family or relatives present? Can the nurses or medical staff try a new technique in an attempt to save the patient's life without consent from someone? Suppose the technique results are more harmful than beneficial and the patient dies or is seriously impaired for life. The researcher is expected to gain informed consent. Are the nurses or medical staff also bound to obtain consent before performing the new procedure designed to save a life? Obviously such emergency treatment is a form of research and it is very easy to criticize research after it has occurred, especially if it was unsuccessful.

Finally, the question of what is research, especially in clinical areas, raises some ethical concerns. In a sense, any nursing procedure is research, even if it has been performed on patients for years.

It seems that the governing issue for ethical research is motive. Some motives such as research grants, performing world-famous procedures, or publishing in a prestigious journal may constitute questionable ethical motives for research.

Do the quality and the creativeness of research decline when it is legislated? Who has the authority to make decisions on what is and on what is not ethical—the government, the funding organization, the researcher, or the professional organization? Many regulations are criticized as being too weak to protect individuals and too restrictive for the researcher. Table 9-1 recaps the major points.

In the final analysis, almost everything done is a form of research, and research in the field of health involves studying and observing human subjects. If we choose to do no research at all on a subject, we have obviously decided that no treatment or experiment is more favorable than treatment or experiment. As an example, in the health care setting, if we continue to do things as they have always been done, we are concluding that the present system cannot be improved; in a sense this too is experimenting. Probably the person who cries loudest against research is also the person who cries, "Why don't they do something?" Unfortunately, in experimental research if a new drug is highly successful, the control group is angry that its members did not receive it. If the drug turns out to be harmful, the experimental group is angry because its members were subjected to it.

SUMMARY

Often in the field of social research the investigator asks questions, takes notes, and pries into the mind of the subject. The situation becomes even more questionable as it relates to what is done with the information. Can the whole world be told the research findings

TABLE 9-1   Ethics in Research

Responsibility of Researcher(s)	Rights of Subject

Privacy
  No revelation of information that could identify
    the subject or organization
  Follow-up in code rather than name
  Sole holder(s) of data; information would continue
    to be confidential and not associated with a
    particular organization or person
Consent
  Must obtain subject's consent without coercion
  Must determine when it is appropriate to gain per-
    mission from volunteers, patients/clients, or
    minors or use the unsuspecting public
  Must allow the subject to withdraw from the project
    at any time for any reason
Rewards/promises
  Must fulfill any promise of payment, reward, or
    information concerning research results
Protection
  Must protect subject from physical or psychological
    harm
Information
  Must inform subject of the use that will be made
    of data, why the subject should participate,
    and any harm or risk involved
Debriefing
  Must debrief subject after experiments or dis-
    tasteful research tactics
Approval
  Must obtain approval from all appropriate research
    review boards
Permission
  Must obtain permission from agencies, institutions,
    and persons owning private materials when
    data are sought
Publication
  Must assure publisher that data were gathered with
    all due ethical consideration and meet the
    ethical standards prescribed by the publisher
	Privacy
	  Anonymity respected as a subject in a
	    research project
	  Confidentiality of information provided
	Consent
	  As a volunteer or willing subject
	  May withdraw at any time
	Rewards/promises
	  May receive them from researcher even
	    though subject does not complete
	    project
	Protection
	  From physical and psychological harm
	Information
	  As to use of research report, benefits
	    or disadvantages from participation
	Debriefing
	  If and when necessary

without revealing personal and private thoughts and ideas of the subjects? The main issue does not concern the findings themselves, but what is done with them.

Closely related to the issue of morals and ethics is the question of methodology. If the subjects are told what the researcher is doing and their permission is gained, will their typical behavior change?

Ethics related to data gathering must answer many questions:

1. What is the risk for the subject?
2. Should the subject know the purpose for the research?

3. Should the subject know the nature of the study situation?
4. What is the secondary effect of the research on the subject?
5. Must the investigator respect the confidence of the subject?
6. What is the nature of the relationship between the subject and the investigator?
7. Should the subject be allowed to see the research results?
8. Does the research design require invasion of privacy?
9. Does the researcher have the right to request subjects to behave in a manner contrary to their profession's code of ethics?
10. Is it ethical to conduct genetic research?

Debriefing is the process of explaining the complete experimental design to the subject. A detailed description is given of the research study along with the reason why the subject was asked to participate. The subject is made to feel as much at ease as possible, is asked to express his feelings, and can offer suggestions for future research.

Concern for ethics in nursing research has been evidence on the national and international levels through the adoption of codes of ethics. National groups, such as the Department of Health and Human Services and the National Institutes of Health, have taken affirmative action to protect human subjects through their guidelines and policies. The American Psychological Association cites concern for the subject's welfare in its standards.

Concerning these ethical problems, we believe that in the interest of good research, information should be gathered in as natural a setting as possible. After the research is completed, if privacy has been invaded, or moral or ethical issues are raised, the material should be publicized only after the subject has given his/her permission. A researcher should never betray the confidence of the subjects. Furthermore, there should be no way for the individual to be identified with the data that he/she provided.

Research is necessary for developing better and more efficient techniques in all areas of life. When we become afraid to use human beings as subjects for research, we are in effect saying, "Our present treatment is best."

DISCUSSION QUESTIONS

1 Why is there a sudden interest in ethics?
2 Are researchers really "tramping their subjects underfoot?"
3 Elaborate on any incident in which participation in a research project was harmful to the subjects.
4 What is your definition of damage as it relates to unethical research?
5 In what ways can the process of debriefing be beneficial to the quality of the research produced by a specific study?
6 Experimental research often uses the phrase "manipulating the independent variable." What do you find offensive or not offensive about the phrase as it relates to experiments involving individuals or groups?
7 Is there any harm done to individuals when their arrest notice is published in a newspaper? Why do the benefits outweigh the negative aspects or the negative aspects outweigh the benefits?
8 What are some of the current ethical issues in the health field?
9 What effects may publishing the name of a research subject have on the individual?
10 What is the effect of stringent ethical guidelines on quantity and quality of research findings?

CLASS ACTIVITIES

Track I

1 Role-play a situation in which a research is contacted by the mother of an interviewee who is upset about the questions that her 20-year-old daughter had to answer.
2 Role-play a situation in which a respondent asks the researcher to discard the questionnaire that the respondent mailed back last week.
3 Role-play a scene in which the researcher debriefs a respondent who was embarrassed by the researcher's questions concerning the respondent's attitudes toward sex.
4 Role-play a situation in which a beginning researcher has discovered that some subjects in his research are obtaining prescriptions for drugs for personal pleasure. He discusses the matter with his advisor.

Track II (Continuous Project)

1 Each student or group writes out the ethical issues that could arise from the conduct of the planned study.
2 List the permissions that must be granted in order to conduct the study.

SUGGESTED READINGS

Allen, Moyra: Ethics of nursing practice, Can. Nurse **70**(2):22–23, February 1974.

Armiger, Sister B.: Ethics of nursing research: profile, principles, perspective, Nurs. Res. **26**:330–336, September–October 1977.

Armington, C.: The right of privacy: cases and research problem, Superv. Nurs **8**:62–64, November 1977.

Aroskar, Mila A.: Anatomy of an ethical dilemma: the theory, Am. J. Nurs. **80**(4):658–660, April 1980.

Aroskar, Mila A.: Anatomy of an ethical dilemma: the practice, Am. J. Nurs. **80**(4):661–663, April 1980.

Barnard, K.E.: Informed consent in research studies, The American Journal of Maternal Child Nursing, **8**(5):327, September–October 1983.

Bergman, R.: Omissions in nursing research, Int. Nurs. Rev. **31**(2):55–56, 1984.

Bergman, Rebecca: Ethics—concepts and practice, Int. Nurs. Rev. **20**(5):140–141, 152, September–October 1973.

Besch, L.B.: Informed consent: a patient's right, Nurs. Outlook **27**(1):32–35, January 1979.

Brink,P.J., and Wood, M.J.: Basic steps in planning nursing research, North Scituate, Mass., 1978, Duxbury Press, pp. 130–136.

The Chronicle of Higher Education **13**(20):1, January 31, 1977.

Code for Nurses—ethical concepts applied to nursing, Int. Nurs. Rev. **21**(3–4):104, May–August, 1974.

Code for nurses with interpretative statements, Kansas City, 1976, American Nurses' Association, ANA Pub. No. G-56.

Code of Ethics as applied to nursing, Int. Nurs. Rev. **21**(3–4):103–104, May–August 1974.

Creighton, H.: Law for the nurse supervisor, Superv. Nurse **8**(11):62–64, November 1977.

Davis, A.J.: Informed consent...ethical issues in research involving human subjects, West. J. Nurs. Res. **1**(2):145–147, Spring 1979.

Davis, A.J.: Ethical issues in nursing research: events in 1980, West. J. Nurs. Res. **2**(1):427–429, Winter 1980.

Davis, A.J.: Research with the mentally retarded and mentally ill: right and duties versus compelling state interest, Journal of Advanced Nursing 9(1):15, January 1984.

Dillman, C.M.: Ethical problems in social science research peculiar to participant observation, Hum. Organization 36(4):406, Winter 1977.

Ethics of controlling brain functions, Times, London, Thursday, September 14, 1978. From Michael Leapman, La Jolla, Calif., September 13, 1978.

Ethics of nursing research, Int. Nurs. Rev., March–April 1977. Reprinted from New Zealand Nursing Journal, March 1976.

Fields, Cheryl M.: Debate over genetic research spreads across the country, The Chronicle of Higher Education 13(20):1, 10, January 31, 1977.

Florio, D.H.: Court upholds confidentiality of research records/date, Educ. Res. 9(5):19–20, May 1980.

Fox, D.J.: Fundamentals of research in nursing, ed. 3, New York, 1976, Appleton-Century-Crofts, pp. 206–212.

Fry, S.T.: Ethics and nursing research, Virginia Nurse L(2):16–21, Summer 1982.

Griffen, A.P.: Philosophy and nursing, J. Adv. Nurs. 5(3):261–272, May 1980.

Group safeguards rights of human research subjects, Am. Nurse 12(6):7, June 1980.

Kelly, K., and McClelland, E.: Signed consent: protection or constraint? Nurs. Outlook 27(1):40–42, January 1979.

Kelman, H.C.: Privacy and research with human beings, The Journal of Social Issues 33(3):169–195, Summer 1977.

Knepper, J.D.: Use of human subjects in experimentation: informed consent, Journal American Medical Research Association 53(6):70–74, December 1982.

Krawczyk, R., and Kudzma, E.: Ethics: a matter of moral development, Nurs. Outlook 26(4):254–257, April 1978.

Krimsky, S., and Ozonoff, D.: Recombinant DNA research: the scope and limits of regulation, Am. J. Public Health 69(12):1252–1259, December 1979.

May, K.A.: The nurse as researcher: impediment to informed consent? Nurs. Outlook 27(1):36–39, January 1979.

Michael, J.A., and Weinberger, J.A.: Federal restrictions on educational research: protection for research participants, Educational Researcher 6(1):3–7, January 1977.

Mitchell, K.: Protecting children's rights during research, Pediatric Nursing 10(1):9–10, 1984.

Monaghan, W.P., and others: DNA recombinant research and you, Am. J. Med. Technol. 44:62–65, January 1978.

Niles, A.G.: Using survey research methodology: an examination of one project, Journal of Continuing Education in Nursing 12:28–34, November–December 1981.

Nursing Life Editors: New research poll on ethics, Nursing Life 2(4):17–24, July–August 1982.

Perspectives on the code for nurses, Kansas City, 1978, American Nurses' Association, ANA Pub. No. G-132.

Polit, D.F., and Hungler, B.P.: Nursing research: principles and methods, Philadelphia, 1978, J.B. Lippincott Co., pp. 303–305.

PROBE, What are your ethical standards? Nursing '74 3(3):29–33, March 1974; 35–44, September 1974; 56–66, October 1974.

Silva, M.C.: Science, ethics, and nursing, Am. J. Nurs. 74(11):2004–2007, November 1974.

Silva, M.C.: Informed consent in human experimentation: the scientist's responsibility—the subject's right, TRIAL 16(12):37–41, 62–63, December 1980.

Stein, F.: Anatomy of research in allied health, New York, 1976, Schenkman Publishing Co., Inc.

Warren, M.P.: Personal ethical responsibility, Physiotherapy 68(11):355–356, November 1982.

Watson, A.B.: Informed consent of special subjects, Nursing Research 31:43 January–February.

Weinberger, J.A., and Michael, J.A.: Federal restrictions on educational research, Educ. Res. **5**(11):3–8, December 1976.

Weinberger, J.A., and Michael, J.A.: Federal restrictions on educational research: privacy protection study commission hearings, Educational Researcher **6**(4):15–18, April 1977.

Weinberger, J.A., and Michael, J.A.: Federal restrictions on educational research: a status report on the privacy act, Educ. Res. **6**(2):5–8, February 1977.

Williamson, J.B., and others: The research craft, an introduction to social science methods, Boston, 1977, Little, Brown & Co.

Wooldridge, P.J., and others: Methods of clinical experimentation to improve patient care, St. Louis, 1978, The C.V. Mosby Co., pp. 184–192.

CHAPTER 10

HYPOTHESES

In the past 300 years, the scientific method has become the trusted and sacred way to gain new knowledge and information. The hypothesis, which is an educated guess, is an important part of the scientific method and research studies. It is a statement of the relationship between two variables which is based on the researcher's rationale.

While it is not absolutely necessary to have an hypothesis to carry out a research study, an hypothesis does serve a purpose.

The scientific method utilizes an hypothesis as a technique for solving a problem. The solution (hypothesis) is then tested by collecting empirical data to determine if the hypothesis is accepted or rejected. An hypothesis is accepted under certain specific conditions, and these conditions should always be stated.

It should be pointed out that hypotheses are not proved, only tested. Any attempt at proving an hypothesis suggests that the researcher is prejudiced toward some particular result and may not be considering conflicting or contrary possibilities. On many occasions an hypothesis is borne out by one study, but another researcher testing a similar hypothesis may obtain findings that are the reverse of the first hypothesis. Whether or not the hypothesis can be accepted is often not as important as how well the hypothesis was tested. The testability of an hypothesis is a measure of the value of the research study. The hypothesis is like a compass pointing the direction in which the researcher is to proceed.

FUNCTIONS

One function of an hypothesis is to provide a statement about a specific relationship between phenomena that allows this relationship to be tested empirically. In other words, with an hypothesis, researchers are provided a basis from which to learn if their speculative statement is probable or not. An hypothesis narrows the field of research to one or two elements. It identifies, in measurable terms, what the researcher believes to be the cause and effect of a given situation. Usually, an hypothesis is a statement of relationship between two phenomena or variables. In a research project at least two variables are being studied or compared, and each of the two variables should be defined as specifically as possible.

Normally, in an hypothesis there are a dependent and an independent variable. The independent variable is considered the cause and occurs before the dependent variable.

Thus, the independent variable is the cause, and the dependent variable is the effect. Usually, then, an hypothesis states some type of relationship between an independent and a dependent variable.

By way of illustration, a simple hypothesis is "Blondes have more fun." We might ask, "How would you measure 'more fun'?" For the purpose of testing, we could way, "More dates." In this instance we are thinking of females rather than males, so we are simply saying that if a woman has blonde hair, she will probably have more dates than a woman with black or brown hair. The independent variable is hair color, and the dependent variable is having fun, or dates. Obviously the variables cannot be transposed; it would be impossible for a person's having fun to determine hair color. The hair color (cause) comes first and the fun (effect) afterwards. Out hypothesis may not be true, or acceptable, but we are subjecting it to an empirical test by finding out if blondes have more dates. The color of hair indicates the tendency, according to our guess or hypothesis, for a woman to have dates.

In the health field, hypotheses often relate to cause of illness. If we find condition A every time we have condition B, we may have discovered a relationship that suggests a suitable hypothesis for testing. Even though two conditions appear to have a cause-effect relationship, we cannot assume that this is the case.

Suppose we find that individuals needing physical therapy for neurological conditions recover more rapidly with music playing than without. Music may be the cause of recovery, and it is necessary to test for the relationship. The hypothesis might then be stated, "Violin music facilitates neurological recovery." In this case, "neurological" must be operationally defined, and different types of music might be tested for their therapeutic value. There may be unknown factors influencing recovery, or perhaps other types of sound would be just as effective. Regaining optimum neurological function could be due to the presence of the staff, the influence of the patient's participation in group activities, certain medications being taken concurrently, subconscious reaction to the rhythm of the music, or individual differences.

Suppose the results indicate that certain factors do seem to occur together. We could test our hypothesis to see if condition A (neurological recovery) ever occurs when condition B (music) does not occur. A well-tested hypothesis provides specific data that determine whether we accept or reject condition B as the supposed cause.

CHARACTERISTICS

A good hypothesis has several basic characteristics.
1. It is testable.
2. It is logical.
3. It is directly related to the research problem.
4. It represents a single unit or subset of the problem.
5. It is factually or theoretically based.
6. It states a relationship between variables.
7. It sets limits of the study.
8. It is stated in such a form that it can be accepted or rejected.

OPERATIONAL DEFINITIONS

The initial statement of the hypothesis is worded so that it expresses the best judgment of the researcher at the moment. It may contain scientific terminology, concepts, or symbols that are meaningless until they are translated into specific definitions. The product of the translation process is called an operational definition. Operationalization is the process of translating a scientific hypothesis into operational terms.

Theories and hypotheses are generally abstract statements that must be converted into precise specific, empirical indicators. Operational definitions are needed since it is impossible to research a construct unless it is measurable. For example, "professional" is a construct whose meaning varies according to the background of the person using the word. If this word were used in an hypothesis, it would have to be operationally defined before the hypothesis could be tested. Suppose we decided to test the hypothesis, "Professionally trained personnel are more capable of assuming leadership than those who are technically trained." As this hypothesis stands, many questions must be answered before the hypothesis can be tested. What is meant by professionally trained? By technically trained? How do we define "capable?" How can the word "leadership" be made observable?

For purposes of testing an hypothesis, the researcher can arbitrarily define all the terms according to self-determined standards. For instance, a professional person can be described as "any individual with at least 4 years of college education." This definition may be unsatisfactory as far as other persons are concerned, but it is specific and easily measured. "Capable of leadership" could be defined as "anyone who has or is in a position of authority over other professionals." A technician, based on the definition of a professional person, would be "anyone with less than 4 years of college education."

Once the terms in the hypothesis are given operational definitions, it is possible to conceptualize a research plan whereby the hypothesis can be tested empirically. "Nurses who have at least 4 years of college education are working more frequently in positions of authority than are nurses with less than 4 years of college education."

The operationalization of concepts must be as extensive as possible to include every situation. For example, "professional" could mean anyone who has passed a state board examination. At the other extreme, it might mean only persons who have at least a master's degree. It could be based on years of practical experience or a combination of experience and education. The point is that within these extremes lies a definition of professionalism that should meet the criteria. Somewhere within the extremes, the researcher must be specific. Rightly or wrongly, for the purpose of an illustration, we have defined the word *professional*. We have arbitrarily set a limit that is measurable. Most researchers experience a similar dilemma when they attempt to make a construct specific.

FORMULATION OF THE HYPOTHESIS

The stating of a research problem through the form of an hypothesis has several advantages. One, it forces the researcher to state the situation under investigation in precise, scientific language. Obviously, the more specific an hypothesis is, the more easily it can be tested, understood, and replicated. If the hypothesis is stated specifically, then the investigator can avoid the confusion of a broad range of selective evidence and can be much more definite in the testing process.

The terms *general* and *specific* have meaning related to hypotheses. A general hypothesis may be so broad that it is difficult to test, and its usefulness may be questioned, whereas a very specific hypothesis may be easy to test or may be something that is already known, in which case the findings may not add to the store of knowledge. If we can test a specific hypothesis, then we might be able to go from a specific to a more general hypothesis; but it is very difficult to begin with and to test a very general hypothesis; but it is very difficult to begin with and to test a very general hypothesis because we become overwhelmed with the large number of variables.

When we formulate an hypothesis, it is necessary that it be conceptually clear. The concept should be something that can be tangibly measured, and all observers should agree on the measurement. For example, let us take the concept *religious*. How can it be measured? We might measure the degree of "religiousness" by how often a person attends a religious service.

Conceptual clarity is the degree to which the concept can be empirically measured. Conceptual clarification is the process whereby we tear down the boundaries of abstraction and isolate the construct to its bare entity. In addition, clarification of the concept should meet the criterion that all observers recognize and agree on whether a condition is present or not. For example, let us take the word *healthy*. How can the word *healthy* be conceptually clarified so that it can be determined if it is present or not? We might start by deciding that persons are healthy if their blood pressure is in the normal range. The range must be predetermined, and then each subject's blood pressure is taken and recorded.

Preferably, an hypothesis should be related to a theory. Often beginning researchers simply find a topic that they are interested in researching and begin to study it without the benefit of a related theory. If an hypothesis is based on previous findings, other hypotheses, laws, models, or theories, then the chance that the findings will be relevant and will provide valuable information is greatly increased.

Hypotheses should be formulated with available techniques in mind. In considering what testing methods to use, investigators should look at their own capabilities as a part of the process of developing an hypothesis.

It is important that the researcher be acquainted with the various research tools that have been developed for use in their discipline and in related fields. If there are no adequate instruments, the researcher may need to develop a new tool for the investigation.

We have cited the necessity for specificity and clarity in wording and in the concepts in the statement of an hypothesis. The necessity for a clear theoretical framework—at least one that the investigator knows—has been pointed out, as well as the necessity for an hypothesis that lends itself to available tools of measurement. In such a process, there are at least two major difficulties. The researcher may lack the ability to utilize the theoretical framework in logical fashion or may have difficulty in remaining objective throughout the research process.

Beginning researchers tend to spend too much time developing an hypothesis and not enough time testing it. They fail to do an adequate library search, lack operational definitions, and in general use loose methodology. The results of a poorly tested hypothesis are not trustworthy and do not contribute to the field of knowledge.

SOURCES OF HYPOTHESES

Although an hypothesis may be based on a hunch that the researcher is interested in studying, a good hypothesis is usually based on evidence.

1. An hypothesis can often be based on astute observation of some phenomenon within the environment, on literature, or on other empirical data.

2. An hypothesis can be a restatement of an hypothesis that has been tested previously and has produced new information that seems to suggest the new hypothesis. In scientific research the hypothesis should be based on other additional facts that have been gathered through research. The sequence, by way of review, is that usually facts or propositions or both are combined to formulate hypotheses.

3. Experience is a source for an hypothesis. Leonardo da Vinci believed that all true knowledge begins with experience. Some of his beliefs are as follows:

> All our knowledge has its origin in our perceptions.
> Wisdom is the daughter of experience.
> Good judgment is born of clear understanding, and a clear understanding comes of reasons derived from sound rules, and sound rules are the issue of sound experience—the common mother of all the sciences and arts.
> Experience never errs; it is only your judgments that err by promising themselves effects such as are not caused by your experiments.[1]

4. Scientific research demands that we have a logical and testable hypothesis. However, we can obtain some relevant and profitable findings by *chance*. But chance is also a matter of hard work because the more effort put forth, the more chances there are that the researcher will come up with serendipity.

5. We cannot express too strongly the importance of a penetrating critical analysis of the problem at hand. One cannot seize the first clever idea or the first suggestion as a research problem, but many hours of contemplation, talking, and discussion are involved in developing hypotheses. A good researcher obviously discusses with other researchers how to go about the research project, and what findings to expect. Perhaps an associate with a different frame of reference will be able to add new insight into the problem. Every discipline or field is a specialty, and professionals from that field are specialists in their own area. For example, in research in nursing, the nurse has some experiences that no other person has. There are certain topics that the nurse should be researching because no one has more understanding of nursing than a nurse. The effectiveness of nursing intervention in specific cases is begging for research.

The culture within which nursing develops or the milieu within which it operates provides opportunities for investigation. Cross-cultural variations provide numerous experiences that suggest hypotheses.

6. Analogies, too, furnish hypotheses. Mauksch states that a hospital is very much like a garage. How patients are treated in hospitals is similar to some of the treatment that

[1] Blake, Ralph M., Ducasse, Curt J., and Madden, Edward H.: Natural science in the Renaissance. In Madden, Edward H., editor: Theories of scientific method: the Renaissance through the nineteenth century, Seattle, 1960, University of Washington Press, p. 13.

is given to automobiles.[2] Such an analogy would provide a useful way of looking at nursing or at hospitals.

7. Individual personal experiences may be sources of hypotheses. The investigator may have a unique background that affords an opportunity to conceive of an unusual research project.

8. The replication of a previous study is always a useful activity. This means that a complete detailed account of the initial research must be available to repeat the entire research project.

Empirical irregularities may not be any more important than regularities, but they at least are less frequent, and their existence provides an intriguing source for an hypothesis. They may be detected by persons who are knowledgeable in the field or by complete strangers to the area of study. For example, the anthropologist is aware of different cultural patterns. In addition, there are some aspects of a culture that cannot be understood until one has talked with its members. Some anthropologists believe that it is necessary to live in a culture for years before the culture is understood.

9. Mathematical implications, that is, adding, subtracting, and combining the theories and hypotheses of other studies, provide interesting stimuli for hypothesis building. While reading the literature, the researcher may notice two or more interesting ideas that could be combined in some way to provide a new hypothesis.

TYPES OF HYPOTHESES

Hypotheses may be classified in many ways. Goode and Hatt, for example, group them into three broad categories based on their levels of abstraction. These are basically common-sensical propositions, complex ideal types, and analytic variables.[3]

The first, dealing with empirical uniformities, may be the study of a problem using common-sensical terms. Quite often, uniformities or stereotypes are bases for investigation. For example, we have the idea that red-haired people have hot tempers. This stereotype provides something that we could research. As another example, we might ask, "What makes the nurse different from other people?" Having taught in schools of nursing and having observed nurses for years, we suspect that somehow nurses tend to be different from other professionals.

This ideal-type hypothesis is a useful comparative approach to research that brings together a series of characteristics typical of some phenomena. An ideal type is perceived as perfection. It is so ideal that quite probably it does not exist out in the real world, but at least it provides a yardstick against which we can measure. We may illustrate by using the concept of a nurse. The ideal-type nurse may be one who is very good in physiology, is concerned with people, excels in interpersonal relationships, is more concerned with

---

[2]Mauksch, Hans O.: It defies all logic—but a hospital does function. In Skipper, James K., Jr., and Leonard, Robert C., editors: Social interaction and patient care, Philadelphia, 1965, J.B. Lippincott Co., pp. 245–251.
[3]Goode, William J., and Hatt, Paul K.: Methods in social research, New York, 1952, McGraw-Hill, Inc., pp. 59–63.

work than with money, and so on. However, this nurse may not exist in society. Rather, a nurse may have one or more of these characteristics but not all of them. We can, however, use the ideal-type concept as a standard against which to measure actuality.

It has already been stated that an hypothesis is concerned with the relationship between two variables. Hypothesizing, which is aimed at explaining a relationship between two variables, is more abstract and sophisticated than simply stating that a relationship exists; it explains why the relationship exists.

Analytic variables offer a deeper level of analysis and consider the relationship of change between one property and another. Hypotheses based on analytic variables are concerned with the quality, degree, or strength of two or more variables on another single variable.

Abdellah and Levine suggest a classification based on relationships in which there are three types of hypotheses: causal, associative, and artificial.[4] In the first type, testing and establishing causal relationships represent a desirable goal of scientific research. If we know the cause, then we can predict the effect. Very few studies ever establish a causal relationship, especially in the social sciences.

Often there is not one cause, but many causes for behavior. In contrast, in the physical and natural sciences where strict experimental control is maintained, it is often possible to establish a causal relationship.

An associative relationship is the continual occurrence of the same variables together. The designation of independent or dependent variable may be difficult to establish. Whereas an associational relationship is potentially useful as a predictive device, it is weak as a diagnostic device. We might quite easily assign to the associational relationship the independent variable or the causal agent, whereas it may be only one of many. A may never cause B; A in relationship with C may cause B; or A in relationship with C and D may cause B. There are any number of possibilities in this type of relationship.

The study of child abuse is a case in point. There is no single factor that causes parents to abuse children. However, parents who were abused as children often abuse their own children. Unemployed parents, unwanted children, and low socioeconomic status are all variables associated with child abuse. Obviously, some children are never abused, even when all these variables are present; whereas other children are abused when none of the variables are present.

The third type, an artificial relationship, is one that is separated by time, distance, or other confounding factors. A crop failure in India may cause a rise or fall in the stock market in the United States. The relationship between the petrel found in Bermuda and DDT poisoning is another example of an artificial relationship. Benchley reported that only 24 breeding pairs of petrels remain in the Bermuda Islands because of DDT residues which were the result of the contamination accumulated in the ocean food chain. The birds had caught fish that had been exposed to DDT even though DDT is not used in Bermuda.[5]

[4]Abdellah, Faye G., and Levine, Eugene: Better patient care through nursing research, ed. 2, New York, 1979, Macmillan, Inc., pp. 140–143.
[5]Benchley, Peter: Bermuda: balmy, British, and beautiful, National Geographic Magazine 140(1):109, July 1971.

Null Hypothesis

The null form of an hypothesis is used when statistical tests are applied to the data. Therefore, if the research design does not include the use of statistics, the null form of hypothesis is not necessary.

Authors and researchers agree on the description of a null hypothesis. However, there is little or no agreement on the proper term for what is sometimes called the theoretical, scientific, literary, or positive form of an hypothesis. The scientific form states the hypothesis in either the anticipated direction of the research findings or the expected relationship between the variables, whereas the null hypothesis states that there is no difference between two variables. We will then "reject" or "fail to reject" the null hypothesis according to our findings.

To make the scientific form of an hypothesis testable, it must be stated in operational language. After the data have been tabulated, they are ready for statistical testing, using the null form of the hypothesis. The literary form seems easier to discuss, especially when we are describing the findings of the study, but the null form is easier to test statistically.

When a null hypothesis is tested and the researcher finds that there is no difference between variables, this does not necessarily mean that there is no relationship. The relationship may exist, but the test of the hypothesis may not have been adequate, there may not have been enough data, or the wrong approach may have been used.

When the hypothesis is actually tested, there seems to be a psychological advantage in stating it in the null or no-relationship format, since objectivity appears to pervade. This does not mean, however, that objectivity will be assured throughout the investigation. It is still necessary for the researcher to be aware of the need for an unbiased attitude in gathering data and interpreting the findings.

Many statistical tests require the use of the null form of the hypothesis. Such tests are designed to measure whether the differences between the variables are "real" differences or the results of sampling error. A null hypothesis states that there is no significant difference between two or more variables. The level of significance for rejection or acceptance of the null hypothesis is arbitrarily determined beforehand by the researcher. Two examples are given to illustrate the operational and null form of hypotheses.

Hypothesis 1

Scientific/literary form
    Nurses graduated from School A in 1981 will indicate a more positive attitude toward continuing their formal education than those graduated from School B.
Operational form
    Nurses graduated from School A in 1981 will indicate a more positive attitude toward continuing their formal education as measured by the _____ test than those graduated from School B.
Null form
    There will be no difference bewteen the nurses graduated in 1981 from School A and School B in their attitude toward continuing their formal education as measured by the _____ test.

Hypothesis 2

Scientific/literary form
    Mothers who bring their children to Clinic A have made fewer prenatal visits than those who bring their children to Clinic B.

Operational form
> Mothers who bring their children to Clinic A have made fewer prenatal visits for health care than those who bring them to Clinic B.

Null form
> There will be no difference in the number of prenatal visits made for health care between mothers who bring their children to Clinic A and those who use Clinic B.

Even though the null hypothesis is commonly associated with the statistical testing procedure, there may be instances when the null form is the anticipated direction of the findings. In this case the results of two treatments or two procedures are expected to be similar. Different treatments (causes) are thought to render the same result. The null form is stated similarly to the scientific form.

The researcher might want to test the hypothesis that there is no difference in the rate of recovery when the client uses a certain home remedy costing $1 and a prescription drug that costs $5. The hypothesis stated in the null form is, "There is no difference in the rate of recovery from malady A using home remedy X or prescription medication Y." The null form happens to be in the direction anticipated in this case.

Quite often, the null hypothesis is used as the basis for the application of a statistical analysis instead of the working hypothesis. As stated earlier, the null version suggests value-free objectivity. However, there is no reason why the working hypothesis cannot be accepted or rejected; at least the wording is less confusing.

When testing an hypothesis statistically, the appropriate formula is selected based on sample size, methodology, and arrangement of data. The hypothesis is then either accepted or rejected based on findings. If a new nursing intervention reduces hospital stay by one day in 60 percent of the cases, the researcher might decide that it is successful and the working hypothesis would be accepted (the null hypothesis of no difference is rejected).

A statistical formula would give a mathematical statement a level of significance such as .05 or .01. This means that only 5 times out of 100 or 1 time out of 100, respectively, such results could have occurred by chance. Further application of statistics will be discussed in Chapter 23.

There are two possibilities in tests of significance: rejecting or accepting the null hypothesis. Often, the authors of research literature state that they failed to reject the null hypothesis of no difference. This indicates that the working hypothesis is accepted. Henkel believes that scientific knowledge is obtained not by finding hypotheses true, but by not being able to ascertain that they are false. Scientific knowledge thus becomes hypotheses and theories which have little chance of being rejected.[6]

Hypotheses in the Social and Physical Sciences

In the physical and biological sciences it is evident that there has been an accumulation of theoretical knowledge. Though the social sciences have not developed an accumulation of knowledge on the same scale, they have uncovered a wide assortment of characteristics that relate to social behavior and that demonstrate a relative constancy of predictable actions. For example, anthropologists have found that males usually do the hunting in most societies. We now know from psychological testing that individual differences are

[6]Henkel, R.E.: Tests of significance. In Uslaner, E.M., editor, Series: quantitative applications in the social sciences, No. 07-004, Beverly Hills, 1976, SAGE Publications, Inc., p. 36.

always greater than racial differences, and that religious beliefs often cause people to react similarly, regardless of the kind of religion they practice. For example, most religions have rules or laws concerning moral behavior such as telling the truth.

Both the physical and social sciences rely on the comparative method of observing, describing, and measuring the relationship between two or more variables in a given situation. The physicist has learned that as the volume of a gas increases, its temperature rises, and that objects move in relationship to the amount of friction present. The biologist has discovered that DNA is the key to heredity.

As we compare the physical sciences with the social sciences, we can note a striking difference. In the physical sciences, if we change one variable and leave all other variables constant, we are able to predict the amount and direction of change. However, this is not true in social sciences. We find that there are extremes and always exceptions to the rule. For example, the statement "the more years of education, the higher the income" may be true in 50% to 80% of the cases. However, there will always be those people who have many years of education but a small income, and there will be people with less than a high school education who earn a great deal of money.

Scientists study, research, compare, and describe the characteristics of their subjects. These characteristics include the quality and quantity of individual units, the quality and quantity of categories, and the cultural and environmental characteristics relating to both units and categories. To illustrate this on the unit level, we could consider the individual differences between two nurses as to their physical size, or their academic grades, or their ability to relate to patients. We could consider the category level by comparing nurses with physicians or with other professionals. Finally, we could compare American nurses with nurses or physicians from another culture.

Historically, those in the health professions were aided by the research done with the methods of the social sciences. Much of the interaction between patients and health professionals has been in personal relationships. The interaction that goes on between a nurse and a patient/client is definitely in the social science arena.

In conclusion, the development of the hypothesis is an important step in the research process. After the broad problem and the purpose of the study is identified, the researcher states the hypothesis that was developed after an extensive library search. This literary statement usually requires restatement in operational terms so that the concepts can be measured and tested. Later, when statistics are applied to the data, the null form of the hypothesis is used. All of these forms are not necessarily reported to the reader of the research process.

RESEARCH WITHOUT HYPOTHESES

It is not always necessary to have an hypothesis to conduct scientific research. However, when there is a basis for prediction, hypotheses should be used, according to Krathwohl.[7] Often, exploratory and preliminary studies do not use an hypothesis. A researcher may

[7]Krathwohl, D.R.: How to prepare a research proposal, ed. 2, Syracuse, N.Y., 1977, Syracuse University Press, p. 27. Permission granted by author.

be interested in learning more about some phenomenon and thus may engage in a fact-finding investigation. It is conceivable that the researcher will initiate a scientific study for the purpose of gathering enough information to develop hypotheses. Perhaps the whole study is a survey to learn the answer to the questions in the mind of the researcher or the project's sponsor.

The following questions could utilize research to provide insight without requiring the development of an hypothesis.

Why do more nurses in group A continue their formal education than those in group B?

How can the quality of patient care be improved in building X?

Why does unit C seem to have more cases of infection than unit D, although they are similar services?

Why do more students fail Nursing 100 than Nursing 101?

Why do members of ethnic group A seem to have more headaches than members of ethnic group B?

These questions could be researched using any of the techniques of the scientific method. If the researcher has enough prior knowledge of the topic to suggest a solution or answer, then an hypothesis should be developed and tested. If the researcher lacks knowledge of the topic, then the steps of the scientific method should be followed, omitting hypothesis formulation. The investigator must clearly state the question to be answered, and conceptualization must be conducted as rigorously as when an hypothesis is to be tested.

According to Marx, there is little fundamental difference between testing an hypothesis and asking a question. A positive statement can easily be turned into a question, or a question can be turned into a positive statement through grammatical means alone.[8]

Hypotheses and the Research Report

The hypothesis is commonly discussed in the third section of a research report. This placement is customary but not mandatory. The hypothesis may have been the inspiration that caused the study to be conducted; however, in the development and conceptualization of the research design, which begins with formulating the problem and reviewing the literature, placing the hypothesis in this section seems the natural order. This section contains the reasoning behind the selection of a particular hypothesis. It also includes a discussion of the selection of additional hypotheses, if the study has more than one.

Hypotheses are often numbered, and it may be that there are major hypotheses and subhypotheses. The author, of necessity, indicates how the testing of the hypothesis answers the problem that was formulated earlier.

The third section also contains an analysis of the line of reasoning running from the formulation of the problem to the hypothesis and the implications of the results. We discussed the use of the null hypothesis versus the scientific hypothesis earlier in this chapter. The hypothesis should be stated in one of these two forms in the research report.

The third section may not be titled "Hypothesis" as such; instead, the researcher may decide to include the hypothesis under the title of "design of the study." For our purpose, the second section is only concerned with the hypothesis.

[8]Marx, Melvin H.: Theories in contemporary psychology, New York, 1963, Macmillan, Inc., p. 20.

SUMMARY

An hypothesis is a tentative answer or an educated guess that can serve to guide a research study. The testing of an hypothesis requires objectivity on the part of the researcher.

An hypothesis is composed of an independent variable (cause) and a dependent variable (effect). Since hypotheses are usually concerned with a comparison of two or more variables, it can often be found that even though two variables may occur at the same time, they may not be cause and effect.

The more specifically an hypothesis is stated, the more easily it can be tested. The more precise the wording, the easier it is to measure. Moral values, however, cannot be tested. The researcher should attempt to relate hypotheses to a tested theory.

Some sources of hypotheses are retesting, restatement of old hypotheses, personal experiences, keen observation and deep understanding of human behavior, and broad background reading.

In addition to the causal relationship, we identify the associative and artificial relationships. For the purpose of testing, an hypothesis may be stated in null form, meaning there is no difference (no relationship) between the two variables.

In the physical sciences causal relationships are easier to establish than in the social sciences where there are confounding variables.

It is not absolutely necessary to have an hypothesis to conduct a research study. If an hypothesis is not being tested, the researcher must clearly state the question that is to be answered. Conceptualization must be rigorous in either case.

DISCUSSION QUESTIONS

1 Is the hypothesis the foundation of the scientific method? Support your response.
2 How many times should an hypothesis be tested before it becomes a theory?
3 Is stating the hypothesis in the null form a biased view? Why or why not?
4 What is the possible value of research without an hypothesis?
5 What are some situations in which an hypothesis would not be needed?
6 When is it preferable to have a research question rather than an hypothesis?
7 When is it preferable to have an hypothesis rather than a research question?
8 What are some factors that should be known about a topic before an hypothesis is developed?
9 Give an illustration of an hypothesis in which the dependent and the independent variables could be interchanged.
10 Give an example in which only one variable could be the independent one.

CLASS ACTIVITIES

Track 1

1 Each student is to develop three hypotheses and then state them in the scientific, operational, and null forms.
2 The class is divided into small groups. An hypothesis is distributed to each group. Members determine the testability of the hypothesis and reword the hypothesis if it needs improvement.

Track II (Steps in Research Project; Work in Project Groups)

1 Each person is to write an hypothesis related to the research project and submit it to the instructor.
2 Exchange the hypotheses so that everyone can read what the others have written.
3 Each group is to select one of the hypotheses to test during the remainder of the course and submit it.
4 Each student conducting a project alone will submit an hypothesis for the selected research project.

SUGGESTED READINGS

Abdellah, F.G., and Levine, E.: Better patient care through nursing research, New York, 1979, Macmillan, Inc., pp. 132–149.

Asher, W.J.: Educational research and evaluation methods, Boston, 1976, Little, Brown & Co., pp. 44–56.

Barnard, K.: Formulating hypotheses, The American Journal of Maternal Child Nursing 8(4):263, July–August 1983.

Cooper, H.M.: The integrative research review, a systematic approach, Applied social research methods series, Vol. 2, Beverly Hills, 1984, SAGE Publications, Inc.

Diers, D.: Research in nursing practice, Philadelphia, 1979, J.B. Lippincott Co., pp. 40, 70–72, 150–151, 182–183.

Duncan, R.C., Knapp, R.G., and Miller, J.C., III: Introductory biostatistics for the health sciences, ed. 2, New York, 1983, John Wiley & Sons.

Gay, L.R.: Educational research: competencies for analysis and application, ed. 2, Columbus, 1981, Charles E. Merrill Publishing Company.

Goode, W.J., and Hatt, P.K.: Methods in social research, New York, 1952, McGraw-Hill, Inc., Chapter 6.

Henkel, R.E.: Tests of significance. In Uslaner, E.M., editor, Series: quantitative applications in the social sciences, no. 07-004, Beverly Hills, 1976, SAGE Publications, Inc.

Jacox, A.: Theory construction in nursing, Nurs. Res. 23(1):7, January–February 1974.

Notter, L.E.: Essentials of nursing research, ed. 2, New York, 1978, Springer Publishing Co., Inc., pp. 57–63.

Pavlovich, N.: Nursing research: a learning guide, St. Louis, 1978, The C.V. Mosby Co., Chapter 3.

Polit, D., and Hungler, B.: Nursing research: principles and methods, New York, 1978, J.B. Lippincott Co., Chapter 7.

Sweeney, M.A., and Olivieri, P.: An introduction to nursing research, Philadelphia, 1981, J.B. Lippincott Co.

Waltz, C. and Bausell, R.B.: Nursing research: design, statistics, and computer analysis, Philadelphia, 1981, F.A. Davis Company.

Wechsler, H., and Kibrick, A.: Explorations in nursing research, New York, 1979, Human Sciences Press, Inc.

Williamson, Y.M.: Research methodology and its application to nursing, New York, 1981, John Wiley & Sons.

Wooldridge, P.J., and others: Methods of clinical experimentation to improve patient care, St. Louis, 1978, The C.V. Mosby Co., pp. 110–112, 169–171.

CHAPTER 11

RELATIONSHIP BETWEEN VARIABLES

DESCRIPTION OF VARIABLES

The relationships between variables is the major theme of research. A variable is anything that can change or anything that is liable to vary. There are several types of variables defined and illustrated in this chapter. The *independent variable* is the variable that stands alone and is not dependent on any other. Grammatically, the independent variable is stated first in an hypothesis, followed by the dependent variable.

The *dependent variable*, of course, comes second in the chain. It is the effect of the action of the independent variable and cannot exist by itself. In experimental research it may be referred to as the predicted or criterion variable.

When studying the relationship between two variables, the researcher sometimes manipulates the independent variable to ascertain if it is the cause of the phenomenon. He/she wonders what will happen to the dependent variable when the independent variable is controlled. The assumption is that the dependent variable will not vary unless the independent variable changes. When working with human subjects, the researcher rarely manipulates the independent variable. It is always possible to get a change in the dependent variable through experimentation.

In the physical world, if there is a rainstorm, the height of the water in a river will rise. The amount of water in the river has no effect on how much it will rain. So, the amount of rain affects the height of the water in the river, but the height of the water in the river does not determine the amount of rain that falls. In this case, the rain is the independent variable, and the height of the water in the river is the dependent variable.

In a nursing situation, if we formulated the hypothesis that the more varied the nurses' tasks, the greater the job satisfaction, then the independent variable is task variety, and the dependent variable is job satisfaction. The researcher could design the study so that the number of tasks could be controlled by grouping them into categories of from one to five tasks. The sample could include nurses who performed from one to five different functions. Then, by means of a questionnaire or an interview, job satisfaction could be ascertained.

An uncontrolled variable that greatly influences the results of a study is called an *extraneous variable*. Extraneous variables are those that lie outside the interest, or, perhaps, the control of the researcher. There are usually a great number of these variables present, and they can often play an important role in affecting research results. Any of the following variables could be the independent or dependent variables for a future research investigation:

The older the nurse, the shorter a refresher course need be.

The younger the nurse, the longer a refresher course need be.

The higher the GPA, the shorter a refresher course need be.

Extraneous variables have often caused invalid research conclusions.

A group of nursing leaders in Nairobi, Kenya, studying research methodology hypothesized that hospital readmission of male tuberculosis patients is caused by the patients' lack of education about their disease. In this case, the dependent variable is readmission, the independent variable is health education. There were numerous variables in the study: age, religion, nationality, the number of times the patients were readmitted, the patients' knowledge or lack of knowledge about tuberculosis on admission to the hospital, and the patients' reports of their symptoms. These variables are considered extraneous because they cannot be controlled by the researcher. Other variables such as academic education and socioeconomic status also could affect the study, but a lack of time prevented their inclusion.

How the researcher approaches a particular problem, the variables that are considered cause and effect, the inclusion or exclusion of other variables, and the relationship between the variables can greatly influence the findings of research (Fig. 11-1).

Another type of variable is the *intervening variable*. This variable comes between the dependent and independent variables. Unfortunately, it cannot be measured with our present research tools, and it cannot be controlled. It is the researcher's responsibility to minimize the number of intervening variables in the design of the study. Such factors as stress, anxiety, and motivation may influence the research findings to a great extent unless the researcher makes an effort to reduce their intensity (Fig. 11-2).

Suppose we were to investigate the relationship between the number of hours a nursing student studied for a test and the student's grade. This investigation does not take into account intervening variables beyond the student's innate ability. For example, the intervening variable of the student's emotional condition at the time of the test is not considered. The hours of study could be controlled because they are an independent variable (cause). The effect is the dependent variable, which in this case is the grade he/she received on the examination. The amount of time spent on study is not necessarily in direct proportion to grades because intelligence, powers of concentration, and general health can all affect the grade. Even if two individuals study the same number of hours, these variables could account for the differences in their examination grade.

Another type of variable is the *organismic variable*. Organismic variables are those that cannot be changed through manipulations. They include such characteristics of the study groups as age, sex, and race. It is customary to report the predetermined organismic variables as background for the reader's understanding. These variables tend to be grouped together, not only for the convenience of the reader, but also for the convenience of the researcher when compiling and analyzing the data and later writing the report of the findings (Fig. 11-3).

Confounding variables are those variables that interfere with the study design and the data-gathering process by influencing the subjects or the dependent variable. They are

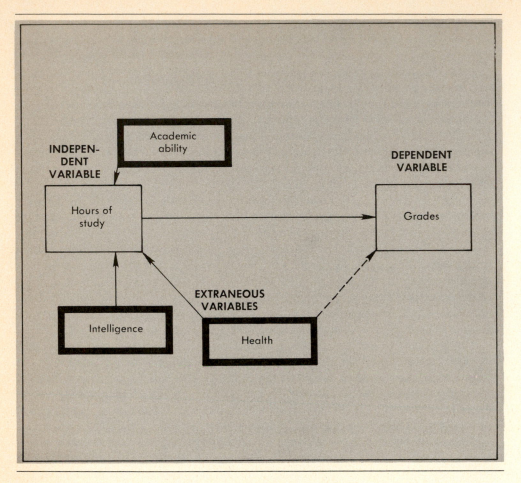

FIGURE 11-1   Extraneous variables.

sometimes referred to as interfering variables or as a type of extraneous variable.[1,2] A great number of variables are always present that can influence the outcome of a study and the confounding variable is one of them. It may influence the dependent variable as much as or more than the one under study. Since it acts in some way to influence both the dependent and independent variables, it is called the confounding variable (Fig. 11-4)

Nurses sometimes comment that one patient responds more favorably to nursing care than others do. Two individuals with the same diagnosis (independent variable), the same age and sex, and the same prognosis recover at different rates. One or more confounding variables may determine the length of institutional care. Some of the confounding variables that may be responsible are home situation, attitude toward recovery, financial resources, and relationships with members of the immediate family.

[1]Simon, Julian L.: Basic research methods in social science, New York, 1969, Random House, Inc., pp. 44–45.
[2]Wandelt, Mabel A.: Guide for the beginning researcher, New York, 1970, Appleton-Century-Crofts, pp. 105–106.

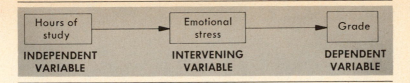

FIGURE 11-2   Placement and relationship of the intervening variable.

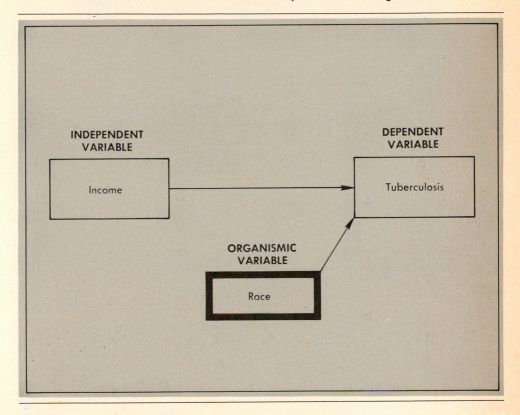

FIGURE 11-3   Organismic variable.

Another type of variable is the *antecedent variable*. This variable occurs earlier than the independent variable and bears a relationship both to it and to the dependent variable (Fig. 11-5).

Two patients, recovering at different rates although given the same health care, may demonstrate the effect of an antecedent variable. Poor general health, predisposition to illness, and living by guidelines of superstition and fads are a few of the possible antecedent variables that the researcher may want to study.

Polit and Hungler suggest six ways to control extraneous variables, but they emphasize the importance of randomization as the best control over unknown variables.[3]

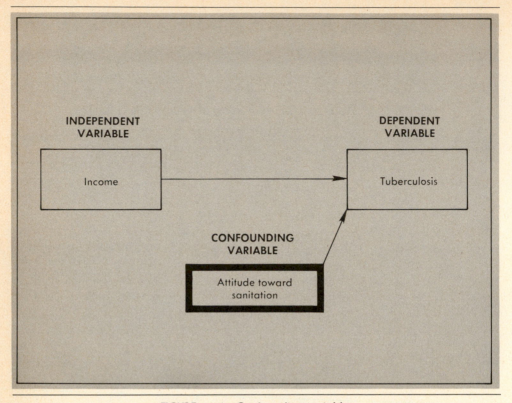

INDEPENDENT
VARIABLE

Income

DEPENDENT
VARIABLE

Tuberculosis

CONFOUNDING
VARIABLE

Attitude toward
sanitation

FIGURE 11-4   Confounding variable.

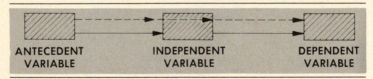

ANTECEDENT
VARIABLE

INDEPENDENT
VARIABLE

DEPENDENT
VARIABLE

FIGURE 11-5   Placement and relationship of the antecedent variable.

IMPORTANCE OF TESTING RELATIONSHIPS

Why is it important to test the relationship between two variables? Suppose we are testing the hypothesis that the more education nurses have, the more likely they are to move away from bedside nursing. Obviously, we are concerned with testing the relationship between education and bedside nursing. We are interested in obtaining data to see if, in fact, the more education nurses have, the less likely they are to take care of patients at the bedside. We are interested in only two variables; however, at the same time we must think about the possibility that there may be other variables at work that make a difference. Yes, there are other influencing variables, and these include such factors as the number of years of experience and marital status. Married nurses are likely to have interrupted career patterns and less dependence on themselves for a livelihood. As a result, unmarried nurses automatically have more years of opportunity for upward mobility. Eventually, they are in the position of being promoted to a leadership role. There is little relationship between marriage and attaining a leadership position, but other factors seem to confound the possibility, so that the likelihood is greater for the unmarried nurse to become a leader.

When the researcher considers relationships between variables, he/ she is interested in learning if a variable with one certain characteristic is associated with the variable being investigated or if an extraneous or intervening variable is confounding the situation. A familiar example is the identification of the cause of juvenile delinquency. We know that there is no single cause of juvenile delinquency. In one case it may be a broken home, whereas in another case it may be the child's association with other delinquents. In yet another case, the reason may be that the young person is a school dropout. At other times, even though children have experienced all of these conditions, they do not become delinquent. Looking at the problem in reverse, we know cases in which children have faced none of these circumstances, and yet they have become delinquent.

When examining the relationship between an independent variable and a dependent variable, researchers are saying that the independent variable causes the dependent variables; but is the cause always the one we think it is? One example is the relationship of sex to the number of accidents (driving ability of men and women).

There is a great deal of discussion about whether women are better drivers than men. Simply making a comparison between the number of accidents men and women have is not enough. If we find some data showing that women have fewer accidents than men, we still have to ask, "What are the number of miles that men and women have driven?" We must compare the percentage of accidents per thousand miles for women and for men, but even this is not enough. We have to compare the time of day that women drive with the time of day that men drive and find out the time of day when most accidents occur. Are there more accidents on freeways or side streets? Who takes more hours of driver's education prior to driving? What percentage of accidents are related to drinking? Also, perhaps women drive more slowly and a little more cautiously. So can we say that women are better drivers, according to our definition of "better?"

The percentage of men and women in each of the variables would contribute to an understanding of driving accidents. A study of driving habits would be a relevant research topic for nurses employed in an emergency room.

This discussion may bring up another question—how do researchers learn all the factors that may affect the results? They really do not know all the influencing factors, which is one of the reasons for the difficulty in arriving at correct conclusions in research dealing with human behavior.

An interesting relationship between variables was used in a program by Blue Cross-Blue Shield of Greater New York. The aim of the project was to reduce surgery by encouraging patients to get second opinions before having an operation. Instead of reducing the number of surgical procedures, second medical opinions reinforced the first physician's advice, and patients were having more operations. From a methodological perspective, Blue Cross-Blue Shield thought that the effect (number of surgical procedures) would be reduced by changing the independent variable (number of opinions), but in reality it increased the effect.[4]

[4]Trends and issues. Blue Cross survey: second opinions increase surgery and hospital costs, Nurs. Health Care **2**(2):62, February 1981.

Cause-Effect Relationships

Scientific research is the study of the relationship between two variables with the primary goal of establishing cause-effect relationships. Obviously, exploratory research can have the aim of investigating a question without looking for cause-effect relationships, but ultimately the researcher will want to know how one or more variables affect each other. Cause-effect relationships come into focus especially at the time of hypothesis development and data analysis.

PURPOSE

Why is it important to know the cause-effect relationship? If we know that specific activities or variables cause a certain effect, then it is possible for us to *predict* and *control*. For example, if we find that medication X can prevent a known disease, then the action can be predicted and the disease may be eradication or minimized. Many communicable diseases are now controlled because of our knowledge of the cause-effect relationship between the disease and its cure or treatment.

Researchers have been studying the relationship between smoking and lung cancer for many years. The results of investigation are so conclusive that smoking, especially cigarette smoking, is increasingly discouraged.

Sometimes we find a relationship so amazing that it is difficult to accept the findings. An example is the story if Ignatz Semmelweis and the rejection of the relationship between handwashing and puerperal fever by his colleagues. Semmelweis decided that there was a relationship between washing the hands before examining each new mother and whether or not a patient contracted puerperal fever. Such a relationship was not accepted by the other medical doctors of his day. They refused to wash their hands; it was too much trouble. They probably felt that it was ridiculous to believe that a possible relationship existed between the two factors.

The stigma of Hansen's disease still carries a fear that affects 50 million lives in the world today. In spite of the scientific work and research of many dedicated men and women, people still shudder at the mention of the word *leprosy*, assigning it a degree of contagiousness unwarranted by scientific evidence.

The danger of alcohol abuse is borne out by numerous scientific studies, and yet an increasing number of people continue to lean on this expensive crutch.

Even in our modern world, we still like to believe in a little magic. What athlete has never worn lucky socks or a lucky t-shirt, taken a good luck charm, or gone through some ritual before the crucial game? They rationalize that it cannot do any harm.

In the world of baseball, the pitcher's skill is much more related to chance than is the outfielder's. The outfielder has a 99.7% chance of catching a fly ball in his area, but the pitcher must be content with considerably less success in his pitching. Therefore, it is usually the pitcher who relies on the good luck charms, not the outfielder.

Remember that the purpose of an hypothesis is to state a relationship between two variables. The quality of the hypothesis depends largely on the extent of the investigator's insight into the most likely link between the dependent and independent variables. The investigator is expected to test the most reasonable cause of the phenomenon under study, based on an understanding of clues from the latest research reports and current publications. Since cause-effect relationships are apparent only to the knowledgeable investigator, it is the researcher's responsibility to be up-to-date in his reading in order to develop a well-conceptualized research design.

Consider the hypothesis that the more education nurses have, the less likely they are to give bedside care to patients. We are saying that in the causal relationship the independent variable is the amount of education. We are hypothesizing that advanced education is the reason that nurses give less bedside care. Critics would quickly reply, "Not necessarily." They would point at exceptions and remind us that different types of education, marital status, and economic needs are factors not to be overlooked.

Individuals without a sophisticated research orientation frequently point to causality from a single event to another single event. In some situations one event may never cause another event. There could be a combination of circumstances involved. At the withdrawal of one or more supposed causal factors, the occurrence may still be observed. A multitude of factors, not simply the A factor, may cause B.

The cause-effect relationship comes into play when the study data are analyzed and the conclusions are formulated. By that time, we have investigated the supposed causative factor and its effects. As data are screened and compiled and as inferences are made, the continual question is, "To what extent are the data and the cause, or the data and the effect related?" The data are the result of an attempt to get at the causative factor by deductive or inductive reasoning. The degree to which the study findings and the conclusions are related is a measure of the accuracy of the cause-effect relationship.

Data may be relatively unbiased so that they are adequate for testing the hypothesis. However, if appropriate conclusions are not drawn, the value of the study is meaningless. All segments of the research process are like links in a chain. The study is no stronger than its weakest investigative process. Are the conclusions that we drew from the relationship factor, as well as from the data themselves, the same as those that we envisioned before the data were collected? In other words, is there a thread running through from the beginning of the research process to the identification of implications for further research and to the population in general?

NATURE OF THE CAUSE

Nature of the cause refers to those components that produce a result or an effect. It is an attempt to identify the mask or alias that is disguising the cause.

There are five general types of disguises under which the cause may be concealed.

First, are there determinants of the cause? Are there circumstances that lead to the cause? If so, what are they? Is it possible to separate situations into categories? If so, what are these categories? In the study of the cause of interrelationships and responses, researchers should investigate the motives of the subjects. They should scrutinize the subject's environment, as well as his/her heredity, when looking for a causal factor. They should explore in both breadth and depth one segment at a time but not necessarily all in one study. In an attempt to discover answers to questions, it is as important to rule out possible determinant factors as it is to hit on the true answer in the first investigation. It is only by eliminating extraneous factors that the cause can be accurately identified.

Suppose we are studying the cause of hyperactivity in children. Some of the determinants might be the degree of hyperactivity, age when the hyperactivity was first noticed, the subject's environment, heredity factors, diet, and stress factors.

Of course a single element in itself may not be a determinant, but a combination of elements, factors, or circumstances may serve as the cause of the phenomenon under investigation. For this reason, it is necessary to study two or more aspects at one time in different proportions, periods of time, or intensities. One attempt may not be sufficient to rule out the suspected cause. It is possible that some error may have occurred to produce the results in the research. Even positive results should be investigated further to give assurance that they will always occur in repetitive studies.

With so many possible combinations of factors, the researcher must select the most apparent as based on any other known investigations. In many types of research it is rather difficult to learn whether one variable causes another variable. In the classical experimental design, with its experimental and control group and before and after test, the introduction of a single variable in the experimental group should produce a difference between the before and after measure. This method is the most effective thus far in establishing a cause-effect relationship in research. The classical experimental design is discussed in Chapter 12.

A second question is, "What are the ideals, the values, the goals, and the philosophical and psychological predispositions of the subjects participating in the project?" If these factors are suspected of having an impact on the effect, either as single or multiple aspects of possible determinants, they should be selected for in-depth investigation.

Human subjects have an infinite number of personality characteristics and philosophical leanings. One person may be gentle, thrifty, kind, and would like to be a leader, whereas another individual may have the same set of characteristics but desires personal recognition rather than leadership. In our research, we might look at one set of characteristics, say leadership potential, as it relates to a limited number of variables. Even though we are looking at one characteristics, all the other characteristics and the philosophical and the psychological makeup of the individual have an effect on the single characteristic we are studying. For example, Miss A, who is overweight and unmarried, is given a medication for hypertension. Mrs. B is of medium weight and not getting along with her husband. She is taking the same medication for hypertension as Miss A. Investigators must realize that Miss A and Mrs. B are different types of individuals, even though they both respond positively to the same treatment. Any nursing research on Miss A and Mrs. B concerning their response to the medication must contend with their multivariate personality predispositions, realizing that they affect every other variable.

Many studied tend to be too broad in scope; therefore the acceptance or rejection of a single variable as a cause or an effect is virtually impossible.

Third, is there an antecedent or predeterminant that should be researched? If we investigated the general topic to the extent that we have identified the cause of a specific effect, then we may decide to go back one step and probe the possible precursors of the known cause. The value of such an undertaking is that we could simply and adequately explain the recognized cause if the antecedents were identified. In fact, research is not complete until the activating cause is identified. Knowledge of the antecedent variable could then lead to the possibility of artificially producing change. If it is found that variable Y causes condition Z only in the presence of certain inherited characteristics (antecedent variables), then the researcher is in a position to modify or eliminate condition Z. Nurses with their skills of observation are well prepared to identify possible antecedent variables.

A fourth area of investigation is the reason for the effect. For example, what is the reason for the patient or member of his family to be anxious? What is the reason for the arrested development of creativity in people? Knowing the causal factor provides an explanation for a phenomenon, but knowing the reason sheds new light on the relationship between cause and effect.

A British friend related the story of an event in his youth that propelled him into a successful career. As a student in elementary school, he was not highly motivated. One day his teacher, in disgust, pointed to a group of men shoveling dirt and exclaimed, "You will never amount to anything except to dig ditches like those men!" Our friend said that he set out to prove his teacher wrong. Many years later, after becoming a wealthy building and land developer, he returned to confront his former teacher. The successful businessman told his teacher that the comment had motivated him to become something other than a manual laborer.

Fifth, what was the person, event, or place that directly or indirectly activated an existing cause? What triggered the situation so that the observed phenomenon occurred? The potential for a cause-effect relationship always may be present, but the actual relationship may never occur unless some triggering factor takes place. A person may have all the attributes and characteristics needed for becoming a nurse but may never make a decision to enroll in a school of nursing until a tragic accident happens to a member of the family. The accident triggers a moment of decision, either to prepare to become a nurse or to stay out of the health-care field entirely. After identifying the cause of the phenomenon, the next challenge is to explore the situation or factor that set the cause in motion. This type of investigation approximates "playing detective"—perhaps the common term for all of research.

Each of the five aspects of the nature of the cause of a phenomenon has its own implications for a discipline. Two major problems for a beginning researcher are selecting a topic of manageable size and studying only one segment of the cause-effect relationship.

ATTRIBUTES OF THE CAUSE

The researcher observes certain attributes of a causal factor, as well as its nature. The question becomes, "What is the extent of the properties of the variable being investigated?" An attribute suspected of being the causal factor may not have been probed in depth or examined with other methodological approaches. Perhaps one investigator utilizes a questionnaire to gather data on a given topic, another researcher interviews subjects, and a third investigator uses a Q-sort in studying the same phenomenon. Results of these varied techniques should be compared to ascertain if they complement or contradict each other. The use of different research procedures may reveal additional properties of a variable.

Conceivably, replication studies can give new insight into the properties of the cause. The first time a study is conducted, the researcher reports any weaknesses in the design. When repeating the study, the researcher can avoid the cited weaknesses and follow the recommendations mentioned by the original investigator or the researcher can ignore them. A replication study can utilize the same population but use a different sample or choose a similar population and similar sample. The value of replication studies are that they may give greater insight into the properties of the cause.

What is said about the cause applies also to the effect. A cause may not always produce the same effect. Is the effect of music on patients in the women's medical unit the same as in the men's unit? Does music affect all patients within the unit similarly? Why or why not?

The nature of the research methodology is often determined by the purpose of the research. Cause-effect investigations require a different type of methodology than descriptive studies.

Casual comparative research (ex post facto) attempts to determine the cause of or reasons for differences. An investigator might be interested in knowing why more nurses specialize in oncology than in pediatrics. It is important to note that the difference between the number of nurses entering oncology is greater than those entering pediatric nursing. Since it is a known fact that a difference exists, the next question is why. Descriptive research could have previously found that differences exist. Causal comparative research can now be utilized to determine why the differences exist. Typically, causal comparative research uses two or more groups and one independent variable.

Experimental research studies the relationship between two variables in an attempt to establish the cause of the independent variable. For example, the researcher asks, "Will nursing intervention Plan A reduce patient anxiety?" and decides to experiment with matched groups. The experimental group receives intervention Plan A whereas the control group receives the usual treatment. Results are compared to find the differences in order to establish a cause-effect relationship.

Descriptive research is usually not aimed at finding cause-effect relationships, but is useful to map out the territory, define the limits, and describe a phenomena or situation. Surveys tend to be descriptive studies. For example, a new health promotion program for the community would require a feasibility study (descriptive) to determine if such a service is needed. Descriptive studies propose to explore and define, not to establish relationships between variables. Chapter 23 discusses rank-order correlation. It explains a statistical technique for finding a correlation coefficient which is significant at some level. Correlations are often expressed by plotting two variables on a scatter diagram (see Fig. 23-20).

QUALITIES OF THE CAUSE

The answer to a question or problem might be found in single factor if the answer provides the identification of the condition that is both essential and adequate for an event to take place. An *essential condition* is a state that must occur if the cause is to occur. If A is the condition that must always occur for B to occur, then B will never occur unless we have condition A. Let us return to our hypothesis concerning nurses and education. If an advanced education was a necessary condition for nurses to withdraw

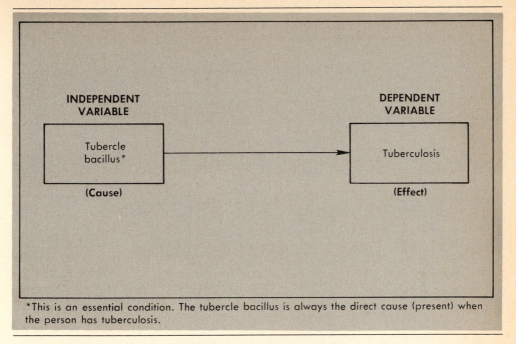

FIGURE 11-6   Essential condition.

from taking care of patients at the bedside, then highly educated nurses would withdraw from bedside nursing every time. But since this is not true, then education is only one of the variables—not an essential one (Fig. 11-6).

An *adequate condition* is one that usually follows the cause. As we can see here, the essential condition is much more important; it is imperative. An adequate condition permits something to happen; but an essential condition must be present for the effect to occur. Essential condition A must be present to cause B. In an adequate condition, A may cause B. We may illustrate this point by stating the hypothesis that the more education nurses have, the less likely they are to take care of patients. This may be an adequate condition, but not an essential condition (Fig.11-7).

OTHER RELATIONSHIPS

Contributory, contingent, and alternative conditions also relate to cause-effect relationships. In a *contributory condition*, A may contribute to causing B, but there may be other factors that also cause B. The possibility that A causes B may be a likely or *contingent* factor. An *alternative condition* means that in some cases A may be the condition that causes B, and in other cases A may not cause B.

We illustrate these statements with an example. In a contributory condition, A (smoking) may cause B (lung cancer), but other factors also may cause lung cancer.

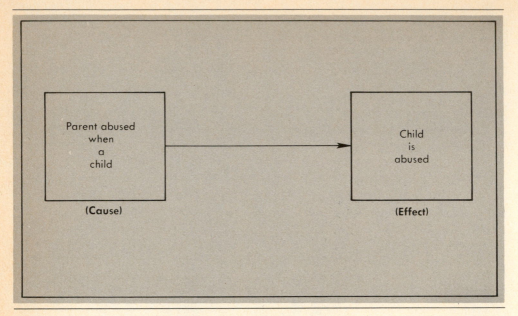

FIGURE 11-7   Adequate condition.

The possibility that smoking is the causative agent may be a likely or contingent factor. An alternative condition means that in some cases smoking may be the condition that causes lung cancer, and in other cases smoking may not be the cause (Fig. 11-8 to 11-10).

In some instances two factors may always be present, although one is not the cause of the other. Such a case illustrates a corelationship between two factors. In other words, if A really does cause B, then A always happens at the same time as B. When such a situation is first researched, the investigator may not be certain that A causes B, but he/she recognizes the fact that there is a corelationship. The investigator is safe by saying that there is at least a corelationship between factors A and B, rather than a cause-effect relationship.

Ackoff suggests that there are three classifications for discussing causes. The first is a deterministic cause, one that is necessary and sufficient to produce a certain effect. A probabilistic cause is nondeterministic, that is, it is necessary but not sufficient for the effect. A correlation exists when there is a relationship between two variables but causality is not known to be involved.[5]

Let us consider another possible relationship. Suppose we give a newly developed paper-and-pencil test to a group of nurses and think our findings show that nurses have a certain type of personality. Now, we must ask several questions. Is it because they are nurses that they have this type of personality? Does nursing have something to do with the development of these characteristics? Or do individuals with a particular kind of

[5]Ackoff, Russell L., Gupta, Shiv K., and Minas, J. Sayer: Scientific method optimizing applied research decisions, New York, 1968, John Wiley & Sons, Inc., p. 16.

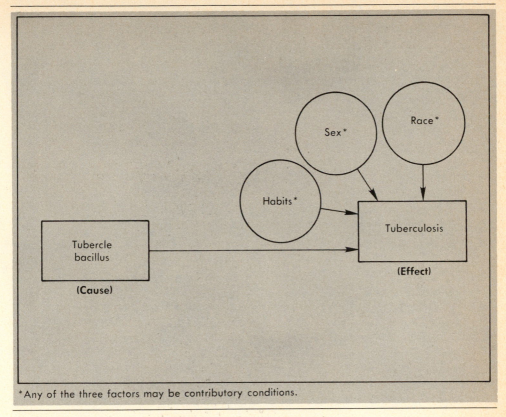

*Any of the three factors may be contributory conditions.

FIGURE 11-8 Contributory conditions.

personality go into nursing? Were they this type of person before they entered nursing? Such questions are timeless and difficult to answer.

In the topic of health, what is the relationship between health and exercise? Does exercise make people healthy or do healthy people exercise?

Still another question we can ask is, "Do skid rows develop because of the area of town, or does this area of town develop because there are men there who desire the types of service that a skid row has to offer?" In solving this puzzle, let us say that when we have variable A, we always find variable B. We recognize that A may cause B. Now suppose we have variables A and C and always find B present. A may still cause B, or A and C in combination may cause B. We might like to see, in this case, how much difference there is between A alone or A and C together in causing B. If we find that variable B is always present when we have variable C, then C may cause variable B. If we have yet another variable, D, and it is not present with B, then we can probably say that D does not cause B. It would be possible to go on at great length suggesting relationships. In conducting health research, beginners must learn to consider numerous possible cause-effect relationships.

After developing a table using letters or numbers, the researcher should substitute the names of variables, events, conditions, or factors pertinent to the study.

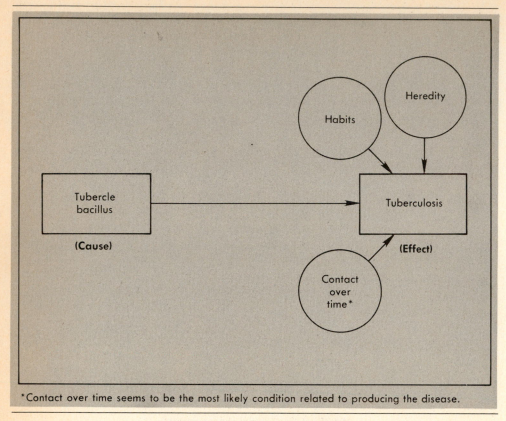

*Contact over time seems to be the most likely condition related to producing the disease.

FIGURE 11-9   Contingent condition.

A few of the possible interpretations of such a table are shown in Fig. 11-11.

A may cause B.

B may be the cause of A.

A and B may both be caused by another unknown variable.

A or B may be the cause of another variable, C or D.

C may cause a variable that is not yet identified.

C may cause the unknown variable simply because it happens to be an accidental occurrence.

Researchers may never be sure of the cause. However, they should try to experiment with as many possibilities as they can to see what kinds of relationships really exišt. If there is time for only one experiment, they cannot conclude positively that one variable causes the other. Researchers must expect to carry out a great deal of experimentation through manipulating and interchanging variables, as we have discussed in this chapter.

SUMMARY

Hypotheses are composed of *independent* and *dependent variables*. The independent variable is the cause and occurs before the dependent variable, which is the effect. The

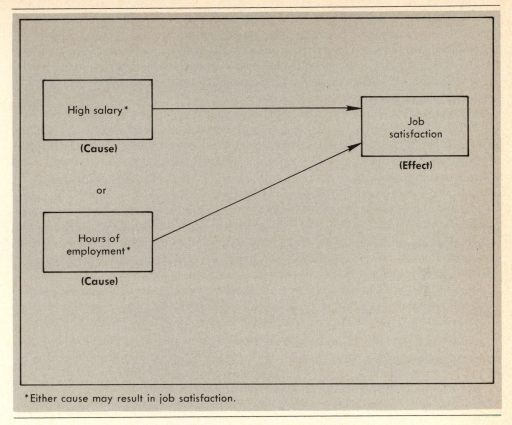

FIGURE 11-10   Alternative conditions.

VARIABLE PRESENT		VARIABLE PRESENT
A	(A may cause B)	B
A and C	(A or C may cause B)	B
C	(C may cause B)	B
D	(D does not cause B)	B not present

FIGURE 11-11   Cause-effect relationship.

researcher usually manipulates the independent variable in attempting to establish a cause-effect relationship.

Other variables are constantly influencing the relationship between the independent and dependent variables. *Extraneous variables*, such as educational level and scholastic ability, are beyond the control of the researcher. *Intervening variables* such as stress, anxiety, and motivation occur between the independent and dependent variable and influence the relationship between cause and effect. *Organismic variables*—for example, age, sex, and race—are attributes that cannot be changed by manipulation. *Confounding variables* include attitudes, relationships, and worries that interfere with the study design and influence the dependent variable. *Antecedent variables* occur earlier than the independent variable, and thus they also have an influence on the dependent variable. General health and predisposition to illness are antecedent variables that are related to recovery. Randomization is the best way for the researcher to counter the biasing of the research results by the variables.

Cause-effect relationships are the heart of human behavior. If the researcher knows the cause, then it is possible to predict and control the effect. Cause-effect relationships are studies through the hypothesis which states a relationship to be tested. In a scientific investigation involving human subjects, there is rarely one single causal factor. The researcher always must consider a multitude of factors. Scientists may start their investigations with either the causal factors or the effects.

The cause of a phenomenon may be either an *essential condition* or an *adequate condition*. An essential condition is necessary and must always occur to produce a given effect. An adequate condition may be sufficient to cause an effect in some cases, but it is not essential. *Contributory, contingent,* and *alternative conditions* are additional factors that should be considered in establishing cause and effect relationships.

Research consists of manipulating variables in an attempt to find consistent relationships in which A will always cause B. Descriptive research must eventually be replaced by experimental research.

DISCUSSION QUESTIONS

1 Why is science interested in establishing cause-effect relationships?
2 Why is multivariate analysis more likely to find cause-effect relationships than univariate analysis?
3 Comment on the statement: True scientific research attempts to establish cause-effect relationships.
4 Comment on the statement: There are always intervening variables in scientific research that affect the independent and dependent variables.
5 Give a hypothetical example of each of the following variables: extraneous, intervening, organismic, antecedent, and confounding.
6 Which of the five variables (item 5) is the most important? Support your response.
7 Give examples of variables based on the students in the class.
8 Discuss cause-effect relationships as a distinguishing feature between library research and scientific research.
9 When, if ever, is it possible to establish an effect with only one cause?
10 Why should the researcher be concerned with antecedent variables?
11 Of what value is the knowledge that variable B is the cause of variable A?
12 Could you learn as much about a phenomenon by studying several variables in great depth as in studying a single causative variable? Support your response.
13 Distinguish between a cause-effect research study and a research paper done in the humanities on the life of a famous person.
14 What is the relationship between an hypothesis and its variables?
15 Give an example of what you believe is a well-established cause-effect relationship.
16 If possible, cite an effect with a single cause.
17 Discuss the relationship between correlation and cause.
18 Why is an essential condition more important than an adequate condition in establishing a cause-effect relationship?

19 Give an example of two or more independent variables that seem to cause a particular dependent variable.

20 Suggest an instance in which there is no apparent single cause for a given effect.

CLASS ACTIVITIES

Track I

1 Copies of a research article are distributed to each group of three or four. After reading the article, each group is to identify as many variables as possible.

2 Each student in the class is to fill out a 10-item questionnaire. The questionnaires are collected and redistributed so that each person receives someone else's. As each item is read by the instructor, the students (representing a living histogram) stand along the sides of the wall in response to the items on the questionnaire that they have received. After completing this process, the students suggest various ways to cross-tabulate the data. For example, how many males have parents who attended college, or how many females have had regular dental checkups?

Track II (Steps in Research Project)

1 Each group identifies the variables in their hypothesis and then lists other types of variables in their hypothesis.

2 The groups who have not presented their hypotheses for class discussion and evaluation are to do so during the remainder of the period.

3 Students working alone are to write out the variables in their hypothesis.

SUGGESTED READINGS

Field, M.: Causal inferences in behavioral research, Adv. Nurs. Sci. **2**(1):81–93, October 1979.

Fleming, J.W., and Hayter, J.: Reading research reports critically, Nurs. Outlook **22**(3):173, March 1974.

Jacox, A.: Nursing research and the clinician, Nurs. Outlook **22**(6):384, June 1974.

Johnson, Barbara A., Johnson, Jean E., and Dumas, Rhetaugh, G.: Research in nursing practice: the problem of uncontrolled situational variables, Nurs. Res. **19**:337–342, July–August 1970.

Lagay, Bruce W.: Assessing bias: a comparison of two methods, Public Opinion Quarterly **33**(4):615–618, Winter 1969–1970.

Light, R.J.: Capitalizing on variation: how conflicting research findings can be helpful for policy, Educ. Res. **8**(9):7–11, October 1979.

Sedlacek, W.E.: Variables related to increases in medical school class size, DHEW Pub. No. HRA76-92, Washington, D.C., December 1975, Association of American Medical Colleges.

Wandelt, Mabel A.: Guide for the beginning researcher, New York, 1970, Appleton-Century-Crofts, p. 69.

CHAPTER 12

APPROACHES TO RESEARCH

Nursing research is conducted under various rubrics depending on the author. Classifications commonly used include the following: (1) descriptive and nondescriptive; (2) historical, descriptive, and experimental; and (3) survey, experimental, case study, and historical. We concur with the third type of classification. Survey research (often called descriptive research) is a study in which a body of data is collected, recorded, and analyzed. It is descriptive nonexperimental research used to answer a question, satisfy curiosity, solve a problem, or establish a cause-effect relationship. This type of investigation is defined by some authors as covering any research not involving experimentation. Other authors limit their definitions to a cross-sectional type of research in which a large number of cases is investigated (surveyed) in a descriptive study. Much nursing research falls under the category of survey.

Experimental research is an approach in which either laboratory or field subjects are used in tests or trials. Research subjects are usually selected randomly and placed into groups for the purpose of manipulation. The experimental group is exposed to a variable whereas the control group is unaltered. The results of tests made on the groups are compared. Experimentation is the most powerful research approach yet designed. It is often used in the physical sciences but is less popular than the survey approach in nursing research. Experimentation often involves ethical considerations when applied to human subjects.

The case study focuses on a single subject or group and can be thought of as an in-depth investigation. Depending on when the subject lived, this could be similar to a survey or historical study. The case study is discussed in Chapter 20 as it relates to qualitative research.

Increasing interest is being shown in historical research in nursing. Historical research is an integrative account of the relationship of people, places, and events in an historical perspective. An historical analysis can be used objectively to investigate almost any topic. Nurses are using historical research to study the lives and contributions of important nursing leaders. However, it must be emphasized that historical research can be extremely subjective. The *approach* to research is the umbrella that covers the basic procedure for conducting research. There are several methods for collecting data, and one or more of these can be used in each approach; questionnaires, interviews, observation, records, and experiments (Fig. 12-1).

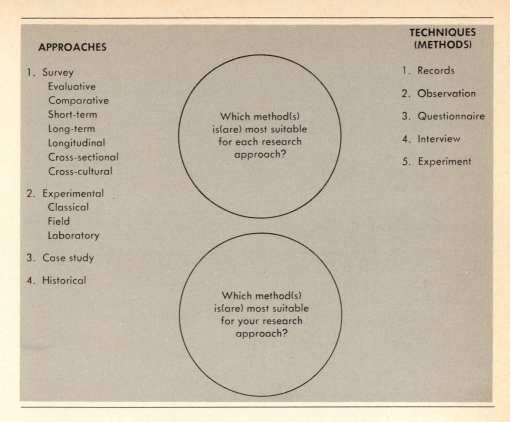

APPROACHES

1. Survey
   Evaluative
   Comparative
   Short-term
   Long-term
   Longitudinal
   Cross-sectional
   Cross-cultural

2. Experimental
   Classical
   Field
   Laboratory

3. Case study

4. Historical

TECHNIQUES (METHODS)

1. Records

2. Observation

3. Questionnaire

4. Interview

5. Experiment

Which method(s) is(are) most suitable for each research approach?

Which method(s) is(are) most suitable for your research approach?

FIGURE 12-1   Approach-method relationships.

SURVEY

Each discipline tends to employ one approach more often than another. Physical scientists emphasize experimental research, whereas social scientists use surveys to a great extent. In the past, descriptive surveys have tended to be the most frequent type of investigation. However, exploratory surveys and clinical experimentation are becoming popular.

An exploratory study might be undertaken to determine the health needs of a section of an urban community. Suppose a group of concerned citizens formed a task force to determine if a new hospital should be constructed in the area. The goal is not the establishment of the hospital per se, nor the establishment of a cause-effect relationship. The goal is to determine the necessity for a new health care facility.

Other surveys are descriptive. These studies are designed to describe specific phenomena or variables or to find relationships between variables. However, they are usually not designed to establish cause-effect relationships.

The survey approach is a nonexperimental study in which the researcher investigates a community or a group of people. This may be done by asking questions, by interviewing, by observing what people are doing, by telephone interviews, and by other techniques.

The survey approach can be an exploratory technique or a learning process for setting up a larger research study. Another name applied to the approach is formulative research. Surveys are not aimed at discovering the cause of a phenomenon but are intended to provide accurate quantitative descriptions. Surveys can sample all or part of a group of people or things. Techniques for obtaining survey data are usually questionnaires or interviews. When a subject cannot read or write because of a language barrier or a physical handicap, it is common practice for the researcher to read the questionnaire items to the respondent and then write in the respondent's answer.

A survey with definite implications was conducted in Canada. In a survey, among the elderly, Snider found that the subject's education and prior health service use accounted for more of their knowledge of health services than any other factors influencing health service knowledge.[1]

Survey research may be a preliminary study in which researchers explore a new situation, new organization, or new group. They formulate questions for a study and pursue an overall description of the situation. Investigators spend time in orientation, looking over the premises, talking with people, and asking questions.

To get a broad perspective, the researcher may need to talk to people at different levels in the hierarchy. In the case of nursing, this might include nursing personnel, hospital or agency administrators, maintenance personnel, allied health personnel, and so on throughout the institution.

Advantages

The survey approach has many advantages. It is a good source for hypotheses, and it can provide information leading to the use of different types of research methods. A survey can provide insight into a situation, suggest kinds of questions to ask, suggest the direction the research should take, and so on. A survey shows the researcher what facilities for research are available, what factors need to be controlled, what variables tend to be confounding, and what might be independent variables. It is useful for the discovery of new insights and methods as well as for pointing out the typical or average response. It may even be possible to find a cause, an effect, or an independent variable. A survey also provides some measure of the value of certain types of research methods for obtaining specific goals.

The survey approach provides data about the present. It tells what people are thinking, doing, anticipating, and planning at this time. It provides the researcher with an opportunity to use his/her creativity, since he/she is the one who determines the area to be surveyed and the method by which the facts will be extracted.

The survey approach has a high degree of representativeness. It usually employs the random sampling technique and, for that reason, is regarded as being representative in proportion to the sample size. In large surveys, the multistage random sampling technique may produce the most reliable data.

Another advantage of the survey approach is the ease with which the researcher can get respondents and information. The researcher can cover a broad range of phenomena in the real world. It is not an artificial setting that yields the possible or probable. Also, the

[1]Snider, E.L.: Factors influencing health service knowledge among the elderly, J. Health Soc. Behav. **21**(4):371–377, December 1980.

researcher can use data accumulated by one researcher to test one variable, and a second researcher can use the same data to provide information on an entirely different subject.

Ebbie Smith encourages the use of surveys to explain the increases and declines in church growth. The strengths of surveys he cites include the following:

1. *Objective.* They are based on quantified data, not opinions
2. *Specific.* They concentrate on a definite sample
3. *Point of focus.* They reveal *why* there has been a gain or loss
4. *Practical.* Surveys have a definite purpose, a known goal
5. *Accurate.* Because of the methodology, results are precise and correct erroneous views
6. *Factual.* They provide actual figures that can be used to suggest change and new goals
7. *Enlightening.* The survey is a way of gaining insight into the present. It probes attitudes, reveals problems, and uncovers strengths in the sample.[2]

Disadvantages

The survey approach offers little control over extraneous variables. Since the researcher is not necessarily working with a single independent variable (just as there may be more than one dependent variable), there is no control over extraneous factors.

Simon states that there are three disadvantages to causal and noncausal relationship research:

> First the crucial disadvantage of the survey method in causal analysis is the *lack of manipulation of the independent variables....* A second disadvantage of the survey is that *one cannot progressively investigate one aspect after another of the independent variable* to get closer to the "real" cause.... Third, *statistical devices are not always able to separate the effects of several independent variables* when there is multivariable causation, especially when two independent variables are themselves highly associated.[3]

One of the problems of using the survey approach is that the researcher may find that verbal responses are unreliable, because people often do not express their true reactions to the questions. Simon observes:

> H. Cantril found that only 86% of people who were interviewed twice at a three-week interval gave the same answer both times about whether or not they owned a car, and only 87% gave the same answer about how they voted in the 1940 Presidential election.[4]

Of course there are other disadvantages inherent in the survey approach. If the instrument lacks validity or reliability, this will be reflected in the survey results.

Types

In this section we discuss several types of survey approaches to research: evaluation, comparative, short-term, long-term, longitudinal, cross-sectional, and cross-cultural.

[2]Smith, Ebbie C.: A manual for church growth surveys, South Pasadena, Calif., 1976, William Carey Library, pp. 5–15. Used with permission of the William Carey Library Publishers, P.O. Box 128-C, Pasadena, Calif. 91104.
[3]Simon, Julian L.: Basic research methods in social science, New York, copyright 1969, Random House, Inc., pp. 243–244.
[4]*Ibid.*, pp. 245–246.

Surveys can include the total population or only a sample. The advantage of a total population survey is that it is inclusive, but the sample survey requires less time and money. When properly carried out, the sample survey may be just as accurate as the total population survey.

The uses of surveys vary. They may be selected for the purpose of discovering causal relationships in a specific area or providing precise quantitative descriptions of some part of the population. In a survey the researcher may observe people, things, groups, and activities, whereas in an experimental design researchers manipulate variables. Other survey techniques are on the borderline between observing and questioning. For instance, subjects may be asked to observe phenomena or to record their activities in a diary or a log.

Surveys are used to obtain demographic data, information about people's behavior, their intentions, future behavior, beliefs, attitudes, opinions, and interests. Surveys are frequently conducted by mail, telephone, or interview.

There are several types and forms of surveys, depending on the authors' semantics. Writers and researchers often interchange the names of similar types of studies.

In the social survey the investigator researches the attitudes and behaviors of different groups of people. Another type is the school survey used to gather data for and about schools and to assess educational achievement and education itself. There are many public opinion surveys or polls, such as Gallup, Roper, Harris, and Crossley. The market survey is aimed at finding out what kinds of people purchase which products, and how packaging, advertising, and displaying affect buying. In motivation research, subjects are asked why they purchased certain commodities. A complete discussion of these and other types of surveys is beyond the scope of this book.

Evaluation survey.   One type of survey approach is the evaluation survey in which the researcher looks back to see what has been accomplished and, with a critical eye, evaluates the results. The researcher using the evaluation survey is particularly interested in finding out the results of some procedure or method already in operation.

Suppose we have tried a new nursing care technique and are wondering if the new procedure has been satisfactory. The new method of patient care has been instituted, so an evaluation survey is conducted by questioning patients, staff, and physicians. From the evaluation survey a larger study could be launched.

The evaluation survey has a relatively small sample, at least initially. This survey approach is usually not a large undertaking, but it may point out directions for the researcher to take for a more extensive study.

The evaluation survey is done for one major purpose: to find if the method in operation meets the criteria stated in the purpose of the original project. The evaluation survey must be conducted with as little bias as possible; therefore, it should not be done by investigators who have a particular benefit to gain from the results.

Suppose two occupational nurses have established an intensive health education program for workers in a foundry. After a period of 1 year they wish to evaluate the effectiveness of their teaching program. Questionnaires and interviews could be used to discover the workers' opinions or to test their knowledge. Records could be studied to compare the amount and kinds of health care that were needed before and after the teaching program was implemented.

Comparative survey.   Another type of survey is the comparative method in which results from two different groups or techniques are compared. In modified terms, Fox says that the effective comparative study has three attributes: (1) it is based on an important professional problem so the resulting data will be significant to the profession; (2) all elements of professional significance are included in the survey; and (3) each element is representative within itself, to ensure complete sampling representativeness.[5]

Comparative data must be collected according to these principles. If we are testing a new patient teaching technique, we have to ask patient teachers and patients about the old technique and the new one. The same inquiries have to be made if we want to compare data.

A comparative study has the advantage of having a standard against which the researcher can measure the effectiveness of a new procedure or two new procedures. However, the study may be too small to really demonstrate differences.

During a seminar on nursing research held in Bogota, Colombia, in 1975, members of each group planned a research project in which the group's instrument would be used in their own areas of the country. Results from each area could then be compared. Not only could the hypothesis be tested in general, but regional differences could be noted.

Field survey.   The field survey is distinguished from other types of surveys by its being conducted in the real world as opposed to a captive controlled environment (laboratory). The researcher or research assistants contact the subjects through the usual sampling procedures. We have noted that in an evaluation survey, subjects are already participants, formally or informally, in the research process. In a comparative survey the focus of attention is on the results, the content, or the effects of a process on two or more groups. In contrast, in the field survey, the researcher is doing an investigative study without prior subject involvement.

An example of a possible field survey comes from Crates. He states that the shocking lack of quality in microbiological specimens taken from patients leads to inadequate diagnosis and treatment of health problems. He contends that one cause for the failure to collect quality specimens lies in the inadequacy of basic microbiological courses in nursing schools.[6] A valuable field survey could involve a comparison of the quality of specimens collected by graduates of the different nursing programs.

Short-term versus long-term surveys.   In a short-term survey, data are collected over weeks, months, or a few years. Any study conducted over more than a 5-year period is usually considered a long-term investigation. The number of times data are collected during both a short-term and a long-term survey may vary. An ideal example of a long-term survey is Terman's study of gifted children. This research project covered nearly 30 years. Terman studied his subjects during their academic careers and on through their adult life to find out if gifted children accomplish any more than normal children.

In both short- and long-term surveys the investigator is observing a sequence of events and has no control over the outcome. Suppose we decide to conduct a long-term study to

---

[5]Fox, David J.: Fundamentals of research in nursing, ed. 4, New York, 1982, Appleton-Century-Crofts, p. 163.
[6]Crates, R.H.: Improper microbiological specimens—a shocking deficit in health care, Lab. Med. **10**(4):234–239, April 1979.

observe the progress of tubercular patients who have been discharged from an institution. The progress and general health of the same persons can be observed 1 year later, 2 years later, 5 years later, and so on.

The long-term survey has a number of disadvantages. It is difficult to maintain contact with all the subjects; some will move, others will have accidents or die, and a few may wish to discontinue their participation. Many factors make it more difficult for the researcher to collect data for a long-term survey than for a short-term survey. Not only is it more difficult to study the sample over time because of attrition, but the study will have to begin with a large sample to end up with the size of sample the researcher desires. The major advantage of the long-term survey is that it gives the researcher an opportunity to observe the subjects' changes over a long period of time. Such changes include physiological, emotional, spiritual, socioeconomic, educational, and marital status. The second advantage is that the researcher can observe the same subjects over time to gain insight into the effects of change. The long-term effects of nursing intervention cannot be adequately understood over a few months' time; therefore a long-term survey has an important place in nursing research.

The advantages of a long-term survey may not offset the much greater additional cost. Before such a survey is begun, cost should definitely be considered.

Longitudinal survey.   According to Simon, the long-term survey and the longitudinal survey are almost the same. The longitudinal method, also called the long view, has different names in the various disciplines. Psychologists and educators refer to it as the longitudinal method; anthropologists and sociologists refer to it as the historical method; and economists refer to it as the time-series method.

A major problem connected with longitudinal surveys is the difficulty the researcher has in studying individuals over long periods of time because some changes are caused by factors other than time. Suppose someone wanted to study the effects of a new treatment for cancer. Perhaps the results of the treatment might show that at the end of the first year there were some good effects, but over a longer period of time, such as 5 to 10 years, harmful effects may develop. When DDT was first introduced, the results seemed so favorable that its use was continued. Now we are aware that it has some harmful effects. The researcher must continue long-range studies for an unknown length of time to accumulate as many facts as possible.

Economists use time-series analysis in which they compare data collected at present with data that were gathered at some time in the past. They do not wait to see how circumstances will affect any given situation. The researcher may carry out such studies by asking the subjects questions about a past event and by comparing the responses to the present state of affairs.

All information concerning the stages that a certain disease goes through may be analyzed by a computer. A computer can provide an analysis simulating the interaction and change that occurs in a normal, real-life situation.

Babbie identifies three primary longitudinal designs for survey research: trend studies, cohort studies, and panel studies. These longitudinal studies are either descriptive or explanatory. In *trend studies* the general population is studied at different points over a long period of time. Participants in trend studies need not be the same subjects each period but rather subjects that are representative of the population at that time. The long-term trends in the use of a particular treatment or medicine could be researched using trend techniques. Suppose we want to learn the attitude of male patients toward a particular nursing intervention. We would sample patients who received this treatment and then continue to sample representative subjects at intervals for a predetermined length of time. Such a method allows the investigator to observe changes, shifts in attitude, and response to health care. The researcher may not collect all the data personally but may use data collected by other researchers for analysis.

Cohort studies focus on the same specific population each time data are collected, but samples may be composed of different subjects. Cohort studies are similar to trend studies except that cohort studies sample a group of individuals with similar characteristics. For example, graduates of a state's nursing schools in 1975 could be studied to find out their opinions concerning nursing practice. Every 10 years a sample could be drawn from the 1975 graduating classes. The criterion would be that the subjects had graduated from the state's nursing schools, not that they had been included in the original sample. Because it would be difficult to collect data from the same subjects every tenth year, for example, any cohort will suffice as long as the subject comes from the same subgroup.

Panel studies use the same respondents at each progressive time period that the data are collected.[7] The panels themselves are groups of subjects composing a permanent or fixed sample. The sample is contacted two or more times at specified periods. Because each panel member is unique, only the original subjects can satisfy the requirements of the researcher. Shifts in attitudes and behavior can be detected more readily as the investigator studies each subject in greater depth than is usually the case in a cross-sectional survey. A disadvantage is the attrition of subjects over time.

The researcher may want to modify or combine some of the features of these longitudinal designs for a particular research study. Variations could be made by studying parallel samples (for example, nursing students, faculty, and nursing service personnel concerning their views toward a specific hospital policy) or the contextual environment of the subject to describe the individual (this necessitates linking the person with his file).[8]

Cross-sectional survey. Another type of survey, called cross-sectional research, is sometimes used in place of a longitudinal study. Basically, the difference between the two is the time factor. In a longitudinal survey, a group may be traced or followed for a long period of time, whereas in a cross-sectional survey several groups in various stages of development are studied simultaneously. Such studies describe or explain the relationship between variables.

If we are interested in studying people who have been smoking for 20 years, and we choose to do a longitudinal survey, we will follow the same people for the full 20 years that they smoke. The sample would include individuals who had been smoking for various lengths of time. With the cross-sectional survey we do not have to wait 20 years to obtain our results, because the sample could include only those subjects who have already been smoking for 20 years. The study will be less expensive, and loss of subjects will not occur. Cross-sectional research is conducted in one short period of time.

If we were studying the effects of smoking from 1965 to 1985, using the longitudinal approach, we would have the advantage of observing individual differences as they

[7]Babbie, E.R.: Survey research methods, Belmont, CA, 1973, Wadsworth, Inc. pp. 63–64.
[8]*Ibid.*, pp. 66–67.

changed year by year. The longitudinal survey would show the progress of cancer in each individual. The introduction of filter-tipped cigarettes and new tobaccos might produce changes that could be studied better by use of the cross-sectional technique. In this case, subjects who had been using filters and certain brands for specific lengths of time could compose the sample. In the longitudinal approach there would be variations within the smoking habits of the sample that could not be controlled.

A cross-sectional survey is no more or less valuable than a longitudinal survey. Both are valuable according to their intended purpose. When doing research, it is better to have a choice of methods for carrying out an investigation than to limit one's methods to a single approach. It is important to remember, for instance, that if the study happens to be one that is investigating change over time caused by maturation or aging effects, then the results of the cross-sectional and the longitudinal designs may differ.

The survey approach is an important type of research methodology. Unfortunately, the term *survey* may be misleading to some individuals who think of it as meaning a shallow type of study—only a survey! Actually, it is a critical inspection of a particular situation, problem, or question. Many research projects begin as exploratory studies. The systematic investigation leads to a general knowledge of the state that exists. An in-depth study follows the initial research, based on the findings.

EXPERIMENT

It is important to differentiate between the experimental approach and the experiment per se. We define the experimental approach as the *process* of gathering data by intentional manipulation. There are numerous experiments the researcher can develop that utilize the experimental process.

The Classical Experimental Design

Fig. 12-2 is a diagram of the classical experimental design. Usually two matched groups are selected through randomization. One group undergoes experimentation and the other is undisturbed. To see what effect the experiment has, tests are administered before and after the experiment. A comparison is then made between the mean differences of the two scores by statistical analysis.

Use of cells 1, 2, 3, and 4 allows the most control of variables possible. It is possible to collect data using any of the various cells, but there is the most control when all four cells are used.

	Before	After
Control group	1	3
Experimental group	2	4

FIGURE 12-2   Classical experimental design.

There are many possibilities for using combinations of the cells in the design. Using cells 2 and 4, we have a before and an after test on the experimental group. The group is tested, an experimental process is introduced, and the subjects are tested again to find out if any change has occurred. However, there is no control group with which to compare results.

Occasionally cell 4 is used alone. Some change is introduced, and then comparisons are made with similar groups to observe differences. An example of this is the research conducted to find out whether or not television violence causes violent behavior in viewers. In this case, cell 4 is used alone, because it is extremely difficult to find subjects who have not watched television.

When cells 3 and 4 are used, there is no before test, but there is an after test and both a control and an experimental group. In the field of medicine, cells 3 and 4 are often used. People with a specific illness are placed in the control and experimental groups. A treatment is given to the experimental group to see if there is any improvement over the control group, who received no such treatment. The before test was not taken, because the participants' conditions had been identified previously.

The classical experimental design in which all four cells are used is an extremely valuable approach. Its worth is probably greater in the physical sciences than in the social sciences; however, in both fields it is the most powerful approach of any known research technique for collecting data, testing hypotheses, and defining cause-effect relationships. The reason for its value in the physical sciences is that there is usually one cause and one effect, whereas in the social sciences cause and effect relationships are complex.

The results of research in human behavior can never be completely controlled because no two individuals or situations are ever identical.

For an example of the classical experimental design in operation, we might study a new technique in patient care. We would select a number of patients in a hospital setting, preferably in the same unit. The patients would be assigned by random selection to either a control group or an experimental group. Then some measure of patient recovery would be made, such as length of hospital stay. A new technique would be tried on the experimental group. We would then evaluate both groups with the measure and compare results. Any difference between the experimental and control groups might be attributed to the new method.

An even more elaborate sampling procedure is called *precision matching*. This requires matching individuals with selected similar characteristics. As an example, for each 50-year-old female with a college degree and in good health in the control group, there must be another female, 50 years old, with a college degree and in good health in the experimental group. Precision matching forces the investigator to ignore some characteristics, because no two individuals have exactly the same personalities or background.

Consideration must be given to achieving balanced groups for both the control and experimental sections. This balance is difficult to attain. It is sufficient to say that the control and experimental groups should be large enough to ensure a broad sample of subjects and should be made up of subjects assigned by random selection. Some researchers attempt to match groups by having the same percentage of women with equal education, from each religious faith, and with other variable characteristics in each group. This is called matching by *frequency distribution*.

The problem of testing hypotheses is always a matter of degree. Science cannot achieve certainty, but it can attempt to eliminate some of the uncertainty of prediction. An interesting example is the present policy of weather prediction by forecasting rain as a *percentage chance of precipitation* rather than saying that it will or will not rain.

Suppose in an experimental research project we were able to obtain the findings we had predicted or a change that was in the direction we had predicted. This does not mean that the variable selected was the reason for the change. There are several reasons why it might have happened. If in testing an experimental patient care intervention technique, using the classical experimental design, we found the experimental group recovering faster, would this mean that we could attribute the cause to the new type of intervention? No, it would not necessarily mean that the intervention had made the difference.

On the other hand, if we found that there was no difference between the two groups in their rates of recovery, it would not mean that the new treatment was ineffective. If we observed that the new technique and patient recovery occurred simultaneously, it could be attributed to other factors, or a combination of factors in addition to the one we are investigating. By chance we might have stumbled on an atypical group of subjects, and therefore the results had been swayed in the anticipated direction or in the opposite direction. These examples suggest reasons why in research it is especially important to test and retest.

Let us use another nursing situation as an example of the experimental approach. Suppose we want to test an innovative method of instruction for teaching nursing fundamentals to a group of subjects. We plan to have a control group and an experimental group on which to test the new method. First, we assign every subject a number, then draw the numbers out of a hat, and divide the subjects into two sections. We pull the first number out and put it in the control group; the next number is placed in the experimental group, and so on until all the numbers (subjects) have been placed. Then all subjects take a pretest that measures the knowledge or skill they have, based on the present teaching method. Lecturing and demonstration have been used in the past, so the instructor continues to use them with the control group; the experimental group is exposed to the "retention" method. After a period of time each group is given another examination developed to test the same objectives as the pretest. A comparison is made of the results from the experimental and control groups to determine if there is any difference in their scores.

The results of the teaching technique study depend to a great extent on whether the same teacher instructs both groups or whether different teachers participate. Such factors as personality, skill, and competency can bias the study results. If we use one teacher, then the question becomes, "Which groups gets taught first in the day?" If the control group receives their instruction first every day, they may talk with subjects in the experimental group or compare methods. If the second group learns that an experiment is taking place, they may unconsciously or deliberately change their usual routine or habits, thus affecting the results.

There is a possibility, of course, that the experimental approach would be so radically different that the subjects enjoy or reject it completely. If the subjects concentrated on the retention method rather than on what they were learning, their motivation might be decidedly affected. For this reason it is best to conduct experimental research under strict security.

An alternative experimental approach uses a control group, an experimental group, and a third group for comparison. The control and experimental groups are pretested, then the control and comparison groups are taught through the usual method, while the experimental group is exposed to the retention method. The three groups take the post-test, and if the comparison group's results are radically different from the control group's, some confounding variables are present.

Advantages

Some of the advantages of using the experimental method lie in the fact that we can select one variable and observe the effects of this variable (the independent variable) on the dependent variable. The experimental approach provides a great deal of certainty and efficiency because it brings together one cause and one effect. There is no perfect way to gather data or to test an hypothesis, but the scientific experiment, using the classical experimental design, is the most powerful of the various methods of collecting data.

Barnes has listed 10 important characteristics of experimental research:

1. Research ideas are restricted by the requirement that they be testable.
2. Theories and speculations are closely related to reality.
3. Simplicity in ideas and conceptualizations is the ideal.
4. Research sets out to test, not to prove.
5. The concept of "failure" is an archaic interference in research activities.
6. The potential value of a research project is directly related to the cogency of the questions asked.
7. The methods of research are intentionally devised to prevent the researcher's deluding himself and others.
8. Values play a legitimate and important part in research activities.
9. The methods of analysis, logical deduction, and statistical inference should fit the limitations inherent in the problem being investigated.
10. The researcher courts recognition through the power of his tested ideas, not through the attractiveness of his rhetoric.[9]

Problem Areas

Several variables must be controlled when the experimental approach is used.

1. The recognition of the causal factor is a major problem. Suppose the researcher believes that periodic bathing in solution X will heal a decubitus ulcer. No doubt some people will recover without the solution, and others will develop decubitus ulcers in spite of the application of solution X. Therefore the researcher needs to recognize the variables that have an effect on the usefulness of solution X.

2. The researcher can control the intensity or number of variables that are believed to influence some end. Continuing our illustration, there is a need to control those variables, other than solution X, that may increase or retard the development of a decubitus ulcer. The researcher must manipulate the variable solution X by using it on the experimental group and by not using it on the control group. Both experimental and control group members may be upset by the experiment depending on the results. If solution X is extremely effective, the control group members will be angry that they were not allowed

[9]Barnes, Fred P.: Research for the practitioner in education, Washington, D.C., p. 13. Copyright 1964, National Association of Elementary School Principals, NEA. All rights reserved.

to receive it. However, if solution X turns out to be harmful or ineffective, then the experimental group will complain. When we discuss manipulation, we are usually considering the independent variable or the cause. The experimental and control groups must be matched as far as possible, usually by three means according to Goode and Hatt: (a) precision matching, (b) matching by frequency distributions, or (c) randomization.[10]

We highly recommend randomization because it is difficult to minimize all the variables in which the control and experimental groups might differ. By randomizing the sample, there is little need to worry about the variables. It is hoped that the sample will be large enough to include some of every variation in both groups. In precision matching an attempt is made to find every type of variable and to match the variables in both control and experimental groups so as to include some members with each variable. If matching is done by frequency distribution, general characteristics are included.

Using age as an example of precision matching, the investigator would have the same variation of ages in both experimental and control groups. When matching by frequency distribution, approximately similar groups would suffice.

3. Causal relationships are difficult if not impossible to establish. The researcher may find that every time patients had pressure on an area for more than 8 hours, they developed a decubitus ulcer in that area. The patients are bedridden, and most of them are over 65 years old. However, the researcher discovers that not all 65-year-old patients who have been in bed for a prolonged period of time have decubitus ulcers. A number of possible causes then exists. The independent variable (pressure) may cause the dependent variable (decubitus ulcer) in some cases, but another variable (age) also may contribute to the cause. When studying the relationship between pressure and decubiti, the researcher should not overlook what has been learned from other cultures. For instance, Auca Indians in Ecuador recovering from polio had no decubiti when they slept in their hammocks in the village. However, preventing skin breakdown in those who were bed patients in the hospital was a challenge to good nursing care.

4. The time element may confound the results of experimental research. Many of the physical sciences are not affected by time, but in nursing research this factor must be considered. The long-range changes observed may be different from the changes observed in a one-time only experiment. Immediate time factors also are related to the experiment. How much have the subjects learned about the experiment between the pretest and the posttest? If a difference is found between the pretest and the posttest in our experiment, does this mean that the independent variable is the cause? Or are there some chance variables?; is the difference simply the result of accidental factors because of the matching of the groups?

5. Another problem is the quantity of change necessary to determine difference. A comparison of the before and after tests with control and experimental groups may demonstrate only a small amount of difference. Campbell and Stanley recommend that posttests be planned for 1 month, 6 months, or 1 year following an experiment, since it has repeatedly been found that long-term effects are qualitatively as well as quantitatively different.[11]

[10]Goode, William J., and Hatt, Paul K.: Methods in social research, New York, 1952, McGraw-Hill, Inc., p. 79.
[11]Campbell, Donald T., and Stanley, Julian C.: Experimental and quasi-experimental designs for research, Chicago, 1963, Rand McNally & Co. Reprinted from Gage, N.L.: Handbook of research on teaching, pp. 171–246.

6. The difficulty of matching subjects is another problem, especially if the experiment involves human subjects. For instance, in our decubitus ulcer experiment, the researcher would need to match the variables in the control and experimental groups under study. To locate individuals of the same age, sex, and who have been in bed the same length of time with pressure on the same areas of the body could be difficult. The size of the sample might be so small that the researcher would be hard pressed to generalize the findings. The matching process becomes even more difficult as the number of matched variables increases.

7. In an experimental laboratory setting, it may be difficult to obtain subjects, especially subjects who are unaware of the experiment. Recruitment of willing participants may be difficult; subjects must be willing to participate and put forth their best effort in an experiment.

8. Obviously, the same test cannot be given to human subjects for the pretest and the posttest in an experimental design; equivalent tests must be developed. Skill is required in writing equivalent items. In some experiments a pretest and a posttest are not appropriate as in the experiment on decubitus ulcers.

9. Quite often the measures, pretests, and posttests are subjective, and their validity and reliability can be questioned. It is difficult to disguise certain aspects of an experiment, and the lack of disguise may bias the results. The posttest results may be cumulative knowledge from subjects having been in the experimental situation or from subjects having transferred knowledge from one to another. The knowledge may build up over the course of the experiment. Finally, the experimental process itself may introduce certain types of variables that interfere with the planned study design. The subject may not like the experiment or the experimenter; the subject may be affected by taking the pretest; the subject may be affected by going through the experiment. The subject may remember the pretest and may answer the same way in the posttest.

10. It is difficult to generalize from the experimental situation to the public at large.

11. There is the possibility of the Hawthorne effect occurring; that is, individuals may act differently just by having an observer around. For example, a researcher was testing creativity in nursing students. Having matched two groups, a control and an experimental group on the basis of a paper-and-pencil creativity test, he then showed the experimental group a film that he thought would stimulate creativity. The control group sat in the classroom and worked on their lessons. Immediately following the viewing of the film, the control and experimental groups were assigned a classroom project to see how creative they actually were. Creativity was judged on the original use of a plastic bleach bottle. Students were given credit for creativity only if no more than two other persons had the same idea. Extra credit was given for unique uses. The experimental group not only had more creative ideas but had more original ones. The creativity of the experimental group exceeded that of the control group by 33%. The researcher had stayed with the control group, while the experimental subjects watched the film with another person. Afterward, when discussing the results of the study, the subjects in the experimental group stated that they had related differently to the person who stayed with them. She was an authoritarian figure, and they said that they were more afraid of her. The experimental group said that they had worked more diligently after seeing the film. This may have accounted for some of the results.

Field Experiment

The experimental approach can be used in the laboratory or in the field. The laboratory setting is an artificial, tightly controlled situation, where subjects, either human or animal, are used for experimental purposes. A field experiment is conducted in any place where normal activity occurs. In a sense, the experimental design used in testing creativity was strictly a laboratory approach. However, this same type of experimentation could be done in the field. In a field experiment, the subjects need never know that they are part of a research study. Often the medical profession uses animals in the initial stages of an experiment. If the results prove successful, the experiment may move into the field. In the field, a true experimental approach, using before and after tests and experimental and control groups, can be attempted.

The field approach to collecting data substitutes a real-life situation for the laboratory setting. In testing a new type of teaching method, two colleges could be used, one as a control and the other as experimental. Though there is less control of variables in the field than in the laboratory, there are advantages. Subjects may be included in the sample who would not consent to participate in a laboratory setting; the responses of the subjects tend to be more spontaneous; situations can be investigated that could not be brought into a controlled laboratory setting; and more varied individuals can be included in the sample, making for greater generalizability of the findings.

Disadvantages include the general lack of control that makes the independent variables difficult to manipulate. The researcher must make sure the experimental and control groups are closely matched to ensure meaningful conclusions. Finally, a field experiment may present so many complex problems that it is not always worthwhile.

The field experiment is still a viable option for testing new techniques and procedures for patient care.

Latin-Square Design

The Latin-square design is an experimental approach for multiple comparisons. Campbell and Stanley consider it effective in achieving a measure of control when subjects cannot be randomly assigned to equivalent groups.[12] The number of groups to be compared equals the number of times each alternative of the independent variable is studied (Fig. 12-3). The Latin-square design also may be set up systematically. Fig. 12-4 demonstrates why there was an error when the Latin-square design was used in an agricultural experiment. Three types of seeds were planted in adjoining plots of land. Plot A always produced a better yield. A stream of water was discovered running under all the A plots, which accounted for the greater yield. It was not the quality of the seed, as first concluded. Had the seeds been planted as in Fig. 12-3 the stream of water would not have influenced all A plots.

The Latin-square is most often used in the physical sciences but can be adapted for use in nursing research. To adapt its use requires only that the multiple comparison be based on cell content, not cell arrangement.

A new teaching method of varying intensity, which uses all levels of nursing education, could be tried (Fig. 12-5). Each cell represents a different level of intensity. Students could be randomly assigned to the four cells, no matter what their program is. The assigned

[12] *Ibid.*, pp. 171–246.

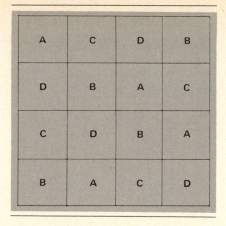

FIGURE 12-3   Latin-square—randomized section.

levels of intensity of the four cells and the use of students from different educational levels demonstrate a possible adaptation of the Latin-square technique. This process enables the researcher to test several variables simultaneously.

Community development on a worldwide basis is an exciting reality. For example, projects are under way in Indian communities in Ecuador. Some of the goals are to provide pure drinking water, improve nutrition, increase the use of latrines, strengthen the vaccination program, and encourage elevated living quarters. The Latin-square design could be utilized by randomly selecting both communities and the order of emphasis of the health variables. Community A might begin with elevated living quarters, community B with a vaccination program, and so on. After all five health variables have been implemented in each community, an evaluation survey could be conducted to determine the most effective order for improving health.

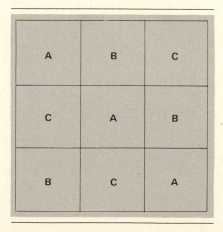

FIGURE 12-4   Latin-square—systematic plan.

TYPE OF PROGRAM	HOURS PER WEEK			
Practical nurse	5	10	15	20
Associate degree	5	10	15	20
Diploma	5	10	15	20
Baccalaureate	5	10	15	20

FIGURE 12-5   Plan for teaching techniques.

Retroactive Design

Another kind of experimental design is called retroactive, or retrospective. Retroactive design refers to a technique using historical literature or recall to find the relationship between events. An event of unusual consequence may stir the imagination of a researcher. To satisfy his/her curiosi y, the researcher can investigate by retrospection.

At what point in time or history was a new variable introduced that resulted in a change that is now noticeable? One of the classic examples of the experimental retroactive process is that done by Max Weber in *The Protestant Ethic and the Spirit of Capitalism*.[13] He noticed that there was a spirit of capitalism among the people (frugality, careful investment of money for a maximum return, hoarding of resources). Weber noticed the frugal handling of money and the hardworking attitude of the people in their attempt to gain capital. Where did this attitude come from, he wondered. Weber began a search back through history and found that John Calvin had introduced the Protestant ethic (salvation is earned by hard work). This Protestant ethic was the independent variable that resulted in the spirit of capitalism among the people. Historians documented that the capitalistic spirit was absent before Calvin's Protestant ethic was introduced but present afterward.

In some situations there may be no particular point or event that can be designated as the cause. For example, a series of social circumstances may have made the times ripe for capitalism to appear, and John Calvin's Protestant ethic may have been the trigger that set it off.

Retroactive studies have both advantages and disadvantages. The advantages are that it is easy to gather data, the data are inexpensive to obtain, and there is much material available. It is a useful technique and provides a great deal of insight. Disadvantages of the retroactive method are that the conditions under which data were collected are unknown, the occurrence of two variables at the same time does not mean that one caused the other, and generalization of the results is less likely.

Suppose an exotic new disease—exotica X—breaks out in Rich Money, a suburb of Millionnaire City. In January there were no reported cases of exotica X. On February 3 the first case was reported. By the end of February, 13 more cases had been reported. In March there were 18 new cases. The retroactive design would be appropriate for finding out what event (variable) occurred on or before February 3 that caused the epidemic. There are numerous variables to consider. The effect (exotica X) may have been developing for some time and the manifest evidence (symptoms) only surfaced in

[13]Weber, M.: The Protestant ethic and the spirit of capitalism. New York, 1958, Charles Scribner's Sons. Translated by Talcott Parsons.

February. The organism that causes the disease may be ever present, but only causes the disease in the presence of another variable. Furthermore, an influenza epidemic also became evident the first week of February. Influenza and exotica X may or may not be related. It is obvious that the retroactive approach is a logical selection, but it is by no means a sure way of discovering the cause of exotica X.

Samples

In the experimental approach, the control and experimental groups should have equivalent characteristics. How do we get samples with equivalent characteristics? As mentioned earlier in the creativity experiment, the instructor was able to obtain a measure of creativity by using a paper-and-pencil pretest. Equally creative people (according to test results) were assigned to both the experimental and control groups. Since creativity was the only variable studied, there was no need to control any other variable such as education, age, or socioeconomic background.

In an experimental design in the health field, it would be very difficult to say that two people were equally ill with cancer. Therefore, it would do no good to match a 60-year-old woman who has cancer with another 60-year-old woman who has cancer, since their degree of illness is unknown. This kind of matching is called stratification matching. It would be very difficult to recognize all the possible variables on which the pairs could be matched. Generally, if we have a fairly large sample to assign to the experimental and control groups by random selection, we need not worry about matching or stratification. There will, no doubt, be some differences between the experimental and control groups, but differences could be evaluated by use of a statistical test.

There is no assurance that any kind of random sampling is going to be completely random. There is always the possibility that a random sampling can be biased or skewed. For example, a randomly assigned sample could conceivably have all women in one group and all men in another group.

Control of the Experiment

It is much easier to control an experiment when dealing with objects rather than with individuals or groups of people. It is often difficult to find subjects who will participate willingly in experiments. Once again, ethics are involved. If we take subjects who are unaware, are we being fair to them? How much can we experiment with human beings? Is there any chance of harming or emotionally upsetting human beings by having them in experimental groups? It has been our experience that we must be very careful about the possibility of students getting upset.

In doing a sociogram, one researcher asked students to name five people with whom they would like to work and five people with whom they would prefer not to work. Some of the students rebelled at the idea of listing five people with whom they would not like to work, and eventually some of the students dropped out of the research project partially for this reason.

We also might ask if the nurses who volunteer to participate in a nursing research study are exactly like the rest of the nurses in the profession. People (including nurses) who will volunteer to take part in a research investigation may be different from the majority. The problems seem to be that either nurses who volunteer are different, or when nonvolunteers are used, their rights may be infringed.

Schultz criticizes the use of college students as representatives of the general population. A great deal of our research uses college students and only a small percentage uses the general population. Eighty percent of research is performed on 3% of the population, and most of these are male college students in psychology classes.[14] Individuals who are studying full time during young adulthood are probably atypical and possibly do not represent the general public.

One study found that participants who volunteered at one institution of higher education did so for reasons of curiosity, money, and to help science—in that order. Other reasons include an interest in the subject matter or the researcher, the pressure to volunteer, having no other choice preferable to volunteering, and the perception that others in a similar situation would choose to volunteer.

Many subjects assume that the experimenter may be trying to trick them or to find out something about them that they do not want revealed. A researcher who is sincere and has a reputation for honesty is more likely to secure the cooperation of subjects.

Role playing also has been suggested as a possibility for experimentation. It would eliminate deception and would involve the subject as a direct participant in data collection. However, role playing can be criticized as being too artificial. There is no emotional involvement in the role-playing situation. When an individual is in a real-life situation involving financial gain or integrity, his/her actions may be very different than when engaging in role playing.

Additional Experimental Designs

A variety of experimental designs is possible. Kazdin reports on a technique known as ABAB design.[15] Descriptively, the design could be defined as the on-again, off-again experiment. As an illustration, suppose it is suspected that soap is the cause of a skin rash. The soap is used to determine the baseline or A phase condition of the rash. It is noticed that the subject has a rash between the fingers a few hours after using the suspected soap. The rash is defined as the baseline condition. In B phase the soap is removed. Assume that the rash disappears. The subject returns to using the soap to see if the rash returns. This stage is the second A phase. Finally, the subject discontinues using the soap and waits to see if the rash disappears. This final stage is known as the second B stage.

The ABAB technique is especially valuable in testing the effectiveness of a new drug, medication, or technique. A single case is used for the research rather than experimenting on a large sample. The diagram of the ABAB design using the skin rash example is illustrated.

In use, this design might require some manipulation. The time periods could fluctuate depending on the condition. A medication might require a long period of time to be effective while the baseline stage could be reached in only a few days. Medication might be needed permanently or one application might be adequate to allow the body to adjust.

Kazdin calls the ABAB an example of intrasubject-replication. Such research is useful in case studies on single subjects who have a problem or ailment which is unique to a

[14]Schultz, Duane P.: The human subject in psychological research, Psychological Bulletin **72**(3):217, 1969.
[15]Kazdin, A.E.: Research design in clinical psychology, New York, 1980, Harper & Row Publishers, p. 172–174.

	Baseline A	B	A	B
Stage	use soap	withdraw soap	use soap	withdraw soap
Condition	rash appears	rash disappears	rash returns	rash disappears

particular individual. Often intrasubject-replication design can be conducted when the outcome is uncertain and some caution is indicated, the sample is small, or the classical experimental design would involve considerable risk.[16]

Kazdin also suggests some types of before-and-after tests which are valuable in experimentation in clinical psychology but have application for nursing or research in general. Some of the tests include projective devices, physiological, psychological or behavioral tests, self-reporting inventories, questionnaires, and other well-known rating scales.

Campbell and Stanley have demonstrated a number of experimental designs which have wide potential use in the health field.[17] Only a brief treatment is offered here to illustrate the extensive variety of possible design.

1. One-shot Case Study.
   group 1   no pretest—experiment—posttest
   One group receives an experimental treatment and a posttest is administered to determine change. A weakness is that without the pretest it is difficult to evaluate the cause or degree of change.
2. One-Group Pretest-Posttest design.
   group1   pretest—experiment—posttest
   A measure of the dependent variable is taken before the experimental variable is applied and then an after-test is administered to denote change. This is a good design, but fails to have a comparison to determine how the results were effected by the pretest.
3. Static-Group Comparison.
   group 1   no pretest—experiment—posttest
   group 2   no pretest—no experiment—posttest
   An experimental and a control group are compared with only a posttest but no pretest. This worthwhile design fails to differentiate between the two groups. However, if the groups are heterogeneous, assumptions might be made that they are similar.
4. Pretest-Posttest Control Group design. This is often referred to as the classical experimental design.
   group 1   pretest—experiment—posttest
   group 2   pretest—no experiment—posttest
   Two groups are given a pretest and then the experiment is applied to one group but not the other. Finally, a posttest is taken of both groups for a comparison of any change, as measured by the posttest compared with the pretests. It is believed that this is the most valuable of the experimental designs and involves the least effort for the most gain in results. It also allows very good control over a number of confounding and intervening variables.

[16]*Ibid.*, p. 172–174.
[17]*Ibid.*, p. 214–218.

5. The Solomon Four-Group design.

    group 1   pretest—experiment—posttest
    group 2   pretest—no experiment—posttest
    group 3   no pretest—experiment—posttest
    group 4   no pretest—no experiment—posttest

    In addition to the classical experimental design, two other groups are included. One experimental group and one control group are added, with neither receiving a pretest, but both being evaluated by a posttest. This design is helpful to determine any holdover effects of pretesting. However, this design is time consuming and consideration must be given to the possibility of interaction between groups, which might contaminate the results.

6. The Posttest-Only Control Group Design.

    group 1   experiment—posttest
    group 2   no experiment—posttest

    A control group and an experimental group are compared with a posttest but not a pretest. A weakness is that differences in the posttests may be the results of the groups and not the experiment since there is no measure of the before differences.

7. Time-Series Experiment.

    group 1   pretest—pretest—pretest—experiment—posttest—posttest—posttest

    A single subject or group is pretested at several periods to see if there is any change or to establish a baseline performance. Then the experiment is introduced and further posttests are administered to determine any change, and to see if the change continues, diminishes, or increases. A major weakness is that social factors may influence the degree of change in the posttest.

8. Equivalent Time-Samples design.

    group 1   pretest—experiment—posttest—posttest—experiment—posttest

    A single group is tested and given an experiment and then tested again several times. It is better to alternate tests and experiments by some random method than to have one following the other each time.

9. Equivalent Materials design.

    group 1   material A test—material B test—material C test

    In operation, the equivalent materials design is similar to the equivalent time design, with one difference. The material factor (e.g., medication, treatment, procedure, dosage, or new technique) replaces "time." Each material change is different, but in the same amount or dosage, and so on.

10. Nonequivalent Control Group design.

    group 1   pretest—experiment—posttest
    group 2   pretest—no experiment—posttest

    This design is quite similar to the classical experimental design (see item 4). The two groups are different but convenient groups which are not randomly selected as in the classical experimental design. For example, a freshman class in introductory psychology could be one group and senior students in nursing research could be another group. This is a very useful technique because it is often easier to handle since the groups are already available and the pretest will give some measure of similarity or difference.

	Intervention A	Intervention B	Intervention C	Intervention D
group 1	5min./posttest	10 min./posttest	15 min./posttest	20 min./posttest
group 2	10 min./posttest	15 min./posttest	20 min./posttest	5 min./posttest
group 3	15 min./posttest	20 min./posttest	5 min./posttest	10 min./posttest
group 4	20 min./posttest	5 min./posttest	10 min./posttest	15 min./posttest

11. Counterbalanced design.

In this design, four groups are exposed to four different treatments at four different times by random assignment. Each of the four groups receives each of the four treatments. The random assignment is usually done in a Latin-square design. For example, the diagram illustrates a nursing intervention with varying amounts of time. No pretest is given but a posttest is administered after each of the 16 treatments.

Some weakness in this design are that it is complex, involves a great deal of time, and lacks pretests which might reveal some differences in the groups. This technique would appear to lend itself to quantities or amounts, and offers controls over experimental variables by measuring increasing amounts of time.

12. The Separate Sample Pretest-Posttest design.

group 1   pretest—experiment—no posttest
group 2   no pretest—experiment—posttest

In this design, two groups are exposed to an experiment but one has only a pretest and the other has only a posttest. This procedure is a practical approach which allows control over several important variables in the experimental design by reducing the need for two tests to only one test. This design has much to offer and reduces the complexity of administering four tests.

13. Separate Sample Pretest-Posttest Control Group design.

group 1   pretest—experiment—no posttest
group 2   no pretest—experiment—posttest
group 3   pretest—no experiment—no posttest
group 4   no pretest—no experiment—posttest

This design is identical to the Separate Sample Pretest-Posttest Control design (see item 12), except that group 3 and 4 are added. Group 3 has only a pretest and no experiment or posttest. Group 4 has only a posttest and no pretest or experiment. This design controls variables well, but involves considerable time and effort.

14. Multiple Time Series design.

group 1   test—test—test—test—test—test—experiment—test—test
group 2   test—test—test—test—test—test—test——test—test

Two groups or sets of subjects are tested several times, but in one group, an experiment is introduced at a randomly selected time. This is an interesting and useful design but requires effort over a period of time. It would seem to offer additional advantages if the tests were administered and evaluated by disinterested judges.

15. The Recurrent Institutional Cycle design. This also is known as a "Patched-Up" design.

group 1   no pretest—experiment—posttest
group 2   pretest—experiment—posttest

In operation, this approach is not specifically refined to the preceding diagram. One advantage of the illustration is that it allows the pretest and posttest to be administered simultaneously. Testing and/or experiments can start or end as money, time, or opportunity demand.

16. Regression-discontinuity Analysis.

        group 1   pretest—experiment or event—posttest

The Regression-discontinuity Analysis design is vague and difficult to explain. It is ex post facto in nature, which means that an hypothesis is developed to explain the cause after an event has occurred. In action it is not known if the experiment or event was in any way affected or measured by either pre- or posttest. Are good nurses the result of a "good" educational institution or do students with "good" potential attend "good" nursing education programs?

Considering the work of Campbell and Stanley in developing experimental design, it is difficult to provide new alternatives. However, the authors suggest some possible alternative designs.

1. Experiment Control Reversal.

        group 1   pretest—experiment—posttest
        group 2   pretest—no experiment—posttest
        group 3   pretest—no experiment—posttest
        group 4   pretest—experiment—posttest

In operation, this approach incorporates the classical experimental design, as is done in the Pretest-Posttest Control Group design, and then repeats the study with the same groups except that the experimental group becomes the control group and vice versa. If the experiment is really the cause of the dependent variable, then when the control becomes the experimental group, the same difference should show up. This technique is often used in experimental laboratory work or in testing new medical interventions or medications.

2. Experimental-Control-Experimental.

        group 1   pretest—experiment—posttest
        group 2   pretest—no experiment—posttest
        group 3   pretest—experiment—posttest

This approach involves the same design as the classical experimental approach, but with an additional experimental group. Groups 1 and 3 are identical experimental groups while group 2 is the single control group. A comparison of the posttest gains of groups 1 and 3 should be enlightening.

3. One Experimental, Two Control with Observational Behavior Scale.

        group 1   pretest—experiment—posttest—behavioral observation scale
        group 2   pretest—no experiment—posttest—behavioral observation scale
        group 3   no pretest—no experiment—no posttest—behavioral observation scale

Operationally, this approach incorporates the classical experimental design in groups 1 and 2. Group 3 is an observation or comparison group. The unique advantage of this design is the behavioral observation scale. This scale is an additional measure to validate the posttest. In the clinical nursing unit, the pretest could be a measure of blood pressure. A new technique for reducing blood pressure is administered followed by the posttest (blood pressure measurement). The behavioral observation scale could be a subjective evaluation by a staff nurse. Ideally, the three groups could be treated by the double-blind method to reduce bias.

Another suggested use is teaching nutrition to the elderly. A pretest of knowledge followed by a teaching session is then followed by the pretest (which serves as the posttest). The behavioral scale would involve observation to determine if the elderly selected nutritional foods as suggested in the teaching session. This method is complicated; however, it tests strength of change as measured by reality and intellectual capacity. If it incorporates the double-blind method, this can be a powerful test of treatment effect.

Reliability and Validity

Chapter 15 contains a discussion of reliability and validity in some depth. However, let us refer to these terms briefly. One method of checking on the internal validity of an experiment is to expose sections of the experimental group to increasing amounts of the variable that is believed to the cause. If the results show change in proportion to exposure, the researcher can assume a measure of validity. If income increases with education, then each educational level from high school on through graduate school should have progressively higher incomes.

Concerning research tools, the researcher must be sure that the measuring tools in both the before and after tests are valid. In the experiment on creativity, both the before tests and after tests measuring creativity could be examined for validity factors such as time of day, fatigue, the number of people conducting the research, the setting, the kind of directions given, and so on. These all raise the issue of reliability and validity.

Other problems arise with the selection of the sample for an experiment or other research: volunteers probably respond differently than nonvolunteers do; there may be a loss of subjects; some people in the experimental group or the control group may be erratic in their participation, especially in a long-term study; and others may get tired of the experiment or for various reasons decide to drop out.

The Hawthorne effect must always be considered. Subjects realize they are being studied but do not know if they are in experimental or control groups. However, the fact that they are involved in a study may be enough to affect their behavior.

If the researcher is personally acquainted with some of the subjects or has information about the experiment that should not be conveyed to the participants, he/she may inadvertently supply them with clues that contaminate the study results. So, too, the study results may be contaminated if series studies are carried out without concern for the effect of carryover. The researcher must recognize that the time span between the first test and the second test can be confounded by age, fatigue, maturation, and increased knowledge. If the subjects have been selected on the basis of their extreme scores, it must be remembered that statistical regression normally occurs.

These are just a few of the problems that threaten external validity. Since there is a possibility that these problems exist, every precaution must be taken to correct or to eliminate them in experimental research.

It seems that no matter how careful researchers are in controlling the variables in an experiment, they can never be completely certain of the validity of the results. There is always the possibility that future research will reveal flaws or failures in the study. A single overlooked factor may make all the difference.

CASE STUDY

The purpose of research is to explain and predict. The case study method is one way of doing so by studying a single unit in great depth. The approach is used when a survey or an experiment is inappropriate, inadequate, or both. The researcher is interested in obtaining a wealth of current information concerning the subjects or problem area.

Stake contends that case studies are a preferred method of conducting research, since they relate to the reader's experience and provide a natural basis for making generalizations. It is through day-by-day events involving people that ideals and values are learned and changed. Therefore, the case study is a popular and valuable way to build theory, add to human understanding, and discover new insight.[18]

A case study is usually directed toward a single case, a limited number of cases, or a certain type of group. A case study probes deeply into factors of interest to the researcher. Data are gathered pertaining to the hypotheses or questions to be answered through the investigation. The researcher can use this method to analyze the interaction between factors bringing about change, usually over a period of time.

Case studies also can be made of individuals from certain recognized groups: drug addicts, alcoholics, juvenile delinquents, professionals, and subjects belonging to ethnic groups, religious sects, and subculture units. Institutions such as colleges, churches, factories, and hospitals have all been the objects of case studies.

A case study is usually a very detailed descriptive analysis of some type of institution, community, group, situation, or individual. The case study describes its subject in depth in the subject's natural setting. It may use past history to report on current events. It is usually a verbal description, but it may also make use of artifacts, records, and question-naires. Anthropologists make good use of case studies. The nursing and health care professions often utilize the case study for a particular type of disease, hospital, hospital unit, or patient. A case study is an introductory approach for a more ambitious future project, but there may be an exploration of a new phenomenon. Anthropologists normally use exploratory approaches to observe the people, their culture, and language.

Denzin considers the case study in the same general category as the life history method of research, since the life history presents the experiences and definitions of an individual, a group, or an organization.[19] Although a life history and a case study of an individual could be the same, the study of a large number of individuals concerning their viewpoints or attitudes is more often considered a survey.

One valuable use of the case study is to compare a known group with an unknown group. Since the known group has certain characteristics and practices, the case study subjects are compared with the known group to observe the differences.

If the case study method is selected, it is necessary to obtain permission from all individuals included in the study. Normally, when studying large institutions, permission from the persons in charge is sufficient to encourage other members to cooperate. If the researcher asks the members of the organization without first gaining the approval of the organizational administration, both groups may give only minimal cooperation. If the

[18]Stake, R.E.: The case study method in social inquiry, Educ. Res. 7(2):5–8, February 1978.
[19]Denzin, Norman K.: The research act, a theoretical introduction to sociological methods, Chicago, 1970, Aldine Publishing Co., p. 220.

researcher can tell the subjects that the administration has given permission, the subjects are usually happy to cooperate with the investigator's plan for research.

Yin believes that a single case is appropriate in several circumstances. It represents a critical case for the test of a theory or hypothesis which might lay the foundation for future research of a broad nature; it affords the opportunity to research an ideal-type case, one of a kind, or a particularly rare example. A revelatory case is another use of the case study which has the potential for revealing a situation or condition that has been unknown and about which it would be difficult to use survey techniques.[20]

Yin suggests special skills which case study investigators need. They include a grasp of the situation, good interview and listening ability, flexibility, and avoidance of biases.[21]

Advantages

1. There are a number of advantages to the case study, one being that researchers may begin or stop the case study at any time. When they have sufficient data, they may stop; even if time runs out or an emergency arises, at least they have some data.

In discussing the case study, Simon says that it is "almost synonymous" with descriptive research. It is the preferred method when researchers want to obtain great amounts of detail about their subjects.[22] Often investigators make up their procedures as they go along. They purposely refuse to work inside a set category of classifications, since they are not certain of the limit or extent of the study.

2. The case-study method has been particularly appropriate to nursing, where so much emphasis is placed on the care of the patient and the relationship of nurse to patient. An example of an appropriate study is an investigation of the effect of a close relationship between nurse and patient on the nurse, the patient, or the co-workers.

3. The case-study approach clearly allows researchers the opportunity to see individuals in their total network of relationships. Good researchers should make use of a variety of approaches, such as political, psychological, biological, health, physical and spiritual aspects of individuals.

4. The case-study approach provides researchers with a rich source of hypotheses and ideas as a result of the in-depth probe into a given situation.

5. Researchers tend to have more freedom in the amount of data to be collected as well as the sources from which they can be obtained.

6. Case studies as a source for generalizations have been defended by Robert Stake. He contends that case studies can be used to test hypotheses, especially hypotheses believed to be false. Further, case studies are a means of exploring and opening up new theories rather than testing old theories. Also, case studies are an experimental approach to research that provides satisfaction and understanding rather than volumes of factual data.[23]

Disadvantages

1. Sometimes the researcher has to decide if he/she will look in great depth at several factors or only one. Phillips points out that learning anything about a society from a

[20] Yin, R.K.: Case study research: design and methods, Applied social research methods series, Vol. 5, Beverly Hills, 1984, SAGE Publications, Inc., pp. 42–44.
[21] *Ibid.*, pp. 55–57.
[22] Simon, p. 277.
[23] Stake, p. 6.

single case is really quite difficult. The single case selected may exhibit a certain characteristic that is not representative, even though it may have been selected at random. If the
researcher uses data from a single case only within the context of discovery and does not
attempt to say anything within the context of justification, then it might be permissible
for him to use a single case.[24]

One way of improving the single-case research study is for the researcher to determine
categories of investigation so that even though there is only one case at one level, other
cases are analyzed at other levels. Another way is for him/her to collect more cases
through personal documents or social systems.

2. Another weakness of the case study is that the researcher can become so close to the
subject that he/she misjudges the amount of depth and insight he/she actually has into
the subject's behavior. When a researcher becomes socially involved with a subject,
objectivity may suffer. In the case-study approach there is a danger of subjectivity
regardless of the effort put forth by the researcher to be objective in drawing conclusions.
It is difficult for one researcher to check another investigator's conclusions because it
requires repeating the study.

3. The cost factor of case studies is another consideration. One or two single case
studies are expensive both in time and money in relation to the amount of knowledge that
is gained. True, the investigator gains valuable insight into a small, single situation, but it
also means that he/she has only one situation from which to generalize to the whole
society. Generalizations made from a single case may be questioned.

4. The researcher must be objective. What is described and what is not described, of
course, are always selected, indicating the particular bias of the observer. However,
objectivity of viewpoint in the case study is very important. The anthropologist who
wants to study a primitive tribe and flies to the region on weekends or stays for a few
hours of interviewing is not going to observe detail with much depth. Malinowski
believed that the researcher should stay in the study area for several years.

5. Data obtained from one source may conflict with data from another source. The
researcher then has to continue investigating the problem to arrive at the truth. Most case
studies rely heavily on memory; inaccurate recall results in inaccurate data.

6. Undesirable traits are frequently the reason for doing a case study and receive the
most emphasis. For example, rather than looking at the positive, we often concern
ourselves with the negative. Persons with serious illnesses are selected for study rather
than those in "perfect" health. If desirable traits were emphasized, the conclusions would
probably be different.

Considerations

Consideration must be given to certain problems in the case-study approach.

If a single individual is being studied, the subject may die before the study is completed.
Likewise, if a group is under investigation, attrition may result from the death of some of
the members. This should be anticipated so that the study will not fail because of
attrition.

The investigator's presence may influence the response of the subject, as in the case of a
participant-observer, so the researcher must constantly be alert to the possibility of such

---

[24]Phillips, Bernard S.: Social Research strategy and tactics, New York, 1966, Macmillan, Inc., p. 129. Copyright
1966, Bernard S. Phillips.

influence. Precautions should be taken as noted in Chapter 19, which deals with observation.

It must be apparent that the case selected for study is representative of the population to which the researcher wants to generalize. Any generalizations, however, must be made with utmost caution. For instance, a single case provides nurses with an example, but it does not provide them with "proof" as it is always possible to find a case to "prove" a particular point of view. Although researchers might want to generalize from a case study, the results do not prove that the case is truly representative.

Two types of analyses are possible when generalizing from case studies. *Nomothetic analysis* is the term for generalizing from a single case to the total population. *Idiographic analysis* is the analysis of the case under study. The researcher is much safer staying within the bounds of the case at hand.

Data and the Case Study

The sources of data in a case study ought to be as extensive as possible within certain limits. For example, an anthropologist cannot rely on records or documents if a tribe has no written language; researchers are not always given permission to read the private records of subjects such as diaries, letters, and bookkeeping accounts. Persons other than the subject can provide data through interviews, verbatim reports, and various records.

The amount of data included in a single case may vary, depending on the purpose of the study. If a single individual is the subject, the amount of data could differ considerably from the amount gathered when a situation of some magnitude is being probed. The researcher must determine the amount and the extent of data that will satisfy the hypothesis, if there is one. A single case itself is not sufficient to test an hypothesis unless the research is limited to the present study or if the control of the variables is assured, making generalization possible.

Usually, if the data are from a single case, they are reported descriptively. The researcher has flexibility in the style of presentation. If the data are quantified, they are analyzed according to the commonly used methods presented in later chapters.

Guidelines for Case Studies

There are sources of potential case studies for the imaginative nurse-researcher. Some general guidelines and suggestions for the beginning investigator follow.

1. Individuals or groups who are moving from one level of nursing to another are on the periphery of both groups and would make a valuable case study contribution. Since they are in between, they are exposed to the conflicting pressures of both groups and offer a number of interesting insights. For example, practical nurses who are continuing their education to become registered nurses, graduates of diploma schools of nursing enrolled in baccalaureate nursing programs, and staff nurses who have become administrators or clinical specialists may all be classified as mobile individuals who would have a great deal of information to offer.

2. Groups or individuals who are new arrivals from one stage of development to the next also would make a valuable case study contribution. Individuals who have been nursing students and are now registered nurses are one example. Students who have had the protection of their instructors and schools find themselves, the day after graduation, giving directions and taking on new responsibilities with no one to protect them as in the past.

3. Case studies could be made of those individuals suited to a given nursing role compared with those who are not well suited. A nurse who is particularly creative, a nonconformist, or too traditional may be good case study material.

4. The reaction of newcomers to a new nursing position or health care facility may point out unusual features that the researcher may have grown accustomed to or may no longer find unusual.

5. Nurses who are radically different from the regular individual in the profession offer possibilities for case studies. For example, nurses who are extremely dedicated to their profession make interesting possibilities for study.

6. Ideal types, although they may not exist in real life, provide a standard from which to make a comparison. They have the perfect features of the variable under study. The characteristics of an ideal type may vary according to the opinions, culture, and biases of those who are identifying it. By studying the ideal type, insight that will contribute to an understanding of case studies can be gained. Florence Nightingale is one stereotype of the perfect nurse.

7. Another case study possibility is to select individuals or groups who represent different specialties in the nursing field. If we chose to study the nursing field in general, we might like to study nurse administrators, educators, staff nurses, clinical specialists, public health nurses, occupational health nurses, licensed practical nurses, aerospace nurses, missionary nurses, and so on. What makes them different from the norm? In what ways are they similar?

8. We, ourselves, are an often forgotten source of information. We should not fail to gather data about our own feelings and experiences. How we feel about a topic is a good indication of how other people feel. if we have questions or anxieties about developments, events, situations, or experiences, then other people probably have them, too.

Evaluating Case Studies

Case study data can be evaluated in several ways. Some authors look at what is known or the dependent variable patterns. They believe that one independent variable will yield several dependent variables. If the dependent variables occur as predicted, it will be possible to make inferences, accept the findings, and assume that the independent variable causes the dependent variable.

To illustrate pattern-matching, one of the techniques for case-study analysis, assume a nurse is doing a case study of the effects of exercise on a client. It would be reasonable to assume the patient's blood pressure would drop, stamina would increase, and pulse rate would slow down. In this instance, a case study is very much like an experiment. But if the three results or effects are not observed, the validity of the study can be questioned. Some authors believe that even if only one of the patterns (or dependent variable) is not present, the whole research design is in question. We believe that all research is relevant whether it confirms or rejects some or all of the pattern variables. The finding will be useful to design a new research study or serve as the basis for a replicating study.

A second type of testing or evaluating results of a case study is almost a reverse type of pattern-matching known as explanation-building. Using the illustration of the nurse studying the effect of exercise, suppose stamina did increase and blood pressure went down but pulse rate stayed the same. According to explanation-building, it is necessary to develop an hypothesis which will explain the two expected results as well as the unexpected results.[25]

An hypothetical explanation might be that pulse rate does not decrease after age 68. At this point the researcher can redesign the study or simply replicate the original study. Perhaps a multiple case study design using one client age 40 and one client age 70 could be investigated.

Another strategy for evaluating case studies is called time-series analysis. The case study is continued over a period of time in which several measures are taken at certain specified intervals. If the results are as predicted at each time, we can expect our finding and assume validity of the results. The time-series analysis is based on a chronology of some orderly arrangement of events. Referring again to our nurse-client exercise study, there is a chronology of events as related to exercise. For example, the client's blood pressure will drop after 1 week, stamina will improve after 10 days, and pulse will drop after 14 days. The three variables will continue their improving trend to a maximum of 2 hours of exercise for a 70-year-old and four hours for a 40-year-old and so on. In using the time-series analysis, it is necessary to be aware that events occur in a chronological order faster or slower depending on other variables, or may not occur at all depending on certain other conditions.

Another technique to evaluate or analyze the results of case studies is a case survey which analyzes results from several case studies by developing a close-ended coding instrument which is applied to each case study. Results are analyzed as in a quantified study.

HISTORICAL RESEARCH

The historical approach to research involves using literature, records, diaries, verbatim reports, letters, artifacts, and other sources of data from the past to arrive at conclusions. Historiography is the science of reconstructing the past from these types of data. Social scientists often use the historical method, and nurses are noting the value of this approach.

Historical research sometimes seems to be little more than a long-term paper based on library resources, but it can be a very unique study using original material. Records that compose the major source of data are often available in great quantity. It behooves the researcher to use discretion in collecting and evaluating the data. Otherwise, the project becomes a subjective description of the phenomenon. Subjective descriptions are not true scientific research.

The effect of historical research on nursing is yet to be discovered. Nurses searching for an identity relating to their roles perhaps through history can gain insight into themselves and their profession.

Ideally, the historical approach uses all the steps of the scientific method. To apply the scientific method, the researcher must consider the problem and possibly develop an hypothesis. It is at the point of analyzing the data that the historical approach frequently

---

[25]From Yin, *op cit.*, pp. 103–119.

differs from other methodologies. Historical data are collected by the researcher, criticized, and then reported. As Newton has stated, in looking at the total picture of historical research, that investigators are not only seeking information about the past but are searching for relationships, developing conclusions, and interpolating between events.[26]

Helmstadter suggests that the historical approach is most frequently used during the review of literature, an important step in descriptive and experimental research, for two reasons. First, the researcher can determine if some other investigator has studied the topic or has solved the problem, and can note the strengths, weaknesses, methodology, and recommendations for future research reported in similar studies. Second, hypotheses are suggested by reviewing the literature.[27]

The historical method has five special characteristics, according to Helmstadter: (1) observations in historical research cannot be repeated in the same manner as in laboratory experiments and descriptive surveys; (2) the researcher must find satisfaction in spending vast amounts of time in the library and in pursuing minute details in relation to the topic under study; (3) a project is usually conducted by one person; (4) an hypothesis is not always necessary in historical research; inferences can be made, more often than not, from the bits of information gathered to produce the general description of the event or the situation; and (5) the writing style of the written report tends to be more flexible, because the researcher wishes to present the facts and information in an interesting manner.[28]

Studies using the historical approach may be longitudinal or cross-sectional in nature. If the events took place a long time ago, and the records are incomplete, the investigator may conduct a longitudinal study by describing some phase of the situation over a long period of time in the past. On the other hand, if the events under study took place in recent history, and the facts have not been compiled yet, the researcher may conduct a cross-sectional study and describe the status of the situation at a particular time.

In most research, the investigator arranges the data quantitatively. However, in the historical approach, data are often ideas, concepts, or opinions. Conclusions, generalizations, and inferences become subjective, and it is possible that no two investigators will reach the same conclusions in a given instance. For this reason, researchers must use the historical approach with the understanding that objectivity is elusive and must be sought throughout the study.

Advantages

There are at least six advantages to the use of the historical approach to nursing research.

1. Historical data are readily available in professional nursing literature, medical literature, secular books, and journals. Additional sources include experts in nursing history, historians in other disciplines, and biographers. Firsthand sources of nursing history and progress can be found in the files of every school of nursing and health care institution. Chapter 18 gives detailed information on the use of records.

2. Some problems can be solved or questions answered only through historical research since the situation cannot be duplicated again. For example, the effect of the

[26]Newton, Mildred E.: The case for historical research, Nurs. Res. **14**(1):21, Winter 1965.
[27]Helmstadter, G.C.: Research concepts in human behavior, New York, 1970, Appleton-Century-Crofts, p. 43.
[28]*Ibid.*, pp. 44–45.

State Board Examination system on the nursing curriculum can only be studied historically. In other instances it would be detrimental to many people if a negative situation were intentionally created simply for the sake of study. The withholding of inoculations from a community to study the results and the rate of infection would not be moral or reasonable.

3. A knowledge of historical events increases the appreciation of nurses for the struggle that has brought nursing its professional status.

4. Nurses can avoid some of the failures of the past and build on its successes as they plan for the future. This points up the pressing need for researchers to report their findings to nurses and to society.

5. Clinical researchers have at their disposal great quantities of data, such as historical, patient, and laboratory records, that can be used to establish cause-effect relationships between health delivery and the state of patients' health.

6. The historical approach can provide the researcher with some predictive insights that are useful to the profession, to the public, and to society in general. In the past, if it took X number of years until a nursing proposal was accepted on a national level, this is some indication of the length of time needed for a proposal to be accepted in the future.

Disadvantages

Several disadvantages are inherent in the historical approach.

1. The historical approach has all the disadvantages of records as sources of data. These disadvantages include not knowing the circumstances under which the documents were written, the extent of their completeness, and the biases of the author.

2. The purpose for which the researcher intends to use historical data can bias the results. For example, an investigator might attempt to show that some well-known person in the history of nursing made a substantial impact on the profession, whereas another researcher might want to conclude that the contribution was actually minimal.

3. Historical data are never complete. There are always facets of information that would be helpful to the researcher if their location were discovered. A nurse cannot be characterized on the basis of one documented letter. Characterization must be based on a variety of documented materials so that recurring patterns may be noted. On the other hand, there may be so much data that the researcher has to be selective in presenting facts. In that case it is impossible to report all the information relating to a given situation, and the researcher must select only those facts that seem important.

4. Related closely to the question of completeness of the data is the problem of sample size. How much data must be collected to make a valid conclusion? The researcher is the only person who can determine the length of time it will take to satisfy the goals of the project—a lifetime or a few weeks. How long does it take to collect an adequate sample?

5. The subjective process of data analysis, present in all research, is especially problematic in the historical approach. The investigator who analyzes historical data must deal with abstract relationships, and must interpret material in prose that sometimes can be disputed.

6. When comparing the present problem with one in the past, the historical researcher has no control over past variables. Therefore, specific cause-effect relationships cannot be definitely determined. Likewise, generalizations from a former situation to the present one can only be made with the utmost caution.

Data and the Historical Approach

Data gathered in historical research come from primary sources (reports of the observations made by an eyewitness, thus directly related to the subject) and secondary sources (reports made by persons not present at the time the event occurred and thus secondhand information). It is important that the researcher utilize primary sources as much as possible rather than depend on the more readily available secondary materials. Patients' charts, autobiographies, diaries, letters, and original research reports are classified as primary sources, whereas biographies, encyclopedias, and most historical accounts fall under the heading of secondary materials. Unfortunately, primary sources are not as organized for easy access to the researcher as are the secondary materials.

The historical researcher must make certain decisions about the sources of data. In the case of primary materials, the investigator must determine if the document is genuine. Is it the true product of the person, group, or organization under study? The historian calls this *external* or *lower criticism. Internal* or *higher criticism* seeks to learn if the information in the document is trustworthy. Was the author of the document competent and able to tell the truth? Is the content of the material consistent with other information that has been found? Does it appear to be accurate? The answers to these questions also help to determine if the document is authentic.

The attitude of the investigator may be positive or negative toward the document at the moment it is studied. For the sake of objectivity, the historian may temporarily assume that the document contains error, is a fake, or lacks consistency and then set out to find evidence that this assumption is correct (negative internal criticism). In contrast, the investigator may assume that the document contains no error, is genuine, and that its author was qualified to make the statements contained in it. In the case of positive internal criticism, the true or literal meaning of the statements is sought.

Secondary materials can be relied on only insofar as they are in agreement with the original documents and products of the person, group, or organization. They should be used to supplement the primary documents rather than to substitute for them.

Libraries become important sources of both primary and secondary materials. Researchers must spend much time taking notes. Helmstadter discusses three types of notes: (1) bibliographical notes (included in bibliographies and reference lists), (2) subject notes (related to evidence and source of information), and (3) method notes (the researcher's thoughts, ideas, and reactions to the literature or to some aspect of the project itself).[29] If the researcher is methodical in taking notes, makes certain that they contain all necessary information, and files them carefully, frustration and loss of time are avoided.

In the historical approach, data may be divided into three major categories: (1) those that are prepared especially for posterity and have been carefully preserved, (2) those that record current events and receive contemporary use without regard for being momentos of the era, and (3) those that seem to be a combination of both. Another categorization of data pertains to their expected use. Public archival records are prepared for the purpose of examination by others, whereas private archival records are not intentionally prepared for the use of others, unless they are in the form of a published autobiography.

[29] *Ibid.,* p. 46.

Nursing and the Historical Approach

When the investigator is conducting research in nursing using the historical approach, it is necessary to meet the standards of good journalism, to practice objectivity, and to critically analyze the research findings. Such individuals should be interested in pursuing truth, in documenting sources of data, and in being specific with details. Facts are preferred over opinions. Objectivity often requires a presentation of facts that allows readers to draw their own conclusions. Some nurses believe that one strength of the historical approach is that it allows for the study of relationship between events. This also becomes a weakness, since personal biases can easily influence interpretations.

The area of research that nurses should be studying is not clear. Much depends on the specialty of the investigator. Clinical research appears to offer valuable insight into improving health care. In the minds of many individuals it seems that clinical nursing research conducted by nurses overlaps medical research. Nor is it clear where historical nursing research ends and where it becomes merely an interesting story about nurses or nursing. Investigators must therefore determine the value of a historical nursing research topic, based on their criteria.

Notter makes a strong appeal not only for nurses to be historiographers and specialists in nursing history but for some who are prepared in the historical method to be in positions of nursing leadership. She advocates preserving historical material such as reports, minutes, manuscripts, speeches, correspondence, diaries, and pictures. Such material will contribute to a historical record of nursing as it evolves. Notter further contends that historical research is not facts, figures, and data, but a study of relationships of events.[30]

One question must be answered by historical researchers before they attempt a project. Who should benefit from the historical approach? Should priority be given to the health of the general public? The nursing profession? Or nurses?

It is our opinion that when beginning researchers attempt their initial projects, they ought to select one of the approaches other than the historical so that they can develop skills in all the steps of the scientific method. Students ought to avoid the historical approach until they have gained skill using methods in which more objectivity is possible.

CROSS-CULTURAL RESEARCH

Cross-cultural research is theoretically necessary and important in considering change. No theory is relevant unless it is applicable and can predict and explain change in the past, present, and future, as well as cross-culturally. Cross-cultural means studying more than one culture at a time. We might do a cross-cultural study of nursing recruitment in the U.S., Mexico, France, Malaysia, Australia, and Argentina. For example, suppose we found that nurses recruited from rural areas are more likely to continue in their nursing career than urban nurses. If this were true in only one hospital or one agency that

[30]Notter, Lucille E.: The case for historical research in nursing, Nurs. Res. **21**(6):483, November–December 1972.

employed a few nurses, the findings would not be considered important. If, on the other hand, these findings tended to be true in the United States in the past and are also true now in foreign settings, then we have information that should be generally beneficial in nursing recruitment.

There are at least four advantages in cross-cultural research.

1. Information gained cross-culturally is more reliable than results from a study in only one country or a study of only one culture.

2. Information gained from cross-cultural studies strengthens nursing theory when hypotheses have been tested and accepted in different cultural settings.

3. Cross-cultural research is valuable to more than one society. Most studies done in single societies benefit only that society, whereas cross-cultural studies benefit several societies.

4. There is a good chance that cross-cultural research will have predictive value, since different societies are in various stages of technological progress.

The three disadvantages in cross-cultural research are major reasons why it is seldom carried out.

1. The time and the method of collecting data in cross-cultural sampling is costly.

2. Language barriers create communication difficulties.

3. Maintaining cultural meanings in an instrument's language is a major problem. For example, if an instrument is developed to note any change in attitude, value system, or judgment, how can the researcher be certain that the tool is actually communicating in a symbolic or verbal language that has equivalent meaning to all the cultural groups?

The *Human Relations Area File* is a cross-cultural collection of ethnographical studies that have been classified, coded, and computerized. In may be used for locating information about many cultural characteristics and qualities. If we trace sexual division of labor, we soon discover that cross-culturally there are almost no jobs carried out exclusively by one sex.

If the researcher decides to do a study in cultural comparisons, the variables to be compared must be universal or must at least exist in all the cultures under observation.

In conducting cross-cultural research, the researcher may investigate a community, or two or more communities, in which cross-cultural variables exist. These variables include age grading (age required to perform a specific task), sexual division of labor, habits of cleanliness, religious ceremonies, courtship patterns, kinship terminology, birth and death rites, and the prevention and cure of disease. In any case the variables must be evident in each group of subjects, and the instrument must produce comparable data from the communities under study.

There are few health workers, if any, who can say that they have only given care or counseling to patients from their own culture. Yet the average nurse has limited understanding and insight into the perceptions, attitudes, and beliefs of persons from other cultures. Nursing tends to be a matter of carrying out routine assignments, as though all patients and clients were born in the United States. The nurse-researcher, then, enters the arena of scientific investigation with little preparation to deal with cross-cultural situations.

Not only have health workers dealt with patients and clients from Spanish-speaking countries in increasing numbers, but in recent years refugees have been arriving from Southeast Asia. Because some refugees are sponsored by individuals and organizations, they may come into communities that have never before had residents from other cultures. Language difficulties may prevent communication, and even after the language barrier is overcome, the barrier of cultural understanding remains. Research is one answer to gaining insight into the cultural differences that exist in a community, and the results can provide data that are valuable for decision making.

When seeking answers to questions concerning cultures where one or more of the groups is illiterate, a means must be developed to communicate what is being asked and to be sure that the subjects can answer without relying on a written response. If the English alphabet is unknown to one of the groups, symbols may be substituted. Such a system needs to be developed and tested for reliability and validity prior to using it in the major study. A pretest and pilot study are invaluable in this situation.

To illustrate the use of symbols, suppose a study is conducted using subjects who neither read nor write English. It is decided that a triangle will mean yes and a circle will mean no. The subjects then mark their answer to each question in the appropriate symbol. For questions that have perhaps three possible answers, a circle, a triangle, and a rectangle could be used to represent the three choices for response. For instance, in some questions a circle might stand for *more*, a triangle for *the same*, and a rectangle for *less*. In items that require an expression of amount or size, graded markings could be used to represent the respondent's estimate of the variable being measured.

The use of symbols in responding to questions is not limited to answering a query; symbols also may be used in place of item numbers. Any system adopted would need to be tested for reliability and validity before it was used in the research instrument. Regardless of the kind and number of symbols selected for the tool, it is of the utmost importance that subjects not be confused by the system. It should be as simple as possible, not unduly tiring to perform, and preceded by a training period for the subjects.

In some cultures individuals do not always respond to questions for themselves. In most extended families there is one spokesman. This means that if the researcher wants to gather data in a community, family members do not respond for themselves; thus the data gathered by the researcher will be a consensus of opinion.

SUMMARY

The survey approach is a nonexperimental type of research conducted as a preliminary study to evaluate a group of people or a situation. This approach is especially valuable as a source of hypotheses and as an exploration for future research. The great strength of the survey approach is in the amount of insight that is attainable with a limited expenditure of money and time.

A survey has minimal control over extraneous variables and must rely heavily on verbal response. Surveys are used to discover causal relationships, to provide precise quantitative description, and to observe behavior. They are frequently conducted by mail, telephone, or interview. Some of the various types of surveys are school survey, public opinion poll, market survey, and motivation research. Surveys provide critical examinations of a multitude of research situations and deserve their high prestige in nursing research.

The evaluation survey is particularly suited to finding the results of a procedure or method already in operation. Its purpose is to test the effectiveness of a new program. It is especially subject to bias, because researchers often have a personal interest in the results.

When the comparative survey is used, two different groups, techniques, or categories are evaluated and compared with each other. The same measuring scale must be used on both units; however, the survey is often too small to show distinct differences between the two situations under study.

Short-term surveys, in contrast to long-term surveys, are 5 years or less in length. Investigators have no control over the outcome of either type. The long-term surveys are particularly effective in observing change over time; however, they suffer from sample attrition and are expensive.

A cross-sectional survey may accomplish some of the same goals as the long-term (or longitudinal) survey. The cross-sectional survey accomplishes its purpose by selecting several representatives at different stages of development rather than following one group for a long period of time, as does the longitudinal survey.

In the experimental design, the investigator highlights the independent variable in an effort to control and minimize the effects of all other variables. The classical experimental design uses four cells containing a control group, an experimental group, a before test, and an after test. Present research is frequently conducted using only one or two of the cells.

An advantage of the experimental method is the ability of the researcher to maintain tight control over confounding variables; it is the most powerful of all research techniques.

When using the experimental method, it is necessary to match control and experimental groups as closely as possible. Matching can be accomplished by precision matching, frequency distribution, or randomization. Of the three, randomization is most highly recommended.

Although the experimental approach is the strongest procedure for research, causal relationships are difficult to establish even under carefully controlled conditions. Many factors combine to account for change. The time element is an important variable in nursing research and sometimes plays a more important role than in the physical sciences. Other variables that must be considered are the quantity of change between control and experimental groups, the recruitment of subjects, and the difficulty of generalization.

An experiment may be carried out in the field, under normal conditions, or in the laboratory, under tight control. One advantage of the field experiment over the laboratory is that subjects do not have to be recruited or motivated, because they are in their natural situation and are available.

The Latin-square design is useful in making multiple comparisons based on randomization. It is possible to use a systematic Latin-square design when cell content or special arrangement is considered more appropriate than random assignment.

In health research, equivalent samples are difficult to obtain, and stratification matching is often used.

The retroactive experiment asks the question, "At what time in history was a new variable introduced that produced a change that is now noticeable?"

Reliability and validity are disturbing factors to the experimental researcher. Human behavior is mixed with social variables and introduces a multitude of unpredictable factors along with ethical considerations that make validity and reliability difficult to establish.

A case study is directed toward a single unit and is often conducted on one individual who seems to be representative of a larger group. It produces data for great insight in depth, but with limited breadth. Hypotheses and ideas may be generated from such an investigation. On the other hand, case studies are expensive, are subject to observer bias, are difficulty to check for accuracy, may rely heavily on recall, and tend to be initiated from negative situations. Subject attrition, the presence of the researcher, and the representativeness of the selected case must be considered.

Historical research uses data obtained from records, letters, recall, artifacts, and literature in the same manner as in other research approaches. The nursing profession can benefit from historical research by gaining insight into nursing roles, seeking information about the past, developing conclusions, and finding relationships between events. Studies may be longitudinal or cross-sectional in nature.

Advantages of historical research include the following: there are many sources of data, an appreciation of the profession's history can be gained, a knowledge of the past can lead to predictive insights, and some of the profession's failures of the past can be avoided.

Disadvantages of the historical approach include such factors as the unknown quality of recorded material (who is the author, what is the purpose, and so on), the subjective nature of the data as well as the researcher's subjective conclusions, the effect of the researcher's bias, the question of completeness, and the lack of control over past variables.

Data used in historical research come from primary or secondary sources, and the historian exercises internal (higher) or external (lower) criticism to determine if documents and various materials are genuine.

Cross-cultural research is extremely important in the development of theory. Cross-cultural, as the name applies, means that sampling is conducted in an international setting. Advantages are that the information gained cross-culturally is more useful, strengthens theory, is valuable to more societies, and has greater predictive value. Disadvantages are, of course, language and cultural barriers. These disadvantages are, nevertheless, offset by the broad, general, nonspecific testing of the research hypothesis. Thus, if an hypothesis is supported cross-culturally, it is more acceptable than if done on a small scale in one culture.

DISCUSSION QUESTIONS

1 What research topic can you think of that could be studied by all four approaches to research?
2 Why is the experiment the most powerful design for testing the relationship between variables?
3 Suggest an hypothesis suitable for testing by the retroactive design.
4 How is the historical approach to research different from writing a term paper?
5 How could the Latin-square design be used in a survey?
6 Is a cross-cultural long-term study feasible? Why or why not?
  Are surveys one of the most popular approaches to research?
7 Why are surveys one of the most popular approaches to research?
8 Suggest a field survey project that you would like to conduct.
9 Suggest a situation in which a case study might include more than one individual.
10 Suggest how all four approaches could be used to test a single hypothesis.

CLASS ACTIVITIES

Track I

1 The instructor is to select a research project and an hypothesis. The student groups are then to suggest ways in which the four approaches may be used.
2 Role play a situation in which a researcher requests permission to conduct a project using the employees of the local school system.

Track II (Steps in Research Project)

1 Each group is to determine the approach it will take in conducting its selected research project.
2 Group members and students conducting individual studies are to develop the research design for the project.
3 Students conducting individual projects are to determine the approach they will implement for their project.

SUGGESTED READINGS

Aday, L.A., and others: Methodological issues in health care surveys of the Spanish heritage population, Am. J. Public Health **70**:367–374, April 1980.

Archives—historical researchers' treasures, (editorial) Nurs. Res. **27**(2):83, March–April 1978.

Avery, D.D., and Cross, H.A., Jr.: Experimental methodology in psychology, Monterey, CA, 1978, Brooks/Cole Publishing Company.

Barnard, K.: Research designs: the historical method, The American Journal of Maternal Child Nursing **6**:391, November 1981.

Barnard, K.: The case study method: a research tool, The American Journal of Maternal Child Nursing **8**(1):36, January–February 1983.

Bauwens, E.E., editor: The anthropology of health. St. Louis, 1978, The C.V. Mosby Co.

Becoming aware of cultural differences in nursing, Speeches presented during the 1972 convention, ANA Pub. No. NP-44, Kansas City, Mo., American Nurses' Association.

Bellman, B.L., and Jules-Rosette, B.: A paradigm for looking, cross-cultural research with visual media, Norwood, N.J., 1977, Ablex Publishing Corp.

Best, J.W.: Research in education, ed. 3, Englewood Cliffs, N.J., 1977, Prentice-Hall, Inc., Chapters 4 and 5.

Bonaparte, B.H.,: Ego defensiveness, open-closed mindedness, and nurses' attitude toward culturally different patients. Nurs. Res. **28**(3):166–172, May–June 1979.

Campbell, D.T., and Stanley, J.C.: Experimental and quasi-experimental designs for research, Chicago, 1963, Rand McNally & Co.

Christy, T.E.: Portrait of a leader: Sophia F. Palmer, Nurs. Outlook **23**(12):746–751, December 1975.

Conners, C.K., and Wells, K.C.: Single-case designs in psychopharmacology, New Directions for Methodology of Social and Behavioral Sciences: Single-Case Research Designs, no. 13, San Francisco, 1982, Jossey-Bass.

Cultural dimensions in the baccalaureate nursing curriculum, National League for Nursing, Pub. No. 15-1662, New York, 1977, National League for Nursing.

de Chesnay, M.: Cross-cultural research: advantages and disadvantages, International Nursing Review **30**(1):21, January–February 1983.

Deets, C.A.: Methodological concerns in the testing of nursing interventions, Adv. Nurs. Sci. **2**(2):1–11, January 1980.

Denenberg, V.H.: Comparative psychology and single-subject research, New Directions for Social and Behavioral Sciences: Single-Case Research Designs, no. 13, San Francisco, 1982, Jossey-Bass.

Dobbert, G.A.: An online system for processing loosely structured records, Historical Methods 15(1):16–22, Winter 1982.

Fleming, J.W., and Hayter, J.: Reading research reports critically, Nurs. Outlook 22(3):174, March 1974.

Foster, S.B., Kloner, J.A., and Stengrevics, S.S.: Cardiovascular nursing research: past, present, and future, Heart & Lung 13(2):111–116, March 1984.

Fowler, F.J., Jr.: Survey research methods, Applied Social Research Methods series, Vol. 1, Beverly Hills, 1984, Sage Publications, Inc.

Garcia, C.: Developing an effective long-term prospective study, J. Gerontol. Nurs. 6:475–479, August 1980.

Garmezy, N.: The case for the single case in research, New Directions for Social and Behavioral Sciences: Single-Case Research Designs, no. 13, San Francisco, 1982, Jossey-Bass.

Gay, L.R.: Educational research: competencies for analysis and application, ed. 2, Columbus, 1981, Charles E. Merrill Publishing Company.

Glaser, W.A.: International mail surveys of informants, Human Organization 25(1):78–86, Spring 1966.

Gortner, S.R.: Knowledge in a practice discipline: philosophy and pragmatics. In Williams, C., ed.: Nursing research and policy formation: the case of prospective payment, American Academy of Nursing papers of the 1983 Scientific Session, Kansas City, 1984, American Nurses' Association.

Hacker, B.: Single-subject research strategies in occupational therapy. Research methods, case study, part I, AJOT 34:103–105, February 1980.

Hockstim, Joseph R., and Athanasopoulos, Demetrios A.: Personal follow-up in a mail survey: contribution and its cost, Public Opinion Quarterly 34(1):69–81, Spring 1970.

Hollingsworth, A.O., and others; The refugees and childbearing: what to expect, R.N. 43(11):45–48, November 1980. Jacobson, S.F.: An insider's guide to field research, Nurs. Outlook 26:371–374, June 1978.

Johnson, H.H., and Solso, R.L.: An introduction to experimental design in psychology: a case approach, ed. 2, New York 1978, Harper & Row Publishers.

Kazdin, A.E.: Single-case experimental designs in clinical research and practice, New Directions for Methodology of Social and Behavioral Sciences: Single-Case Research Design, no. 13, San Francisco, 1982, Jossey-Bass.

Kazdin, A.E. and Tuma, A.H., editors: New directions for methodology of social and behavioral science: single-case research designs, no. 13, San Francisco, 1982, Jossey-Bass.

Kovacs, Alberta R.: The personality of Florence Nightingale, Int. Nurs. Rev. 20(3):78–79, 81, May–June 1973.

Krieger, Dolores: Therapeutic touch: the imprimatur of nursing, Am. J. Nurs. 75(5):784–787, May 1975.

Leedy, P.D.: Practical research planning and design, New York, 1980, Macmillan, Inc.

Leininger, M., editor: Transcultural nursing concepts, theories and practices, New York, 1978, John Wiley & Sons.

Light, D., Jr.: Surface data and deep structure: observing the organization of professional training. In Van Maanen, J., editor: Qualitative methodology, Beverly Hills, 1983, Sage Publications, Inc.

Lutz, F.W., and Ramsey, M.A.: The use of anthropological field methods in education, Educ. Res. 3(10):6, November 1974.

Majchrzak, A.: Methods for policy research, Applied Social Research Methods Series, Vol. 3, Beverly Hills, 1984, Sage Publications, Inc.

Matejski, M.P.: Humanities: the nurse and historical research, Image 11:80–85, October 1979.

Mathis, B.C.: Evaluating the effectiveness of teaching. In Loveland, E.H., guest editor, New Directions for Program Evaluation, Measuring the hardmeasure, No. 6, 1980.

Mills, Lenore Isobel: Quality of nursing care measured by audits of nursing records and patients'
     perceptions, Research abstracts, Can. Nurs 70:42, October 1974.
Monteiro, Lois: Research into things past: tracking down one of Miss Nightingale's correspondents,
     Nurs. Res. 21(6):526–529, November–December 1972.
Newton, Mildred E.: The case for historical research, Nurs. Res. 14(1):23, Winter 1965.
Norman, E.M.: Who and where are nursing's historians? Nursing Forum 20(2):135, 1981.
Nursing research under way, Health Professions Educators Exchange of Research, August 1974, p.
     7.
O'Barr, W.M., and others, editors: Survey research in Africa, its applications and limits, Evanston,
     IL, 1973, Northwestern University Press.
Overholt, G.E, and Stallings, W.M.: Ethnographic and experimental hypotheses in educational
     research, Educ. Res. 5(8):12–14, September 1976.
Phillips, Bernard S.: Social research strategy and tactics, ed. 2, New York, 1971, Macmillan, Inc.,
     pp. 128–129.
Pless, I.B., and others: Apparent validity of alternative survey methods, J. Community Health
     5:22–27, Fall 1979.
Ragucci, Antoinette T.: The ethnographic approach and nursing research, Nurs. Res. 21(6):486,
     November–December 1972.
Riecken, Henry W., and Boruch, Robert F.: The purposes of social experimentation, Educ. Res.
     3(11):5–9, December 1974.
Rosenthal, R., and Rubin, D.B.: A simple, general purpose display of magnitude of experimental
     effect, J. of Educational Psychology 74(2):166, 1982.
Salancik, G.R.: Field stimulations for organizational behavior research. In Van Maanen, J., editor:
     qualitative methodology, Beverly Hills, 1983, Sage Publications, Inc.
Scully, Malcolm G.: The 55 sheepish goals of Dr. Fox, The Chronicle of Higher Education 8(4):1,
     5, October 15, 1973.
Simon, Julian L.: Basic research methods in social science, New York, 1969, Random House, Inc.,
     pp. 242–251.
Sjoberg, Gideon: Project Camelot: selected reactions and personal reflections, ethics, politics, and
     social research, Cambridge, Mass., 1967, Schenkman Publishing Co., Inc.
Smith, M.C., editor: Implications of research for nursing practice, education, and policymaking.
     Proceedings of the second annual SCCEN research conference, Southern Council on Collegiate
     Education for Nursing and The University of Alabama in Birmingham School of Nursing,
     December 3–4, 1982, Birmingham, AL.
Spector, R.E.: Cultural diversity in health and illness, New York, 1979, Appleton-Century-Crofts.
Wechsler, H.: Approaches and methods for data collection. In Wechsler, H., and Kibrick, A.:
     Explorations in nursing research, New York, 1979, Human Sciences Press, pp. 173–177.
Weisenberg, M., and others: Children's health beliefs and health behavior, J. Health Soc. Behav.
     21(1):59–74, March 1980.
Williams, Lillian B.: Evaluation of nursing care: a primary nursing project. Part I, Report of the
     controlled study, Supervisor Nurse 6(1):39, January 1975.
Yin, R.K.: Case study research: design and methods, Applied Social Research Methods Series,
     Vol. 5, Beverly Hills, 1984, Sage Publications, Inc.

CHAPTER 13

THE SAMPLE AND SAMPLING

THE SAMPLE

It may sound like an oversimplification to suggest the following definition of a sample: a sample is a part of the whole. There are certain circumstances or situations in which we can assume that any given part of a whole (sample) is the same as the remainder. For example, if we are sampling a jar of liquid, we would assume that if the liquid was well stirred and thoroughly mixed, any sample we removed would be of exactly the same quality and content as the liquid remaining in the jar.

In the physical world it is possible to obtain samples that are representative of the whole. By taking part of the grain from one boxcar or each boxcar of a single shipment, we are obtaining a true sample of the total contents of the boxcars. However, the social world has so many complex variables that sampling is an integral part of the methodology of research. For example, Wilson reports there was a time when the inoculation of children against diphtheria was thought to protect them against a second disease, chicken pox, as well. This belief was based on a study in which the sample of children had a low incidence of chicken pox after they had been inoculated against diphtheria. It was found later that the incidence of chicken pox was related to the nature of the sample rather than to protective action of the inoculation. The parents of the children in the sample were better educated and more careful than those of average families in general, so the researcher concluded that they had more effectively protected their children from exposure to chicken pox.[1]

Researchers seldom observe the whole (total population) for a given study. It becomes necessary then to obtain a sample that is representative of the total population with which the researchers are dealing. It may be difficult to know if the sample is truly representative of the whole. The researcher must select a sampling technique that most accurately reflects the characteristics of the population being studied.

The term *population* refers to the entire number of units under study (the whole), for example, all the inhabitants living in city X including every man, woman, and child living within the city limits. The researcher takes a sample of the inhabitants of city X before making a statement about the people who compose the total population.

[1] Wilson, E. Bright, Jr.: An introduction to scientific research, New York, 1952, McGraw-Hill, Inc., p. 154.

The researcher utilizing the sample finding wants to say something about the population that the sample represents. Thus, it is of the utmost importance that the population be clearly defined, so that the sample can be accurately identified.

TYPES OF SAMPLING

Various types of sampling are possible. One type is, of course, the simple random sample that we have already discussed. The use of *a simple random sample* means that the selection of the units in the sample is chosen by some sort of chance. The alert researcher is aware that it is impossible to see all the pertinent points of view, but tries to make the sample as representative as possible. In analyzing the situation, the researcher attempts to randomize his/her ignorance in all conceivable areas. If no endeavor is made to control any particular factor except by simply taking units for the sample by pure chance (such as drawing names out of a hat, one by one), the researcher is able to overcome variables and problems that might otherwise bias the study.

Stratified sampling or stratified random sampling involves taking certain areas of the population, dividing the areas into sections, and then taking a random sample from each section. For example, we might want to know how people in the United States would vote on a particular health issue. To accomplish this polling, we might decide to take the same percentage of people from each of the 50 states. A number of factors must be considered in designing plans for a stratified sample. Certainly we would be interested in including both men and women, and the opinions of people of various ages, socioeconomic backgrounds, and occupations.

Although we have treated it separately, a stratified sample still employs randomness. In fact, stratification incorporates randomness as the additional measure calculated to increase representativeness. This additional effort is to ensure that important variables will be sufficiently represented. The homogeneity of the sampled strata will be increased, since subjects in each category are alike in relation to the selected variable.

The basic consideration involved in stratified random sampling is the fact that a homogeneous universe requires a smaller sample than a heterogeneous universe. There are two requirements for a homogeneous sample: first, its divisions must be correlated with the variables being studied, and second, the criterion must not provide so many subjects in the subunit that it increases the required sample over that required by simple random sampling techniques.

The word *stratified* comes from strata, meaning various sections of, or layers. Stratified sampling is better than completely random sampling if the members that compose sections or strata are more uniform in each property studied than the whole population. For this reason, it is necessary that the characteristics of the total population be studied before stratified sampling is undertaken.

Cost is a major factor in the decision to utilize stratified sampling. Another factor to consider is that stratification allows for efficient use of the researcher's time and is an effective method for approximating the mean and other parameters of a population.

In this type of sampling, known factors are used to divide the population into groups, so that the units in the sample are more alike than the units in the population as a whole. It is by stratified sampling that the person doing research can reduce the chance of obtaining a nontypical sample. If, for example, we are interested in studying the dating habits of nursing students, we will find that some are married, some are going steady, and some may or may not be dating. This means that we would have four types of people to include in our sample. We might decide to limit our sample to those nursing students who are actually dating, or we might decide to study the habits of dating and nondating in nursing students.

The question of sample size becomes an important consideration in stratified sampling. Do we take the same number of each subclass, or do we choose a representative number of them? If 50% are dating and 10% are not dating, should the sample percentage be 5 daters to each nondater? Or do we have the same number of daters and nondaters for comparison? The proportions can be selected in advance for stratified random sampling according to whatever subdivision or stratum seems best. Random selection should be used for the actual sampling procedure. Continuing our example, if we used an equal number of daters and nondaters, the responses from the nondaters would be more varied than if there were five times more daters than nondaters. The nondaters would overrepresent the population in the case of equal-sized samples.

Another type of sampling is called *quota* or *purposive sampling.* In this procedure the researcher selects some special group because there is good evidence that it is representative of the total population he/she wishes to study. An example of this technique is the study mentioned earlier in which the researcher investigated the attitudes of the student body on certain religious factors. He learned that there were two required courses that could be taken any time during an academic career. Further checking revealed that the two courses were composed of students from various majors and from all class levels. It was assumed that there would be proportional numbers of men and women, so the two classes were sampled. The investigators checked the percentages of men and women, the types of majors, and the percentages in each class level in the institution. The figures were later compared with those of the sample, and although there were small differences, it was concluded that the sample was basically representative. The purposive sample was valuable to the college administration for planning future changes.

When its use is appropriate, the purposive method is an efficient and effective manner of sampling. The technique is left up to the researcher. If he/she is told by the funding organization that certain characteristics are to be studied, such as age, sex, economic status, or race, the researcher must carry out the organization's desires. When the purposive method is used in the field, the researcher must select the subgroups of subjects and attempt to represent each type of the desired characteristic. At the end of the day or the week, the researcher will total the number in each subgroup category and then purposely include more or fewer of the subgroup categories as sampling continues. Such a procedure could lead to biases (in the researcher) such as not wanting to go to certain kinds of places, talking with certain age groups, and so on. It also might lead to biases that are unintentional or unobserved.

In the use of any method other than the random sample, there are too many variables to try to select all the characteristics; but the random sample is not subjected to variations. Therefore, a large sample should be representative of the total population. This would not be the case in any other sampling technique.

Another type of sampling is *systematic sampling*. The systematic sample includes every n^{th} name from a roster of names, or, for example, every fifth house on the block, or every third patient on every floor.

Frequently, problems arise that must be anticipated in planning for the sample. For example, if the telephone book is chosen as representative of the population, not everyone may be listed in a given directory. The investigator may go through a city and select every fifth house, but it may be that the blocks are arranged so that the fifth house is located on a corner. Built-in bias may occur, possibly because people living in corner houses have more money.

Wilson suggests that in systematic samplings, rather than take the same n^{th} number every time, we might start with 6 one time (taking every sixth one), and continue 12, 18, and so on. Another time we might start with 4, and continue 10, 16, 22, and so on throughout the sampling. Care must be taken to avoid round numbers such as 10, 100, or 1,000 because there might be some sort of multiple of these numbers that may have been purposely set apart when the numbering system was instituted.[2] For example, the first house in the block usually has an even hundred number (400, 500, 600, and so on).

If the researcher decides to use a systematic random sample, Simon advises that it is better to use two or more systematic subsamples that originate in different randomly chosen places rather than one systematic sample of double size. This procedure results in reducing the danger of an unrepresentative start, such as the use of corner houses just mentioned, as well as permitting rapid inspection of the subsamples for estimating the amount of sampling error that might be present. There is practically no extra cost in this useful procedure.[3]

The *cluster sampling* technique is one in which a small sample of various sections of a larger sample, or various sections of the total population, are taken. A single subject can appear in only one cluster. As an illustration, suppose we desire to conduct a study of nurses' attitudes within the state, but it is too expensive to contact all the nurses. The next best method is to include a few nurses from each county in the state for the sample. There are several advantages in doing this: the cost is reduced; such a procedure is easy to administer; and a large selection is made, which might not be chosen otherwise. At the same time, the entire state is sampled. The use of cluster sampling decreases transportation time and reduces the cost of interviewing or mailing questionnaires.

The researcher may well consider use of the cluster sample in gathering responses from 200 nurses in a large hospital. He/she might question 5 persons from the same hospital unit or 5 nurses who are taking their coffee break. The advantage of using a cluster sample in this instance is that the 200 subjects can be obtained in clusters of 5 rather than obtaining 200 individual subjects. There is no certainty of the accuracy or advantage of a completely random sample of 200 individual cases versus 40 subsamples of 5-cluster size. Although some randomness or representativeness may be lost, the overall saving in cost and time may be worth the loss in accuracy.

Multistage sampling is undertaken by randomly sampling a percentage of a population and then within each of its selected areas randomly sampling smaller subunits. If we

[2] Wilson, p. 163.
[3] Simon, Julian L.: Basic research methods in social science, New York, 1969, Random House, Inc., p. 41.

wanted to take a survey of the nurses in state Y where there were 30,000 registered nurses, we could use multistage sampling as follows. Assume that we decide that a sample of 1,000 is adequate, based on time and cost. If there are 50 counties, then each county should be represented by 20 randomly selected nurses. However, since some counties have more nurses than others, each county should be sampled on a percentage basis. If 60 registered nurses live in county X, a 1 to 30 ratio would yield a sample of 2. The 2 registered nurses would be selected randomly. If we wanted representation from particular cities within each county, they would be selected in the same manner. The sample could be selected on a percentage basis or simply by random sample.

Cluster sampling can be part of multistage sampling, or the various stages can be eliminated, and a number of individuals can be chosen in a unit. For example, we could select clusters of 5 individuals from 4 different townships as a cluster sample; or we could divide the state into counties, selecting 5 counties and then dividing each county into township or census tract areas. One individual is then selected from each township. This is known as multistage sampling because the sampling has been conducted by dividing the population into units that are of decreasing size.

Most authors agree that a complete listing of the population is not necessary in multistage sampling. However, we feel that a complete listing of the population is always advantageous to the investigator. The more knowledgeable researchers are about the population, the more intelligently they can select their sampling procedure and perform the other steps of the research process.

Multistage sampling is valuable and fairly accurate for any population that lacks a complete listing. In addition, the cost of multistage sampling is much less than for most other types of sampling.

Sequential sampling is another technique used in certain instances. In this procedure, the investigator examines subjects in turn, until the results are adequately satisfying, from a statistical viewpoint, to warrant ceasing the collection of data.[4] For example, in sequential sampling, test results of the octane rating in gasoline would be continued until the predetermined rating has fallen outside some selected critical limit.

In the health care setting, the researcher hypothesizes that procedure X will relieve patient anxiety. It is decided that 7 out of 10 favorable responses will be sufficient to adopt procedure X. If after 4 trials there is no improvement, the researcher can cease testing because there is no possibility that the hypothesis can be accepted.

Incidental sampling utilizes readily available subjects. As a means of obtaining a sample of the organization's employees the researcher might question respondents who come to the coffee shop at break time. Obviously, this leaves something to be desired. For example, two shifts would not be included unless the researcher decided to go to the coffee shop during each shift. Management may go to another coffee shop, and some individuals may not choose to go to the coffee shop at all.

The only way it would be possible to generalize from the sample obtained in the coffee shop would be to describe and explain how the results were obtained. All conclusions and generalizations from such a sampling would have to be based on a description of the sampling technique.

---

[4] Wilson, p. 163.

LONGITUDINAL VERSUS CROSS-SECTIONAL TECHNIQUES

Longitudinal sampling can be contrasted with cross-sectional sampling in that two different time periods are used. The techniques, however, may be somewhat the same. The longitudinal sampling technique follows a given group of subjects for an extended period of time, whereas the cross-sectional technique observes subjects at only one point in time. Let us consider an illustration of each technique with vocational choice as the focus of our interest. Vocational choice is the selection of one's regular field of employment. Important work in this field has been done by Eli Ginzberg, Donald Super, and David Tiedeman.

In the longitudinal approach, the sample is selected at a period in time (such as junior high or senior high school) in which the study group is asked, among other questions, what vocation they wish to follow. Then at predesignated time periods, each participant is questioned again about various facets of his vocational choice. These contacts may be made on a yearly basis at first and then every fifth year later on. Or the study may begin when the students are completing junior high school, senior high school, and the sophomore and senior years in college, or a vocational school of some type. Later contacts may be made to see if they remain in the field they have selected. The researcher chooses time periods based on an understanding of the variables in the research study. The longitudinal study technique would be better in this case for noting how the subjects' choice of vocation changed or remained stable over time.

In the cross-sectional approach, the subjects are asked at the time of the study when they made their vocational choice. Instead of following the same group of subjects for 40 years, the researcher has at least two alternatives: recently retired subjects may be selected to provide data based on recall about their vocational career, or subjects categorized into different age groups may be asked to provide data about their current vocation.

Advantages and Disadvantages of the Longitudinal Technique

The advantages of using the longitudinal approach are as follows:
1. The data are more accurate since the subject does not have to reply by recall.
2. Each individual is followed separately, and it is possible to observe and interpret any variations near the time they occur.
3. The observer will be able to make more objective observations about a given event than the subject who simply makes a subjective recall.
4. The researcher can pursue in depth a particular point of interest.
5. Early apparent trends can be investigated in depth at forthcoming data collection points.
   Disadvantages of the longitudinal approach include the following:
1. It may take many years before the results of the study are known.
2. There is the danger of a loss of participants. Both researcher and subjects may lose interest, they may move to a different location, funds may be depleted, and so on. There are always fewer subjects in the sample at the end of the study than at the beginning.
3. It is costly in time and money.

4. There is a confounding of variables because the subject is aware of being under investigation. Repeated collection of data may even influence the actual behavior of the subject.

Fig. 13-1 is a hypothetical example of a longitudinal study made over a 15-year period, showing the attrition of subjects. Fig. 13-2, in contrast, is a cross-sectional study of 100 people who have smoked from 1 to 15 years. All 100 cross-sectional subjects can be questioned, whereas the longitudinal sample has been reduced over the years to 61 subjects. The cross-sectional study is much less expensive, has no opportunity for attrition, and takes a short period of time to collect all the data.

The National Longitudinal Study of the High School Class of 1972 is an example of longitudinal research. The focus of this study was on the graduates' access to higher education.

In the spring of 1972, a national sample of 19,136 seniors from 1,070 schools was first contacted. Follow-up surveys were repeated in October 1973, October 1974, and October 1976. For this research project, respondents were added from additional schools to replace losses. Follow-up was accomplished through questionnaires and interviews. The results of the data contributed to an understanding of the trends and the changes in college attendance.[5]

It should be noted that in Fig. 13-1 there is no replacement for subjects who moved, died, or for other reasons were lost from the study. Replacing missing subjects has the advantage of maintaining the sample size, but, as in the case of the longitudinal study,

[5] Peng, S.S., Bailey, J.P., Jr., and Ekland, B.K.: Access to higher education: results from the national longitudinal study of the high school class of 1972, Educ. Res. **6**(11):3–7, December 1977.

Year 1 (1970)*	Year 5 (1975)	Year 10 (1980)	Year 15 (1985)
Study begins with 100 subjects	— Study continues with 91 of first subjects. (9 subjects have died, unable to locate, etc.)	— Study continues with 77 subjects. (Attrition continues for same reasons as previously.)	— Study continues with 61 subjects. (Attrition continues for same reason.)

*Data collected January-February 1970, 1975, 1980, 1985.

FIGURE 13-1 Longitudinal study on the effects of smoking.

DESCRIPTION OF SUBJECTS*

100 subjects
    Ages 20 to 25 years.
    Have been smoking from 1 to 15 years.

Number	Years smoking
25	1
25	5
25	10
25	15

*Data collected January-February 1981.

FIGURE 13-2 Cross-sectional study on the effects of smoking.

replacements have had 1 year to mature before entering the study. They also do not know what questions were asked and in some ways might be different from the original sample. This may or may not add a new dimension to the longitudinal study.

In following up the subjects of longitudinal studies, it is obviously necessary to match the names with the data. This could be considered a breach of confidentiality. Astin and Boruch report on the "link" system for assuring confidentiality in longitudinal studies. In this system unrelated identifying numbers are substituted in the name and address file. To further ensure confidentiality, a "link" file is created, containing two sets of numbers, the original set of numbers substituted for the names and the new set of identifying numbers. This third file is deposited at a computer center in a foreign country. The foreign country is under an agreement not to allow anyone to see or use the two sets of identifying numbers. Such a system protects the information from congressional or judicial subpoena[6] as well.

Longitudinal studies in nursing are conducted by professional organizations. One such study is the Longitudinal Study of Nurse Practitioners. Baseline data were gathered from students who graduated between May 1974 and June 1975. Data also were collected from the nursing programs involved. The initial group of students was to be followed in phases II and III of the study.[7]

A longitudinal study may be extended if the researcher determines the need for such an extension. The dates for collecting follow-up data may vary according to the study design. Longitudinal studies are appropriate for nursing organizations, educational institutions, and patient and client followup.

[6] Astin, A.W., and Boruch, R.F.: A "link" system for assuring confidentiality of research data in longitudinal studies, vol. 5, No. 3, American Council on Education, Office of Research, Washington, D.C., February 1970, ACE Research Reports.
[7] Sultz, H.A., Zielezny, M., and Kinyon, L.: Longitudinal study of nurse practitioners, phase I, DHEW Pub. No. (HRA)76-43, Washington, D.C., March 1976, Department of Health, Education, and Welfare.

Advantages and Disadvantages of the Cross-Sectional Technique

Cross-sectional sampling is much more common than the longitudinal approach to research. Some of the major advantages of this approach are as follows:

1. It can be completed in a relatively short time.
2. The variables will not be confounded by time.
3. It is relatively inexpensive as compared with the longitudinal approach.
4. The results are known immediately without the researcher waiting for years to complete the study.
5. The researcher is able to have a larger sample; that is, sample loss is minimal.
6. All subjects respond at approximately the same time. For example, they all respond to the same mailing, interview schedule, experiment, and so on.
7. The researcher does not have to be concerned with contacting the members of the sample again.

   The disadvantages of cross-sectional sampling include the following:

1. The researcher must be content with biased recall on the part of the respondents.
2. The method does not allow for a composite picture of the respondents' feelings and emotions but must rely on a single incident or time when the subjects may have been emotionally upset or ill.
3. The researcher cannot tell if change is the result of a personality characteristic or a series of circumstances beyond the control of the subject.
4. The method can only consider the present and the past, whereas the longitudinal approach can deal with the past, present, and future, thereby showing changing trends or patterns over a period of time.

MEANS OF OBTAINING TRUE SAMPLES

There are a number of ways of obtaining samples. The process by which sampling is done is called *sampling variation*. There are negative and positive aspects to all kinds of sampling, but random sampling is best done through random choice. *Random sampling* is a process by which the researcher obtains the sample without aiming for specific individuals, objects, or conditions. Random choice allows every member of the population equal chance to be included in the sample representing the total population.

Wilson suggests that an ideal method for selecting a random sample is a perfect roulette wheel. All the subjects in the population are assigned a number along the edges of the roulette wheel in equally spaced intervals. The wheel is spun, and the persons whose numbers are selected by the pointer are included in the sample. The process of spinning the wheel is repeated until the desired size of the sample has been reached; every person in the population thus has an equal chance of being included in the sample.[8] There is no process for selecting a sample that allows better representation than does some method of random choice.

In obtaining a random sample, it is necessary to know the total population. A clear definition of the subjects is necessary so that everyone knows exactly who or what should

---

[8] Wilson, p. 155.

be included in the sample. For example, in a study investigating the background characteristics of people living in a certain area of the city, it was necessary for the researcher to develop precise definitions to differentiate rooming houses, household dwellings, apartment buildings, and apartment houses.

On occasion, it is possible to test a sampling against known factors. For example, if we were sampling a group of nursing students, we might want to see the percentage of seniors in the population as compared with the percentage of seniors in the sample. We also might want to know the percentage of individuals in the sample who came from a farm versus the percentage who came from urban areas. We could then compare those figures with the figures for the population to test the representativeness of the sample. It is certain that our sample could not be representative of every background and characteristic. There might be a single individual with an exceptionally high intellectual ability, or another born into a wealthy family. If there was only one individual uniquely different from the remainder of the subjects, that person might or might not be included in the sample.

If we wanted to study the effectiveness of patient teaching in a large inner-city hospital, and our concern was to compare the learning successes of two ethnic groups, we would need predetermined percentages of each group in our sample. This ought to be commensurate with the total population in the area. On the other hand, if the total number of patients from both ethnic groups is small, the researcher might decide to include the total hospital population of both ethnic groups or he/she might extend the data-gathering period until a larger number of subjects from each ethnic group is contacted and included.

Sampling requires a degree of insight into the background characteristics of the population area under investigation. The more knowledgeable the researcher is about the topic being studied, the better equipped he/she is to recognize the variables involved in selecting a representative sample. For example, how accessible are individuals for inclusion in a study? The student may decide to administer his instrument to patients on the third floor of the hospital. He plans to spend Monday through Thursday gathering data on individuals having at least a 3-day hospital stay. Instead of having at least 75 subjects in the study (there are 90 beds on the third floor), the census drops, and it takes longer to administer the instrument than anticipated because of interruptions by physicians, nurses, the telephone, and laboratory personnel. The discharge of patients eliminates 20 prospective respondents, and 4 patients are too ill to participate. The student had given his attention to the size of the sample and the quality of his instrument but had neglected the pattern of patient admission-discharge, possible hospital interruptions, patient attitudes toward research, and the number of patients who might be too ill to participate.

There are various ways to get a random sample. As mentioned previously, the roulette wheel is one method. Another method for selecting a random sample is to list the population, assign each a number, and throw these into a hat. The numbers are mixed thoroughly and then withdrawn one at a time until the desired sample size is obtained.

This method of random selection raises the question of whether or not to replace the number into the hat after it has been withdrawn and listed. There are important implications involved with this decision of whether or not the number is placed back into the hat. Suppose the researcher wishes to study a group of 20 adults, 15 of whom are females and 5, males, The sample is to be 5 of the group. If sampling with replacement is followed, after sex is determined, the male is returned to the population where he can be selected again. If Z equals the number of males in the sample, the possible values for Z are 0, 1, 2, 3, 4, 5. The probability of choosing a male each time is given by $P(M) = n(M)/N(S) = 5/20 = 1/4$. The probability of choosing a female each time is computed by $P(F) = n(F)/N(S) = 15/20 = 3/4$. Legend: P, probability; M, males; F, females; N, number of population; n, number of sample; S, sample. Sampling in this case is independent because one selection is not affected by the next selection.

Let us look at the same problem, this time drawing a sample *without* replacement. This time the probability of choosing a male does not remain constant. For example, if a male is selected first, the probability of choosing a male during the second selection is 4/19. But if a female is selected on the first drawing, the probability of choosing a male on the next drawing is 5/19. It is not 5/20 in either case. This explanation of the probability of outcomes is based on the concept of equally likely events.[9]

Another method of obtaining a random sample is by the use of a random number table (Fig. 13-3). The researcher enters the table at any position and proceeds in orderly fashion row by row or column by column until the required sample is obtained. For example, a sample of 10 students is desired from a class of 80 seniors. Each student is assigned a number from 1 to 80. The researcher arbitrarily decides where to enter the table and which direction to go. Let us suppose that he decides to move from left to right in the row selected. He then moves to the row underneath and again proceeds from left to right, and so on. To enter the table, he could close his eyes and place his finger on the table and start at this point. Suppose the number he touches is the twelfth set of digits in the second row (23). He needs the first 10 numbers of 80 or less for his sample. Thus, the following numbers make the sample: 23, 14, 11, 66, 63, 24, 70, 34 (00—cannot use), 71, (99 and 92 are too large to use since the entire class is only 80), and 49. This particular table works well for small samples. If several hundred numbers were needed, it would be inadequate, because it does not provide for 3-digit numbers in the case of hundreds or 4-digit numbers in the case of thousands.

Population lists have been used at times as a source of a representative sample. However, usually such lists are nonexistent, incomplete, or out of date. If the population is relatively small in number, it is more likely that a list of the members is available, and it is hoped that the list is accurate.

The U.S. Census Bureau is one of the groups that often uses the multistage area-sampling technique. This is a process whereby randomly selected areas of the population are chosen to be included in the survey. The technique is further described on pp. 218–219.

Researchers enjoy telling stories of investigations in which the samples have prejudiced the findings. One well-known study dealt with the number of people of each religious faith who were having weddings. June was selected since it is usually thought of as the month for weddings. The investigators did not know that persons of the Jewish faith do not have weddings during the seven weeks after Passover nor during the three weeks prior to Tishah b'ab day (which is a day of mourning). This time period usually covers at least

[9] Marascuilo, Leonard A.: Statistical methods for behavioral science research, New York, 1971, McGraw-Hill, Inc., pp. 99–100.

```
20 09 54 18 10 49 53 20 29 11 61 32 52 06 56 20 10 38 29 96 05 01 37 99 11 32
37 42 44 92 89 62 39 80 96 99 86 23 14 11 66 63 24 70 34 00 71 99 92 49 13 74
20 80 24 12 87 56 56 05 70 10 46 61 70 51 58 22 96 40 59 60 86 65 36 87 31 10
15 68 56 48 84 93 02 49 15 78 73 46 26 22 37 84 02 31 64 22 73 94 31 90 71 46
93 15 26 67 10 63 99 16 81 49 73 44 24 67 32 47 66 86 08 14 33 44 78 97 18 30
03 71 18 44 50 31 48 18 23 96 48 21 06 89 23 63 00 09 97 85 58 35 66 61 28 25
84 31 97 89 14 96 13 61 83 59 79 12 87 04 18 40 20 11 50 28 61 48 87 44 06 53
26 06 24 52 95 01 65 30 06 10 84 92 93 22 20 56 57 72 57 99 25 70 69 19 98 43
07 09 38 25 04 65 17 20 75 07 69 63 69 10 37 31 44 66 12 39 85 54 52 02 82 33
95 03 87 65 81 03 86 59 16 03 62 88 19 19 63 32 93 05 72 94 52 78 13 63 91 30
61 94 07 43 67 25 66 92 74 77 97 32 69 76 58 25 79 15 44 55 02 38 73 19 96 62
56 81 76 05 32 62 69 99 94 05 05 85 17 10 73 59 62 22 60 68 44 93 55 92 48 59
86 72 78 41 95 08 67 30 65 95 44 50 40 29 08 65 67 45 27 81 33 16 96 58 09 52
54 75 26 06 31 52 40 70 99 12 26 35 99 71 63 18 52 50 09 02 24 57 12 03 02 01
38 94 08 93 95 38 06 71 72 80 30 74 21 08 10 91 85 70 90 68 03 75 10 86 10 78
07 80 46 11 90 58 89 94 97 21 12 25 05 73 71 32 03 11 66 37 44 29 42 75 75 76
88 50 51 24 19 33 41 09 86 10 94 70 74 99 39 58 64 53 70 07 09 62 50 56 67 81
15 97 57 96 75 56 68 65 97 29 19 47 17 22 81 21 35 81 94 46 23 41 39 54 26 78
54 79 88 81 42 21 91 38 47 51 36 25 79 78 24 43 12 59 38 22 80 04 56 74 65 66
75 85 66 33 52 21 89 44 90 49 26 74 40 83 67 37 14 74 66 61 70 22 58 66 18 53
00 13 21 22 16 00 98 72 65 81 58 01 73 67 19 36 06 65 54 55 11 24 37 30 06 11
71 94 55 21 12 81 23 78 46 98 03 40 97 49 61 62 54 35 65 65 36 37 05 82 24 82
57 58 60 36 59 97 02 01 71 64 38 67 03 17 93 92 15 20 68 65 85 27 44 28 04 80
79 79 71 49 24 15 99 69 00 36 20 23 01 29 94 54 29 66 69 26 29 88 91 43 94 34
47 98 26 41 63 08 11 99 04 76 38 61 88 05 66 44 54 92 10 89 39 17 60 78 97 71
05 64 93 40 12 20 75 35 34 63 96 36 93 43 65 14 19 36 54 78 91 51 63 94 01 77
00 84 17 34 41 10 40 47 60 98 94 26 10 54 59 05 66 26 27 72 65 43 49 18 93 76
18 65 50 05 76 03 82 95 54 20 92 77 57 54 38 45 01 73 64 62 05 58 11 51 20 20
60 60 76 75 12 92 87 41 97 28 53 75 19 93 06 08 57 15 31 56 44 15 33 46 55 14
17 67 54 91 82 94 59 46 43 98 77 30 34 89 98 64 61 28 27 25 69 28 71 14 07 16
74 13 15 78 81 02 98 91 18 06 86 15 37 27 96 71 62 44 42 89 89 70 38 37 66 92
32 93 57 33 80 92 07 48 75 39 95 93 81 04 03 75 56 18 67 25 28 08 71 75 01 04
74 01 40 47 25 97 77 31 10 73 78 68 45 55 45 17 59 52 81 94 33 38 46 27 26 30
69 36 01 63 85 62 50 52 53 95 15 76 59 20 79 06 21 23 65 60 34 29 68 18 77 16
01 53 85 65 34 40 65 14 27 22 21 79 68 95 22 20 35 49 26 49 43 20 28 73 79 49
42 55 14 47 79 69 04 42 73 12 76 41 70 23 59 65 03 69 46 59 55 41 12 02 00 14
07 31 98 53 15 89 75 07 05 25 04 14 80 89 30 64 42 85 16 05 57 20 17 22 72 75
61 04 37 16 72 47 78 91 33 70 31 21 95 10 08 23 21 63 35 03 47 19 94 90 28 06
44 96 38 19 06 14 05 56 06 06 92 86
```

FIGURE 13-3   A small table of random digits.
From Wilson, E. Bright, Jr.: An introduction to scientific research, New York, copyright 1952 by McGraw-Hill, Inc. Used with permission of McGraw-Hill, Inc.

part of the month of June. Therefore, when the study was completed, the researchers found many Protestant and Catholic weddings in June, but few Jewish weddings in June during the 10-year coverage.[10] Had they been aware of the Jewish custom, their sample would have been considerably different. When any kind of alteration in sampling procedure is followed, except for pure random sampling, it is possible to unexpectedly alter the results in some unforeseen manner.

Another biased sampling technique involves using the telephone book to obtain a random sample of the population of a city. In one study predicting the election of Tom Dewey to the presidency, a telephone sample was used. The findings were invalid, because not everyone in the community, especially poor residents, had a telephone. Using the telephone book had provided an unbalanced sample.

Even today an increasing number of people has unlisted telephone numbers, including the wealthy, the famous, the harassed, single women, political figures, and people in hiding. Low-income families may not be able to afford a telephone and therefore are not available to be contacted by researchers. In our mobile society about one fifth of all American families move each year, so their names are not listed in the current telephone directories for at least part of the year.

Creative sampling techniques are certainly valuable and desirable, but it is expedient to do some careful checking and comparing of methods and sampling.

SAMPLING ERROR

Sampling error is defined as the error (differences, variations) between the means (averages) of two samples or between the mean of the sample and the mean of the total population if it were available. We do not assume that the sample mean is truly representative of the mean of the total population; it is only an attempt to approximate by taking a portion of the whole. If we are interested in the average age of nurses employed in state X, we can take a sample from two counties to see how their average ages compare. The means for the two groups would probably differ, just as each mean would differ from the total population mean. These differences in means are caused by sampling error. Such error occurs when a sample is not truly representative. For example, suppose a researcher is taking a sample of the students in a given school. It happens that 60% of the student body is male. If it is found that 50% of the sample is male, this is a sampling error in which females are overrepresented. A truly random sample, if large enough, should minimize errors of this kind.

Wilson has suggested that sampling errors are caused by inadequate instruments, personal errors, mathematical mistakes, and random variations.[11] Instrument failure could be caused by an inaccurate stopwatch or a poorly worded questionnaire; a personal error includes those errors resulting from poor judgment, incorrect reading of instruments, and inadequate training; random variation involves chance occurrences that are beyond the control of the researcher.

[10] Goode, William J., and Hatt, Paul K.: Methods in social research, New York, 1952, McGraw-Hill, Inc., p. 218.
[11] Wilson, pp. 232–234.

Sampling error is defined in terms that make possible the quantification of error in a study. Specifically, it is "the ratio of the variation of the values of the measurements among the sampling units of a target population to the square root of the number of sampling units in the sample," according to Abdellah and Levine.[12]

FACTORS THAT LIMIT SIZE

A sample is used in research when it is not feasible to study the whole population from which it is drawn. Other factors, such as cost, limited time, and lack of accessibility, prohibit a direct study of the total population.

Some researchers say that we should take as large a sample size as is financially possible. Sometimes budgets are allocated according to the size of the sample; at other times, the sample size is dictated by the size of the budget. Even in the case of small studies done by students, cost may dictate the sample size. Before we decide what the sample size should be, it is important to select a small trial sample to determine patterns or characteristics that are representative of the total population.

Another factor that may determine the size of the sample is the amount of time available. If time is limited, or if subjects in the population are difficult to contact, the researcher will necessarily limit sample size to availability. For example, a researcher and his students in a methods course were interested in obtaining a sample of a group of 1,000 students to determine their religious beliefs. Attending chapel was defined as the criterion in the study. Preliminary investigation revealed that three required courses had a wide representation of students from many study disciplines and all educational levels. A questionnaire was completed by 180 students in these three courses. The question that had to be answered was, "Is the sample representative?" If 60% of the student body were men, then the sample was partially representative if it also contained approximately 60% male respondents. Other factors considered were educational level, major, marital status, place of residence, and home town. Percentages of these factors were computed for the whole student body. The sample had similar percentages and it was concluded that the sample was fairly representative of the total student body, based on the variables under study. It is evident that we cannot cover long periods of time in the sampling process. It may be that our sample will include people or units available only at present, not during the past or in the future.

The size of the population is a factor in determining the size of the sample. A measure or value that describes the characteristics of a sample is called a statistic. Similar measures or values of the population are called parameters. Since it would usually be time-consuming or costly to determine the parameters of the population, the researcher uses samples and works with statistics.

Suppose we want to find out the attitude of students at a local college toward certain types of nursing programs. All the students are the population; any quantity of students less than the total number is the sample. In certain instances, 10% of the total population might be a feasible sample size for a population of 1,000 units. A sample of 10%, however,

[12]Abdellah, Faye G., and Levine, Eugene: Better patient care through nursing research, ed. 2, New York, copyright 1979, Macmillan, Inc., p. 347.

is obviously too small if our total population is only 10. On the other hand, a 10% sample of the inhabitants of a city with a population of 1 million people would be too costly and time-consuming to undertake under normal conditions. A much smaller sample (such as 2%) would still include a wide enough variety of variables and characteristics (extreme cases on both ends) to cover almost every conceivable type of deviation.

The gain in accuracy from including all the members of a population in a research study is often not worth the time and expense required. For example, in national surveys where attempts are made to forecast the popular vote, experts are often able to predict accurately the total vote for each candidate by using a small sample of people. During the reporting of the actual voting in a presidential election, it may have seemed at times that the predictions were incorrect; and yet when the final tally was made, the predictions were relatively accurate. Likewise, it would not be necessary to include the total population of 5,000 adults if we were interested in the clients' opinions about hypertension screening. A sample of 200 would probably be sufficient.

In some studies sampling rather than researching the entire population will better control the Hawthorne effect, which is the influencing of the actions of the subjects by the study itself. If the entire population was polled to determine anticipated voting preference, the citizens might be influenced to vote at the actual election as they said they would; whereas in reality people often change their minds many times before making a decision about a candidate. It seems easier to control such bias through the sample than through the entire population.

Again, when certain types of experiments are done, it may be more desirable to study a few persons' reactions rather than those of the total population. This is especially true when experimenting with a new drug or an unusual technique. It is more feasible to try a new drug on a few subjects and observe their reaction than to try it initially on a whole population before the consequences are known.

Finally, when we are using nonhuman subjects in a study, the subject is often destroyed; thus it is cheaper to sample or work with just a few subjects. Animals are frequently used in research, and they must be cared for adequately (food, housing, and so on) prior to and during the research process. Such maintenance may be costly in time, effort, and materials for the researchers. Humane consideration, as well as cost factors, dictates smaller samples.

SAMPLE SIZE INFLUENCED BY TECHNIQUE

Walker and Lev state that the decision on how large a sample should be is related not only to the matters of cost and time but also the plans for an investigation. If there is a small difference between two populations, a large sample is needed to show this difference.[13] An example of this is never more clear than in the U.S. presidential election. Quite often in a close presidential election, the largest number of votes will sway back and forth from one candidate to another. Only when the last state has reported will the final result be known. What if there was one more large state such as California? Would this swing the

[13] Walker, Helen M., and Lev, Joseph: Elementary statistical methods, rev. ed., New York, 1958, Henry Holt and Co., Inc., pp. 163–164.

election the other way? This is the problem that the researcher must consider when looking for differences. The rule is that there should be a fairly large sample size if the difference is small.

When the difference observed by the researcher is not significant, he/she may wonder how to interpret the findings. Is the real difference zero, or is the sample too small to find out if any difference actually exists? If the researcher has decided in advance how large the sample size should be to find a difference of predetermined size, the case is stronger than if the researcher has not decided in advance. Also, if the researcher has determined the sample size in advance and finds that there is no difference between the two, the statement can be made, with some confidence, that there is no difference.

Several decisions must be made to determine the size of the sample. The investigator must answer the following questions before the sample size is determined.

1. How big a risk do I want to take in deciding what the significant difference is going to be? Will it be at the .01 or .05 level? Here again we are considering type I or type II error and the risk involved in making a decision. Suppose, for example, that we find there is some risk involved in using a new medication. How much risk do we want to take? If a researcher finds that of every 10,000 women taking birth control pills, 2 die, whereas 3 die through complications of childbirth, should the use of birth control pills be continued? Someone will have to make a decision on whether or not to continue using the pill.

2. How much difference between the study group and the population will we accept as important?

3. What is a reasonable estimate of population variation? Perhaps studies that have been done in the area by other investigators will provide us with at least a hazy estimate of what the difference really is.[14]

Sample size depends on the research topic. Only one crash would be necessary for the Federal Aviation Administration to decide to ground a plane. Because the loss is so great, the FAA cannot take a chance on adding one more accident to the sample. However, a mechanical failure on a kitchen appliance or washing machine would not be considered serious unless perhaps 10% of all the appliances were found to have flaws. When research results establish some chemical additive as a cause of cancer in rats, a large sample may be needed to determine its effect on humans.

Against a background of cost, time, number of available personnel, size of the total population or subpopulations, and the purpose of the study, the researcher must decide what sample size is reasonable. Simon suggests that we take a guess at the sample size. If we get less accuracy than is desired, we know that we must increase the sample size, and if we oversample, we have wasted some money but have obtained a representative sample.[15]

Fig. 13-4 provides interesting insights into sampling variations. The data are results of a 135-point exam given to 35 students. The left column represents the student number. The number could be the result of alphabetical order, order of finishing the exam, or ascending order of identification numbers.

The second column represents the score the students received out of 135. Column three is the cumulative score which is the total score of all grades before, plus the specific score. The fourth column is the mean of all scores to that point.

[14] *Ibid.,* pp. 163–164.
[15] Simon, Julian L.: Basic research methods in social science, New York, 1969, Random House, Inc., p. 425.

Some points to observe:
1. The mean score of all scores is 102.25.
2. The mean of the first five scores is 108.60.
3. The mean begins to move toward the eventual total mean by score 25.
4. Fluctuations, even extreme scores higher than 124 or lower than 39, would have little effect on the total mean by score 25.
5. By the time score 31 is reached the mean is relatively stable.

Observe that Sample A, which was chosen randomly, has a mean of 108.20. Further notice that Sample B, which is every fifth score, has a mean of 98.57. Every seventh score was chosen for Sample C and has a mean of 97.30. None of the three samples is representative of the population mean. In such a small population the sample size needs to be larger than five to be representative. Observe that Sample B, which has seven scores, is closer than either A or C which have five scores each.

It has been concluded that a sample of 38 is quite representative of the whole regardless of the population. The representativeness of 38 is dependent on several factors. In relationship to the 35 scores in Fig. 13-4, it must be assumed that if more students took the exam the approximate mean of 102 would hold only if the same exam was given, the same teaching procedure used, the same textbook used, and the same calibre of students involved. If all variables were the same, the same approximate mean should prevail. However, a different teacher, test, text, or school would probably result in a different mean.

Rewards

"Why should respondents participate in a study?" Experimentation has been done with rewarding respondents. One medical sociologist doing research with medical doctors was told by a physician that if there was a $10 bill enclosed with each questionnaire, the physical could afford the time to fill it out. This advice was tried, but the investigator found that the rate of response was no greater than when the money was not included. When some of the physicians who had not returned the questionnaire were questioned, the researcher was informed that physicians are so busy that they just do not have time. They could make as much money taking care of a patient as they could filling out a questionnaire, so there was really no monetary gain. And time spent treating patients, they felt, is more worthwhile.

One of the national magazines included a tiny pencil with each questionnaire. This made it easier to fill out the form, and the pencil became a souvenir.

Rewards may motivate some people to answer questionnaires. However, most students doing research will not have money to offer as a reward. The least that the investigator can do when asking someone to fill out a mailed questionnaire is to include a self-addressed stamped envelope in which to return the questionnaire.

SUBJECT PARTICIPATION

Why should an individual agree to participate in a study? The potential respondent should be told the benefits of participation. If we are doing a research project on nurses,

Student	Score	Running Total	Mean
1	97		
2	115	212	106.00
3	105	317	105.67
4	118	435	108.75
5	108	543	108.60
6	88	631	105.17
7	116	747	106.71
8	124	871	108.88
9	108	979	108.78
10	99	1078	107.80
11	86	1164	105.82
12	119	1283	106.92
13	106	1389	106.85
14	113	1502	107.29
15	115	1617	107.80
16	118	1735	108.44
17	89	1824	107.29
18	88	1912	106.22
19	89	2001	105.32
20	59	2060	103.00
21	38	2098	99.90
22	100	2198	99.91
23	117	2315	100.65
24	116	2431	101.29
25	103	2534	101.36
26	96	2630	101.15
27	112	2742	101.56
28	120	2862	102.21
29	84	2946	101.59
30	107	3053	101.77
31	114	3167	102.16
32	82	3249	101.53
33	111	3360	101.82
34	120	3480	102.35
35	99	3579	102.26

$$\bar{X} = 102.26$$

Sample A Random Sample N = 5		Sample B Every 5th Student N = 7		Sample C Every 7th Student N = 5	
	88		108		116
	108		99		113
	116		115		38
	113		59		120
	116		103		99
	541		107		486
			99		
			690		
	$\bar{X} = 108.20$		$\bar{X} = 98.57$		$\bar{X} = 97.30$

FIGURE 13-4   Table of running means.

then we hope the results obtained from the study will benefit nursing in general and patient care in particular. If respondents understand the purpose of the study and also understand that it is meant to benefit their profession, an organization, or the health of the consumer, as well as the individual carrying out the project, they are more likely to participate. These informative facts may be included as part of the instrument or as part of a cover letter accompanying the instrument.

Disadvantages for the participant in a research project must be recognized: (1) it takes his/her time, (2) his/her attitudes or feelings may be misunderstood, (3) policy changes may result that seem to be disadvantageous to him/her, and (4) he/she must go out of his/her way to favor the researcher by participating in the project.

Potential participants in a study must be made aware of the importance of their contribution to the research project. In one study done at a local college for a class in research methodology, a student put a questionnaire in every student's mailbox. Approximately 50% of the students opened their mailbox, pulled out the questionnaire, looked at it for a few seconds, and dropped it in a nearby wastebasket. At least half the recipients could see no reason why they should answer the items. How would they have answered the items if they had taken the time to fill out the form? Would their responses have influenced the research findings?

If the president of the college had signed his name to a cover letter and requested the students to cooperate with the research project, no doubt there would have been a higher proportion of completed returns. If the benefits and purpose of the study had been described briefly before the instrument was read, cooperation would have been even more likely.

If a beginning researcher has a good reason for requesting information from the potential sample participants, a cover letter will enhance the project's image. Sending questionnaires to friends or acquaintances will probably increase the number of returns. So that the researcher may not be discouraged, it helps to know that it is sometimes difficult to get a high rate of returned questionnaires.

A sample composed solely of volunteer respondents may provide the researcher with a different kind of data than if the sample had been composed of individuals at random. Researchers should make every effort to obtain a representative (unbiased) sample if they wish to make generalizations from the findings. Still, it is the responsibility of the researcher to report how the sample was obtained and how permission was granted.

SAMPLING AND THE RESEARCH REPORT

The research report must give detailed information regarding various aspects of the sample. Nursing research, along with research in the social and behavioral sciences, is closely tied to the process of sampling. Many variables influence the findings in nursing research. The following nine topics are all important to the reader's understanding of the research method and should be included in the discussion of the study sample.

1. Discuss the process used to select a random sample, if one was used.
2. Describe the proportion or percentage of the total population that participated in the study.
3. Tell which subjects or respondents were included and the kinds of follow-up used.

4. Define the sample limits, and explain any relationship between sample size and the desired statistical level of significance.
5. Explain the reasons for the cutoff date beyond which the instrument returns were not accepted.
6. List specific background information about the sample subjects who returned the instrument or who participated in the research.
7. Describe the time span for the research as related to the sample.
8. Give information on how the sample subjects were contacted.
9. Include any description unique to the particular study sample.

SUMMARY

Sampling is a procedure inescapably tied to the scientific method. A sample is a representative part of the whole. Samples are relatively easy to obtain in the physical world but are much more difficult to obtain in the social and behavioral sciences.

A representative sample, which is a small part of the total, should contain all the variables, values, and characteristics of the population. Sample size is limited by such factors as time, cost, and accessibility of sample participants.

The researcher considers the size of the total population in determining the sample size.

Generalizing (that is, extending conclusions and meanings from a small study to the population) is the aim of researchers; generalizing can be done only on the basis of the specific study that has been undertaken. The larger and more extensive the study, the greater the possibility of generalizing about the whole. It is only on the basis of replication that the researcher will be able to extend both the quantity and the quality of generalizations. Small studies that include many exceptions have little power to produce generalizations. The more homogeneous the population, the more beneficial the sample becomes in terms of true representation of the total population.

There are a number of sampling techniques, but none is more effective than the random choice method of selecting the sample. The random technique involves assigning all subjects a number and then, by means of a chance process, selecting a sample. A random sample should have all the characteristics of the total population. A test for representatives may include checking the percentages of selected variables found in the population against those of the sample (for example, ratio of men to women). Two simple procedures for selecting the sample are random number tables and drawing numbers from a hat.

Major types of sampling include such categories as stratified, purposive, systematic, cluster, multistage, sequential, and incidental, sampling.

1. Stratified sampling. The population is divided into areas or sections, with a random sample taken from each section.

2. Purposive (quota) sampling. The researcher selects a special group of sample members because there is evidence that it represents the larger population.

3. Systematic sampling. The researcher arbitrarily selects every n^{th} number in a list of names, of houses in a block, or some other variable.

4. Cluster sampling. Rather than study the individuals or participants singly, readily available small groups are studied in sufficient numbers to make up the desired sample size.

5. Multistage sampling. A random selection of small units is made from randomly selected large units of the population. The process is fairly accurate and is valuable when a complete list of the population is not available. The cost is relatively low compared to most other types of sampling.

6. Sequential sampling. The researcher collects data from his subjects to the extent that he feels that further sampling will not change the direction of the data.

7. Incidental sampling. Data are collected from anyone available, such as people on a street corner or in a coffee shop.

Research carried out in a longitudinal study follows the subjects for a long period of time to observe change. Two disadvantages are loss of subjects and the lack of readily available data from which to draw conclusions before the study is complete. In contrast, cross-sectional studies are those that take information at one time and probably require subjects to recall past events or feelings, which may contribute to a loss of accuracy and may support bias. In spite of these disadvantages, the cross-sectional method is the most often used.

DISCUSSION QUESTIONS

1 What is a *large* sample?
2 When is a large sample preferable to a small sample?
3 When is a small sample preferable to a large sample?
4 What is the process you would use to identify every n^{th} member in your professional organization? Support your response.
5 How could a random number table be biased?
6 How could a random sample be biased?
7 What variables should be represented in sampling a population of 209 pregnant women?
8 Why is random sampling the most effective (representative) of all sampling techniques?
9 How large should a sample be to represent the inhabitants of a city of 50,000 people?

CLASS ACTIVITIES

Track I

1 Divide the class into groups of three or four members. Each group is to develop a list of characteristics that they believe should be represented in a matched sampling project using two different ethnic groups.
2 Members of the class suggest variables they would include in developing matched samples for a research project using the members of the class.

Track II (Steps in Research Project)

1 Each group is to describe their project sample as to its size, social and physical characteristics, subject occupations, and contact setting.
2 Each group is to decide which sampling procedure it will use when conducting its research.
3 The recorder from each group is to relate to the class the basis for the decisions that were made in items 1 and 2.

4 Each student conducting a project alone is to describe the project similar to items 1 and 2.

5 All students are to write a description of the sample and sampling technique that are planned for the intended project regardless of whether they are working alone or in a group. Submit it to the instructor for evaluation advising.

SUGGESTED READINGS

Abdellah, Faye G., and Levine, Eugene: Better patient care through nursing research, ed. 2, New York, 1979, Macmillan, Inc., Chapter 8.

Barnard, L.: Research designs: sampling, The American Journal of Maternal Child Nursing, **7**:15, January—February, 1982.

Best, John W.: Research in education, ed. 3, Englewood Cliffs, N.J., 1977, Prentice-Hall, Inc., Chapter 8.

Brewer, James K., and Knowles, Ruth Dailey: Some statistical considerations in nursing research, Nurs. Res. **23**:69—70, 1974.

Daniel, W.W., and Longest, B.B., Jr.: Statistical sampling and the nurse-researcher, Nurs. Forum **16**(1):36—55, 1977.

Fleming, Juanita W., and Hayter, Jean: Reading research reports critically, Nurs. Outlook **22**(3):174, March 1974.

Guilford, J.P.: Fundamental statistics in psychology and education, ed. 3, New York, 1956, McGraw-Hill, Inc., p. 159.

Hsu, L.M.: On why many hypotheses in educational research are supported and on the interpretation of sample effect sizes: a comment, Educ. Res. **9**(5):6—8, May 1980.

Overholt, G.E., and Stallings, W.M.: Ethnographic and experimental hypotheses in educational research, Educ. Res. **5**(8):12—14, September 1976.

Phillips, Bernard S.: Social research strategy and tactics, ed. 2, New York, 1971, Macmillan, Inc.

Shelley, S.I.: Research methods in nursing and health, Boston, 1984, Little, Brown & Company.

Simon, Julian L.: Basic research methods in social science, New York, 1969, Random House, Inc., pp. 170, 257, 355.

Sultz, H.A., and others: Longitudinal study of nurse practitioners, phase 1, DHEW Pub. No. HRA 76-43, Bethesda, MD, March 1976, Health Manpower References.

Treece, Eleanor Walters: Vocational choice and satisfactions of licensed practical nurses, 1969, The League Exchange No. 87, Publication no. 38-1351, New York, 1969, The National League for Nursing.

Wilson E. Bright, Jr.: An introduction to scientific research, New York, 1952, McGraw-Hill, Inc., p. 162.

CHAPTER 14

THE INSTRUMENT

An instrument in research refers to the tool or equipment used to collect data. It may take the form of a questionnaire, an interview schedule, a projective device, or some other type of tool for eliciting information. Often the term *instrument* is not used by authors or researchers; but rather, they call the instrument by its proper name, such as questionnaire, check-off list, interview schedule, or Q-sort.

In this chapter we focus attention on the instrument used in research. We do not include a lengthy discussion of each type of instrument, since the major types are dealt with separately in each of the chapters in Part Four. Other sections of the book also refer to many of the instruments commonly used by researchers. We first consider the tools and categories of scientific research; second, we suggest a number of guidelines that the researcher should follow when developing the instrument; third, we present several practical tips for developing a research tool; and fourth, we offer suggestions for writing the research report.

TOOLS OF SCIENCE

The scientific method requires certain materials that we will call tools, or instruments, which are used for measuring the phenomena we have under investigation. The physical sciences have a great number of tools to simplify and record precise quantities of data.

There are two broad categories of tools; mechanical devices and clerical materials. A tool may be identified as a measuring device or a facilitator of the measuring process. Two important components of a measuring device are its accuracy or, more specifically, its reliability and validity. Mechanical devices include almost all tools (such as microscopes, telescopes, thermometers, rulers, and monitors) used in the physical sciences. The social and behavioral sciences use such mechanical devices as tape recorders, cameras, film, video tape, and computers. Clerical tools are helpful when the researcher studies people and gathers data on the feelings, emotions, attitudes, and judgments of the subjects. Examples of clerical tools are filed records, histories, case studies, questionnaires, and interview schedules.

Both mechanical and clerical tools have wide potential for collecting data. Mechanical tools allow precise measurement that can be replicated with accuracy. Clerical tools are more difficult to use because they are less reliable, less accurate, and less precise than mechanical tools. For example, it is easy to use mechanical tools to measure weight, height, and blood pressure. Two researchers can agree on the exact height or weight of a person. However, it is difficult to use clerical tools to measure abstract concepts such as prejudice, pride, and humility. The two challenges that researchers in the health sciences face are (1) to develop clerical tools that are as precise as their mechanical tools, and (2) to define concepts so that they are amenable to the measuring tools.

The research project should be set up with replication in mind. The study should be stated with such precision that another researcher can duplicate it in exact detail.

It is often less time consuming and more valuable to use a tested instrument than to design a new one. However, for the beginning researcher, the struggle to develop a new tool is a learning experience. Often, the process of carrying out each step of the scientific method is of greater value than the findings. As one student said, "I learned more from my mistakes than from anything else."

It would be difficult to imagine any research project that would not need a tool for collecting or measuring data. Even the case study, which pursues a single situation in great depth, requires an interview guide or other instrument to record data.

Sources of Tools

There are several ways of searching for tools. First, the researcher can read professional journals to learn what kind of instruments are being used for similar studies, their format style, and how they were used by the writers. Second, a researcher can read books that provide a description or an actual copy of various instruments for the reader. Third, a researcher may talk with other researchers who may know of certain tools, have developed tools themselves, or may have used tools developed by others. Fourth, the researcher can combine or adapt one or more tools used by other researchers. Fifth, the researcher may develop his/her own instrument to fulfill a specific need. One note of advice and caution is that the researcher should always try out the tool in an actual setting prior to launching into a full-scale, data-collecting expedition.

When developing or locating existing tools for a research project, it is important that researchers conceptualize the whole data collection process. That is, if they want to observe nurse-patient relationships, they must project themselves into a situation and imagine all the circumstances that might develop during patient contact. This technique of thinking through the whole process applies whether the investigator is developing an interview schedule or questionnaire, conducting a content analysis, or searching for a record file. All of these techniques require the researcher to have thoroughly conceptualized not only the procedure, but also the form in which the data will be organized in the final presentation.

Beginning researchers frequently need assistance in selecting an instrument for studying their problem. There may be no *best* instrument, since all have both strong and weak points. The individual must make an arbitrary decision as to which tools and methods are most appropriate.

For example, a beginning researcher desiring to see if married students get better grades than single students wants to know how to begin, and what instrument or tool to use. There are several ways to approach this problem. The researcher might simply compare the average score (mean score) of an equal number of married and single students in a given situation. If the sample were large enough, this method might service the purpose. Another way is to have a matching sample that compares single and married female senior students who ranked in the upper 60th percentile of their high school class. This may be done with students in all levels of the educational program. Or we might take 75 married seniors, as an illustration, who were single when they enrolled as freshmen. We could look at their grade point average (GPA) during their freshman year and compare it with their GPA at some point after marriage. This does not consider the variable of the major, nor the fact that students tend to get better grades in their major than in their nonmajor courses.

There are strengths and weaknesses in all these approaches. Which one should the student use? A very skillful researcher might conclude that one method is better than the others, but for a student, a better solution is to do further library searching and learn the method used by other researchers for similar studies. Also, the researcher must determine how much time is available for research, how many subjects are available for the project, and how accessible the various types of records are. It is important to consider how the data will be analyzed and the types of tables and graphs that will be used to present them. All these factors will have a bearing on the tools and methods the investigator should use.

Beginning researchers usually develop the tool for their research project in order to gain skill in instrument development. However, by evaluating available instruments, new researchers become aware of what is considered a good format, the variety available in instrument design, the cost of instrument duplication, the time required for instrument administration, the language level used, the necessity for clear directions for completing the items, and the types of groups that have used the instrument previously. Once acquainted with available instruments, the researcher has attained a foundation for developing or purchasing a tool suitable for the current study.

Uses of Tools

Usually some training is necessary if anyone other than the researcher is to use a tool for gathering data. More training is required to use such techniques as interviews and observations than to administer questionnaires. The researcher who organized and conceptualized the project is the likely person to conduct training sessions. Training is necessary to ensure that all factors relating to the administration of the tools are kept constant.

When using a mechanical technique such as a tape recorder, the researcher should become familiar with the equipment so that there is no delay in gathering data and no chance of making errors. For example, in the picture-taking process there is no opportunity for a retake of a situation until after the film has been developed. It may then be too late to recapture the same event or situation.

In using mechanical equipment, test runs should always be made before the actual experiment is done. It is easy to operate equipment in familiar surroundings, but it is much more difficult to operate it in the presence of strangers and in an unfamiliar situation.

If the researcher is able to handle the mechanical tools easily and efficiently, the respondents will be much more at ease and less distracted by the researcher.

Other disciplines often develop specialized tools that are appropriate for more than their own field. It is important, therefore, that researchers become familiar with them.

For example, sports medicine is an expanding field that often uses experimental methods and equipment that are applicable to a wide range of health research.

CATEGORIES OF DATA ELICITED FROM THE SUBJECT

Instruments are developed to gather many kinds of information. Some data are already available, having been compiled for other uses. Such data would have to be collected with an instrument the researcher devised to help categorize and arrange the data in an order suitable for analysis. It is the researcher's prerogative to decide by which method these data are to be compiled, compared, and analyzed for a particular study.

Rather than use available data, the investigator may want to develop a new data-gathering instrument appropriate for a particular study. When data are elicited directly from the subjects, the instrument is designed to collect information in a form useful to the researcher. Regardless of the research purpose, the investigator will want to gather information about the respondents in addition to the material needed for testing the hypothesis. Opinions have little value unless we know whose opinions they represent. If we know that 80% of our sample is in favor of socialized medicine, it becomes very important to know if the sample is composed of medical personnel or state legislators. It is important to know the characteristics of the respondents for purposes of description and cross tabulation.

The kind of data to be gathered from individuals or inanimate objects may require the use of the same or different types of instruments, depending on the format and appropriateness of the tool. Nevertheless, such data may be fitted into the category of factual information that will provide material for gaining insight into the attitudes and feelings of the respondent. It will also help the researcher to make judgments about situations or conditions, the extent of selected psychomotor skills, or tests and experiments.

Facts

The purpose of a specific research study may be to gather data based on historical recollections alone. The investigator, then, may want to include facts on the activities and personal background of the respondent, his/her likes and dislikes, information he/she can supply about other people, his/her observations and perceptions, or statements about lifestyle, plans, and motivations. An entire research investigation may be limited to such types of information, or to fact-gathering items that may make up one or more sections of the instrument.

Researchers are responsible for determining the level of the intellectual processes they wish to probe. They may decide to go beyond mere factual knowledge and explore the comprehension of the subject. Researchers may even intend that their subjects use intellectual processes that demonstrate the subject's ability to apply, analyze, synthesize, or evaluate the factors being studied. Investigators are free to make whatever decisions deemed necessary to fulfill their research design.

Some types of factual information are reported as numbers, ages, quantities, time periods, amounts, qualities, dates, places, and sources. Examples are as follows:

In 1981, 15,208 clients received attention in the outpatient clinic.

Of the books signed out in the library, 20% were not returned within the 2-week checkout period.

On July 26, 1979, 10 boys and 5 girls were vaccinated against yellow fever.

Attitudes and Feelings

The purpose of some studies is to learn the attitudes and feelings of subjects toward themselves, other people, events, circumstances, their environment, or profession. The respondent may be expected to answer direct questions about his/her thoughts on the items, or the researcher may choose to develop an instrument that will provide insight into the subject's attitudes or feelings—of which the subject may or may not be aware. An effective *back-door* (indirect) approach is difficult for a beginning researcher, since it necessitates using carefully laid plans based on principles of psychology, learning, and testing.

Data from a single study may include both subjective and objective information. When data are subjective, they are derived from the subject's own ideas and thoughts on a topic. Such data give the researcher information as to whether the subject is aware of the area of focus being studied, his/her values concerning the topic, and his/her personal feeling about the worth of the idea being investigated. The instrument may be constructed to reveal the extent to which the subject has internalized the factor being studied.

As an example of subjective information, a nursing authority in another country commented, "Nurses are not as dedicated as they were in the past. They are only interested in their salaries." Such a statement is the personal opinion of one individual. However, it could serve as an hypothesis to be tested if the word *dedicated* were operationally defined.

Objective data are factual information that is beyond the subject's personal preference; that is, he/she has no personal involvement with the data. Objective data, such as age, place of birth, education, and so on, can be rated or categorized similarly by different observers. Other sources include letters, documents, diaries, pictures, taped records, and video tapes. Objective data have greater empirical value than data contaminated with emotions or interpretations.

As an illustration, suppose we are interested in studying nursing dependability. The instrument may contain items that reveal the subject's feelings about dependability. We could define dependability as "recording every medication on the patient's chart after it was administered." Then, by observing the subject and checking the patient's chart against the pharmacy records, we would be able to verify actual behavior (objective).

Subjectivity and objectivity are closely related and often overlap, depending on who is talking about whom. The program planners grumbled, "Not many nurses showed up at the seminar after all the hard work we went through." The nurses, on the other hand said, "The program topic wasn't interesting to us so we skipped it," or "We admitted a lot of emergencies this afternoon so we had to forget about the seminar this time." Each of these comments is subjective. However, each statement also can be interpreted objectively. The researcher could compare attendance at last year's seminar with this year's attendance; a survey of the nurses could reveal the degree of interest in the program topic; and a count of emergency records would reveal if there was in truth, "a lot of emergencies." By verifying the facts through research methodology we could make objective statements relating to the seminar. Of course, an evaluation of the facts could still be interpreted subjectively by both the program planners and the prospective participants.

Developing a cross check for the detection or interception of bias is not always possible. Any instrument can be biased. Sometimes researchers ask questions on only one side of the issue or appear to see only their preference. Individuals may say that they are against cheating when answering items on a questionnaire, but given the right circumstances, they may indulge in cheating and justify their behavior by defining the activity as acceptable in that situation. Students sometimes justify taking reserve books out of the library on the pretense that it was the only way they could gain access to them.

Humans tend to be biased whether they are subjects or researchers. In all of our dealings with other human beings, we are probably wrong about 50% of the time; therefore we should design our research studies with this in mind.

Summers and Hammonds say that bias can be grouped into six types: sampling bias, instrumentation bias, nonresponse bias, respondent bias, interviewer bias, and processing bias.[1]

Henerson, et al. give attention to the value of self-reports as the most direct method of assessing attitudes, whether they are in written or oral form. They point out that if the researcher does not believe that subjects are willing or able to provide the data sought, then another procedure should be selected.[2] This could include attitudinal scales and projective devices.

Judgments

There are times when the purpose of the research instrument is to elicit a judgment from the subject. The instrument must then be designed so that it provides sufficient information for the subject to make a decision.

Judgments relating to quantity and quality might be set up on a five-point scale from strongly agree to strongly disagree. The subject must have sufficient knowledge of the topic to make a valid judgment.

1. What should be the extent of a child's injuries before the police are notified of child abuse?
2. How appropriate is nursing as a career for men?
3. Should fathers accept half the responsibility for their children's care?

Researchers must decide if they want data that provide the subject's opinion or his actual behavior. Is the study dealing with what is or what should be? Is the ideal state the standard of measurement?

The instrument developed for use in eliciting judgments may be in the form of a paper-and-pencil tool, photographs and questions, interviews, or an observation in an artificial or real setting. The levels of judgmental skill may be in sequence or independent of each other. Beginning students can only be expected to make basic judgments concerning a program curriculum, whereas the professional in the field can more accurately recognize its strengths and weaknesses. Whatever the purpose of the instrument,

[1]Summers, Gene F., and Hammonds, Andre D.: Toward a paradigm for respondent bias in survey research, Sociological Quarterly **10**(1):113, Winter 1969.
[2]Henerson, M.E., Morris, L.L., and Fitz-Gibbon, C.T.: How to measure attitudes, Beverly Hills, 1978, SAGE Publications, Inc.

the context as well as the incident being judged must be the same for all respondents or groups for purposes of comparison.

Psychomotor Skills

The next type of instrument is developed to gather information about psychomotor activities. It may be the researcher's intent to observe, to ask questions about, or to test the muscular coordination (dexterity) of the subject. He/she may wish to involve more than one individual in the study situation while observing the subject's adroitness. For example, how well is the nursing student able to perform at the patient's bedside? Has the student mastered certain manipulative skills? The researcher may decide to require that certain objectives be met (such as correctly administering a medication). These objectives may be available from other sources or developed for a particular investigation.

A researcher might be interested in relating psychomotor skills to cultures and customs. Some of the early research in social psychology centered around subjects who used psychomotor skills alone or in groups. It was found that subjects usually perform at a higher level in groups than when alone.[3] Runners tend to go faster when running with others than by themselves, and the slower runners are motivated by the faster ones, resulting in improved performances.

Again, it is up to the researcher to determine the level of accomplishment that the subject is to achieve. Will it be just an observation of activities, a trial, or a discovery of accomplishment? Will it be a broad survey investigation or an in-depth analysis of some identified problem? Will one or all five of the senses be studied? Is the subject expected to perform a new skill or one that has been learned and practiced in the past? Finally, is there to be a sequence of activities for the participant to perform; if so, is the order an important consequence to the study?

An instrument can be designed so that the observer simply checks off whether the psychomotor skill is used or not. Another variation records varying degrees of competency through the use of a continuum scale. In certain instances the time necessary to reach a functional level of performance may be measured. The investigator determines the specific levels to be attained and tests the length of time necessary to attain the skill. Many aspects of health require the development of psychomotor skills for professional performance. The learning of such skills is mandatory and often expected to be mastered within a specific time.

Tests and Experiments

Researchers may decide to develop their own test or select a standardized one as the instrument they prefer for data collection. If the test has been normed, the researcher knows that it was administered to large numbers of individuals and the distribution of their test scores were graphed and based on a construct or broad areas. The test items were submitted to an appropriate group of subjects, and both item discrimination and the difficulty index were computed. Norm-referenced scores are commonly reported as percentiles, z-scores, and T scores, and usually reflect the performance of the individual as compared with others in the group.

[3]Zajonc, Robert B.: Social psychology, an experimental approach, Belmont, Calif., 1966, Brooks/Cole Publishing Co., p. 2.

Tests that are published usually are standardized. An accompanying manual that presents such information as the norm group, validity and reliability of the instrument, administration, scoring, and interpreting results, provides the researcher with the basis for judging the relevance of the tool for data collection. After reading the manual and observing the test items and procedures used in the testing process, the investigator should be prepared to determine if the test is suitable for the present study.

Norm-referenced tests are not, however, suitable for all situations. If the researcher wants to establish how much the individual knows about the subject matter rather than how his/her scores compare with those of others in the group, a criterion-referenced test is more appropriate. Criterion-referenced tests have a cutoff score that determines if the person has mastered the information or skills.

If students are expected to master certain information before proceeding to the next grade level, a criterion-referenced test is appropriate. If the student's scores must be above the 50th percentile, then a norm-referenced test is useful.

An instrument may be based on factors related to the subject's education or current educational program. Standardized tests may be selected as the study instrument. These include achievement and aptitude tests, self-inventories, rating scales, checklists, and tests of psychomotor skills and physical performance.

New experiments may be developed or old experiments repeated by the researcher in an attempt to discover what behavior the respondent will display. The subject's power to accomplish a certain feat may be the aim of the investigation in certain instances.

After the respondents have completed the experiment, the results may need to be judged by other individuals or professionals to reduce the possibility of bias. The researcher will probably need assistants to help him/her with tests and experiments, especially if the study is large. Assistants will need a period of training before the research data are gathered.

Frequently, the instrument used in an experiment is the pretest and the posttest. The teacher instructing nursing students in a new procedure or the dentist trying a new type of drill must compare the old method with the new. Several variables should be controlled. The instrument can be designed to measure length of time to reach a level of competency, the effectiveness of the teaching process, and so on.

Weisenberg and others report a study dealing with children's health beliefs and health behavior in which the Health Belief Model was used along with a pretest and posttest to see how useful the instrument is for predicting the long-term health beliefs of children. Previously the instrument had been used with an adult sample.[4]

GUIDELINES FOR DEVELOPING AN INSTRUMENT

The instrument used in a research investigation should, as far as possible, be the vehicle that will best elicit data for drawing conclusions pertinent to the study and, at the same time, add to the body of general knowledge in the discipline. Therefore, great care must be taken throughout the planning and developmental stages of the instrument (conceptu-

[4]Weisenberg, M.S., and others: Children's health beliefs and health behavior, J. Health Soc. Behav. 21(1):59–74, March 1980.

alization). If certain guidelines are followed, the researcher can expect that problem areas will be minimized or eliminated entirely.

1. The instrument must be suitable for its function. Whatever the designer's aim in the study, the research tool will be effective only as it relates to its particular purpose. For example, an instrument meant to gather data on the subject's extent of dexterity would be inadequate if it only provided means for recording statements from the subject about his/her skills rather than obtaining evidence at the same time. In other words, the instrument should be constructed to contain components that get to the heart of the problem and that tap the vital elements of the question being studied. After the purpose of the instrument is determined, the characteristics can be decided and then made to permeate the construction of the instrument.

2. The instrument must be based on the theoretical framework selected for the study. The researcher may need to read extensively to identify which aspects of the theory are appropriate for investigation. On the other hand, the researcher may already be acquainted with a theory and will only need to review the literature. The researcher's theoretical framework is separate from, and in addition to, theory-based research. The two should be integrated into the investigation. Background information points to other studies that may suggest a research design, instruments, hypotheses, and so on.

3. The researcher, through the instrument, must be able to gather data that are appropriate to test the hypothesis or to answer the question under investigation. If the researcher has an hypothesis based on theory, then the instrument should be constructed in line with the concepts and rationale of the theory. The format of the instrument should elicit information about the factors being tested. For example, if the hypothesis deals with a cause-effect relationship between A and B, then the instrument will have to contain statements or conditions about both A and B in addition to other possible causes (such as C, D, and E) to ascertain the real cause. It is important to note that the more variables on which information is collected, the more possible causal relationships the investigator can consider when running cross-tabulations, because more combinations are possible.

Researchers may not have an hypothesis for their study—instead, they may want to learn the answer to a question that seems to be important enough to occupy their time and effort and that will contribute to their discipline. If an answer to a question is sought, then only those items that are relevant should be included. Nonessential data only increase the cost and take the researcher's time and effort that could be used for other purposes. All items in the instrument are to be directly related to the study and planned so that the data will be useful to the investigator. However, it may be wise to include a question, problem, or situation for the purpose of gaining rapport with the respondent; but even these contribute to the study if carefully planned.

The sequence of items may contribute to gaining or maintaining rapport. Personal questions may be somewhat offensive to some respondents, so they may be asked at the end, rather than the beginning, of certain questionnaires and interviews. Eye-catching items or situations are likely to spark the respondent';s interest and help to establish rapport early in the data-gathering process. One of the major difficulties beginning researchers have is that they make their instrument too long or too comprehensive to handle in a single investigation.

4. The instrument should be valid. The content of the instrument must be appropriate to test the hypothesis or answer the question being studied. Furthermore, the data gathered should yield information relevant to the study. It is important that the instrument itself does not become a problem to the subject so that it biases the response. If respondents do not understand how to handle or complete the instrument, the data will not give a true picture of the respondent's ability, ideas, or feelings about the item. The instrument is valid to the extent that it does not influence the subject's answer or performance. A good instrument elicits the data that it was intended to elicit with a minimum of influence.

The beginning researcher may not have time to test the validity of his/her instrument, but by being careful, known factors or variables that would affect the data can be eliminated. The important question is, "Will the instrument test what we want it to test?"

5. The instrument should be reliable. The devised research tool should provide comparable data every time the subject uses (or answers) the instrument. That is, if he/she were to fill out the questionnaire, answer the interviewer's questions, perform a skill, and so on, on two occasions without time to remember the items or gain greater proficiency through practice of the skill, he/she would provide a similar response both times.

An instrument can be highly reliable without being valid, but it cannot be valid without being reliable. It may be reliable and valid for senior students in a baccalaureate nursing program and reliable for students in an associate degree nursing program. But it cannot be considered valid if it was meant to elicit data from students who had gained the greater depth of understanding that an advanced nursing education provides. Instrument reliability does not guarantee validity in all cases.

6. The instrument should be free of bias. It should be prepared in such a way that the respondent has no idea of the researchers attitude toward the topic under study. For example, questions should not be stated with built-in bias. "Don't you think that physicians' orders are often unimportant?" suggest the investigator's attitude toward physician's orders. The researcher should neither assume nor suggest any attitude or response to the subject. Forcing the subject to give a "yes" or "no" answer also may bias the data. When the subject is required to answer "yes" or "no" to some idea, we may be forcing him/her into a trap without permitting qualification of the response. In another instance the respondent may approve of an activity but for a different reason than the researcher has suggested in a list of alternative responses.

The setting for an observation should not of itself encourage an emotional response from the observer. If the researcher happens to be uncomfortable when in the presence of ongoing surgery, there will be difficulty observing nurses in the operating room. Data may be more accurate if instead an assistant is assigned to making the observations there. The researcher should certainly investigate any possibilities of subjective bias when the study site may contaminate the findings.

7. A good instrument is free of built-in clues. The instrument should not contain measures that function as hints for desired responses. In an experiment, for example, there should be no direct suggestion to the experimental group through wording, the order of questions, or behavior that assists them in responding to the question or

problem. If it is possible that clues have been inadvertently given to the respondents, this should be discussed with those who participated in the pilot study. Unintentional clues may invalidate a portion of the data and lead to erroneous findings.

A group of students objected to the dismissal of a faculty member. They developed a questionnaire that they hoped would produce evidence to show that the professor taught some valuable courses and that he was a good teacher. All items were aimed at obtaining positive responses about the professor. Those persons who were in favor of his dismissal refused to answer the questionnaire because it had built-in clues. If they returned the instrument, the professor might be rehired, so they thought it wiser not to return the questionnaire. If the subjects had been asked to rate the professor with an impartial instrument, the study findings would have been more representative of the total population.

8. The researcher should gather a group of items from such sources as persons knowledgeable in the field, accepted theories or hypotheses, personal experience, or material from studies reported in books and professional journals. Care should be taken to ensure the appropriateness of items, their clarity, continuity, and level of reading difficulty.

9. An instrument should include an item that directly asks the hypothesis. For example, suppose in an international development project the researcher suspects that the women are not preparing food at home as they have been taught in a nutrition course. As part of a systematic investigation the researcher tests the hypothesis, "The nutrition course is ineffective because the women are still not convinced that diet and health are directly related." The research instrument includes the following three items:

1. How do you prepare rice at home?
2. Which is more important, the kinds of food you eat or the amount you eat?
3. Does your diet affect your health?

10. The research tool should be designed and constructed in such a way that cheating is minimized. The response given by each respondent in the research study should be solely his/her own. There should be no contamination through outside influences, such as someone else's ideas or products. Therefore, the respondent who agrees to participate in a study is responsible for supplying information or for exhibiting behavior that is truly his/her own. Cheating should be minimized whether the instrument is administered to a group or to an individual. It is especially important when comparisons are to be made of skills or where the results of an experiment are involved.

An experiment was performed in one of the group sessions at a professional convention. Responses were tallied and reported back to the group for discussion. One of the convention participants purposely attempted to invalidate the data. How can we prevent such incidences from occurring? If respondents are not aware of the exact nature of the research until after the data have been collected, some cheating can be eliminated.

11. Simple directions should be included with the instrument for the respondents, as well as for whoever is to administer it. Each section of the instrument that asks for a different type of response should provide explicit directions concerning what is expected of respondents. Are they to check off all responses that apply to an item or only one of them? Should they sign their names to the instrument? Should they add comments if

they do not understand an item, or leave the space blank? Here again pretesting and the pilot study should reveal problems concerning the directions. If the instrument is administered to several groups, care must be taken to ensure that the same directions are given each time. Questions raised by the respondents concerning any experimentation or the instrument must be carefully answered to avoid supplying one group with more information than another.

Those who administer the instrument should know exactly the extent and limitations of their roles. They must have guidelines to follow so that the instrument will be used as intended by the researcher. For this reason, the researcher should make certain that assistants understand and carry out their roles adequately.

12. The instrument should be as easy as possible to administer. While developing the tool, the researcher must decide the sequence of steps to be taken. Depending on the type of research, much of the administrative process may be more or less routine. Suppose a new method of patient care is being studied. The observation instrument, interview schedule, or other recording device, or all of these should require a minimum of attention so that the observer can concentrate on the particular event under scrutiny. The observation process should not be hampered by the observer's recording process to the extent that he/she is distracted from the assigned task. There should be concentration on the event rather than on recording the event.

PRACTICAL APPLICATION

Several considerations must be made when preparing an instrument. By way of review, remember that the instrument may be of one's own design or someone else's. It may be one that has been adapted from various sources. By taking part from one source and part from another, it is possible to develop an appropriate instrument. One advantage of doing a library search first is that the review of literature will provide information about instruments other people have used and how they have used them.

Suppose you are doing a study about schools of nursing, and you want to know how they vary on entrance or graduation requirements, curriculum, or other specific areas. According to your hypothesis, you decide to develop an instrument for compiling information from college catalogs. From the catalogs you could learn such facts as the requirements for enrollment or graduation, the number and academic preparation of the faculty, general information about the curriculum, and the philosophy of the school.

Suppose that even though you have decided to develop your own instrument, you discover that there seems to be no instrument available for measuring such data. By reading more broadly you notice that similar research has been done in other disciplines at other institutions of higher education. By studying and observing their instruments, you might get some ideas on how to set up your own tool.

It is important to remember that your research is no stronger than the instrument you use. The instrument is one area of research over which you have some control, so take every precaution to see that it will test what it was designed to test.

After the instrument has been put into its final form, a pretest of the instrument should be undertaken using subjects similar to those who will be in the final sample.

Be sure to have the results of the pilot study evaluated by someone experienced in research before attempting the major study. Furthermore, be sure to answer the following questions. Was the instrument really testing what you wanted it to test? Are the data collected by your instrument precise? Does the instrument detect any significant differences among subjects on the variables under consideration? As you analyze the data gathered, do the findings appear to have practical value? If so, what application may be made with the results?

Other questions you will want to ask include the following: Does the instrument seem to have a built-in bias? How long did it take the average subject to complete the instrument, or how long did it take to make an observation? Did cheating seem to take place among the participants? Were the directions easy to follow? Was it difficult to administer the instrument? Did any unexpected problems arise during the administration of the instrument or gathering of the data? Were the data easy to compile and to analyze? Do the data fit into the tables, charts, and graphs that you have prepared for them?

Writing the Instrument

The researcher should list concisely the criteria for the instrument. All of the following guideline questions for criteria construction must be answered.
1. Why was the particular format selected?
2. How are the data gathered by the instrument pertinent to the study?
3. How much time did it take the subject to complete the instrument?
   Examples of weaknesses included in the report are as follows:
1. The questionnaire should have taken no longer than 30 minutes to complete.
2. The items should have included opinions and should not have been offensive.
3. The questionnaire should have been coded to facilitate transfer of responses to datapunch cards.

The developer of the research tool should report the reason for the inclusion of each item in the instrument (Fig. 14-1); however, major studies for publication usually delete this information.

If the researcher conducted any tests of reliability or validity (see Chapter 15) on either the instrument as a whole or on individual items, this information should be presented. The pretest and the pilot study conducted prior to the major study should also be described. A description of preliminary studies is important to the reader's understanding of the entire research process. Since a discussion of each individual change made as a result of the pretest and pilot study makes for a lengthy report, the researcher need only provide general information. In some instances only a particularly interesting or unusual alteration of an item is included, if the information is deemed important to the reader.
1. Describe the cover letter. Include a copy of this letter in the appendix.
2. List the dates of mailings or other administrative details.
3. Provide a complete description of the control and experimental settings, if there has been experimentation.
4. Describe any type of follow-up that was carried out.
5. Tell about rewards to subjects, if any were given.
6. State the response.

QUESTION NO.

1. Have you ever been a patient in the hospital before?
    Yes ____ No ____
      This question could readily and quickly be answered by every patient, and
      was used to gain rapport with the patient.

2. Did student nurses care for you at that time?
    Yes ____ No ____
      This question was not asked if the patient replied negatively to question 1.
      If the first answer was positive, this was an indication that the patient
      might be aware that there was a school of nursing in the hospital.

3. Have you had x-ray films taken or lab work done?
    Yes ____ No ____
      This was a lead question so that a reaction could be obtained to question
      4. The answer would almost surely be yes, and the patient could give
      expression to his feelings if he so desired.

FIGURE 14-1   Reasons for including items in a questionnaire.

7. Tell how many respondents participated in the investigation.
8. State the cutoff date and tell why it was selected.
9. Attempt to answer who, what, where, when, why, and how in writing up the administrative process.

For the benefit of those who might want to repeat the study, every detail relating to how the study was designed and administered should be included in this section of the report.

SUMMARY

In research, the instrument is the tool or equipment developed for collecting data. The term *instrument* may not be used in every study published; rather the researcher frequently refers to the proper name of the instrument, such as questionnaire.

Data may already be on file somewhere, or the researcher may decide to gather new data for the study. The investigator may use an instrument that has been developed by someone else or one that is newly designed. Parts of one or more previously tested instruments may be borrowed to develop a new instrument.

The kinds of data gathered in a research project include facts, attitudes and feelings, judgments, psychomotor skills, and tests and experiments. The researcher may decide to use one or more classifications within a single study, depending on its breadth and depth.

Certain guidelines should be followed to minimize problem areas and errors.

1.   The instrument must be suitable for its function.

2. The instrument must be based on the theoretical framework selected for the study.
3. The researcher, through the instrument, must be able to gather data that are appropriate to test the hypothesis or answer the question under investigation.
4. The instrument should be valid.
5. The instrument should be reliable.
6. The instrument should be free of bias.
7. The instrument should be free of built-in clues.
8. The research tool should be designed and constructed in such a way that cheating is minimized.
9. Simple directions should be included with the instrument for the respondents, as well as for the research assistant if someone other than the researcher is to administer it.
10. The instrument should be as easy as possible to administer.
11. The instrument should ask the hypothesis directly to the subject.

The beginning researcher must remember: *your research is no stronger than the instrument you utilize*.

DISCUSSION QUESTIONS

1 What is the advantage of discussing the instrument separately from the research approach?
2 Comment on the importance of emphasizing opinions in an instrument.
3 Illustrate why some research projects require a more extensive use of tools than others.
4 If you were conducting a research project, how would you decide whether to develop your own instrument or to use one already developed by someone else?
5 What is the relationship between the hypothesis and the instrument?
6 Would available data ever be preferable to new data?
7 In what way is the library search helpful in developing an instrument?
8 Comment on the statement "An instrument that is valid in one research project may not be valid in a similar project."
9 Discuss how psychomotor skills can be evaluated using an instrument.
10 What advantage is there in asking subjects a question directly related to the hypothesis?

CLASS ACTIVITIES

Track I

1 Members of the class are to design the format of an instrument that elicits response to questions dealing with health.
2 The class is divided into groups of two or three students. Each group is to develop a few items that could be included in an instrument dealing with student health.

Track II (Steps in Research Project)

1 Each group or student is to (a) identify one or two instruments that would be appropriate for study, (b) determine the cost and length of time it will take to gather the necessary data when using the selected instruments, and (c) identify problems and the permission that must be granted if the instruments were used.
2 All students are to begin development of the selected instrument by determining the format, content to be covered, directions for its use and method of administration.

SUGGESTED READINGS

Ackoff, Russell L., Gupta, Shiv K., and Minas, J. Sayer: Scientific method optimizing applied research decisions, New York, 1968, John Wiley & Sons, Inc., p. 209.

Bond, John: The construction of a scale to measure nurses attitudes, Int. J. Nurs. Stud. 11(2):75–84, July 1974.

Chamorro, Ilta L., and others: Development of an instrument to measure premature infant behavior and caretaker activities: time-sampling methodology, Nurs. Res. 22(4):300–309, July–August 1973.

Cornell, Sudie A.: Development of an instrument for measuring the quality of nursing care, Nurs. Res. 23(2):108–117, 1974.

Dickoff, James, James, Patricia, and Semradek, Joyce: 8–4 research. Part I. A stance for nursing research—tenacity or inquiry, Nurs. Res. 24(2):85, March–April 1975.

Dunn, Margaret A.: Development of an instrument to measure nursing performance, Nurs. Res. 19(6):503–5095, November–December 1970.

Fox, D.J.: Fundamentals of research in nursing, ed. 4, New York, 1982, Appleton-Century-Crofts, Chapter 17.

Henerson, M.E., Morris, L.L., and Fitz-Gibbon, C.T.: How to measure attitudes, Beverly Hills, 1978, Sage Publications, Inc.

McFarlane, Jean K.: Study of nursing care—the first two years of a research project, Int. Nurs. Rev. 17(2):107, 1970.

Morris, L.L., and Fitz-Gibbon, C.T.: How to measure achievement, Beverly Hills, 1978, Sage Publications, Inc.

Wallston, Kenneth A., Wallston, Barbara S., and Gore, Susan: Development of a scale to measure nurses' trust of patients, Nurs. Res. 22(3):232–235, 1973.

Ward, M.J. and Fetler, M.E.: Instruments for use in nursing education research, Boulder, January 1979, Western Interstate Commission for Higher Education.

CHAPTER 15

RELIABILITY AND VALIDITY

After an hypothesis is developed, the researcher must decide what should be measured and how it should be measured. It is imperative that the instrument selected for data gathering be as accurate and consistent as possible. The theoretical basis for research is limited to the extent of the accuracy of the measurement. In this chapter we discuss in depth reliable and valid measures for the phenomenon under study.

We use the term *reliability* as the proportion of accuracy to inaccuracy in measurement. Reliability is usually defined as the ability of the data-gathering device to obtain consistent results. *Validity* refers to an instrument's ability to actually test what it is supposed to test. If we were referring to an intelligence test, obtaining reliable results means obtaining similar results time after time, because intelligence does not vary from day to day. However, blood pressure does vary and a sphygmomanometer must accurately measure these variations to be considered reliable.

A measurement technique must be accurate and valid if it is to be useful. If a test is valid, it will measure what the developer is actually trying to measure; but just because the intelligence test is accurate does not mean it is valid. To establish validity, there must be some evidence that relates the scores on the test to behaviors such as academic ability, success on the job, and abstract reasoning ability. Behaviors that should be related to test scores depend on the theory of the trait being measured. Abstract reasoning and success on the job are known correlates of intelligence, so valid intelligence tests should predict these behaviors. The color of a person's eyes is not part of our theory of intelligence, so we would not expect a valid test to predict eye color.

Objectivity affects both reliability and validity and is therefore an important factor in all research. The researcher must be objective to ensure that personal preference does not influence the interpretation of reliability or validity.

Evidence from data is only reliable to the extent that one can confidently affirm that similar findings would be obtained if the collection of data were repeated under identical circumstances. As so often occurs in human behavior studies, one researcher collects data in a given instance and obtains certain findings. Another researcher will conduct a study in exactly the same manner and report conflicting results. In such circumstances, the reliability and validity of each researcher's methodology must be closely examined.

Stinson cites several reasons why nursing research may not be valid and reliable: (1) its character is exploratory, and the findings are not definitive; (2) the weak design of some studies makes findings and conclusions untrustworthy; (3) unwarranted generalizations are made on the basis of an inadequate sample; (4) statistical methods may be inappropriately used; and (5) conclusions are sometimes unsound.[1] Another author further contends that at least 50% of the data in scientific journals is wrong or based on so little evidence that readers are unable to trust its reliability.[2]

DIFFERENCE BETWEEN RELIABILITY AND VALIDITY

Reliability and validity can apply to a broad area of topics. They may apply to questionnaires we develop, tests we construct, conclusions we arrive at, or other research-related activities. Certainly in research methodology, it is necessary to consider the factors of reliability and validity. Tests, questionnaires, interviews, instruments, and various research techniques are all concerned with these two factors. What a measurement technique intends to measure, and what it actually measures may not be the same; therefore, data may not reveal what we think they reveal. If a measurement technique measures any factor accurately, even though it may not be the factor we want to measure, the technique is still reliable. If a technique is inaccurate and its measurements are inconsistent (unreliable), then it is not valid.

For example, a patient was going to an ophthalmologist for treatment of an eye problem and at the same time to an orthopedist for a leg condition that the patient had developed. One day the two specialists happened to eat together at a restaurant and started discussing their patients. As the conversation continued, they each described what turned out to be the same patient. From their pooled knowledge they were able to diagnose what they had not been able to diagnose individually. Their patient had multiple sclerosis. Each physician had measured the man's physical condition accurately but limited it to a particular part of the body. The data were actually only partial. It took information from both specialists to obtain a valid diagnosis.

An easily understood example of the difference between validity and reliability is in the grading of test papers. Suppose a teaching team asks students to write a paper that tests the student's understanding of patient care. Even though the instructors are interested in the students' understanding, they may include questions that require recall, association, and opinion. Rather than eliciting information that demonstrates each student's level of understanding, the test results depend largely on memorization and writing skill. Some of the instructors notice the legibility of the handwriting, the length of responses, and punctuation and grammar. When the teaching team compares grades on the papers, they find that there is a wide variation in the grades assigned to each paper by different instructors. The test is invalid because many factors other than understanding patient care enter into the grades the students received. These factors include recall, association, and opinion. The test is unreliable because of the variation in the grades given by different instructors for the same paper.

Let us use the example of firing a gun. Having locked the gun in a vise, we aim it at a target. We are assuming that the vise holds the gun perfectly steady even after recoil.

[1]Stinson, Shirley M.: Staff nurse involvement in research—myth or reality? Can. Nurse **69**(6):30, June 1973.
[2]Boffey, Phillip M.: Scientific data: 50 pct. unusable? Chronicle of Higher Education **10**(1):1, February 24, 1975.

Assuming, too, that the gun is aimed exactly at the center of the target, suppose we fire 10 rounds. All the holes in the target appear in the lower righthand corner on the outer edge (Fig. 15-1). The gun is reliable because it performed the same way every time. We fired 10 rounds all hitting the same area of the target. But is the gun valid? No, it is not valid, because it did not do what we intended it to do. We wanted to hit the center of the bull's eye, where it was aimed. If we are certain that the gun is reliable, then something is in error. Either we did not aim exactly at the center of the target, or something is wrong with the sighting mechanism. Perhaps we can test another gun, lock it in the vise, aim it at the target, and fire 10 rounds. If this gun, too, shoots into the same areas as before, we may assume that the person aiming the gun is not accurate. Once we find the problem, and the gun puts all 10 rounds right in the bull's-eye, then we can say that the gun is reliable, and also valid; it shoots where we want it to shoot consistently.

This is what a faculty would like to do with all of its tests. Teachers want their tests to give consistent results time after time and also to test for certain educational objectives that they decided on when they developed the course. The test may be used to diagnose, to grade, to increase learning, to improve teaching, or to place students, but it still should meet the requirements of validity and reliability.

When the researcher develops a questionnaire, designs an interview technique, or gathers data for a research study, the technique or method of obtaining data and the data themselves need to be reliable and valid.

Suppose we have a test that measures those abilities (aptitudes) that an individual must have to be successful in achieving the goals of nursing education. If we are able to ascertain that those who score high on our test also will achieve high scores in their college courses, then our test has validity. Obviously it is also reliable. But suppose our test shows some potential nurses to have low scores and some to have high scores, and in college some of the low scorers go on to do well and some of those with high scores do not achieve high scores in college. Then we can question both the validity and the reliability of our instrument.

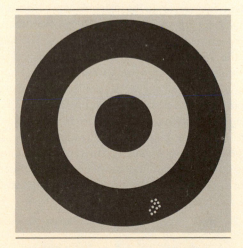

FIGURE 15-1   Target (reliability).

Many studies have been done on the accuracy of clinical thermometers. Pourintun and Bishop report a study on the accuracy of clinical thermometers in which 11 of 48 thermometers were found to be inaccurate at specified levels ranging from 0.40 F to 3.0 F.[3] Differences like this should make one check for accuracy when purchasing a clinical thermometer.

Accuracy in measuring blood pressure is always a concern. Sphygmomanometer accuracy, faulty technique, and physiological variation are three variables that can affect blood pressure readings, according to one study.[4] A test of 133 sphygmomanometers in four acute-care facilities found 22% were inaccurate in all six pressures tested (50, 80, 100, 150, and 200 Hg). The National Bureau of Standards allows a deviation of ±3 mm Hg, so a deviation of ±4 mm Hg was considered inaccurate. Only 44 of the instruments were accurate at all six readings.

Batten discusses the "scratch test," which is used to determine hardness of material. If one of the materials can scratch the other but not vice versa, then we assume that the first material is harder. This test is quite reliable; it gives the same results consistently, and no doubt all independent observers would agree. But is the test valid? If we decide to run a series of other tests to detect erosion, water solubility, and breakability, and the material that scratches all others is also the least soluble and least breakable, then we would say that this scratch test for hardness is valid. It is valid as well as reliable. However, if the material that scratches all others did not survive any of the other tests, then it could be called a reliable test but not a valid test.[5]

What we are saying is that it is easy to check the reliability of a tool or piece of equipment, but to check both the validity and reliability of an achievement test or an aptitude test is more difficult. Human behavior is not as easily measured.

RELIABILITY

Reliability refers to the accuracy of a measuring instrument. There are two basic sources of inaccuracy: one is deficiency (error) in the instrument itself, and the other is inconsistency between different individuals who are taking readings from the instrument.

Inconsistencies between measurers can be minimized by training them in objective methods of utilizing the instrument. For example, the blood pressure cuff should be placed on the patient in the same fashion every time. Suppose a nursing student is taking a blood pressure and consistently getting a different pressure reading than the instructor. Probably the student is in error, because supposedly the instructor is competent and has acquired skill in taking blood pressures. This more than likely means that the student is inaccurately reading the sphygmomanometer, although a hearing defect may confound the problem. Although inaccuracy is usually due to the instrument or the measurer, we must not overlook the possibility that instability occurs in the measuree. In this case, the patient's blood pressure or rate of heartbeat may fluctuate because of the presence of one

[3]Purintun, Lynn R., and Bishop, Barbara E.: How accurate are clinical thermometers? Am. J. Nurs. **69**(1):99–100, January 1969.
[4]North L.W.: Sphygmomanometer accuracy, Am. J. Nurs. **79**(10):2004, November 1979.
[5]Batten, Thelma F.: A guide for social science methods reasoning and research, Boston, 1971, Little, Brown & Co., pp. 116–117.

of the measurers, so it is important that the two readings be taken simultaneously. The same problem of inaccuracy could occur in other nursing functions.

Researchers usually discuss reliability in terms of a reliability coefficient. This term refers to the correlation between two measurements that are obtained in the same manner. Some of the basic principles that apply to the interpretations of reliability coefficients are that the coefficients report the proportion of the test variance that is nonerror variance and that they depend on the number of observations and the spread of the subjects' test scores.[6]

Testing Reliability

In this section we discuss different ways of estimating the accuracy of the measurement techniques themselves. Several procedures have been employed to test the reliability of questionnaires, interview techniques, observations, experiments, and other methods for gathering data. We discuss four methods for testing the reliability of an instrument or scale. Beginning researchers should become familiar with these methods so that they can select an appropriate one for testing their instruments.

One method for testing reliability is a *test-retest*. A test is administered to the subjects, and after a period of time it is administered again. If the test is reliable and the trait being measured is stable, the results will be consistent and essentially the same both times. One problem with this method is that the individuals may remember some of the test items from the first administration. The measurement of any ability that depends on learning or recall is liable to be biased. Another point is that people change over time; so inconsistent results, especially if there has been a long time period between testing, may be because of actual changes in the trait being measured. Intelligent use of the test-retest reliability depends on a knowledge of the trait being measured. Test-retest reliability should be high for traits that are stable, such as intelligence. Unstable traits, such as current mood (joy, boredom, or depression), may produce low reliability estimates, but this is because of the nature of the trait rather than the inaccuracy of the test (Fig. 15-2).

Another test for reliability is the *equivalent* test. In this method, two forms of the test are developed using the same specifications but requiring separate samples of behavior in the area under study. In other words, both tests contain the same types of items based on the same kinds of material, but the particular references and items are different. The same subject may be given the first test, followed immediately by the second, or a period of time may be permitted to lapse before the second one is given if stability over time is being studied. These parallel forms of the test supposedly reveal a high correlation in results if the tests are reliable. Unfortunately it is difficult to develop sufficient items to construct two tests or scales of the desired length (Fig. 15-3).

The third type of reliability test, the *split-half* method, is carried out at the time of scoring the results. Separate scores are given for the even-numbered and odd-numbered items. The results from each half of the test are compared to determine the internal consistency of the test. If the two halves of the test produce approximately equal scores, this suggests that the test is reliable. Before the split-half method is selected for use, we must consider whether the length of the test or scale is long enough to permit each half-test to contain sufficient items to be reliable in itself. We must demonstrate, too, that

---

[6]Cronbach, Lee J.: Essentials of psychological testing. New York, 1970, Harper & Row Publishers, pp. 165–166.

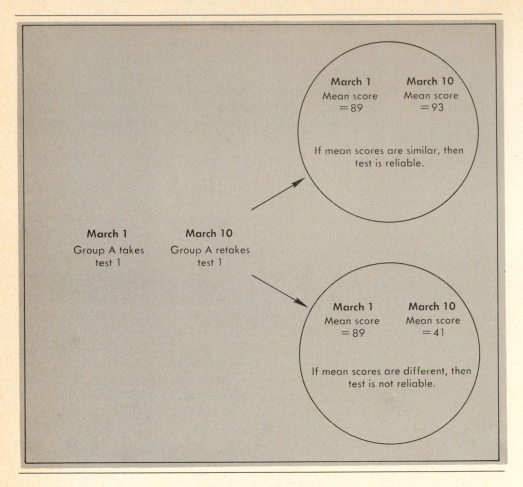

FIGURE 15-2   Test-retest.

the entire group of items actually makes up a single unity. This test has generally been replaced by the Kuder-Richardson test. The Spearman-Brown formula, found in statistical books, has been used to obtain a coefficient for the full test (Fig. 15-4).

The *Kuder-Richardson* reliability coefficients are a measure of the internal consistency or the homogeneity of the items in a test. In the Kuder-Richardson procedures, we assume that the items in the test are accurate to the extent that they are alike or related to each other. The Kuder-Richardson formula 20 (KR 20 coefficient) gives an estimate of item intercorrelation as does the more simplified KR 21 formula (Fig. 15-5). The latter is less accurate but easier to compute. For mathematical reasons the Kuder-Richardson method is preferred to the split-half method.

After the test is given, the formula is applied to the test results to determine the reliability of the test (Fig. 15-6). Two testing periods are needed for the test-retest and equivalent test methods, whereas a single test is administered in the split-half and Kuder-Richardson methods. Both the Kuder-Richardson and split-half methods are

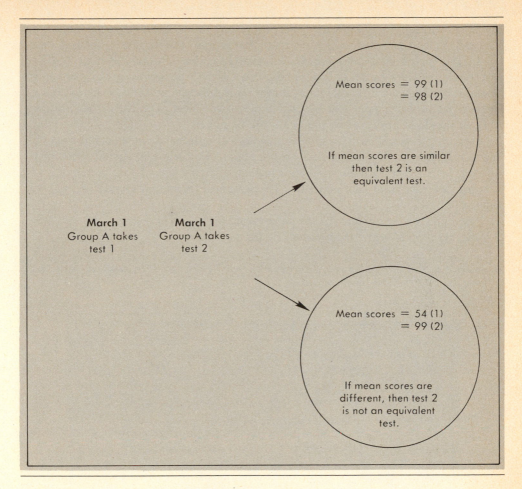

FIGURE 15-3 Equivalent test.

inappropriate for speed tests. Also the Kuder-Richardson method makes no provision for the possibility of variation in the subject from one time to another.

Item Analysis

If the investigator develops a test for his/her research, every item should be both reliable and valid. Each item should discriminate between the subject who is a high achiever and the one who is a low achiever. If knowledgeable subjects are likely to miss the item and least knowledgeable subjects tend to get it correct, then the instrument discriminates negatively.

If every item on a test is found to be reliable, then every item would be checked in the way we had anticipated. If we have a scale or test that predicts the responses of both poor and good subjects on every item, then the poor subjects will tend to miss the item and the good subjects will tend to answer it correctly. If the test has been developed to the point that every item discriminates highly, it is a good test. If a 100-item, highly discriminating test is given to a group of individuals with the result that the knowledgeable subjects do well and the least knowledgeable subjects get low scores, then the test is probably valid.

Another factor to be considered in item analysis is *item difficulty*. A discriminating test should include items at all levels of difficulty. Here, too, we expect that the knowledgeable participant will be able to answer the more difficult questions, whereas the least knowledgeable participant will be unable to answer them. The items that are least difficult should be answered by practically all the subjects.

According to Stecklein, it is a rare test that has a discrimination index of more than 70. Individual items that have a difficulty index about 80 or below 20 should probably be deleted. Tests whose total discrimination index is approximately 50 are preferred, since they provide maximum discrimination.[7] The procedure for making an item analysis is as follows:

1. Based on the total score, rank the papers from highest to lowest.
2. Select the top 27% and the bottom 27% for analysis.

[7]Stecklein, John E.: How to make an item analysis of an objective test, Bulletin on classroom testing, no. 8, Minneapolis, 1957, University of Minnesota.

March 1   Group A takes test 1   100 items

Teacher grades test 1. She scores even-numbered items and odd-numbered items separately. The total number of possible points in each half of the test is 50.

Situation 1: Final scores for each half.
        Odd items = 50 correct
        Even items = 49 correct

Test 1 is reliable because scores are similar.

Situation 2: Final scores for each half.
        Odd items = 23 correct
        Even items = 49 correct

Test 1 is not reliable because scores are different.

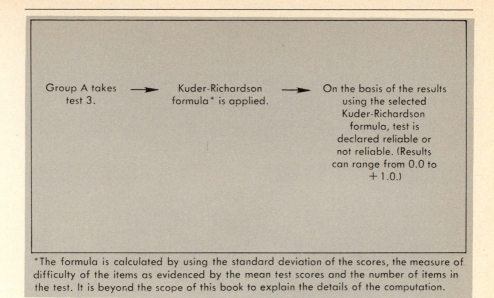

FIGURE 15-5   Kuder-Richardson reliability coefficients.

3. Tally the response made to each item by the subjects.
4. Compute the percentage of each group that answered the item correctly (Table 15-1).
5. Average the two percentages from step 4 to obtain the *difficulty index* of each item.
6. Subtract the percentage from the two extreme groups to obtain the *discrimination index* of the item.

VALIDITY

It is much more difficult and important to establish validity than to establish reliability; but the research instrument must have validity if a study is to be meaningful and worthwhile. If the instrument is valid, it can be used for prediction, as a representative of that which is to be measured, and to tell us something about the subjects. In this section we identify and discuss several types of validity. We must understand that an instrument or measure that is valid for one purpose may not be valid for another. Therefore, it may measure what it is supposed to measure with one group of subjects but not with another group of subjects. No evaluation instrument should be used in research until its validity has been ascertained.

Predictive Validity

An instrument possesses predictive validity to the extent that its predictions of future behavior are found to be accurate. If we develop a new scale to predict which potential students will successfully complete their education and advance in their nursing career, we will have to wait a specified length of time after administration of the scale to see how well it has predicted for us. If, on the basis of our instrument, we find that it has predicted

	A	B	C	D	E	F	G	H	Total Correct	Less Mean	Squared Deviation
April	R	W	R	R	W	R	W	R	5	.20	.04
Bobi	R	W	R	R	W	R	R	R	6	1.20	1.44
Cristi	R	W	W	R	W	R	W	R	4	− .80	.64
Debra	W	W	R	R	W	R	W	W	3	−1.80	3.24
Gina	R	W	R	R	R	R	R	R	7	2.20	4.84
Jan	R	W	W	W	W	R	W	R	3	−1.80	3.24
Kim	R	W	R	R	W	R	R	R	6	1.20	1.44
Vani	R	W	R	R	W	R	W	R	5	.20	.04
Mimi	W	W	R	R	W	R	W	R	4	.80	.64
Nan	R	W	W	R	W	R	R	R	5	.20	.04
	.80	.00	.70	.90	.10	1.00	.40	.90	48		15.60
	.20	1.00	.30	.10	.90	.00	.60	.10			
	.16	.00	.21	.09	.09	.00	.24	.09	.88		

Mean = 48 ÷ 10 = 4.8
Variance = 15.60 ÷ 10 = 1.56
Standard Deviation = 156 = 1.25

FIGURE 15-6   Kuder-Richardson K-R20 Example

successfully for 70% to 85% of those who completed the new scale, we might decide that all applicants should complete the instrument in the future. If we decide that we want to be sure of success in at least 95% of the cases, then we must refine the scale until it meets our requirement (Fig. 15-7).

Content Validity

Content validity is the extent to which the instrument samples the factors or situations under study. The content of the instrument must be closely related to that which is to be measured. Someone must judge if the content of the instrument is appropriate, and in this case a jury opinion is better than a single individual. The jury, of course, should be composed of individuals who are experts in the field under study. Perhaps in one case we would want a group of head nurses, several physicians, nursing instructors, and two or three staff nurses to look at the items in the instrument. If they agreed that the items were valid, we would have a jury opinion. In another instance, the jury might be limited to community health nurses, school nurses, and occupational health nurses or members of a single group. The number of individuals selected to act as a jury (sometimes also called judges) would be determined by the investigator.

Content validity is an important characteristic of inventories, checklists, evaluation instruments, questionnaires, and interview schedules. It is sometimes secondary to other types of validity, but it is reasonable to expect the instrument to include a balanced sample of items to test the hypothesis. Every item should be related to the hypothesis and to the focus of the study, or it is meaningless and costly in time and effort to both the researcher and the subject (Fig. 15-8).

Concurrent Validity

The third type of validity is concurrent validity, or status validity. Predictive validity is future oriented, whereas concurrent validity is present oriented. The behavior that it reveals can be demonstrated at the present time. Concurrent validity is important when there is concern for placement, achievement, adjustment, judgment, and attitudes. Various aspects of the topic under study may be broken down for in-depth investigation, but there is always association with the present behavior of the individual. The research tool has concurrent validity if data resulting from its use are related to behaviors in the current situation. If the performance of the nurse or student in the clinical setting is similar to that in a practical test, the practical test has concurrent validity to that degree (Fig. 15-9).

Construct Validity

Construct validity is the interplay between theory and the measurement of the constructs that make up theory. Construct validity is often difficult to understand because the term *construct* is given a hazy definition, or because it deals with the intangible. A construct is an hypothetical definition used in our theory. For example, intelligence is a construct that is used in the theory of human abilities to explain differences. Human characteristics that are examples of constructs may be such traits as flexibility, poise, integration, insecurity, and professionalism. Construct validity is of importance where such elements as values, reasoning, intellectual skills, and personal adjustment are concerned. The term *construct* frequently refers to the phenomena of concepts that are not directly observable. The construct or human characteristic that can be observed in human behavior must be defined so clearly that it is possible to verify inferences from it.

If an instrument is developed to identify a certain construct, then it must be tested for construct validity. Two methods frequently used for testing construct validity of an instrument are (1) to correlate results from the instrument with that of one believed to measure the same construct and (2) to utilize a group of independent judges who observe and record evidence of the subjects' behavior in situations that spell out the concept in operational terms. An example of the second method might be in a case where insecurity is being studied.

Suppose we have a theory that insecure people are ill at ease in interpersonal situations. We develop and give a test to a group of nurses with the result that some have

TABLE 15-1   Difficulty Index and Discrimination Index

	Percent Correct	Difficulty Index	Discrimination Index
Item A			
Upper 27%	100 ⎫	85	30
Lower 27%	70 ⎭		
Item B			
Upper 27%	60 ⎫	50	20
Lower 27%	40 ⎭		
Item C			
Upper 27%	88 ⎫	59	58
Lower 27%	30 ⎭		

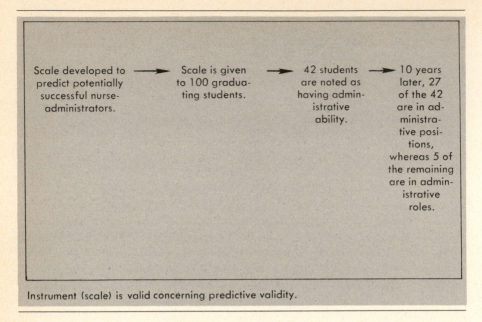

Scale developed to ⟶ Scale is given ⟶ 42 students ⟶ 10 years
predict potentially   to 100 gradua-   are noted as   later, 27
successful nurse-   ting students.   having admin-   of the 42
administrators.   istrative   are in ad-
                                                 ability.   ministra-
                                                                     tive posi-
                                                                     tions,
                                                                     whereas 5 of
                                                                     the remaining
                                                                     are in admin-
                                                                     istrative
                                                                     roles.

Instrument (scale) is valid concerning predictive validity.

FIGURE 15-7   Predictive validity.

high scores of insecurity and some have low scores. Then we observe their behavior during organizational meetings, while they talk with patients and physicians, and while they attend social gatherings. Next, we make a comparison between our observations and the responses on the instrument. If our theory was correct and the test was valid, then we would expect nurses scoring high on the test to be rated as more insecure in these three situations; but if they are not, then either our test is invalid or our theory is wrong. Perhaps they are uneasy in large crowds, rather than having general insecurity. On the other hand, insecure nurses may only be insecure in professional relationships, not in social relationships.

If a research hypothesis concerns a concept and an instrument that is intended to measure the concept has been devised, then it is necessary that the instrument be tested for construct validity. Construct validity and construct validation procedures are theory oriented. For nurses, construct validation is important because it can lead to theories that can predict or explain aspects of nursing and nursing education.

In another example suppose we develop a rating scale to measure insecurity in a patient, and our hypothesis is that insecure patients are more demanding than other patients. However, we discover that this is not the case. One of two things appears to be wrong: our instrument is wrong or our theory is wrong. If we do not get positive results from the use of our instrument, we must ask, "Is it the test or the theory?" We use our instrument again, and this time our hypothesis is that insecure patients change physicians more frequently than secure patients. Depending on the results of this study, we may say that our theory is wrong again or that our instrument is inappropriate. Either the tool needs refinement, or other hypotheses must be tested.

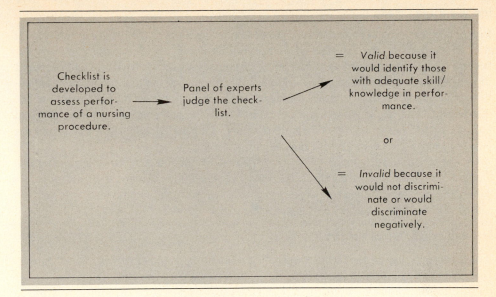

FIGURE 15-8   Content Validity.

In another instance we may wish to study variables involved in teaching a diabetic patient to care for himself. We want to find out if there is a relationship between how fast a diabetic patient learns and his level of intellectual ability. We administer one of the standardized intelligence tests to our subjects and find that there is no difference between the diabetic and nondiabetic groups. In this case, we would conclude that our theory was not accurate, because intelligence tests have been studied for many years and are known to be valid measures of intellectual ability. Perhaps intelligence is not a factor; then we begin to think of other factors, such as nervousness or anxiety, that may interfere with the rate of learning. (See Fig. 15-10.)

Face Validity

Face validity, or logical validity, involves an analysis of whether the instrument appears to be a valid scale. This procedure calls for a high degree of subjectivity. By just looking at the instrument, the investigator decides if it has face validity. Of course, a second researcher may disagree, just as a panel of judges may disagree among themselves.

Suppose we developed a questionnaire that we expected to elicit information identifying nurses' perceptions about certain competencies. If, when we look at it, the questionnaire seems to focus on the selected topic and the values of nurses who demonstrate the competency, then the questionnaire would seem to identify those perceptions. However, this does not mean that we have a valid instrument. (See Fig. 15-11.)

Face validity is a questionable criterion to use for testing validity, but it is perhaps the least time-consuming of all the methods. Therefore, it should be included in every test for validity.

Independent Criteria

Independent criteria are another method of validating an instrument. If our instrument was developed for the purpose of identifying students who have the potential for becoming successful (according to our definition) nurses, we could check other independent measures such as their absentee record and their errors in giving treatments and medications. Such records could be used as a means of checking or confirming the results of the instrument. The investigator must be careful that the independent criteria are good indexes of the factor being studied. If they are, then independent criteria provide a powerful means of validating the instrument.

An observation instrument could be validated by the independent criteria method. Suppose we have observed muscle atrophy in a bedridden patient. Furthermore, we notice that the patient has a loss of coordination. An instrument could be developed that will verify these observations in measurable terms.

Internal and External Validity

The terms *internal* and *external* are applied to validity in the experimental situation. Internal validity refers to interpretation of findings within the study, experiment, or data. External validity is concerned with generalization beyond the study, relating to the use of the findings. The researcher, of course, attempts to determine if the studied variable is actually the causal factor or if there are extraneous or intervening variables unaccounted for in the study setting. The degree to which he/she is able to accomplish this is called internal validity. The extent to which he/she can make a generalization

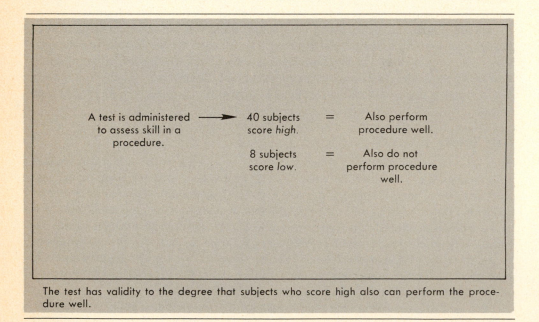

The test has validity to the degree that subjects who score high also can perform the procedure well.

FIGURE 15-9   Concurrent Validity.

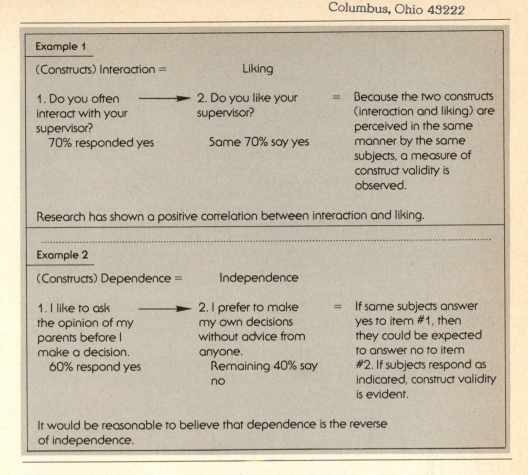

Example 1

(Constructs) Interaction =   Liking

| 1. Do you often interact with your supervisor?
70% responded yes | ➔ | 2. Do you like your supervisor?

Same 70% say yes | = | Because the two constructs (interaction and liking) are perceived in the same manner by the same subjects, a measure of construct validity is observed. |

Research has shown a positive correlation between interaction and liking.

- -

Example 2

(Constructs) Dependence =   Independence

| 1. I like to ask the opinion of my parents before I make a decision.
60% respond yes | ➔ | 2. I prefer to make my own decisions without advice from anyone.
Remaining 40% say no | = | If same subjects answer yes to item #1, then they could be expected to answer no to item #2. If subjects respond as indicated, construct validity is evident. |

It would be reasonable to believe that dependence is the reverse of independence.

FIGURE 15-10   Construct validity.

about the relationships identified in the experimental setting is a measure of the external validity of the study. This suggests that if we introduce into an experiment some independent variable, and it does in fact influence or cause the dependent variable, then the experiment may have internal validity. (See Fig. 15-13.)

If the independent variable works within the experiment group, will it work externally? Will it work on a group outside of the experimental setting? To be more specific, suppose that in a test on creativity, we design a film that causes nursing students in an experimental setting to respond more creatively. Tests have now shown that the film appears to be valid with the experimental group; but will the same film stimulate creativity in another class, or in mathematics majors, physic majors, or art majors? Will they be able to understand math better, draw scenes with more imagination, and so on? Will the instructor be able to note they have been stimulated and are more creative? This information would yield verification of external validity. (See Fig. 15–14.)

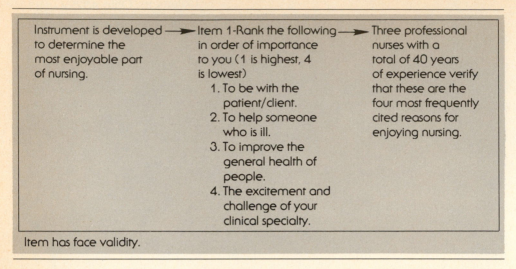

FIGURE 15-11   Face validity.

Best suggests that several problems are threats to external validity. Maturity may result in the subjects' being wiser, fatigued, or bored, or in the subjects'; trying to outguess the experimenter. Perhaps those in our experimental group have been subjected to unusual experiments that now cause them to react differently. The fact that they are in an artificial situation and are being tested may cause the subjects to react differently. Some changes in recording or instrumentation may result in a loss of validity. The subjects or the judges may become tired, the equipment may not work well, the lighting may be inadequate, or it may be a stormy day. All of these variables may affect responses.

Another point is statistical regression. All examples of any subject tend to regress toward the mean. For example, exceptionally tall parents usually have children who are shorter than they are, and exceptionally short parents quite often have children who are a little taller than they are. All things are regressing toward the mean (average).[8]

[8]Best John W.: Research in education, ed. 4, Englewood Cliffs, N.J., 1981, Prentice-Hall, Inc., p. 81.

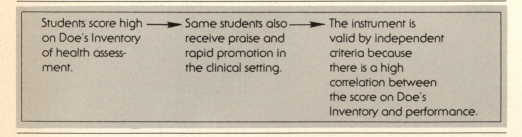

FIGURE 15-12   Independent criteria.

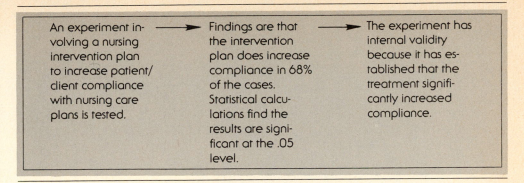

FIGURE 15-13   Internal validity.

All of the problems just discussed represent threats to the validity of research. However, the multitude of problems confronting the researcher should not be threatening, but challenging.

MISCELLANEOUS TERMS

Other terms are frequently used when validity is discussed from different points of view. An instrument is *experimentally valid* to the extent that it achieves the purpose for which it was developed. The *empirical validity* of a test is established later through evaluation and statistical reasoning.

We have already referred to obtaining a *jury opinion* about the validity of an instrument. This is somewhat better than face validity, but only slightly better. To test against *known groups*, we might ask a group of nurses who have demonstrated competency in an area to provide data with which to test the sample. We would compare their answers with those of individuals who have not as yet enrolled in a school of nursing. If we find that the answers given by the nurses are discriminating, and the instrument appears to be a valid scale, then we can assume that we have developed a good scale, and we may use it for predicting competency. Or we might have a medical nursing test, and we are wondering if it is really testing what the students are supposed to have learned. We might have a group of medical nursing instructors take the test, having made certain that the test meets its objectives.

Because of the importance of validity, it is imperative that we apply as many types of validation to the instrument as possible. At a minimum, face validity plus one other measure should be used. In addition to our discussion of reliability and validity, other factors indicate the sensitivity of the instrument. Appropriateness and facility are two characteristics for judging the worth of an instrument.

The usefulness of the instrument is of concern in *pragmatic validity*. Does the instrument work, or could we have gotten along without it? The approach to answer these questions may be taken through the avenues of concurrent and predictive validity.

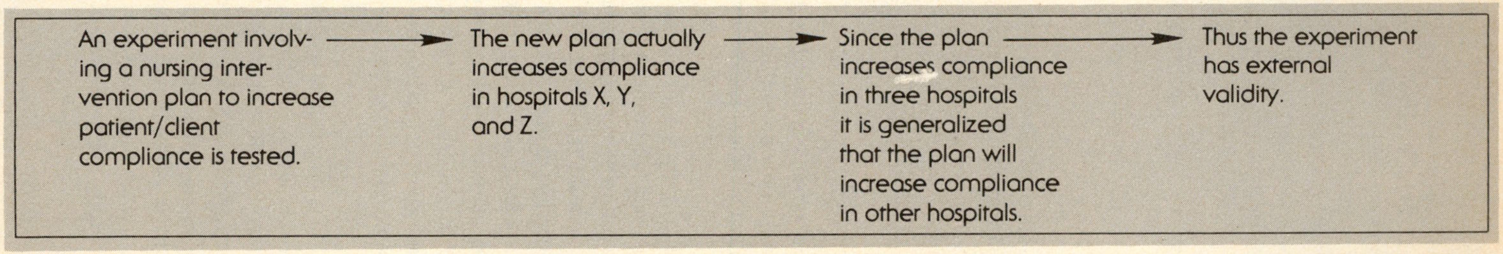

An experiment involving a nursing intervention plan to increase patient/client compliance is tested. → The new plan actually increases compliance in hospitals X, Y, and Z. → Since the plan increases compliance in three hospitals it is generalized that the plan will increase compliance in other hospitals. → Thus the experiment has external validity.

FIGURE 15-14   External validity.

A questionnaire has been developed to assess patient satisfaction with nursing care in Hospital D. The patients are complaining to the nurses that their food is always cold, no one ever stops to check on them, and their signal lights are on for 20 minutes before anyone answers. The instrument should contain questions that elicit complaints about the food, about signal lights being answered, and about personal attention. Further, the instrument should provide some opportunity for open-ended replies. If the instrument does not offer evidence of patient dissatisfaction, it does not have pragmatic validity.

A number of threats to reliability and validity can bias research results:

1. Failure to include topics or items in instruments which might influence the results if they had been included.
2. Poor operational definitions or assuming that operational definitions are understandable.
3. Quantifying data into categories by dropping neutral values, redefining qualitative variables such as good or poor into numerical values, and reclassifying abstract dimensions of data into Likert-type scales.
4. Assumptions which may be opinions rather than facts.
5. Contamination of control and experimental groups by subject interaction, attempts to outwit the researcher, differences in directions to subjects, and difficulty in maintaining equal conditions.
6. Carryover from pretests to posttests, unanticipated events that occur between pre- and posttests, and maturation or changes in subjects between tests may bias the results.
7. Analysis of data errors can result from inappropriate or too lengthy intervals, failure to consider other variables, statistics not suitable for the data, and incorrect interpretation of findings or statistical results.
8. Summary and conclusion not justified by the results, sample, tables, and evidence.

SUMMARY

Reliability is the proportion of accuracy to inaccuracy in measurement. The concept commonly refers to the consistency of the data-gathering instrument in obtaining the same results in similar situations even though the subjects and environment differ. *Reliability coefficient* refers to the correlation between two measurements that are obtained in the same manner. *Validity* refers to an instrument or test actually testing what it is supposed to test. A measurement technique must be accurate and valid if it is to be useful. There are different ways of estimating the accuracy of the measurement techniques themselves.

The *test-retest* method of determining reliability requires that a test or instrument be administered twice to the same subjects. If the test is reliable and the trait being measured is stable, the results will be consistent and essentially the same both times.

Equivalent tests also can be used in the same manner as the test-retest method. Equivalent tests contain the same types of items based on the same material, but the particular references and items are different. Parallel forms of the test reveal a high correlation in results if tests are reliable.

The *split-half* technique compares the results of one half of the items (perhaps odd-numbered versus even-number) against the other half. If the results are approximately equal, the test is probably reliable. The split-half technique has generally been replaced by the Kuder-Richardson method.

The *Kuder-Richardson* reliability coefficient is a statistical formula that gives an estimate of item intercorrelation (KR 20). The more simplified version (KR 21), is less accurate but easier to compute. These formulas are applied to the test results to determine their reliability. These are measures of the internal consistency or the homogeneity of the items in a test; the items are assumed to be accurate to the extent that they are alike or related to each other.

Item analysis operates on the assumption that a test should discriminate between good students and poor students (or with or without the trait under investigation). If items discriminate well, then the test is considered reliable.

Content validity refers to the extent that the data-gathering tool reflects the factors under study. It is ascertained by submitting the instrument to a group of judges or experts who estimate validity on the basis of their experience.

Concurrent validity is established by checking to see if subjects actually are presently engaged in the activity or able to exhibit the quality measured by the instrument. In contrast to *predictive validity*, which is future oriented, concurrent validity is present oriented.

Construct validity is the interplay between theory and the measurement of the constructs that make up the theory. A construct is a hypothetical definition that is used in a theory. Construct validity is of importance where such elements as values, reasoning, intellectual skills, and personal adjustment are concerned.

Face validity is judged on the basis of visual scrutiny. By observing the instrument, a decision is made that it is or is not testing the variable under consideration. The instrument looks valid.

Validity may be established by comparison with a group known to have the variable being considered or by comparison with other *independent criteria*.

When we use independent criteria, we compare one variable with another similar variable of the same quality. If the considered variable is confirmed by the second variable, validity is assumed.

Internal and *external validity* are applied to validity in the experimental situation. If the variable performs as expected within an experimental group, this suggests internal validity. If the experimental variable also performs as expected beyond the group (in real situations), the experiment is viewed as having external validity.

DISCUSSION QUESTIONS

1 Why are reliability and validity important?
2 If you could select one test of reliability, which would you choose and why?
3 If you could use only one test of validity for your research, which would you select and why?
4 Explain how item analysis could be useful with a questionnaire.
5 Validity and reliability are often discussed in relation to testing procedures by educators. How are reliability and validity related to an experiment in testing a new cold remedy?
6 If a mathematical test is both valid and reliable, can we assume that it is a good test? (Explain your definition of good.)
7 Why are examples of validity and reliability usually related to tests rather than to a research tool?

8 What would you look for in face validity?

9 What are the similarities between face validity and content validity?

10 Define construct validity in your own words.

CLASS ACTIVITIES

Track I

1 Copies of instruments are distributed to groups of three or four students. Each group is to analyze the instruments for face validity and content validity.

2 Old or prepared examination papers are distributed to groups of students. Each group tests the reliability of its instrument using the split-half method or item analysis.

Track II (Steps in Research Project)

1 All students are to test the instrument individually that they are developing for face validity and content validity whether they are conducting the project alone or as part of a group project.

2 Students are to continue refining their instruments after exchanging them with classmates for suggestions and/or comments.

SUGGESTED READINGS

Ackerman, W.B., and Lohnes, P.R.: Research methods for nurses, New York, 1981, McGraw-Hill, Inc.

Barnard, K.: Measurements: reliability, The American Journal of Maternal Child Nursing 7:101, March–April 1982.

Barnard, K.: Measurement: validity—keys to research, The American Journal of Maternal Child Nursing 7:165, May–June 1982.

Boffey, P.M.: Scientific data: 50 pct. unusable? Chronicle of Higher Education 10(1):1, February 24, 1975.

Byrne, B.M.: The general/academic self-concept monological network: a review of construct validation research, Rev. of Educational Research 54(3):427–456, Fall 1984.

Cooper, H.M.: The integrative research review, a systematic approach, Applied Social Research Methods Series, Vol. 2, Beverly Hills, 1984, Sage Publications, Inc.

Cronbach, L.J.: Essentials of psychological testing, ed. 3, New York, 1970, Harper & Row Publishers, pp. 142–149.

Henerson, J.E., Morris, L.L., and Fitz-Gibbon, C.T.: How to measure attitudes, Beverly Hills, 1978, Sage Publications, Inc.

Kazdin, A.E.: Single-case experimental designs in clinical research and practice, New Directions for Methodology of Social and Behavioral Sciences: Single-Case Research Design, no. 13. San Francisco, 1982, Jossey-Bass.

Krueger, J.C., Nelson, A.H., and Wolanin, M.O.: Nursing research, development, collaboration, and utilization, Germantown, MD, 1978, Aspen Systems Corporation.

Morris, L.L. and Fitz-Gibbon, C.T.: How to measure achievement, Beverly Hills, 1978, Sage Publications, Inc.

McBride, H., Littlefield, J., and Garman, R.E.: A simulation method measuring psychomotor nursing skills, in Evaluation & Health Professions 4(3):295–305, September 1981.

News, Experts agree valid approach not yet found to measure quality nursing care, Int. Nurs. Rev. 23(3):94, May–June 1976.

North, L.W.: Sphygmomanometer accuracy, Am. J. Nurs. 79(10):2004, November 1979.

Polit, D., and Hungler, B.: Nursing research: principles & methods, Philadelphia, 1978, J.B. Lippincott Co., Chapter 20.

Walberg, H.J., Gordon, W., ed.: Quantification reconsidered, In Review of Research in Education, 11, Washington, D.C., 1984, American Educational Research Association, p. 369–402.

Waltz, C. and Bausell, R.B.: Nursing research: design, statistics and computer analysis, Philadelphia, 1981, F.A. Davis Company.

Westwick, C.R.: Item analysis, J. Nurs. Educ. **15**(5):27–32, January 1976.

Williamson, Y.M.: Research methodology and its application to nursing, New York, 1981, John Wiley & Sons.

PART FOUR

COLLECTING DATA

Part Four is divided into six chapters. Chapters 16 through 20 deal separately with the major types of data-collecting methods. These methods include the questionnaire, the interview, records, observation, and other techniques. An introduction to qualitative research as contrasted to quantitative research is included in this section.

Chapter 21 focuses on the pilot study and pretesting the research instrument. Both of these steps are essential parts of the research process. The construction of tables also is discussed since their trial use is part of the pilot study process.

CHAPTER 16

THE QUESTIONNAIRE

The questionnaire is the most common research instrument. It comprises a series of questions that are filled in by all the participants in a sample. Questionnaires may be distributed directly to the respondents in the classroom, on the streets or on campus, in the dormitory or at home, or at work. It is necessary to mail them to respondents who live in a large geographical area, since handing questionnaires directly to the participants is too costly or time-consuming for the researchers.

In a single study, questionnaires may be used in conjunction with other instruments or techniques. The investigator may wish to elicit information from the subjects to supplement findings, to compare with other observations, or as one method of investigation.

ADVANTAGES

The use of questionnaires as the study instrument has several advantages.
1. Questionnaires are a relatively simple method of obtaining data. Items can be constructed rather easily by beginning researchers.
2. They are a rapid and efficient method of gathering information.
3. The researcher is able to gather data from a widely scattered sample.
4. They are inexpensive to distribute.
5. Data from close-ended items are relatively easy to tabulate, especially if there are check-off responses.
6. Respondents can remain anonymous.
7. The questionnaire offers a simple procedure for exploring a new topic.
8. Questionnaires can be flexible concerning the type of item, the order of items, and the topics covered by the researcher.
9. The questionnaire is one of the easiest tools to test for reliability and validity.
10. The subject has time to contemplate his/her response to each question.
11. Measurement is enhanced because all subjects respond to the same questions.
12. Analysis and interpretation of data can be easily accomplished.

DISADVANTAGES

There are also several disadvantages in the use of questionnaires.

1. The instrument is unable to probe a topic in depth without becoming lengthy.
2. The respondent may omit or disregard any item he/she chooses, without giving an explanation.
3. Some items may force the subject to select responses that are not his/her actual choice (forced-choice items).
4. The amount of information that can be gathered is limited by the subject's available time and interest span. Usually respondents do not like to take more than 25 minutes to answer a questionnaire.
5. Printing may be costly if the questionnaire is lengthy and is printed on high-quality paper.
6. Addressing outside and return envelopes and postage are time-consuming and expensive, respectively.
7. Data are limited to the information voluntarily supplied by the respondents. Not all members of the anticipated sample may comply with the request to participate.
8. Some items may be misunderstood.
9. The sample is limited to those who are literate.
10. Subjects who return their questionnaires may not be a representative sample of the total population.
11. The researcher cannot observe the subject's nonverbal cues.
12. If the respondent is promised anonymity, it is impossible to know who returned the questionnaires in case follow-up is needed.
13. A special effort must be made to test for reliability and validity.
14. The researcher does not have the opportunity to interact with the subject.
15. Subjects usually are able to express their opinions or their views more easily when speaking than when writing.

It must be emphasized that questionnaires are often only opinionnaires. Even factual data are not always reported accurately. Hodgkinson and Edelstein illustrate the notion that facts from questionnaires cannot always be accepted as such. During May 1972, Hodgkinson and Edelstein received questionnaires from 1,873 institutions of higher education. In a follow-up, it was found that 25 institutions had returned an extra questionnaire. None of the 25 questionnaires had less than 7 disagreements; the mean number was 14 with an extreme of 23. The errors usually resulted from two people from the same institution each filling out a questionnaire.[1] Information obtained from a questionnaire may be only an opinion, a misinterpretation, a guess, a bias, or an error.

TECHNIQUE FOR DEVELOPMENT

After the study is designed and the type of instrument selected, the researcher decides the specific information that is needed and then develops the research tool. Frequently the instrument is a questionnaire. Respondents have great amounts of information, but unless the items in the questionnaire elicit this information, the knowledge goes untapped. One of the secrets of meaningful research is asking good questions.

[1] Hodgkinson, Harold L., and Edelstein, Stewart: Questionnaires: in fact there is error, Educ. Res. **1**(8):9, August 1972.

There are several sources of ideas the researcher may explore. He/she may read the literature to learn how other investigators developed their questionnaires, look through available questionnaires, talk with those knowledgeable about the field of interest, obtain help from an expert, or devise an instrument through interviewing several typical subjects.

Open-Ended Questions

An open-ended question allows the subject to complete the questionnaire items with an appropriate response in his/her own words. Open-ended questions may be broad or narrow. Frequently they ask why, what, and how: "What do you think?" "In your opinion...?" "How do you feel about...?" "What is the reason that...?"

A broad question suggests a topic and requires the respondent to answer from his/her point of view. For example, "In your opinion, what is the most important health care problem today?" The narrow question allows only limited flexibility in responding.
Why did you select the care of children as your specialty?
What was your reason for enrolling in this school of nursing?
What was your career goal when you graduated from high school?
List the three main satisfactions your nursing profession has provided.

Suppose we want to find out if people know what is meant by overstimulating the cardiovascular system. We may provide space for the respondent to write in such terms as walking, running, tennis, and weight lifting. If the respondents are given five responses from which to choose, they may only guess at the correct answer. As a result, the investigator cannot be sure of the response. If, however, the respondents are required to fill in the answer, we are then sure that they know the correct response.

Another method of developing an item is to give people a variety of responses and, in addition, leave a space for their own answer in case none of the others applies. This may be done even in a "yes or no" response.

Did you hold a full-time or part-time job in an occupational field related to nursing prior to enrolling in a school of nursing? ☐ Yes ☐ No If yes, please specify job(s)

_____

_____

An open-ended question can be used to develop responses for close-ended items, to test the respondent's knowledge of the topic, to explore a topic in depth, to arouse the subject's interest, and to collect opinions.

It must be kept in mind that different responses are obtained when broad questions are asked instead of narrow open-ended items. For this reason, it is important that the researcher have a specific purpose for including each question in the instrument.

The response to an open-ended item demonstrates the respondent's knowledge and opinions.

Broad
What are some reasons why the freshmen selected X School of Nursing?

_____

Narrow
Why did you enroll in X School of Nursing?

_____

Broad
What are some of the academic advantages of attending X School of Nursing?

Narrow
What has been the most important academic advantage for you in being enrolled at X School of Nursing?

Broad
What problems do registered nurses face in their profession?

Narrow
What is/was your greatest problem as a registered nurse?

Open-ended questions have the advantage of permitting respondents to express their feelings. In addition, their responses may trigger new insights for the researcher.

The chief disadvantage to the use of open-ended questions is that they are difficult to tabulate. The researcher must categorize the responses subjectively and thus may introduce bias.

Close-Ended Questions

A close-ended question is one in which the respondents' answers are limited to the choices offered them. In other words, the respondent has no opportunity to express an opinion unless a special provision is made (Fig. 16-1). Close-ended questions are sometimes called forced-choice questions. Choices may include ascending or descending scales, quantity and quality checkoffs, a variety of opinions, or a "yes" or "no."

In your opinion, were two 3-week rotations better than one 6-week experience?
☐ Yes ☐ No

Subjects may be asked to differentiate on the basis of some quantity or quality.

All nursing students should be members of their State Student Association. (Please check at the appropriate point.)

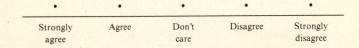

| Strongly agree | Agree | Don't care | Disagree | Strongly disagree |

How would you evaluate this convention? (Please check at the appropriate point.)

| Well organized | Fairly well organized | Disorganized |

Subjects may be allowed to check a response from a variety of reasons for believing a certain way. The choices may represent the most popular open-ended responses taken from an open-ended questionnaire. Unfortunately, in close-ended questionnaires, the respondent may be forced to choose between answers, none of which he feels is correct. By adding a category called "other," he/she has the opportunity to express an accurate opinion. For an example, see Fig. 16-1.

An advantage of the close-ended question is that the researcher can provide a number of alternative responses to fit a situation. The same question can be used in two different settings and allow for answers that can be compared.

Disadvantages are that the researcher must provide enough alternatives from which to select an answer, and care must be taken to offer realistic choices.

Asking Questions

Lunstedt states that there are four major considerations for good questions: (1) Is the answer to the question important, and would it add substantially to already known facts? (2) Does the question get to the basic issue? (3) What is the historical background of the issue being penetrated? (4) Is the question logical, and does it meet the grammatical standards of the language?[2]

Asking good questions takes practice. Suppose we decide to ask the question: "Should nursing students have an internship similar to the one medical students must serve, or not?" If someone answers "yes" to the question, is he answering "yes" to the internship or "yes" to the "or not"? A better question would be, "Do you think nurses should have an internship similar to that of medical students? ☐ Yes ☐ No"

The manner in which a question is worded will make a difference in the answer received. For example, Payne reports that there was a 19% difference in the responses

[2]Lunstedt, Sven: Explorations in methodology: the scientific question as a schemapiric dimension, J. Psychol. **72**:85, May 1969.

What reason would most influence your decision to attend the same school again? Please check one.
___ 1. I like the teachers.
___ 2. I liked the educational program.
___ 3. The school was conveniently located.
___ 4. I could afford it.
___ 5. I would not attend this school again.
___ 6. I agreed with the emphasis placed on theory.
___ 7. The school has a good reputation.
___ 8. Other, please specify _____

FIGURE 16-1   Provision for the subject's particular response.

given when might, could, and should were used. This is the same percentage as that missed by the Literary Digest Poll in calculating the outcome of the 1936 presidential election.[3]

The U.S. Bureau of the Census found that quite often people are omitted from the census because the interviewees forget to include babies as members of the family. Such errors should be anticipated while writing an item to ensure that similar oversights do not occur in the instrument.

Understandably enough, people often try to give an answer that enhances their image in the eyes of the researcher or give answers aimed at pleasing the interviewer. We might ask nursing students if they have read the current best seller. If they think their names will be connected with the response, or if they want to appear well-read, they might answer yes. Other students might not want to be associated with the book if it was deemed questionable. Certain students might be confused if the title was similar to that of another well-known book, and might erroneously state that they have read it.

It is not certain how many respondents hedge on such categories as age, income, qualifications, or experience. Some respondents may overstate or understate their qualifications if they think that it is to their advantage to do so. Prospective employees sometimes overstate their job preparation hoping to get a job, whereas others may not admit having special skills because they do not want to perform certain tasks or to take more responsibility.

Dillehay and Jernigan experimented with biased and controlled questionnaires and found that they could influence subjects' responses. They administered questionnaires that were constructed to elicit harsh, lenient, or actual opinions regarding people who commit crimes. One form of the questionnaire was administered, followed by a standardized attitude scale. Respondents displayed more lenient attitudes after they were exposed to the lenient questionnaire. The people who received the neutral and the harsh forms of the instrument showed no change. The authors concluded that the way a question is worded can influence the results.[4]

In a study by Hagsburg, the subjects reported attendance at classes conducted by their union. The subjects' reports of their attendance were then compared with the instructor's record. Only 36% accurately reported their attendance, 52% overreported their attendance, and 12% underreported their attendance. The overreporting suggests that the respondents were interested in meeting the requirements of the educational program.[5]

Respondents may misunderstand a question if it is not explicit. When asked in a survey, "When you speak of profits, are you thinking of profit on the amount of sales, on the amount of money invested in the business, on year-end inventory, or what?" more than a third of the public admitted that they had no particular concept of profits in mind. The result was even more revealing when almost as many respondents said they thought of a year-end inventory base (14%) as said they thought of the investment base (18%).[6]

[3] Payne, Stanley L.: The art of asking questions, Princeton, N.J., Copyright 1951, Princeton University Press, p. 4. Reprinted by permission of Princeton University Press.

[4] Dillehay, Ronald C., and Jernigan, Larry R.: The biased questionnaire as an instrument of opinion change, Journal of Personality and Social Psychology 15(2):144, June 1970.

[5] Hagsburg, Eugene C.: Validity of questionnaire data: reported and observed attendance in an adult education program, Public Opinion Quarterly 32(3):456, Fall 1968.

[6] Payne, p. 19.

Items that may frequently be answered with "Don't know" or "No opinion" should not be included in a questionnaire. Such responses yield no insightful data. There are times, however, when a respondent does not answer the item because of hazy recall.

Items left blank are of even less value. They are classified as "No response" and must be coded and counted. Even though the responses are counted, they have not provided quantitative data for testing the hypotheses (Table 16-1). A question that forces people to answer with a "yes" or "no" provides no reasons for the response and sheds little light on the hypothesis or question.

A telephone call was made in which the caller asked if the respondent knew what the Super Oil Company manufactured. The response was, "Oil." The conversation continued:

"Do you know any other products?"

"I can't think of anything."

"Did you read this week's _____ magazine?"

"Yes."

"Do you remember the Super Oil Company ad?"

"No."

"You don't remember seeing the ad?"

The questioner related the context of the ad; Super Oil Company manufactured a great number of products. Following the mentioning of these articles the respondent said, "Oh, yes, I remember that." This conversation illustrates the fact that people may not be aware of the commonplace, or they may be aware but are unable to recall such events readily.

The response to a health history item may be incorrect, because the question was not worded to elicit the correct reply. Diseases must be named using common terms as well as the scientific if they are to be understood by most people.

The fact that people are not aware of many everyday terms in a locale was brought to attention when a young lady commented, "I'm afraid to ask anyone else this question because it is so dumb, but can you tell me what DFL stands for?" The "dumb" question turned out to be more difficult to answer than expected. No one seemed to know that DFL signified the name of the Democratic party in Minnesota (Democratic-Farmer-Labor). Finally the group had to consult the telephone book for the correct answer.

The amount of space provided for the response might suggest something to the respondent. If space is left for only one or two words, this suggests a short answer; if space is provided for several lines, this may mean that a longer answer is expected. Even though

TABLE 16-1   Occupational Level of Respondent's Parents

Occupation	Father		Mother	
	Number	Percent	Number	Percent
Nonprofessional	200	80.0	76	30.4
Professional, semiprofessional	8	3.2	25	10.0
At home only	0	0.0	77	30.8
Unemployed, retired, ill	11	4.4	4	1.6
Deceased	23	9.2	10	4.0
No response	7	2.8	58	23.2
Don't know	1	0.4	0	0.0
TOTAL	250	100.0	250	100.0

a question is declared to be open ended, a variety of clues will determine, influence, or condition the quantity and quality of the answer.

Notice what happened when two possible alternatives were used, as reported by Payne in 1951.

Do you think the United States should allow public speeches against democracy?
Do you think the United States should forbid public speeches against democracy?
Certainly the opposite of "allow" is "forbid." We should expect directly opposite replies to these questions, but this is what happened?

First question		Second question	
Should allow	21%	Should not forbid	39%
Should not allow	62	Should forbid	46
No opinion	17	No opinion	15

Evidently there is something very forbidding about the word "forbid." People are more ready to say that something should not be allowed than to say that it should be forbidden.[7]

The possibility of a middle-ground statement is also important. We might ask some nursing students, "Do you think the tuition at X School of Nursing will be higher or lower next year?" This may not give them enough alternatives, so we might ask instead, "Do you think the tuition at X School of Nursing will be higher, lower, or about the same?" When we give them the opportunity to say "about the same," we give them a safe answer—the middle answer—and it allows an area between "higher" and "lower." When respondents are allowed to choose the middle area, definiteness is sacrificed, but broader replies are gained. Respondents are given a forced choice or an opportunity to dodge the issue.

In item development there is the possibility that uncomplimentary choices may have to be made.

Poor
    Do you think the salaries of nurses, like yourselves, are too low or too high?
Better
    Do you think the salaries of nurses like yourselves are too low or about right?

Probably very few nurses would say that their salaries were too high but they would think they were a little above average. Another variation of this item is:

Better
    Do you think the salaries of nurses like yourselves are
    (Please check at appropriate point.)

Much too low	Somewhat low	About right	Somewhat high	Much too high

---

[7] Payne, p. 57.

Fig. 16-2 is another type of item format that yields quantitative data.

Some questions are so open that any kind of answer is almost no answer at all: "Is nursing service better or worse now than it was a year ago?" Only part of the question should be asked, "Is nursing service better now?" or "Was nursing service better a year ago?" The term *better* requires clarification if such an item is used.

It is possible to test the wording of items to ascertain if the word order influences people. Two forms of the items could be prepared. For example, form A would be given to half of the group and form B to the other half. Then we could compare the differences between the two. If there are differences we might have to say that the true response falls somewhere in between. This situation would suggest that the word order of the question may be influencing people.

Payne provides an example of the split ballot.

Form A wording	Form B wording
1 ( ) Higher	3 ( ) Lower
2 ( ) About the same	2 ( ) About the same
3 ( ) Lower	1 ( ) Higher
4 ( ) No opinion	4 ( ) No opinion[8]

It has been suggested that if there is a choice of answers, especially numerical answers such as, "What is the average score that nurses get on their State Board Examination?" the correct answer should be one of the extremes rather than one in the middle.

	•		•		•
SCORE	300		400		500

[8] *Ibid.*, p. 73.

FEELING OF ACCEPTANCE	WELL ACCEPTED	FAIRLY WELL ACCEPTED	NOT ACCEPTED
By staff physicians			
By staff nurses			
By underclassmen			
By auxiliary personnel			
By technical personnel			

FIGURE 16-2   A format for soliciting opinions.

In what order should the name of products be listed? Or, in the case of elections, are there implications for voting when the individuals running for office are unknown? Which product or which candidate should be listed first?

One experiment presented several ideas in different order to matching samples of respondents.

> *Idea A was selected by—*
>   27% when it appeared at the top of the list,
>   17% when it appeared near the center, and
>   23% when it was put at the bottom of the list.
> *Idea B was selected by—*
>   11% when at the top,
>   7% when near the center, and
>   7% when at the bottom.
> *Idea C was selected by—*
>   24% when at the top,
>   20% when near the center, and
>   21% when at the bottom.
> *Idea D was selected by—*
>   23% when at the top,
>   16% when near the center, and
>   18% when at the bottom.[9]

Notice that in every case the most frequently selected idea was at the top of the list rather than in the other two positions. Generally, the top position was 6% higher than the middle position and 4% higher than the bottom position.

The ability to write good questions increases with practice. The items become less biased and have the same meaning for all respondents. The researcher is able to keep the instrument briefer while eliciting the amount and type of information needed.

Direct versus Indirect Approach

The direct and indirect approaches also may be called *coming in the front door* versus *coming in the back door*. Perhaps the researcher would like to ask a group of nursing students, "Why did you choose X institution of higher education for your nursing education?" This is a straightforward question, and the response will probably be straightforward. If, however, the respondent has some reason for hesitancy (the information may be turned over to administration, or trouble may result from answering), he/she may decide to evade the issue.

There are other possibilities for gaining information about the respondent's admission in this particular institution. Questions may be asked, as in the following examples?

1. Did you ever attend any other institution of higher education? ☐ Yes ☐ No
   If so, did you like the other school? ☐ Yes ☐No
2. Did you like the other school better than this school? ☐ Yes ☐No
3. How would you rate this school with other collegiate schools of nursing? (Circle one on the following page.)

---

[9] *Ibid.*, p. 84.

1	2	3	4	5

(Lowest)   (Highest)

These are brief examples of an indirect approach to obtaining desired information. A great number of possible questions can be asked to obtain the information being sought. As suggested earlier, the value of responses can be checked by asking a direct and an indirect question and then comparing the answers. If both questions are eliciting the same type of response, then it can be assumed that they are good questions and, furthermore, that there is some measure of reliability to the questions.

There are instances when the back-door approach will not be effective, and a direct question is the only satisfactory way to get the desired information. As an illustration, suppose we have a hypothesis: "Nurses who graduate from a 3-year nursing program will be more efficient nurses in the eyes of the physician than nurses who graduate from the 2- or 4-year nursing programs." Many varied types of questions around the whole area of efficiency might be asked by the investigator, but a direct question using the wording of the hypothesis should not be avoided. Unfortunately researchers may not get the answer they are looking for if they use the direct approach; however, they may misinterpret the response if they use the indirect question.

The researcher cannot assume that asking questions related to the hypothesis will replace a direct question concerning the hypothesis. We recommend asking the indirect question first; later, after the respondent is accustomed to the topic, the direct question can be asked. The time lapse will serve to cloud the researcher's purpose for the two questions.

Evidence of Misleading Questions

1. "All-or-none" responses. If answers are all given in the same direction (such as all "yes" or all "no"), then we can suspect that our question has provided us with only a stereotyped response or cliché. Everyone is against sin, and everyone is in favor of adequate health care, so responses that elicit this type of information have really told us nothing.

2. Considerable difference in responses when the order is changed. This may be a change in the word order of an item or a change in the order of the questions.

3. High proportion of omission or "no response." The reason a respondent does not answer every question may be unclear. Perhaps he does not notice the item and inadvertently skips over one or more. Often a question is placed in an unstrategic spot on the page and is overlooked. If lines are drawn for the respondent's answer, he is more likely to see the question than if there is only blank space for the response. On the other hand, he may refuse to answer an item because it offends him or the wording is not clear to him. If more than 5% of the items are left blank because the respondent has omitted answering the question (whether in a questionnaire or other tool), then it is important that the reason be discovered. A pilot study should point out excessive "no response" questions before the major study is undertaken.

4. High proportion of "don't know" or "don't recall." Such responses as these indicate that the items are improperly stated or inappropriate. It is hoped that these are discovered when the instrument is pretested. The questions may be revised or eliminated.

5. High proportion of "other" answers. If the choices for selection are inadequate or inappropriate, there is a great possibility that many of the respondents will decide to write in their own independent responses. These must then be compiled under the title of "other." Unfortunately, these answers require subjective interpretation and are difficult to classify and tabulate. Here again, the pilot study should point out difficulties that respondents seem to be having with the item.

6. Considerable number of added comments. If a great number of comments are added in the margins or at the end of the items, it indicates enthusiasm on the respondents' part or weakness in the items. These comments should be carefully studied to note the cause. If the comments are irrelevant, the items are either unclear, or the alternatives are inappropriate.

To sum up the results, the influence of poor question wording and questionnaire design is no doubt underestimated in many research projects. Ir split-ballot field experiments were carried out on questionnaire and interview wording, there is strong reason to believe that the efficacy of much of the research carried out by beginning researchers would be enhanced.

Appearance

To expect a high percentage of response from research participants, the items should appear answerable, neat, and not too lengthy in number. The quality of the questionnaire should be considered. Items should be well-spaced with printing of appropriate size. A questionnaire that has been done haphazardly, has typing errors, and lacks neatness and readability does not seem important.

If cost is a major factor in doing a study, the least the researcher can do is be sure that the questionnaire contains no misspelled words, strikeovers, or smudges. At best, a mimeographed questionnaire does not give the respondent a good impression. One that is well printed on high-quality paper is likely to be answered and returned.

PROBLEMS IN CONSTRUCTION

There are several more problem areas in the construction of the questionnaire. In this section we include suggestions for the solution of these problems.

1. Not enough alternatives. We might ask the question:

Why is it that nurses do not want to work at Hospital Y?
☐ a. The pay is too low.
☐ b. The working conditions are unpleasant.

Additional responses should be included, since the real reason may have to do with their feelings toward administrative personnel, the hospital policies and regulations, or lack of in-service education.

2. Inadequate knowledge or careless responses. A *sleeper question* is a question containing a fictitious name or nonexistent idea put into the list of alternatives to serve as a control measure. Surprisingly, some respondents do check these if they seem to be

authentic. If the same proportion of persons check the fake choice as the answer, we can conclude that the respondents really did not know what they were talking about.

3. Forced alternatives. There are some questions, such as, "Do you still beat your wife?" "What is Mickey Mouse, a cat or a dog?" that force the respondent into a difficult position. Be sure the alternatives are appropriate for the intended respondents.

4. Double negatives. An item related to nursing that would be difficult to answer is, "Are you against not allowing nurses to strike?" The double negative confuses the respondent, and he/she is not sure how to answer.

5. Nonspecific items. The question, "Is the quality of nursing better than it used to be?" is confusing. A specific time should be included in the wording. A better item is, "Is the quality of nursing care better now than it was 5 years ago?" Of course, even this item does not indicate what is meant by "quality of nursing care," and "quality" should be defined somewhere in the questionnaire.

6. Lengthy questions. It has been suggested that questions should be limited to about 20 words or less to avoid confusion.

7. Suggested answers. The item should not be worded so as to suggest the answer that is expected. A question such as, "You don't approve of strikes, do you?" suggests that the respondents should answer "No."

8. Personal questions. If a very personal question is being asked, some reason should be given as to why the answer is needed. Otherwise, the respondent is apt to omit the item, give a vague answer, or lie.

9. Length of questionnaire. Questionnaires should not take more than 20 to 25 minutes to complete. There are two reasons for this: first, respondents may not take the time to answer a long questionnaire, and second, they may become fatigued and not give accurate responses. However, Champion and Sear found that long questionnaires tended to be returned more frequently than short ones. Their distinction between short and long was three and nine pages.[10] In their study of attitudes, Marin and Howe found that questionnaire length affects response rates. More than three-fourths of the subjects responded to a 1-page questionnaire in contrast to slightly more than one-half who returned 8-page questionnaires.[11]

It is important that the investigator be truthful when stating the amount of time it will probably take to complete the instrument. One questionnaire received from a researcher took nearly 6 hours to complete, although the investigator suggested that 20 minutes would be the average length of time required. To answer some items with any degree of accuracy, it was necessary to compute the cost of the factor being studied. Other items required much thought and reflection, so they could not be answered rapidly. This questionnaire should have been shortened, or an accurate statement made concerning completion time.

10. Problem words. Payne, among others, has suggested a number of problem words. One of these is "you." For example: "How many patients did you care for last week?" The

[10] Champion, Dean J., and Sear, Alan M.: Questionnaire response rate: a methodological analysis, Social Forces **47**(3):335–339, March 1969.

[11] Marin, J. and Howe, H.L.: Physicians' attitudes toward breast self-examination, a pilot study, Evaluation and the Health Professions, **7**(2):193–204, June 1984.

respondent might not be sure if the items refers to himself, to all employees in the institution, or to nursing employees working in one of the units.

About

What percentage is "about 95%?" Is it 75%, 80%, 85%, 90%, or 95%?

All

"Is the school of nursing doing all it can to help the students?" Few would say that any person or organization was doing "all it can." Some respondents may be of the opinion that a great deal was being done, but certainly not all.

Country

Does this mean a nation as a whole or the portion of it in which the respondent lives?

Dr. John S. Hoyt, Jr., University of Minnesota, did a study on word meanings. Forty percent of a sample of 2,900 people returned questionnaires dealing with quantifying adjectives. *Several* ranged from 3 to an average of 11.94. Words such as *lots* and *many* were most frequently defined as 40.[12]

Other confusing words are always, may, large, many, important, better, no, never, none, some, could, anyone, get, most, much, near, several, generally, and often.[13] Some words present problems because they have become a part of American slang and have taken on a different meaning.

ORDER OF QUESTIONS

A questionnaire will appear less confusing and be easier to complete if it is carefully planned. Responses given by subjects will tend to be more accurate and representative of the participant when certain principles are followed.

1. Every item in a questionnaire should relate to the topic under study. However, it is wise to have a variety of other related questions included as long as their purpose is predetermined. Suppose the question being asked concerns the hypothesis that "Associate degree program graduates have as much technical and theoretical knowledge as diploma school graduates." It would be possible to ask questions limited to this specific area. But it would also be valuable to ask various other questions, since there may not be a relationship between the two variables in the hypothesis under study. Socioeconomic background questions may suggest other factors that influence results more than those included in the original hypothesis. Or, they may explain why the original hypothesis can or cannot be accepted. We must be sure that there is a valid reason for the inclusion of each particular item in the questionnaire.

2. Items should be organized into units. Although each item must be considered individually, they should fit together as a unit. There should be a progression from one type of item to another and from one group of items to the next. First, the respondent's interest must be awakened; second, items should progress from those that are simple to answer to those that are more complex, difficult, and thought provoking. Those questions dealing with the same topic should be placed together in the same unit or section.

[12]Smith, R.T.: Minneapolis Tribune, p. 1B, November 7, 1972.
[13]Payne, pp. 158–176.

3. General questions should lead to specific ones. The investigator may think that questions should ask for such information as name and occupation, but these questions are not very interesting to the person receiving a mailed questionnaire. (Frequently, identifying data and socioeconomic items are placed at the end of the mailed questionnaire.)

4. There should be a logical progression in the order of items within a unit and between units. If the instrument designer goes through the order of thinking required by the items, he/she will probably not jump around from one kind of question to another. The researcher should not mix the types of items; instead check-off items should be placed together, completion items together, essay items together, and so on.

5. One question should not influence the next. Although it might deal with the same general topic, the response to one item should not provide a clue or bias for the next item.

6. Personal background information such as the age, educational level, and marital status is usually included in questionnaires. The number of items depends on the purpose of the study, the hypothesis being tested, or the research question being investigated.

Questionnaires are not complete without an introduction. Subjects have the right to know the purpose of the study and why they are being questioned. Confidentiality and anonymity should be assured. Directions for completion of the items should be explicit and unambiguous so that the respondents understand what the researcher wants.

CODING

Coding is an important part of questionnaire development. All items should be stated in such a way that some classification of answers is possible. By coding, responses may conveniently be punched into IBM-like cards or tallied by hand if the study is small.

Each alternative in an item should have a consecutive number, and these numbers are placed in a space that is provided in the righthand margin. By numbering the coding spaces, it is possible to identify an item rapidly. In addition, identification of the school, class, institution, type of employment, clinical area, and so on also can be coded. For example, if 10 schools are participating in a study, they may be numbered 1 through 10 in the space provided. Furthermore, students may be identified by class level; for example, freshman classes may be numbered 1, sophomore 2, junior 3, and senior 4, depending on how many classes are included in the program.

It is important that coding be simple to carry out. Definite categories are easy to code; however, if categories are not definite—as occurs in an open-ended questionnaire—it may be extremely difficult to categorize responses. Perhaps the only solution in an investigation is to lump the responses into some codes. People who say, "seldom," "almost never," and "occasionally" may be included in one grouping, and those who say "often," "a great number of times," or "a great deal," might be placed into a category at the other end of the scale.

Note the coding and format for one commonly used social factor in Fig. 16-3. The coding space is labeled number 61, because it is the 61st item in the questionnaire. Alternative number 5 was checked by the respondent.

A code number should be provided for subjects who respond "Don't know" and for those who fail to answer the item (Table 16-1).

B. Where did you spend most of your preadult years (age 14-17)? Please check one.

_____ 1. Farm

_____ 2. Village

_____ 3. Small town (2,500 to 10,000 and over 15 miles from nearest large city)

_____ 4. Suburb (outside city limits but within 15 miles of large city)

__X__ 5. Small city (10,001 to 50,000)

_____ 6. Medium-sized city (50,001 to 100,000)

_____ 7. Large city (100,000 or more)

FIGURE 16-3   Coding.

DISTRIBUTION

Questionnaires may be distributed directly or through the mail; there are endless ways and places to hand out questionnaires. For one research project, the investigator hitchhiked and asked the people offering rides to fill out a questionnaire about picking up hitchhikers. Another researcher asked people shopping in a downtown area to fill out a short questionnaire. Other investigators may go from house to house asking residents to fill out the instruments.

When opinionnaires are placed in mailboxes in educational institutions, the response is sometimes as low as 25% or as high as 60%. A great number of factors influences the rate of response. For example, the time of year may be important. When questionnaires are handed out near the end of the academic year, students are too busy studying to respond. Questionnaires distributed earlier in the term may be returned in higher proportion.

Personal experience in distributing a short questionnaire to every third house in a selected area of the city produced a 93% return. The length of the questionnaire and the ease with which the items could be answered contributed to this high proportion of return.

Members of an organization may be handed a questionnaire when they come to a meeting. Frequently, questionnaires are handed out in church, in a coffee shop, or any place that people gather together. The investigator ought to be creative in selecting the locale for obtaining participants.

Mailing

There are advantages and disadvantages in mailing questionnaires to respondents rather than distributing them directly. There are advantages in effort, time, and the anonymity of the response. If the investigator wishes to obtain information from nurses who graduated from a specific school of nursing, effort can be saved by mailing the questionnaires rather than personally searching for those who have moved or have married. However, if alumni records are not up to date, it may be very difficult to trace all members of a particular class. When a questionnaire is mailed to the most current address on hand, the post office does part of the searching, instead of the investigator.

A second advantage is the time factor. The respondent can complete the questionnaire in a few minutes, whereas if the researcher had to be present, it would take the time of both investigator and respondent.

The third advantage is the guarantee that responses will remain anonymous. Respondents may feel more free to write their answers than to talk with the researcher in person. Some personal questions may be asked and answered through the mail if the respondents think that they will not be identified.

Even though mailing the research tool is probably the easiest method of gathering data, it is, at the same time, probably the poorest method. A disadvantage of the mailed questionnaire is that some items may need clarification. If the question is ambiguous to the subject, the answer is probably invalid or ambiguous to the researcher. Other questions are, "Was the respondent given enough choices?" "Was the respondent joking when he/she gave certain answers?" "Was he/she trying to outguess the item developer to throw off the results?" "Why were some of the questions not returned?"

What percentage of responses can be expected from a mailed questionnaire? If a questionnaire asking about life insurance is mailed, probably only a very small percentage of the recipients would respond because they would be afraid that a sales representative would contact them to buy insurance. However, if the questionnaire is simply an opinion poll, there might be a 50% to 60% response. Any questionnaire sent through the mail that produces 75% to 85% response is doing extremely well.

Andreasen indicates that researchers have explored the effectiveness of a wide range of variables in an effort to increase the response rates for mailed questionnaire surveys. These have included such variables as the number and timing of mailings, stamped or metered reply envelopes, cash and prize rewards, printed versus mimeographed forms, and various types of cover letters. A personally typed letter only increased the response rate over a form letter by 7% to 8%. It was concluded that the cost of personalization did not justify the benefit.[14]

One study, reported by Joseph Alutto, dealt with the rate of response based on destination. Questionnaires were sent to a sample of workers. Half were mailed to their homes and half to their places of employment. The rate of response was the same for both groups; however, differences did occur according to whether the items were open-ended or closed-ended. Open-ended items received a significantly greater number of completions when the questionnaires were received at the place of employment. The 64 close-ended questions were completed by the same number in both groups.[15]

When a high percentage of subjects fails to return the instruments, the researcher cannot draw valid conclusions. By providing a deadline for return of the instrument which gives the researcher time to contact the subject again, the validity of the findings is increased. Unfortunately, it is usually impossible to identify respondents who fail to return questionnaires.

[14] Andreasen, Alan R.: Personalizing mail questionnaire correspondence, Public Opinion Quarterly 34:273–277, Summer 1970.
[15] Alutto, Joseph A.: A note on determining questionnaire destination in survey research, Social Forces 48:251, December 1969.

Cover Letter

When the questionnaire is mailed, it should be accompanied by a cover letter stating the purpose of the questionnaire, who is sanctioning the study, what will be done with the information, the reason that the respondent should answer, and the deadline date for the return of the questionnaire. The investigator also should include a guarantee of anonymity or confidentiality of information. He/she should thank the respondent for participating in the study and make an offer to inform the respondent of the results if he is interested.

The more personal the letter looks, the more likely people are to take an interest in answering the questionnaire. The letter should be neat and printed or typed on good quality paper. Also, a personal signature (not mimeographed) should be used.

FOLLOW-UP

A number of techniques can be used to ensure that a questionnaire will be returned. One method is for a letter signed by a well-known or important figure in an organization to accompany the questionnaire. The letter should state good reasons why the questionnaire should be returned. In one instance the reason that questionnaires were not returned by the sample participants was because the return envelope was a small, personal letter envelope, whereas the questionnaire had been mailed in a large business envelope. The respondent had to fold the questionnaire so many times to get it into the small envelope that some individuals did not feel that it was worth all the bother.

The question arises, "How do you do follow-up work in case the respondent has been told that his answer will remain anonymous?" Follow-up (a second communication is mailed to the respondent) is a difficult problem. The investigator may mail a special letter to everyone in the study sample if he has no way of knowing which respondents returned their questionnaire. If he has designed some type of informal code that identifies the person by town or some mark on the outside of the envelope rather than on the questionnaire, then he knows which participants have not returned their study instrument. The questionnaire would not need to be numbered if it has an identification mark. The ethics of this procedure are sometimes questioned, however. A telephone call can be made to participants living in the same area as the investigator to learn if the questionnaire was received or returned. In a mailed research investigation, a small percentage of envelopes can be expected to get lost in the mail.

What should be done about people who do not return their questionnaires? Are they going to sway or bias the results of the study because they did not return their questionnaire to the researcher? Possibly the persons who do not answer their questionnaires have some difference in attitude or personality from those who submit returns. Most studies seem to indicate that there is little difference in responses between those who return the question- naire and those who do not. This fact has been verified by seeking out and interviewing those who did not return their forms. Among the reasons given for not returning them were that they did not like the organization, they were unhappy, they had lost the questionnaire or put it aside intending to fill it out later, they had forgotten about it, or they had laid it aside and still plan to return it. However, some said that they *had* returned the questionnaire, a fact that suggested it had been lost in the mail.

How soon should a follow-up questionnaire be sent out? How soon should a letter of inquiry be mailed? These are questions open for debate. From our experience, the largest proportion of returns, especially mailed returns, are sent back to the researcher in the following mail. Most respondents answer the questions the same day the form is received and return it directly. Each day from then on, fewer and fewer questionnaires will be returned. If a cut-off date is not made explicit, some questionnaires may not be returned until 2 or 3 months after they were sent out. If data are needed before this time, a cut-off date is essential. Questionnaires received after the cut-off date are not included in the study.

It is safe to say that if a questionnaire has not been returned within 4 to 5 weeks, some type of follow-up is required. A second wave of questionnaires should be mailed to anyone in the sample who possibly may not have returned the questionnaire. This wave may be followed by a double postal card if there are one or two items of information that the researcher still wants to obtain, which are pertinent to the study.

If the investigator does not want the recipient to suspect that some type of identification record of returned questionnaires has been kept, he might add a statement to the second questionnaire such as, "If you have not returned your questionnaire, please return this one." Or, the respondent might be asked to check a specific category on a postal card stating the reason he did not return the first questionnaire. It is important to the study that as many instruments as possible be returned so that the investigation results will be accurate.

SUMMARY

The questionnaire is the most popular research instrument and the most easily distributed. However, the items are plagued with problems of wording and meaning. Questionnaires may be mailed or distributed directly to the respondent. Mailed questionnaires have a lower rate of return, whereas personally distributed questionnaires may lose randomness and lack anonymity.

In developing items for a questionnaire, the researcher must have a good understanding of the respondents' background and be willing to expend a substantial amount of time and energy. Questionnaire items may be borrowed from other sources or developed initially by the investigator. Background reading of literature in the area to be researched is extremely important. A good way of developing questionnaire items is to interview typical sample subjects who will not be included in the final sample.

There are two types of questionnaire items: open-ended and close-ended questions. Open-ended questions allow the respondent complete freedom in answering, whereas close-ended items restrict answers to check-off items. Open-ended questions are a good preliminary technique in developing close-ended items.

Anyone can ask questions, but asking the question that will elicit the respondent's knowledge or feelings is difficult. Questions must be asked that do not suggest the answer.

Alternate wording of items, word order, item order, or similar words may all influence the respondent's answer. A direct, straightforward question may be valuable in one situation, while at other times an indirect one seems more appropriate. "No response" and "do not know" answers indicate poor questions that should be analyzed when they appear in the pretest or pilot study.

Checks, which test the value of the item, can be built into the questionnaire. Such techniques include sleepers (nonexistent possibilities) and the same question stated differently.

Certain problem areas to be avoided in question construction include the following: not enough alternatives, forced alternatives, double negatives, compound questions, and qualitative wording. Questionnaire items should follow a logical sequence, should not be too long, should be organized into units, and should lead from general questions to specific ones.

Coding is the process of classifying answers so that they may be punched on IBM-like cards or tallied readily by hand. Therefore, all questions should be stated in measureable terms. Rating (assigning values to a variable) should proceed in the direction anticipated by the hypothesis.

Return of questionnaires is facilitated by a cover letter from the governing organization or supporting persons (such as faculty advisor or organization president). Mailed questionnaires take less time and effort than interviews; however, the response rate is lower. Mailed questionnaires should be accompanied by self-addressed stamped return envelopes for the participant's convenience.

Follow-up techniques such as a postal card or another questionnaire, mailed after a reasonable waiting period to nonreturners, will increase the total number of questionnaire returns.

DISCUSSION QUESTIONS

1 Why is a questionnaire only an opinionnaire in many cases?
2 Defend or criticize the statement: A questionnaire is still the most efficient means of gathering information from human subjects.
3 Illustrate the coding for a 10-item questionnaire.
4 Word a question in several different ways.
5 Select the most valid wording of the question in item 4. Justify your response.
6 What is a valid questionnaire?
7 What would you do to improve a questionnaire in which many respondents failed to answer some of the questions?
8 How could you use a questionnaire when the subjects are illiterate?
9 How could you develop a questionnaire on the attitudes of your classmates toward research?
10 How would you list the names on a ballot in a professional election to ensure that each candidate has an equal chance of winning?

CLASS ACTIVITIES

Track I

1 Members of the class are to develop a five-item open-ended questionnaire and devise a system to code the responses.
2 Members of the class are to write five questionnaire items for each of the following categories: socioeconomic factors, education of respondents and their families, opinions concerning health issues, and personal professional goals.

Track II (Steps in Research Project)

1 Each group member or student working alone is to develop open-ended and close-ended questionnaire items to gather data for the research project.
2 Select the most appropriate items to use in the research project.
3 If a different type of instrument is selected for the research project use Track I suggestions for practice and continue to develop the other instrument.

SUGGESTED READINGS

Alutto, Joseph A.: A note on determining questionnaire destination in survey research, Social Forces **48**(2):251–252, December 1969.

Andreasen, Alan R.: Personalizing mail questionnaire correspondence, Public Opinion Quarterly **34**(2):273–277, Summer 1970.

Bradburn, N.M., and others: Improving interview method and questionnaire design, San Francisco, 1979, Jossey-Bass.

Brandt, P.A.: The PRQ—a social support measure...personal resource questionnaire, Nursing Research **30**:277–280, September–October 1981.

Burosh, Phyllis: Physicians' attitudes toward nurse-midwives, Nurs. Outlook **23**(7):453, July 1975.

Dunning, Bruce, and Cahalan, Don: By—mail us. Self-administered questionnaire, Public Opinion Quarterly **37**(4):618–624, Winter 1973–1974.

Glaser, William A.: International mail surveys of informants, Hu. Organization **25**(1):86, Spring 1966.

Godwin, K.: The consequences of large monetary incentives in mail surveys of elites, Public Opinion Quarterly **43**(3):378–393, Fall 1979.

Henerson, J.E., Morris, L.L. and Fitz-Gibbon, C.T.: How to measure attitudes, Beverly Hills, 1978, Sage Publications, Inc.

Lagay, Bruce W.: Assessing bias: a comparison of two methods, Public Opinion Quarterly **33**(4):616–617, Winter 1969–1970.

Nehring, Virginia, and Geach, Barbara: Patients' evaluation of their care, why they don't complain, Nurs. Outlook **21**(5):317–320, May 1973.

Noelle-Neumann, Elisabeth: Wanted: rules for wording structured questionnaires, Public Opinion Quarterly **34**(2):191, Summer 1970.

Payne, Stanley L.: The art of asking questions, Princeton, N.J.: 1951, Princeton University Press, pp. 8–9, 100–101.

Paynich, Mary Louise: Why do basic nursing students work in nursing? **19**(4):242, April 1971.

Rosse, J.G. and Rosse, P.H.: Role conflict and ambiguity: an empirical investigation of nursing personnel, Evaluation and the health professions **4**(4):385–405, December 1981.

Schuman, H., and Presser, S.: Question wording as an independent variable in survey analysis, Sociological Methods and Research **6**(2):151–170, November 1977.

Snelling, W. Rodman: The impact of a personalized mail questionnaire, J. Educ. Res. **63**(3):126, November 1969.

Vaughn, R.A., and others: Tracking respondents: a multimethod approach, Lexington, MA, 1981, D.C. Heath & Co.

CHAPTER 17

THE INTERVIEW

The interview is probably the second most common method for gathering information in research. (The questionnaire is most popular.) To quantify results, the researcher may use an interview schedule for recording the discussion, or a tape recorder or video tape so that he/she can analyze the interview content later. Sometimes the researcher develops an interview guide to be used when recording the respondent's answers to questions during the interview. In this chapter we focus first on the interviewing process itself, then on the interviewer, and finally on the interviewee. Tools developed for the interviewer's use, as well as suggestions to aid the beginning researcher in carrying out an effective interview, are included.

ADVANTAGES

The interview schedule, interview guide, and questionnaires are similar types of instruments in that they all require factual recall or presentation of opinions. There are advantages in doing an interview to gather data for a research project.

1. Data from each interview are usable, whereas this may not be true for each questionnaire returned. Reasons for unusable questionnaires include blank items, misunderstandings, late arrival, incorrect completions because of poor directions, and so on. The researcher may have to mail a large number of questionnaires to obtain a sufficient number of usable ones.

2. Depth of response can be assured, since the researcher can pursue any question of special interest. The interviewer can ask questions of the respondent that were not included initially but that will add to the richness of the interview content. such information may be added to the data, or it may be recorded by the interviewer for his/her own understanding of the situation.

3. In an exploratory study, the researcher may decide to use the interview technique to determine which questions would be most valuable in a questionnaire. Combining the questionnaire and the interview in the same study quite often enhances a research investigation.

4. If the interviewee does not understand one of the questions during the interview, he/she may ask to have it repeated. The interviewer on the other hand may ask, "*Why don't you understand it?*" By rewording the item, the researcher can make the question more meaningful to other interviewees.

5. No items are overlooked by the interview method. The interviewer is more likely to be sure that all questions are answered than is the person who fills out a questionnaire.

6. A higher proportion of responses are obtained from potential respondents. Some persons in the research sample fail to return mailed questionnaires, but most will consent to an interview.

7. Another advantage of interviewing is its flexability. Objections can be pointed out and rapport established so that the respondents are able, or more willing, to respond and cooperate.

8. The interview offers an opportunity to appraise the validity of the report, because the interviewer is present to observe what is taking place. Verbal and nonverbal cues that would not appear on a questionnaire can be noted.

9. The interview is a suitable technique for probing complex situations and sensitive issues. Even though the topic may not be conducive to open, frank discussion, an atmosphere that encourages confidentiality will help the researcher to be more successful in obtaining information than will the more or less rigidly structured questionnaire.

10. The interview procedure may save time for the interviewee, because he/she does not have to go through the process of returning the instrument.

11. Generally, an interview can be used to elicit information from a broader group of individuals than can the questionnaire, since the respondents do not have to know how to read or write.

12. The respondent cannot be influenced in answering the current questions by looking ahead to other items as often occurs with the questionnaire.

13. The amount and variety of information that can be elicited is increased at times.

14. Telephones may be used for soliciting some types of interview data, especially when the time period for gathering information is short. The response rate will probably be better than for mailed questionnaires dealing with the same issues.

DISADVANTAGES

1. One major disadvantage in selecting the interview as the method for obtaining data is the time element involved in carrying out the procedure. A thousand question-naires can be mailed in a relatively short time, whereas a thousand interviews would require many long hours of effort and would probably entail the assistance of a specially trained staff, which would add to the cost of the project.

2. It may be difficult to make a comparison of one interviewer's data with another interviewer's data unless a rigid procedure is followed at all times. Bias may result because of differences in question order, which would invalidate some of the information obtained. Word order in interviews has the same effect as word order in questionnaires.

3. The cost of interviews depends on the number and length of the interviews. If much traveling is required, the cost of transportation could be exorbitant. If, on the other hand, there is easy access to the sample and they are few in number, expenses may be minimal.

4. The interviewee usually has little or no choice in the date or the place of the interview. The investigator has limited time in which to complete the research project; therefore, it may not be possible to provide subjects with a choice of time for the

interview. In contrast, the subject may complete a mailed questionnaire at his/her convenience.

5. In a large research project, the director will need to hire interviewers and suitable persons may not be readily available. A training program, of course, adds to the expense of the project.

TYPES

Interviews can be categorized into five groups, depending on the point of view of various authors. These include standardized, nonstandardized, semistandardized, focused, and nondirective types. Investigators may become partial to one or two types and use them in most studies.

Standardized.   Interviewers are not permitted to change the specific wording of the interview question schedule. They must try to conduct each interview in precisely the same manner, and they cannot adapt questions for a specific situation or pursue statements to add to the data. Another name for the use of prearranged specific questions is structured.

Nonstandardized.   Interviewers have complete freedom to develop each interview in the most appropriate manner for the situation. They ask a few general questions and list a few probing comments to encourage the interviewee to continue talking.

Semistandardized.   Interviewers may be required to ask a number of specific questions, but beyond these they are free to probe as they choose.

Focused.   The focused interview is much like the nonstandardized type in that no specific questions are asked of all respondents. Rather, researchers ask a series of questions based on their understanding and insight into the situation. Special attention can be given to specific topics or ideas. The interviewer asks questions within a limited range of interest but in more depth.

Nondirective.   In this type of interview, the subject is allowed an opportunity to relate personal feelings without fear of disapproval. Subjects can express their opinions and beliefs without waiting to be questioned. There is freedom to discuss a topic without pressure from the interviewer.

The clinical interview, done for the purpose of developing an understanding of a client's motives, may be classified as nondirective. When nondirective interviews are used in psychotherapy, patients are encouraged to express their feelings without any suggestions from the interviewer. The purpose of the nondirective interview is that it results in a comprehensive picture of the interviewee's values and thoughts and, therefore, provides a larger context in which respondents can express themselves. Such results can occur only when there is an atmosphere of freedom, interest, and understanding. The interviewer should, as far as possible, resist the temptation to offer advice or to pass judgement.

Perhaps the greatest difficulty in nondirective interviewing is that of getting the subjects to talk about their feelings rather than about what they think the investigator wants to hear. Another serious problem is that the question the investigator asks to initiate the conversation may influence the subject's point of view.

INTERVIEW INSTRUMENTS

The interview guide and interview schedule are two instruments used in conjunction with the interview. They are literally sets of questions, which can be either structured or unstructured. An *interview schedule* is a questionnaire that is read to the respondent, whereas the *interview guide* is one that provides ideas but allows the interviewer freedom to pursue relevant topics in depth. In other words, it is a loosely structured interview schedule. The items provide for flexibility in the manner, order, and language of questioning. The interview guide is frequently used in a pretest or in an exploration of possible questionnaire items.

The interview guide is an effective tool for studying areas that the investigator wishes to explore in depth. The more information known about a particular topic, the more structured the items can be. Thus the interview schedule is appropriate when the investigator is informed about the facts and the situation involved, and the interview guide is appropriate for general probing.

There are instances when questionnaires are read to interviewees and the researcher records their responses. This may be particularly true if the respondents are unable to read or write. Even with literate subjects it may be easier for the researcher to write in responses. For example, the elderly may not be steady enough to write or may not see well, arthritis may hamper an individual, and temporary disabilities or injuries may prohibit the subject from filling out the questionnaire. Interviewees may request that items be read to them and their responses recorded, when they are occupied at the moment, such as a housewife who has her child in her arms, the man painting a house, or the person who is getting ready for bed and answers questions through a closed door. Fig. 17-1 illustrates an interview schedule that was used in an area survey.

An interview guide is sometimes used to interview job or nursing school applicants. Whether or not it is followed closely depends on the policy and attitudes of the interviewers. Fig. 17.2 is an example of a loosely structured guide. Its purpose is to obtain the impressions of the interviewer as well as certain facts.

Problems

Results may be unreliable when an interview schedule or guide is used. The reason may be in the use of the selected instrument or the choice of the interview as the method for obtaining research data.

1. An interview is effective for obtaining opinions, attitudes, values, and perceived behavior. However, it is usually an ineffective procedure for obtaining actual behavior patterns.

2. Depending on the sample, some of the interviewees may have faulty memories and either cannot remember a certain fact at all or guess at what seems to be a reasonable response.

3. Subjects may consciously give responses that seem to be what the interviewer wants, may lie, or may give answers representative of a group rather than their own ideas. These responses are invalid and bias the data.

4. The presence of the interviewer may influence the subjects so that they answer the questions differently than they would if filling in a questionnaire by themselves. Also,

---

INTERVIEW SCHEDULE

1. Sex   Male _____   Female _____

2. Where are you from? _____

3. Reasons for moving to _____. Please check all that apply.
   ___ Lack of work in another area
   ___ To see new things
   ___ To get away from parents
   ___ To continue education
   ___ Other _____

4. Go back and check the most important reason a second time.

5. Why do you live in this section of _____? Please check.
   ___ Close to work
   ___ Near friends
   ___ Reasonably priced rent
   ___ Near relatives
   ___ Other

6. Go back and check the most important reason a second time.

7. Date of arrival in _____ Month _____ Year _____

8. If you have moved here from out of town, what did your parents think of the idea of your leaving home? Check the one best answer.
   ___ They suggested the idea.
   ___ They encouraged the idea.
   ___ Little or no comment was made.
   ___ They discouraged the idea.
   ___ They were displeased.

9. High school graduate? Yes ___ No ___ If "yes," what year? _____

10. Have you had any education beyond high school? Yes ___ No ___ If "yes," please
    list _____

11. What type of work do you do?
    ___ Clerical   ___ Professional
    ___ Mechanical   ___ Waitress
    ___ Sales   ___ Secretary
    ___ Manual   ___ Other _____
    ___ Technician

FIGURE 17-1   Interview schedule.

respondents might answer differently than they would in an informal conversation with a friend or fellow worker.

   5. Not everyone in a chosen sample may be available for an interview; thus the response rate is less than anticipated. However, the response rate cannot be determined before the interviewing process is completed. This may lead to the overrepresentation of some of the sample and the underrepresentation of the others.

INTERVIEW GUIDE

Name _____   Date _____

Address _____

         _____

Appearance:

Education:

Health problems:

Professional goals:

Comments:

FIGURE 17-2   Interview guide.

6. Some of the interviewees may not be qualified to answer certain questions asked of them. They may not recognize their own lack of knowledge, of insight, or of the facts. They may also be prejudiced to the point that their answers are strongly biased.

7. The interviewer may become so concerned with the mechanics of using an interview schedule or guide that nonverbal cues are overlooked.

8. Subjects may become nervous about the fact that their answers are being written down or recorded on tape, adding a degree of bias to their responses.

9. Time is lost when the interviewer has to write down the interviewee's responses. In haste, mechanical errors may be made.

10. Interviewees may lose their trains of thought while waiting for the interviewer to finish writing their responses. Thus, some of the data may be lost.

11. Subjects may be difficult to locate for an interview, whereas data could be obtained more conveniently through the mail by questionnaire.

TYPES OF QUESTIONS

There are several methods by which researchers can arrive at questions to be used in interviews. (1) They can devise them personally; (2) they can talk to other people who are experts in the field; (3) they can obtain an already prepared interview schedule; and (4) they can make an adaptation of other researchers' instruments or improve one that has been used previously. After the items are selected and, when necessary, improved, they should be tested in the field under the circumstances in which they will be used in the study.

We discussed briefly in Chapter 16 the open-ended question as used in a questionnaire. The open-ended or unstructured question also may be used in the interview situation. One of its primary advantages is its flexibility. If a respondent says something that sounds interesting, the interviewer may be able to pursue the topic further. However, it is difficult to categorize answers to open-ended questions. For example, suppose we want to ask a nurse working in surgery if she enjoys working there. One nurse may answer, "Yes, I enjoy working with Doctor A." Another nurse may respond, "Yes, now that I don't have to be on call." And a third nurse may say, "Definitely, I find it very rewarding." How should these responses be categorized? If the interviewer has definite check-off slots, a structured questionnaire, or a closed-question type of instrument, the interviewer can check off the identical responses. By giving every subject the opportunity to select from the same responses, the investigator can easily carry out a quantitative analysis.

The closed question, sometimes called the fixed-alternative question, has the same advantages and disadvantages as when found in a questionnaire. Choices are limited to those suggested by the interviewer and are not always appropriate for all interviewees.

In generating interview questions, the researcher must consider the approach, interests, maturity, vocabulary, and preconceived ideas of the interviewee. Within this context the amount of time allotted for each interview will determine the extent to which opinion polling, consumer-performance surveys, or probing interviews can take place.

SEMANTICS

Language is used in all interviews, but not every word has the same meaning for every person. It is important, therefore, that the most comprehensible questions be formulated. The problem under study must be stated so that it permits scientific investigation. Furthermore, the formulation of any questions used in the study must be constructed so that they may be tallied, coded, and analyzed as accurately as possible. In interviewing, researchers must ask these questions in a similar fashion throughout the data-gathering process if they are to systematically study the responses.

Whether one individual does all the interviewing, or whether there are trained interviewers, it is important that both researcher and assistants put an accent on the same word in a sentence. In a simple question such as, "Do you enjoy working here?" by putting the emphasis on various words, the interviewer drastically changes the meaning. Variations in emphasis should not occur during an interview.

There are obviously no right or wrong answers in an interview. In an unstructured situation, interviewers should not express surprise, disagree, or give a personal opinion. Instead *they should make every effort to see that their statements are value free.* They should simply ask a question (such as, "Where were you born?") without adding a value judgment. Interviewers do not necessarily care where the individual was born. When they ask the age of the respondent, they are not asking the question because of a personal interest. Rather, the response is meaningful only as it adds to the data. There should be an attempt in all interview questions to have this impartial and unbiased approach. An unbiased attitude, of course, comes through conscious effort.

RAPPORT

The art of establishing a rapport, of putting the interviewee at ease, is really not difficult. The beginning researcher may feel a little uneasy approaching the first subject each day, but after the initial interview it is easier to walk up to the second individual. As the interviewer gains confidence, smiles, and shows enthusiasm in the interviewing task, the subject will usually respond positively.

It is important that interviewers begin by identifying themselves and by giving the reason for the research. They should ask for permission to interview and show their credentials if they have any. Every potential subject should be told the name of the study's sponsor and the purpose of the interview.

Rapport is established by creating a friendly and pleasant atmosphere for the subject. Interviewees should be promised confidentiality, and told that their frank opinions are needed. They should be assured that it is safe to put their confidence in the interviewer. There are no right or wrong answers, only an interest in the subject's feelings and thoughts.

Most people seem happy, curious, and sometimes quite pleased to be interviewed. If researchers establish a rapport with their respondents, they may often be invited to sit down and talk for a while. Interviewing can be a pleasant experience for both, as well as a method of obtaining useful information.

Interviewers should not be timid or aggressive. They should not pressure the individual into answering the questions; but by being pleasant, friendly, and courteous they should try to establish a rapport with the subjects and secure their cooperation. An informal interview is much better than one that is rigid and staid.

Interviewers are reporters. However, they should not snoop or pry. They should never show surprise at any answer the respondent gives. Nor should they encourage or show open approval of any answer.

Obviously, if anyone says that he/she does not care to participate in the survey, the interviewer should say thank you simply and leave. Undue pressure is not conducive to reliable research.

In gaining rapport with subjects, the researcher should tell them that their responses will be anonymous. How can the interview be anonymous if the interviewer is sitting face to face with an interviewee, writing down the answers? First, subjects can be reassured that their responses will be anonymous since their names and addresses are not being taken. Also, the interview schedule can be put in a box or folder of completed forms so that the respondents can slip it in anywhere they choose.

There is no need for the researcher to be afraid or shy about interviewing, because people usually like to express themselves. Remember, the focus of the conversation, their attitudes and life experiences, is important to the respondents. Very few individuals will resist the temptation to talk about their own interests or problems.

It is true that interviewers must be friendly to the subjects, but not so friendly as to lose their objectivity. Researchers want the respondents to express themselves as subjects and not necessarily as personal friends.

Another consideration that must be made when gaining rapport with a subject is that there will probably be other interviewers in the future. If the subject is treated shabbily or his confidence betrayed, he may not respond positively to the next researcher. Science and knowledge in general suffer through the unfair treatment of subjects.

Most researchers agree that the interviewer should never give personal opinions. However, if a respondent is interested, after the interview is completed the interviewer may express a personal opinion. People are frequently interested in learning the interviewer's ideas about certain questions.

SUBLIMINAL CUES

Subliminal cues are behavior or attitudes that are covertly displayed. They include inflections in the voice; manner of speech, such as how hesitant the speakers are and how much enthusiasm they display when they speak; how subjects sit on a chair; mannerisms such as frowns, movements of the head and hands; statements subjects make when other people are around; hesitancy in answering certain questions; and eagerness to talk about some topics while ignoring others.

Birdwhistell states that there is an infinite variety of body movements that have specific meaning. The human face alone can make approximately 250,000 different expressions.[1] This is not to suggest that researchers must become body language experts to be efficient researchers, but they should be aware of this rich source of information. Interviewers should be considerate of their subjects. They must be aware of such nonverbal cues as nervousness or the fact that the subject may want to get up and stretch or have a drink of water. When the interviewee is allowed to move around the room to relax or compose himself if necessary, rapport is apt to be maintained.

Beginning researchers should develop skill in reading subliminal cues. They may mention such cues to the respondent as a check on their interpretation of the subject's behavior and as a means of alleviating tension. Interpretations and predictions based on nonverbal cues must be accurate; otherwise they will bias data.

Inflections in the voice serve as cues to the interviewer. It is often said that in interviewing, how we say something is as important as what we say. For example, if we ask somebody, "Would you like to go for a cup of coffee?" and the person replies, "Mmmm, I guess so," the inflections in the response are as important as the actual words themselves. A good interviewer is able to gain insight into the response by watching for these types of cues.

There is a danger that researchers may misinterpret nonverbal cues from subjects, because the researchers are not aware of cultural differences. One culture may have practices, attitudes, and values that are quite contrary to another. For example, people from the United States stand farther apart when talking to each other than people do in some other cultures. Shaking hands, gesturing, and other physical behavior have different meanings in other cultures.

[1]Birdwhistell, Ray L.: Kinesics and context, Essays on body motion communication, Philadelphia, 1970, University of Pennsylvania Press, p. 8.

TRAINING THE INTERVIEWERS

In the interview situation there may be one or more persons doing the interviewing. If more than one researcher is involved, training of the other interviewers is required. Often the size of a survey determines the number of interviewers, the amount of time needed, and the cost. If there are many variables and much data to be gathered, it may be necessary to tabulate and analyze data by computer, although some may have to be done by hand. The amount of data gathered may depend solely on how many people are interviewing.

As Phillips points out, the large survey, especially when based on a probability sample, has some important advantages within the context of justification. But it also has several difficulties. One major obstacle is, of course, administration when a number of interviewers is involved. It is difficult to hire people for just a few days or weeks for the interviewing phase of the research. However, obtaining and processing data may require assistance, and those employed will have to be trained. Unfortunately, the researchers who are responsible for directing a large survey often spend more time working on administrative duties than on the technical problems.[2] Another difficulty is inadequately trained interviewers who have little motivation. They can have an adverse effect on the quality of the data obtained. Fowler suggests that volunteers usually are unsuccessful interviewers for probability sample surveys.[3]

Generally, the shorter the time span for the study, the less chance there is for intervening variables to influence the results. Therefore, it is more desirable to employ 10 interviewers to gather data in 1 week than to have one interviewer gather data for 10 weeks. During the 10-week period, a new law or a major event could more strongly influence the results of the first interview than the results of the last interview. An additional advantage in employing several interviewers is that it randomizes individual biases.

The interviewers should be mature and intelligent. They must be able to maintain rapport and receive satisfaction from the work and pay. Interviewers should be methodical and capable of following directions and winning the subjects' confidence.

The first interviews are important because the interviewers may bring back information that points out future difficulties requiring changes in either the wording of the interview questions or in some of the techniques used in its administration. It may be difficult at this time to detect some interviewers who cheat in their reporting. An interviewer may not only cut corners but also may make up a number of interviews. This problem is discussed at more length in the section on the biased sample.

As an illustration of the training of interviewers, suppose the interviewer is to estimate the income of the patient's family. Now, if we were to have all the interviewers look at the same family, we would probably find a great deal of variation in their reports. But if we have the interviewers investigate more specific factors such as the type of car the subjects drive, what section of the city they live in, and whether or not their home is mortgaged, it

---

[2] Phillips, Bernard S.: Social research strategy and tactics, New York, 1966, Macmillan, Inc., p. 116.
[3] Fowler, F.J., Jr.: Survey research methods, Applied Social Research Methods Series, Vol. 1, Beverly Hills 1984, Sage Publications, Inc.

might be possible to learn, through the socioeconomic background, something about their income without asking a direct question about it. The place of employment of family members or the kinds of jobs they hold also would be some indication of their income.

If we are to train our interviewers to look for this information, each interviewer must know in advance what questions to ask, and then everyone must use the same wording. This brings to mind a research project that a student carried out some time ago. The beginning researcher wanted to test the friendliness of several cities in America. He proposed having some friends who were going home on vacation stand on the main street of their hometown on a Saturday morning between 10 AM and noon. They were instructed to say, "Hello" to everyone who came along and then to record how many responded.

A discussion of the variables involved in such a study led to the discovery that many problems would be encountered. What effect would the sex and the personality of the researchers and their subjects have on the greeting? Would the weather make any difference? Would there be different types of people out at that time of day? Are people more friendly in a small town than in a large city? Since these variables would be very difficult to control, the best that the student could do was to bring all his assistants together and tell them how to say, "Hello," demonstrate what kind of smile to display, go through the process with them, and test them until everyone was doing the same thing. This was one step toward making the data more reliable, making it more objective, and, at the same time, training the interviewers so they would all act and react the same way.

Sometimes interviews must be conducted through an intepreter. In one instance, a nurse working in a refugee camp was requested to ask four basic questions of the refugees about themselves. The questions were actually symptoms of tuberculosis. For example, Have you lost weight? Do you spit? These questions were asked to the heads of families living in selected units. One person in each unit was under treatment for tuberculosis and the physician wanted to know if other persons in the group also had the disease. the interpreter soon memorized the questions and the responses expected. Another volunteer was assigned to observe the living quarters to note if the persons housed there were following the health measures they had been taught. while the nurse was occupied, the volunteer had to observe if friends, relatives, and small children might have been overlooked. In this instance, both the interpreter and the volunteer needed to be trained so that important decisions could be made concerning the health of the unit groups as well as the thousands of refugees living in the camp. Responses and observations were carefully recorded under the supervision of the nurse team director until she was satisfied that all members of the team were consistently performing their roles.

Considerations for the Interviewer

Interviewers should be aware that their subjects may belong to a subculture. For example, when subjects are from a certain ethnic group, or from a particular religious background, or have a certain political viewpoint, this problem arises—how shall the interviewers best adapt themselves to this new culture or to the individuals to whom they are speaking? Suppose they are talking with subjects who belong to a specific profession such as nursing. It would be important that they use and understand certain words. Slang or abbreviations are used for some areas of the hospital and for patient care procedures, OR, OB, Peds, CCU, PAR, and ICU are just a few examples. Symbols and letters that represent a patient's condition may not be known outside the nursing profession. Every health care agency can be expected to have its own phraseology that employees use almost absentmindedly. Interviewers would be wise to familiarize themselves with such language. Likewise, if the interviewer is familiar with the phraseology associated with nursing, then care must be taken not to use it when interviewing someone from another discipline.

When anthropologists begin working with people in a different culture, they may find that some words in their language have no equivalent in another culture. Perhaps the people in the other culture have no need for the missing words. If nurses wish to use a medical term, then the word must be defined in the language understood by the people.

Untranslatable terms become a problem for many individuals who travel to another country to study or live. A nursing student from the Philippine Islands was listening intently one beautiful May morning as her roommate explained the meaning of *spring fever*. It took many sentences to explain spring fever, a rather difficult idea to grasp for someone from another culture, particularly from a land of constant mild temperatures—perhaps the explanation was not very clear either.

After interviewers have been in the field for a while, idiosyncrasies may be picked up that will demand changes in interviewing techniques. Again, the pilot study tends to point out such problems.

CONTENT OF QUESTIONS

Quite often people do not offer an interviewer all the information he/she may need to know. It may be because the interviewer does not know enough about the topic under study to ask the best questions for eliciting information. Asking good questions about any opportunity, organization, or situation involves having some knowledge of the topic beforehand.

In one study, the researcher was making a survey of a community. He was unable to discover any cracks in the facade of community solidarity, and yet he thought there must be some dissension in the group. It was not until later, while talking with an outsider, that he discovered that the group had had a split at one time; part had left and formed a new unit. The researcher then began asking the members about the split, as he continued interviewing them. He was told, "Oh, yes, that's right. It did happen." When they were queried as to why they had not mentioned it before, the reply was, "You never did ask." The researcher responded, "Yes, but I didn't know what to ask. Why didn't you just tell me?" To this statement they replied, "Well, we didn't know you were interested in that sort of thing."

Interviewers must have some knowledge of the topic or theme before they can ask an intelligent or essential question. If they are unaware of many of the ramifications of the situation being explored, important data will be missed that perhaps would have a significant bearing on the case.

The focus of the interview does not mean the same thing to all interviewees. There are times when subjects do not think the topic under discussion is polite. They may not be knowledgeable about the problem being explored, or they may be insensitive to it. They may even think the topic is unimportant. It has often been said that if you want to take pictures when you visit a new country, do it right away before things become commonplace and no longer seem unusual. This is somewhat true with interviewees. They may become so accustomed to certain events that they do not perceive them as unusual.

If interviewers gain rapport with their subjects, these individuals often feel free to confide in the interviewer. They may begin to relate personal facts or feelings that they would not reveal to their family or friends.

The interviewing process may make a positive contribution to the interviewee. Through the interview technique the researcher may increase the subjects' understanding and insight into the question and into themselves. The researcher may even be able to gain information from the subject concerning a point neither had been aware of until then.

A BIASED SAMPLE

The researcher also faces the problem of bias. As an example, several interviewers go out to interview a group of people during the morning. It may be that all the interviewers are married women and they select mornings for conducting interviews because their husbands have gone to work and their children are at school. Consequently, these interviewers are only interviewing other married women who are at home when they knock on the door. Perhaps if they had selected evenings for their interviewing sessions, they might have gotten an entirely different sample, yielding a different kind of data.

It is not always possible to determine initially what kind of biases will be faced in a study. Until the investigator has had a little experience in interviewing or until the interview returns begin to come in, no one may be aware of all the problems to be overcome. Consequently, the first interview results should be tabulated, analyzed, and observed as quickly as possible. If the hypothesis is not supported, and there was a strong belief that it would be, perhaps the reason is a bias.

We mentioned earlier the possibility of some of the interviewers cheating, perhaps faking whole interviews. It might be possible to prevent cheating by telling the interviewers beforehand that periodic checks with the subjects will be made, such as sending letters, making telephone calls, or conducting follow-up interviews. Another inquirer is sometimes sent to check interviews to see if the information was actually collected. The threat may be sufficient to convince the interviewer to carry out all the questioning. Spot checks might be made if necessary.

Hauck reports having used postcards as an effective check. Thank you letters and postcards were sent to persons who had and had not been interviewed. "Of the interviewed sample (587), about one-half (49.1%) returned the postcard while for the not-interviewed sample (580) only about one in ten (9.5%) returned the postcard....[4] Later, some of the sample said they had been interviewed when they had not been and vice versa. The reasons why some of the people who had been questioned reported that they had not been interviewed were that they had forgotten about the interview, or that someone else in the family who was unaware of the interview had completed the postcard.[5]

[4]Hauck, Mathew: Is survey postcard verification effective? Public Opinion Quarterly **33**(1):117–120, Spring 1969.
[5]*Ibid.*, p. 119.

Doob and Ecker describe another type of bias, stigma and compliance. They found that the interviewer has a great deal to do with how people answer questions in an interview. In this study some of the interviewers wore black patches. It was found that their appearance had made a difference in the responses given by the interviewees.[6]

Often interviewer bias is not a matter of prejudice or premeditation; rather, it is accidental, unintended, and often unknown. Instances of bias can actually be detected by comparing the results of the interviews in the present study with other studies and noting differences. For example, differences between the subject and interviewer in age, status, and education may influence both individuals at the time of the interview. In recording long responses, the interviewer may be selective for the sake of brevity or because of fatigue.

We must realize that interviewers are prone to bias by some of their own prejudices and must attempt to reduce such bias. this can be accomplished by such techniques as standardizing instruction, classifying answers, role playing, giving *dry run* interviews, and giving the interviewer less chance to make individual choices. As the interviewer's freedom is limited by rules, so too is the opportunity for probing and for gaining new insight. It is in the pretest and the pilot study that some freedom can be allowed. By basing a decision on knowledge learned in the pretest and pilot study, researchers can restrict their freedom to gathering material that seems most relevant and, at the same time, is free of bias. It must be remembered that bias is present in all kinds of data, and should not be thought of as limited to the interview method.

Bias is sometimes initiated by the subject. It has been noticed that if a certain nursing class decides that specific instructors or physicians are "out to get them," then this attitude can permeate the whole class until the students become biased, in spite of the fact that empirical data may not justify their attitude. For example, a student once asked, "Why is this school so difficult? Half the junior class is dropping out." On investigation, it was learned that only 5 of the more than 80 students were actually dropping out and only one because of academic difficulty. The remainder were leaving of their own accord for marriage or other reasons. Nevertheless, a number of the class members continued to complain that the courses were too difficult. It is important that the interviewer learn to detect biased attitudes to strengthen the data-collecting aspect of the study.

HELPING PEOPLE RECALL

Several factors can help interviewees to recall information the investigator would like to glean from them. For example, if the interviewer is asking someone, "Where were you going to school 2 years ago?" "What were you doing a year ago on this date?" or "What date did such and such an event happen?" there are ways to help the subject recall the answers. One can help the subject reconstruct the events that were taking place at the time. Almost everybody can remember where they were working or what they did to celebrate a particular holiday.

Another technique is to ask if the subject remembers what day of the week it was, whether he/she was going to school at the time, whether it was morning or evening, and if

[6]Doob, Anthony N., and Ecker, Barbara Payne: Stigma and compliance, Journal of Personality and Social Psychology 14(4):302–304, April 1970.

it was before a holiday or on a weekend, so that he/she may be able to focus more closely on the particular event. Certain individuals are helped to recollect incidents by being asked where they were working at the time, what kind of car they were driving, or what time of year it was. Looking at the calendar is sometimes helpful. Diaries, checkbooks, and appointment books, not only the subject's but close relatives', will aid in recall.

Although an effort should be made to assist the interviewee in recalling events, it is important that they not be made to feel that they must remember the circumstances, events, people, or incidents. This may put them under such stress or discomfort that rapport is weakened or lost. If it is apparent that the interviewee really cannot remember, then the investigator should move on to the next topic.

ASKING QUESTIONS—PRACTICAL APPLICATION

If possible, the interview should take place in a quiet atmosphere. Often, when we enter a building tenants have the television set on. If they are watching a particularly interesting program, it may be wise for researchers to wait until the program is over or to suggest to the subjects that the researchers return in a few minutes.

The subject should be seated in a comfortable position and should be told beforehand approximately how many minutes the interview will take. This is known if a schedule has been set up beforehand and a pilot study run. If the interview is part of the pilot study, this fact may be told to the interviewee along with the fact that the interview will take approximately _____ minutes.

In recording answers during an interview in which the subject talks very rapidly, it is impossible for the interviewer to take it all down in longhand. In this case, it may be more feasible to use a tape recorder or some other electronic device. If a tape recorder is used, the subject should be reassured that the information will not be used for any purpose other than that stated or any purpose that will be detrimental to the subject. The individual may be nervous during the recording session, but there are certain advantages in this method. The tone of the voice and the emotional impact are preserved by the tape, providing additional clues. In addition, the entire message is recorded—something that seldom is accomplished when paper and pencil are used. Hesitations and inflections in the voice are preserved in tape recordings but are usually not recorded in the written notes of a conversation. If it is absolutely necessary to write down every word that subjects say, it may be necessary to ask them to speak slowly.

If there are specific questions that the subjects do not want to answer, they should not be pressured into responding. If the subjects do not want to answer embarrassing questions, they should be told that they need not answer unless they wish to do so. If embarrassing questions are left until late in the interview, after a rapport has been established, it is usually easier for the interviewee to answer them.

If it seems important that direct questions be asked of the interviewee, then a simple straightforward approach should be used. It is found that if the researcher first brings up topics close to the issue at hand, this will sometimes reveal the person's attitude without having to ask the question directly. If it appears that the subject may refuse to answer, a second approach is to confine the discussion to various questions on the periphery.

OTHER IMPORTANT FACTORS

At what time of day should we interview a subject? At what time of month should we plan to interview subjects? What day of the week would be best to interview the sample? These are all interesting and important questions. Once, when surveying homes in a certain area, we found that Monday evening was a very good time to interview the age group we were seeking. We found most residents at home after 7 PM and before 9:30 PM. this particular time during the week seemed to be best because the subjects were single young people who often went home on weekends. If they did not go home, they often had dates and so were not in their apartments on weekend evenings. Before 7 PM they were usually involved with the evening meal or were getting ready for a date. They seemed to be available for interviewing on Monday evening because they were tired and wanted to get to bed early. We discovered that if we arrived after 9:30 PM, often they were getting ready for bed and did not want to answer questions. For this particular research project, the best time to interview subjects was between 7 and 9 on a Monday evening.

Weeks and others presented some interesting results from a study done on the optimal times to contact sample households, covering the years 1960, 1971, and 1976. They found that in 1976 there was a declining number of homes in which at least one person aged 14 or older was present. There were the largest number of people at home in 1960 and the smallest number at home in 1976. More people were in the house from 5 PM to 8 PM than at any other time during the 12-hour period from 8 AM to 8 PM.[7]

Concerning research on telephone answering time, it was found that 16 seconds is needed for a phone to ring three times (ring, pause, ring, pause, ring). It was also found that 88% of the people will answer within three rings if they are at home. After four rings 96.7% will answer and after five rings, 99.2%. The researchers felt that four rings was sufficient for contacting anyone at home.[8]

It may require quite a number of interviews before the prime hours and days for interviewing are determined. Every type of interviewing situation may involve an entirely different set of variables in terms of deciding when and where interviewing should take place. Ideas may be gleaned from other studies, but an exact repetition of the study results cannot necessarily be expected in a different interviewing situation. Again, it is important to remember that a pilot study or an interview pretest may yield an extremely important clue as to what to expect in the major study.

RELIABILITY OF THE INTERVIEW

As is often said in social research, how you obtained your data may be more important than what you found. This is borne out time and time again when a study is replicated, resulting in almost the exact opposite findings.

[7]Weeks, M.E., and others: Optimal times to contact sample households, Public Opinion Quarterly, pp. 101–114, Spring 1980.
[8]Comments and letters, Public Opinion Quarterly, pp. 115–116, Spring 1980.

If several interviewers are assigned to gathering data, the results each interviewer brings in should be checked from time to time. If all the interviewers seem to be getting generally the same results, we may assume that there is some reliability in the findings. However, if one interviewer consistently brings back results different from the others, perhaps a seasoned interviewer should discreetly accompany that interviewer so any differences in method will be identified.

Interview data from a certain geographical area that differs markedly from data collected in other areas also is a cue that the interview results may not be accurate. At least there should be a close examination of both the interview process and the results. It may be wise to continue training the interviewers throughout the course of the data-gathering process if difficulty continues.

If the research hypothesis has been well thought out and seems satisfactory, but continued review of data fails to confirm the hypothesis, something may be wrong with the interviewing process. Analysis of the interviewing technique and the instrument is in order.

Reliability of the interview instrument depends on the wording of the questions and scales. the questions should mean the same thing to all respondents. At the same time the interview presentation should be uniform. Validity of the interview is increased through the use of reliable questions and a follow up to discourage cheating.

SUMMARY

The interview is second only to the questionnaire as a popular process for gathering information from subjects. By using an interview guide, interview schedule, or a tape recorder, or by simply writing down the answers to questions, sometimes verbatim, the interviewer obtains information pertinent to the study. Questionnaires and interviews are two methods for answering questions. Many of the techniques used in designing a questionnaire are appropriate for the interview.

Advantages of using the interview technique for obtaining raw data are numerous.
1. Data are usable.
2. Misunderstandings can be minimized when questions are explained by the researcher.
3. Some topics can be pursued in depth.
4. No items are omitted, accidently or purposely.
5. A higher percentage of response is possible.
6. Greater flexibility is provided in the interview than in the questionnaire.
7. It is useful for developing a questionnaire.
8. The subject need not be literate.
9. Verbal and nonverbal cues can be noted.
10. The interviewee's time may be saved.
11. There is more opportunity to appraise the validity of the report.
Disadvantages in using the interview are few but important.
1. It requires more time for the researcher to locate and interview each person individually.
2. The interpersonal relationship between subject and researcher is different for each interview.

3. The cost in time and effort is greater for the interview than for the mailed questionnaire.
4. The interviewee usually has little or no choice in the date or place of the interview.

There are five types of interviews: standardized, nonstandardized, semistandardized, focused, and nondirective. In standardized interviews the inquirer is held to specific wording during the interview. In the nonstandardized type, there is freedom to develop each situation. Semistandardized interviews require a specific number of questions, but there is freedom for probing. A focused interview is directed toward specific topics. Finally, in the nondirective interview, the subject has complete freedom to express his/her feelings without regard to topic.

In the less structured interview, the subject is not only more able, but more likely, to reveal personal feelings than in a structure interview. The nondirective interview requires an atmosphere of freedom that can only be acquired by a permissive and understanding interviewer.

Interview guides and interview schedules are the usual instruments for questioning a subject. The interview schedule can be read to the respondent (structured), whereas the interview guide only suggests ideas, thus allowing the interviewer more freedom (unstructured). The interview guide is often used as an exploratory tool for developing either an interview schedule or questionnaire items. The interview schedule is appropriate when specific answers are required, whereas the guide is beneficial for probing feelings and attitudes. Interview guides are frequently used for potential job applicants and students.

Several problems arise with the use of interviews in the data-gathering process. Some of these problems are as follows:
1. Responses may be only opinions.
2. Subjects may not be able to recall.
3. The subjects may be seeking the approval of the interviewer.
4. The interviewer's presence may affect the interviewee's response.
5. Not everyone wants to be interviewed.
6. Some people may not be qualified to participate in an interview.
7. The interviewer may become preoccupied with recording the responses.
8. The subjects may be nervous because his answers are being recorded.
9. The researcher needs time to write out responses.
10. The interviewee must wait until the answers are recorded.
11. A subject is more difficult to find in person than through the mail.

Interview material can be devised by the researcher, suggested by an expert, or found already prepared from other studies, or combinations of these may be used. Responses from open-ended questions, such as those found in the interview guide, are difficult to categorize but are valuable for developing the interview schedule.

The semantics of asking questions determines the type of response that will be given. Therefore, it is important that the interviewer does not suggest answers to questions, favor one answer over another, or influence the response in any way.

Interviewers should begin by identifying themselves and by stating the purpose of the study and the length of the interview. They should establish rapport with their subjects by being pleasant, friendly, considerate, and enthusiastic. Undue pressure on the subject to participate in the study or to answer the questions should be avoided. All subjects should be assured of anonymity. Researchers should treat subjects with respect because they are willing participants in the project, because their cooperation is appreciated, and because it is important to leave them with a good impression of scientific research.

Subliminal cues are nonverbal behaviors such as voice inflections, facial expressions, body movements, hesitancy of speech, enthusiasm, and so on. Videotapes and tape recordings of an interview provide a record of subliminal cues.

If there are several interviewers, they will need training. Each interviewer must be trained regarding approach, the exact words to use, and inflections in the voice, so that no bias is introduced because of the way the interview is conducted. If the interviewers are required to make judgments about socioeconomic factors pertaining to the subjects, the interviewers must be trained to develop a high degree of correlation between interviewer's judgments, which is necessary for reliability.

Many factors influence the results of interviews. These include smiles, sex differences, socioeconomic background, dress, and so on. The interviewer should be informed about the topic and understand slang or colloquial phrases. The interviewer should develop the art of asking questions and giving cues that will elicit the subject's feelings about the question under consideration. The researcher, in asking questions, must use the proper cue to elicit the respondent's true feelings.

A trained interviewer should be able to help the subject attain depth and insight into both the topic and himself/herself. Biased data can result from the time of the interview, dishonest interviewers, unknown variables, oversights, and prejudices. Interviewers may be subject to their own biases, so the results from one interviewer should be compared with those gathered by another interviewer. Follow-up can be used to prevent cheating and to check accuracy.

When subjects are unable to recall desired information, reminders may help them remember. Such reminders include diaries or checkbooks. Another method is for the interviewee to recall the day of the week, important events that took place near the time of the incident under study, occupation when the event occurred, and time of day.

The research should include checkpoints, at which time the data are scrutinized for weaknesses. Such measures make for productive data gathering.

DISCUSSION QUESTIONS

1 If you could choose either the interview or the questionnaire to gather data, which would you select and why?
2 Comment on the statement: The only difference between the interview and the questionnaire is that one is written and the other is oral.
3 Subliminal cues may offer additional insight into a subject during an interview. Do you think it is possible or impossible to interpret body language (nonverbal) accurately? Support your response.
4 Comment on the statement: A questionnaire is a more appropriate instrument for asking personal questions than an interview schedule.
5 Give an example of how you could use the retroactive design in an interview.
6 How can you discover the best time for an interview?
7 How would you go about obtaining permission to interview five employees of agency C?
8 Give an example of when you would use an interview guide.
9 Give three different meanings for the statement "Everyone here is satisfied with working conditions."

CLASS ACTIVITIES

Track I

1 The class is divided into small groups. Each group develops a brief interview schedule dealing with a selected topic. Each person then interviews one individual within walking distance and returns to share the collected data.
2 Class members decide on a topic and the appropriate questions to be asked. Each individual then interviews someone randomly or as directed by the instructor. Interviewing experiences are shared at the end of the hour.

Track II (Steps in Research Project)

1 Each group or individual students are to develop an interview guide for gathering data for the course research project.
2 Group members or individual students are to develop an interview schedule appropriate for the research project, for practice or project.
3 Have a friend or relative try out the project instrument and write a brief description of the weaknesses, flaws and problems. Submit to the instructor or share orally.

SUGGESTED READINGS

Bauleke, J.K.: Promoting change through nursing research, Minnesota Nursing Accent 43:16–17, January, 1971.

Bozett, F.W.: Practical suggestion for the use of the audio cassette tape recorder in nursing research, West. Can. Res. J. 2(3):601–605, Summer 1980.

Bradburn, N.M., and others: Improving interview method and questionnaire design, San Francisco, 1979, Jossey-Bass.

Burgess, A.W., and Holmstrom, L.L.: Crisis and counseling requests of rape victims, Nurs. Res. 23(3):196–202, May–June 1974.

Harrison, A.A., and others: Cues to deception in an interview situation, Soc. Psychol. 41(2):L156–161, June 1978.

Henerson, M.E., Morris, L., and Fitz-Gibbon, C.T.: How to measure attitudes, Beverly Hills, 1978, SAGE Publications, Inc.

Holder, J.M.: Research abstracts, Can. Nurse 70:42, October 1974.

Klecka, W.R., and Tuchfarber, A.J.: Random digit dialing: a comparison to personal surveys, Public Opinion Quarterly 42(1):L105–114, Spring 1978.

Masterson-Allen, S., and others: Terminally ill patients' and families' responses to participation in a research study 18(1):83–92, March 1985.

Taylor, S.J. and Bogdan, R.: Introduction to qualitative research methods, the search for meanings, ed. 2, New York, 1984, John Wiley & Sons.

CHAPTER 18

RECORDS

Records are a valuable and lucrative source of nursing research data. Questionnaires, interviews, observation, and experimentation all require the researcher to interact with the subject to obtain information, but records are an ever-present source of material.

Records are found everywhere, in homes, offices, and places of leisure. Students keep records even though they may be only names of persons with whom they correspond and bank account records. Most people keep some types of records—recipes, receipts, sales slips, or business transactions. The hospital is no exception. Records are available in every department. The medical profession has become a careful record keeper, especially in recent years.

It may come as a surprise to learn that there are records dating back to the Romans. These records contain names such as those of the captain of the guard and his lieutenant who were placed around Jesus' tomb. The Roman rulers were careful keepers of records.[1]

DEFINITION

Records are compilations of writings and figures that individuals have collected. It is necessary to distinguish between research that uses records (including those found in libraries) and a research term paper. This chapter is concerned with research that uses records. It is *not* concerned with using books, periodicals, pamphlets, and other publications to write a term paper. True scientific research makes use of all the basic steps of the scientific method.

Differentiation must be made between primary research and secondary research since records fall into both types of investigation. Stewart defines primary research as that which is designed, implemented, analyzed, and summarized by the researcher. The sources of data can be original or produced for another purpose. Secondary research, on the other hand, begins after the data has been collected and the researcher analyzes information that is already available. The two types of information usually complement each other rather than substitute.[2]

[1] McIntosh and Twyman, translators: The Archko volume, or the archeological writings of the Sanhedrin and Talmuds of the Jews. From manuscripts in Constantinople and the records of the senatorial docket taken from the Vatican at Rome. Grand Rapids, Mich., 1954, The Archko Press, pp. 144–145.
[2] Stewart, D.W.: Secondary research, information sources and methods, Applied Social Research Methods Series Vol. 4, Beverly Hills, 1984, Sage Publications, Inc., p. 12.

SOURCES

The use of records as a source of data for research is as broad as the imagination. Someone has said that creativity is mathematics: you either add to what you already have, you subtract, you divide, or you multiply. The same is true with records. Researchers may take records from two different sources to make a comparison; they may add the data, subtract them, or use parts. A creative investigator is able to look beyond written records to artifacts and cultural data for research material.

Many sources of records are used as research data. One of the richest accumulations of records is published by the U.S. government.

Census tract data are a valuable source of numerical information. A city, for example, is broken down into areas of a few square blocks each; then each time the census is taken, comparisons can be made with the last census results. Changes that have occurred in each tract can be compared. All census tracts and their data are listed in a census tract publication, distributed by the U.S. Department of Commerce, Bureau of the Census. Some of the general characteristics of the population include race, marital status, where students attend school, number of years of education, and income. Labor force characteristics include such categories as type of employment, means of transportation to and from work, structure of the house, number of rooms, and types of heating. Both a census tract map and the statistics are included in a single population and housing report. Such data are extremely valuable, not only because they are used in many scientific investigations, but because creative uses for the data are limited only by the creativity of the researcher.

One study done on a section of a city is an example of how government records can be used. A comparison was made between the investigator's findings and the census tract data on such factors as age and population. It proved to be a useful process because the findings from the research study agreed with the tract data, suggesting that the research data were accurate.

Census tract data can be a valuable source of information enabling the health professionals to better understand the people living in specific areas of the city. It might be important information for a public health nurse to know the racial composition and income level of an area.

In the nursing profession, educational records are extremely important. Suppose we are interested in learning, for purposes of recruitment, the number of potential nursing students graduating from high school. This information would be available in records, either in compiled forms from an appropriate organization or from the individual schools. By checking the number of entrances into elementary schools during the past 10 years, for example, we could predict the rate of graduation increase or decrease. Furthermore, such information might serve as a basis for future projections.

That almost no one keeps enough records becomes evident if we begin to do a geneology search. It becomes difficult to learn the birth date of many individuals—even those born in the 1890s. The exact data may be missing from military records, and searching comes to a halt when the exact date is unknown and cannot be located in courthouse records (vital statistics) or family records.[3] Such problems must be addressed

[3]Each of us should keep more and accurate records. We would be wise to write a brief history of our lives to be carefully filed away for future use. Someone might want to use it someday in doing research.

by nurse-researchers who are becoming increasingly interested in the historical background of nursing and the leaders who have made contributions to their field.

Health care facilities are particularly geared toward keeping records. It is absolutely necessary that histories, backgrounds, treatments, medications, diagnoses, and prognoses be recorded. Any attempt to relate social variables within the framework of epidemiology requires careful historical data.

Suggestions for places where one may find records in a hospital or health care institution are numerous. Every hospital has medical records. If there is a school of nursing affiliated with or sponsored by the hospital, it will have educational records. The business office has financial records, and the personnel office has records of the employees. The diet kitchen keeps records pertaining to the cost, preparation, and consumption of food by patients and personnel per day, month, and year. The maintenance department keeps records of the types of fuel and their use throughout the year, as well as equipment needed to run the physical plant. Every department in the hospital or health care agency keeps records that may be useful for research purposes.

There are even original or primary sources of unpublished materials. These are available if sought diligently enough. Old church records are often very good sources of dates of weddings, funerals, baptisms, and so on. If an historical study were being made on the life of a famous person or group who lived in a particular community, many facets of their lives could be substantiated by searching through church and institutional records. Cities often have historical and reference libraries. Museums and state archives are devoted to collecting and maintaining records and documents from past generations. The librarian can usually assist in finding materials and information needed. At times, the librarian will say, "No, we don't have it." But personal investigation may unexpectedly reveal sources of information. Perhaps the librarian did not understand what was wanted, or the wrong title was used when the request was made. A no from the librarian should never be taken as the final word. Researchers more than anyone else know the value of a given piece of data; they should search for the material personally.

Not to be overlooked are the repositories located throughout the U.S. In 1973 the nursing profession established a repository at the National Library of Medicine, Bethesda, Maryland. Boston University is an example of a university that has designated an area for nurses to store original documents, letters, materials belonging to individuals of note, and important papers in the history of the profession. In the case of the national repositories, two guides covering all these acquisitions have been published: *A Guide to Manuscripts and Archives in the United States*, edited by Philip M. Hamer[4] for the National Historical Publications Commission, New Haven, Yale University Press, 1965, and *National Union Catalog of Manuscript Collections*, prepared at the Library of Congress, 1981.

Professional societies preserve their own archives, as well as collect private papers. Private research libraries are located at the major universities or private foundations. *The New York Times Index, Facts on File, Facts about Nursing*, and the *Vertical-File Index* are examples of research data. There are monthly publications, leaflets, and pamphlets currently available from a wide variety of sources at every library.

Four of the useful yearbooks are *Information Please Almanac, World Almanac, Statistical Abstract of the United States*, and *Statesman's Year Book*. These all contain

---

[4]Brooks, Philip C.: Research in archives, the use of unpublished primary sources, Chicago, 1969, The University of Chicago Press.

some U.S. statistics. Medical references and encyclopedias should not be neglected when searching for data. WHO publishes official records concerning health information and some statistics on numerous countries, concerning such topics as demographic data or other statistics, hospital services, environmental sanitation, medical and allied personnel, and training facilities.

An even more comprehensive source is *Guide to Reference Books* by Constance M. Winchell. This is a listing of reference books on specialized subjects with a supplementary update every 2 years. Two other excellent directories that list library specialty holdings are *Directory of Special Libraries and Information Centers* and *American Library Directory*. These are organized according to subject and names of categorized libraries that have unusually large collections of books and other reference material on a particular topic. The *Science Citation Index* is an international interdisciplinary index to the literature of science, medicine, agriculture, technology, and the behavioral sciences.

A directory to government documents is *Government Reports Announcements* (GRA), which includes business and economic data as well as scientific and technical report literature.

W.I. Thomas and Florian Znaniecki made an interesting use of records to write the book *Polish Peasant in Europe and America*.[5] For this unique study they advertised in a large newspaper that they would pay cash for letters either to Polish immigrants from Poland, or from Polish immigrants to those back home. The feelings and attitudes of the writers were analyzed, producing some interesting and unique research findings.

The possibilities for doing nursing research studies from records is only as limited as the researcher's imagination. Berthold, for example, reported on a study made to compare the 136 approved proposals and 192 disapproved proposals on the basis of the records consistently kept by the National Institutes of Health (NIH) Division of Nursing and the American Nurses' Foundation. Comparison was made on all dimensions that were available in the records.[6]

ADVANTAGES

There are certain advantages to using available records for research.

1. Records are unbiased. The person who collected the data had no knowledge of their future use. He did not expect that beginning or professional researchers would be delving into files or storage rooms to look through the records that were collected. Therefore, the records are unbiased as far as the researcher is concerned—for the purposes of a particular project.

2. Records quite often cover a long period of time. This is a valuable feature. In many research studies, especially cross-sectional ones, the investigator is only collecting data over a brief time span; but with the use of records, researchers can discover events and trends covering many months or years.

[5]Thomas, William I., and Znaniecki, Florian: The Polish peasant in Europe and America, vols. 1 and 2, New York, 1958, Dover Publications, Inc.
[6]Berthold, Jeanne S.: Nursing research grant proposals, what influenced their approval or disapproval in two national granting agencies, Nurs. Res. 22(4):292, July–August 1973.

3. Records are inexpensive. All the data are available at one time. Numbers or statistics are in tables or other convenient forms readily accessible to the researcher. Pertinent information can even be selected by assistants who have been trained.

4. Records are convenient and time-saving. Little work is required on the researcher's part after they are located, except for processing the data. Records are available in their pure form, compiled in neat (it is hoped) and orderly fashion. After gathering data from subjects, the researcher must do a great deal of work to put it into some form for analysis. However, at least the records provide readily available data.

5. Records have already been collected; the researcher cannot bias the subjects. In other forms of data gathering, the process itself may upset the subjects, or the investigator may have some effect on the sample population.

6. The existence of a large quantity of records often allows the researcher a considerable choice of data. It may be possible to validate or cross-check recorded data from one source with another source. Cross-checking in traditional methods, such as comparing responses from interviews and questionnaires, requires considerable time and effort.

7. Data are obtained by an unobtrusive method.

8. Records can supply personal information about the subject's beliefs, attitudes, and feelings concerning the topic of interest.

9. Records do not rely on recall but were recorded when they occurred.

DISADVANTAGES

The use of records as data sources has several disadvantages.

1. The amount of information is limited to what is available. Researchers cannot obtain any more data because the subjects are not present. If the record is incomplete, there is no way that it can be completed. Any omissions have to remain; they cannot be recovered.

2. No one can be sure of the conditions under which the records were collected. Was more than one person involved in compiling the data? How careful were the people who handled the facts and figures? Were the records collected for more than one purpose? It is possible that the records were stated in such general terms that their meaning is questionable?

3. There is no assurance of the accuracy of the records. Quite often, dates written near the beginning of the new year may be wrong since the writer was used to dating written reports with the past year. At best, both written records and artifacts may only be circumstantial evidence.

4. The people who preserved the original records had no idea that they would be used for research; therefore the researcher is forced to admit any error into the study that was built into the original records.

5. There may be some serious drawbacks in the material of which the researcher is not aware. The person who recorded the data may have recorded only one type of data or may have been interested is only one factor. The collector may have had some personal bias that affected the material, but there is no way of knowing if some of the material is actually irrelevant to the researcher's purpose; it may still be necessary to sift through the data to glean what information is really needed.

6. Extracting the exact information sought for a study can be time-consuming. Once obtained, it must still be categorized and prepared for interpretation.[7]

7. Requesting persons not otherwise involved in a research project to keep records for data input may be an imposition on or intrusion into their work schedule.

PROBLEMS

The foremost problem in using records as research data is locating the place where they have been stored. Where does the researcher go to search for records? How does the researcher gain access to the records? Not everyone is permitted to look through the files. It may be necessary to obtain permission from several individuals before final access is possible.

Records are often stored, published in books that may be located in libraries, or put in files. Whether they are written or artifacts it may be difficult to access them for several reasons. Time is a major factor. Perhaps an office has a series of records in its files, but the people working there do not want to allow an outsider to come in and disturb their office routine by going through rows and rows of the various files and pulling out information.

Another problem is that there may be a reason why the organization or institution does not want anyone other than selected individuals to go through its private files. The organization may permit the researcher the use of the information if arrangements are made to retrieve the data without exposing individual names. If a computer printout form is available, it may be possible to gain access to the stored information. If data are not available in anonymous form, the assistance of office personnel may be required to retrieve the information. Often the organization does not have time for one of its employees to assist. However, if absolutely necessary, the researcher may pay one of the employees to collect the data.

A research reported his experience collecting data from records in a large university. He spent almost one entire day visiting various people and getting permission. Finally, when all the people were satisfied that the request was in order, they gave the researcher a secretary's services to help pull out all necessary information.

Often records are in such a form that it would be difficult to understand them. The researcher may require help in interpreting the meaning of words, figures, and symbols. With computer printouts, it may be quite difficult for the researcher to understand the data until they are explained.

Another problem with records is item equivalency. Suppose a researcher wants to compare information about how clients are served by one nursing center with another. Are their record items equivalent? Are records based on the same criteria? In comparing client histories, if one institution used type A form and the other institution used type B form, would they yield equivalent information?

Record research may be a disagreeable task. Records are often stored in boxes covered with dust. They may be stored in old basements or attics. It may be known that

[7]Henerson, M.E., Morris, L.L., and Fitz-Gibbon, C.T.: How to Measure Attitudes, Beverly Hills, 1978, Sage Publications, Inc., p. 37.

information is available, but no one seems to be able to locate it. The investigator may be looking for records from a certain year, and it may be difficult to find them.

Some records are seldom used after they have been compiled. The people who originally compiled the records may have left the organization, died, or moved away, and after a few years the records' value is forgotten. So far all practical purposes they are actually lost.

Some records, on the other hand, may be available, but the researcher is unable to gain access to them because permission is not granted. It seems that one of the big problems in the use of records is that people who own them do not want personal names revealed. If the researcher can assure the owners that names will not be made public, access will be granted more readily.

Organizations will usually allow the use of their records if the researcher presents a copy of the final report of his/her study. The researcher may be required to show the organization a copy of the paper before it is presented in final form for publication or other intended use. At the same time, the organization will check for accuracy or point out some fact they prefer not to reveal.

It is very important that the integrity of the research field be upheld. Integrity involves maintaining strict standards of anonymity, privacy, truth, and accuracy, and a consideration for the personal preferences of the individuals involved. We cannot jeopardize future research because we were unscrupulous in handling other persons' data.

SCIENTIFIC USE

Objectivity must be considered when records are gathered and analyzed. It is ethically unfair to select only the records or data that support the opinion of the investigator.

The purpose of any science is to predict and explain. The researcher can never include all the facts and information; he/she only includes those events or items that he/she feels are relevant and important to the viewpoint presented. Therein lies the problem of subjectivity.

Let us illustrate the reporting of information in a familiar context. A man, on arriving home in the evening, is greeted by his wife with the question, "Who did you talk to today who was interesting?" The man answers, "Oh, the boss at work."

"How long did you talk?"

"Ten minutes."

"What did you tell him?"

"About our vacation."

"What did you say?"

"Oh, I told him we went out West and visited relatives."

"Is that all you talked about? If you talked for 10 minutes, then you haven't told me all you said to him."

The historian is like the man who cannot repeat every detail of his conversation with his boss. Just as the historian leaves out some of the details, the original record-keeper omits selected details.

In a police investigation, every tiny event is important. The smallest clue, unimportant as it may appear to be, may be all that is needed to solve a case. No detail can be tossed aside without being given some attention.

To argue for the validity of record material, we have noticed that in recent years records tend to be carefully written. Many records are observed, recorded, and checked several times. For instance, courthouse records are meticulously filed; boundaries are surveyed completely; sales and transactions are carefully recorded, and copies of the deeds are retained; before land is bought or sold, its true ownership is carefully investigated again; and corporations, businesses, and organizations have their books audited periodically. At the same time we recognize that records are often lost through fire, floods, aging, theft, accidental destruction, or when moving. However, many records are reliable, having met rigorous standards of authenticity, truthfulness, and accuracy. Such scrutiny is rarely available in many of the methods of research (such as questionnaires and interviews), which may not be nearly as accurate as many records are. Educational records are usually correct since they are under constant checking by both the student and the institution personnel. Such records are often transferred from one institution to another, which makes further demands on their accuracy.

Through the use of records, the researcher can formulate hypotheses that can be tested by data from the records just as well as data that have been collected especially for research. Logic, probablility, and statistics can be used with the same results.

CLASSIFICATION OF RECORDS

There are two classifications for records, written and artifact. Some of the written sources are diaries, deeds, letters, old photograph albums, newspaper clipping files, records of business transactions, daily ledger accounts, patients' charts, formats of periodicals, and so on. The other type of record is the artifact. Material objects include paintings, phonograph records, coins, clothing, and art objects. Archeologists frequently use combinations of these to substantiate or strengthen theories, or for dating purposes. For example, clothing on a skeleton would indicate a certain period when the individual died. If coins with dates are found with the body, this would also help to substantiate the era in which the person lived.

A subclassification of records is primary and secondary. Primary records are the original documents or products of an author. Examples include original copies of authors' works (as opposed to photocopies), authors' quotations from their own books (as opposed to a quote in another's book), and a nurse's notes and signature on a chart (versus a microfilm of the chart). Secondary data refers to published facts and statistics not originally intended for the researcher's project and varies in format and scope.

Secondary sources have gone from the creator to a second person who has made a contribution in the form of copying, quoting, analyzing, critiquing, enlarging, or altering the original some way.

Primary sources are preferable to secondary sources. If only secondary data are available, then the researcher should cross-check the accuracy of the records.

AUTHENTICITY OF RECORDS

In an effort to establish authentic and accurate data, three major criteria apply; authorship, body, and function of the data. The author is the person who conceived the material. In the case of a painting, it would be the painter; in the case of a book, the author. A painting might simply be perceived as oil on canvas until someone discovers that the painter's name is Rembrandt. The body of the material is the outward form. In the case of a painting, it would be the actual work of art. Finally, the function of records refers to the purpose or reason for them. Again, using painting as the example, the purpose of the painting may be to decorate the ceiling of a great cathedral or palace.

In the field of nursing these three criteria still apply to any records available. In searching for nursing records, the researcher needs to know where they came from (for example, the state or a school), and perhaps who kept the records and that person's official capacity (authorship). The body is the form in which the data are found. Are they consecutive (arranged serially)? Are the data meaningful? Are they well labeled? What is their form—what is the meaning of the figures after the names, for example? Are they IQ scores, grades, or what? By function, we mean the purpose for which the data were collected originally. Suppose we found a list of names with a series of numbers following them. We would need to know the purpose of the numbers. Are they entrance or exam scores? Were they used to screen applicants?

So before researchers can make use of data, they must know the authorship, body, and function of the available data. Frequently, these three criteria are discussed under the titles internal and external criticism. What we have classified as authorship and body is called external criticism, and function is known as internal criticism. There are times when these lines of demarcation are not strictly held, however. Biblical scholars are especially concerned with these types of criticism. External criticism asks questions about the data when a document was written, the author, and the conditions under which it was written. Internal criticism attempts to verify authorship and purpose through the content.

VERIFYING DATA

As with all data, there is the constant need for verifying, cross-checking, and evaluating the findings. Often the records themselves serve as internal checks, much like a system of double entry bookkeeping of credits and debits. Perhaps there are two different sources of the same kind of data that can be checked against each other.

In dendrochronology (the science of tree ring dating) a system of cross-checking is available by comparing one type of tree growth with another type of tree growth. It so happens that trees have different growth cycles, requiring varying amounts of moisture and temperature during the seasons. If the evidence of age and climate can be determined by looking at pine trees, and the results are verified by observing oak trees, we have a system of cross-checking.

If the researcher can find two sources of records that will serve for cross-checking (such as patients' charts, and laboratory or x-ray reports), these sources can be used to verify the accuracy of the data. In education almost no college uses only one criterion as a measure of ability in entrance requirements. Usually, high school percentile rank and at least one other test score are used as predictors of college performance. A single criterion has no guarantee of accuracy. It is not trusted as a valid indicator of success. Rather, two or more criteria must be successfully met.

Most researchers make few attempts to cross-check their data regardless of which method they use. When only one source of data is considered as the basis for accepting or rejecting the hypothesis, the study is weakened.

AVAILABLE AND NEW DATA

Available data are material that was not collected with research in mind. They were kept to record the business and transactions of organizations or agencies and may not be suitable for a researcher's use. Such data may be found in any of the various stages of research processing, from raw data to data already coded and prepared for computer use. Some available data may even have been studied by other researchers. In this instance, these studies would have to be reanalyzed and reinterpreted for use in the new study. Data that have not been collected for research purposes may be found as statistics in yearbooks, medical records, and so on.

New data are material that researchers gather themselves, with their own objectives in mind. In other words, new evidence or facts are drawn from original sources. Information is elicited from the individuals being studied or is discovered in an experiment. New or available instruments may be used to gather these data.

Frequently, a research project may include available and new data, yielding important findings. This combination of data sources is another possible database.

Advantages of Using Available Data

The obvious advantages in choosing data that have already been collected include the following:

1. The use of available data makes for greater efficiency. The researcher save time, effort, and cost, since he/she can go directly to the first stage of data processing rather than searching out the subjects, developing the instrument, collecting the data, and compiling it for use.

2. Available data are often the only source of some kinds of information. In the past, groups that were located in distant lands were difficult to include in studies. Now the researcher has access to the *Human Relations Area File*, which is a huge compilation of valuable ethnological data. It would be impossible, of course, to collect much of this information oneself, because the tribes are already extinct or irreversible changes have taken place in them. It would be impossible to gather these stored data in a current cross-sectional study.

3. Great masses of data are available that would be beyond the scope of a researcher to collect. For example, the Bureau of the Census or the vital statistics section of a health department has a collection of facts and figures that could not be compiled by an individual researcher. Files of the health professions organizations also contain compilations of records that should not be overlooked.

4. Directories of organizations and agencies provide names and addresses of members. These lists could provide subjects for questionnaires or interviews. They may even provide the researcher with all the data needed for a research project without having to contact the subjects.

Disadvantages of Using Available Data

Available data have a number of disadvantages that must be considered before their inclusion is made a part of the research study design.

1. Available data are often incomplete. They were not originally compiled for the present researcher's use, so they may not contain all the information desired for the project.

2. The researcher cannot know the exact conditions under which available data were collected, that is, how they were collected, when they were collected, or over how long a time period they were collected. It is not possible to go back and ask questions of the respondents or to check the reliability of their responses.

3. Available data may not clearly fit the conceptual framework for the present study. Unless the researcher is familiar with the profession, culture or lifestyle of the group or with the process being investigated, he/she may misinterpret the responses of the participants.

The researcher will, therefore, have to base his/her interpretations and analysis of the findings on the recognition of the limitations inherent in such data.

VERBAL AND NONVERBAL DATA

Available data may be divided into two categories: verbal and nonverbal. Verbal data are found in such written forms as diaries, letters, poems, documents, novels, speeches, sermons, and case records. Much effort has been given to interpreting or to learning what the underlying attitudes and values were of those who wrote the materials. Furthermore, organizational patterns and professional trends can be better understood when such data are dealt with systematically.

Nonverbal data include such materials as medical and nursing equipment, works of art, musical compositions, paintings, artifacts, household furnishings, clothing, and dwellings. Much of research has left the nonverbal data available to it unexamined. What secrets do these data hold which could add to nursing theory and improved patient care? What contributions could they make to the nurse's understanding of nursing trends? Among these unwritten forms of communication, expressed in their own medium, are the beliefs and attitudes of the creator or composer about the importance of the preservation of life.

DATA IN GENERAL

In considering data in general, it must be pointed out that the reasonableness of the results should be examined. Simon has warned beginning researchers about the dangers of erroneous data.

> If the results are not reasonable, there may be an error. Novices laugh when they hear economists or psychologists say, "If the data don't agree with the theory, check the data." But, indeed, the data are often found to be in error when they disagree with the hypothesis.

The stronger the theory, of course, the more likely you are to put your money on it when it quarrels with the data. But watch out—danger ahead! If you recheck your data when they do not agree with your hypothesis and do *not* recheck the data when they *do* agree with the hypothesis, you are loading the dice in favor of getting data that agree with your hypothesis. The only solution is always to recheck your data.[8]

Old data should be verified by such means as cross-checking with other material. Experts in the field, computer searches, and professional organizations or similar agencies may provide helpful assistance. The researcher should use every means possible to gain confidence in the data collected, regardless of the source and method used to collect it. If there is doubt as to the reliability of the data, it is better to take the time necessary to verify the data than to assume they are sound.

SUMMARY

Records, one of the five methods of collecting data, provide a readily available and valuable source of information for research. Records are numerous and are found in such places as libraries, offices, homes, and institutions. More specifically, records are diaries, correspondence, checkbooks, patient charts, government statistics, census tract data, and so on.

Some of the advantages of using records are as follows:
1. They are unbiased.
2. They often cover a long period of time.
3. They are inexpensive.
4. They are convenient and time-saving.
5. They have already been collected, so the researcher cannot bias the subject.
6. There is considerable choice of data.
7. They are obtained by an unobtrusive method.
8. They can supply personal information.
9. They do not depend on recall.

Some of the disadvantages of using records include the following:
1. The researcher cannot add to the record if it is incomplete.
2. The conditions under which the records were collected are usually unknown.
3. The accuracy of the records is unknown.
4. The records were not collected for this specific study.
5. The researcher is forced to admit into the study any bias that was built into the original records.
6. Extraction of needed information can be time-consuming.
7. Requesting others to keep current records may be an imposition on them.

Some of the problems related to gaining access to records are as follows:
1. Collecting data may upset the routine of the organization. The employees may not want an outsider searching through their private files.

[8]Simon, Julian L.: Basic research methods in social science, New York, copyright 1969, Random House, Inc., pp. 317–318.

2. Files contain names of individuals that the administration may not want revealed.
3. Records may require special help in interpretation.
4. Two sources of data may lack item equivalency.
5. All the records of an organization may not be available.
6. To gain permission to use data, the researcher often may have to guarantee anonymity, or may have to present a copy of the research findings to the organization for approval.

The use of records also involves the question of validity. Historical records are biased since all the material can never be presented. Therefore, any decisions to include or exclude certain facts are based on the subjectivity of the researcher.

As for record validity, many records have met rigorous standards because they are constantly in use (such as courthouse records and business transactions).

Records can be classified as written and artifact. Written sources include patient charts, letters, deeds, and diaries. Some examples of artifacts are coins, paintings, clothing, and photographs.

Data are available in primary (original) and secondary forms (collected by others). Primary forms are usually preferred for research purposes.

Three major criteria are necessary to establish authentic and accurate records. These are authorship, body, and function. Authorship is the identity of the person who conceived the material; the body is the outward form of the material; and the function is the purpose for which it was compiled.

There is a pressing need for cross-checking the reliability and accuracy of data. A scholarly investigator will not be satisfied to generalize on the basis of one set of records. Cross-checking is possible internally and externally in many instances.

Both available and new data have advantages and disadvantages. Records, for example, are more convenient and inexpensive to obtain than new data, but may lack completeness. Furthermore, the conditions under which the data were collected are unknown. Available data can be categorized as verbal (such as diaries and letters) and nonverbal (such as artifacts and nursing supplies).

DISCUSSION QUESTIONS

1 Why are records, as a source of data, not as popular as questionnaires and interviews?
2 What records are kept in your home that reveal many aspects of your lifestyle?
3 What could an investigator learn from checkbook stubs or cancelled checks, income tax returns, diaries, files, desk calendars, or photo albums that could be a possible research topic?
4 Why do the health professions keep so many records?
5 Why do many records seem available to numerous individuals but not to the person involved (for example, work and credit records)?
6 Explain why you would or would not use records as a source of data.
7 Propose a research project using records from *The World Almanac.*
8 Propose a research project using records from your local Red Cross chapter.
9 What would you do if you were refused permission to use the records of organization X for a research project?
10 How would you cross-check the reliability and accuracy of data from patient history records?

CLASS ACTIVITIES

Track I

1 Each student is to design a form containing items useful in screening employees for possible occupational health hazards.
2 The instructor provides the class with records. After studying the data, the students evaluate their usefulness, completeness, and value as a source of available data.
3 Members of the class are to list the types of personal records that they keep and those to which they have access. How many of the records would be appropriate for research purposes?

Track II (Steps in Research Project)

1 Each project group or individual student is to determine the types of records that could be used as a second source of data to test their hypothesis(es). Are the records readily available? Which records would be the most appropriate? Whose permission would have to be granted to gain access to the records? Identify the person(s) who has the authority to grant permission in each case.
2 Finalize research design and literature search.

SUGGESTED READINGS

Archives—historical researchers' treasures, (editorial), Nurs. Res. 27(2):83, March–April 1978.

Bryant, F.B., and Wortman, P.M.: Secondary analysis, the case for data archives, Am. Psychologist 33(4):381–387, April 1978.

Florio, D.H.: Court upholds confidentiality of research records/data. Educ. Res. 9(5):19–20, May 1980.

Morse, G.W.: The concise guide to library research, New York, 1966, Washington Square Press, p. 62.

CHAPTER 19

OBSERVATION

Observation is one of the basic research methods by which data are gathered. It is a two-part process: (1) someone is observing, and (2) there is something to observe.

In observation it is usually assumed that data are collected by some means other than asking people questions. The interview technique involves some observation also, but the verbal response is the focus of attention. Even the experimental technique involves observation, but basically observation means collecting all the data through occurrences that can be observed visually.

A variety of observation methods are discussed later in this chapter, but the following uses, advantages, and disadvantages outline the basic idea of the technique. One or more observers may be involved, or there may be participant observers. There also can be field experiments in which the observer records events when a given variable is present in a situation and absent in another.

Observation is one of the oldest forms of gathering data. It is through the observation of events that hypotheses are suggested.

Just as observation has been useful for evaluating instruction in the classroom, it also can be useful in nursing education. According to Rosenshine, some of the uses are "(a) assessing the variability of classroom behavior within or between instructional programs, (b) assessing the agreement between classroom behavior and certain instructional criteria, (c) describing what occurred in the implementation of the instructional materials, and (d) determining relationships between classroom behavior and instruction outcome."[1] Teachers also may be observed to determine if they are using an instructional package as it was intended.

ETHICS

Ethics are an important factor in the observation of human beings. Should we observe human beings without their permission? For example, consider the one-way mirror

[1] Rosenshine, Barak: Evaluation of classroom instruction, Review of Educational Research **40**:288, April 1970. Copyright by American Educational Research Association. Washington, D.C.

technique in which the researcher observes through a mirrorlike glass, while subjects only see what appears to be a mirror. Should we observe people without their knowing it? Is it permissible to inform the subjects that they are being observed? Will we get the same results if they are informed of the observation procedure? Is it ethical to have a planned experiment in which an individual feigns a heart attack to observe the reactions of persons in the vicinity?

Concerning concealed research, if someone may be hurt by the research results, permission should be obtained from the subject after data has been collected. However, the authors do not know of a case in which any scientific observers have identified subjects by name or caused them embarrassment.

Denzin makes the point that if it is mandatory to obtain permission to use an individual in a research project, research is limited to studying volunteer subjects.[2]

ADVANTAGES

Observation studies can produce large quantities of data with relative ease. Researchers do not need to wait for replies to be returned, as with mailed questionnaires, and subjects need not be recruited, as in the experimental approach. In the observation technique any bias is shifted from the subject to the researcher. Questionnaires are criticized as being merely opinionnaires, since respondents may not actually act as they said they would in their questionnaires. When data are collected by observation, the subjects are acting as they would normally, but the researcher may misinterpret the meaning of their actions. All data obtained by the observation technique are usable, whereas information from questionnaires is often irrelevant because the subjects misunderstood the question asked of them.

Other advantages of the observation technique are listed as follows:
1. Observation is an important technique for studying human behavior.
2. Observation techniques are relatively inexpensive to use.
3. The researcher is not dependent on subjects who consent to answer. All subjects are potential respondents.
4. Subjects are usually available. Other research techniques are dependent on questionnaire returns, volunteers for experiments, and so on, which limit the quantity of data.
5. The observation technique is most open to using recording devices such as tape recorders and cameras.
6. The instrument is quite simple to develop as compared with a lengthy questionnaire.
7. Observation allows the researcher to view the complete situation firsthand as it develops and also affords the inclusion of a sequence of events.
8. The observation technique can be begun or stopped at any time.
9. Observations may be recorded at the time they occur, eliminating biased recall.
10. Observations made and reported by persons not involved in the research project can add to the credibility of the research.

[2]Denzin, Norman K.: On the ethics of disguised observation, Social Problems 15(4):504, Spring 1968.

11. Observations made with checklists permit the accurate recording of rapid interaction and movement on the part of subjects.
12. The training of observers to use recording devices and checklists is relatively simple.

There is no better way to obtain data or to describe a type of behavior than to watch the person behaving. Observation is also an excellent method for evaluating or appraising the actions of individuals.

For example, it might be desirable to observe nurses' reactions to certain types of patients. In answering a questionnaire, the nurses might say that they would react negatively, but when we observe them, we find that they react positively. Do we believe what they say, or do we believe what we see them do? We can observe people in their activities and can describe the events, but we cannot be sure of the reasons or motives behind their actions. The presence of the researcher is always a factor that will influence the study, the results, and the subjects. Marascuilo states:

> This is a very common problem of observational studies in which the researcher has not deliberately manipulated the external conditions of the investigation...it only means that the researchers who conduct observational studies have a greater responsibility to be attuned to the assumptions that are required for certain statistical tests employed in the analysis.[3]

The rigorous methodology advocated by Marascuilo is commendable, but rarely attained in most research utilizing the observation technique.

DISADVANTAGES

There are at least ten disadvantages in using the observation technique.
1. The time and duration of an event cannot be predicted usually. The observer must wait until an event happens. Therefore, it is difficult to know when to be present to observe key events.
2. Interviewing selected subjects may provide more information, economically, than waiting for the spontaneous occurrence of the situation.
3. The presence of an observer gives the subject(s) a quality normally absent. It also creates an artificial situation.
4. Observed events are always subject to the bias of the researcher's cultural background and personal interpretation.
5. Unless cameras and tape recorders are used, events often occur so rapidly or suddenly that it is impossible to record every detail.
6. Extensive training is necessary if more than one observer is used to gather data.
7. Some situations are not open to observation (for example, jury discussions, counseling).
8. Results may be unreliable because different observers may not see and record a particular event in the same manner.
9. The observers may lose their objectivity by becoming personally involved in the situation.

[3]Marascuilo, Leonard A.: Statistical methods for behavioral science research, New York, Copyright 1971, McGraw-Hill Inc., p. 314. Used with permission of McGraw-Hill, Inc.

10. Regardless of the role the observers take, they limit their range of observation by placing themselves in only one position.

11. The observer has little control over the number of observations that will be available in a given period of time or in the categories under study.

12. At the observation site, persons not involved with the research may become annoyed with the interruptions that result from an extra person(s) in the area.

We must be suspicious of the observation technique because it relies on the observer's interpretation of the subject's behavior. If we observe people at a demonstration, we are prone to evaluate the situation from our own personal perspective. Some of the people may be present simply because it is exciting to be there, others may be curious to find out what is going on, and some may have infiltrated the organization to oppose the movement. At the same time, the purpose of the demonstration may be misconstrued. If the researcher were to interview the participants in the demonstration, would it be better to accept what seemed to happen or what the interviewee reported?

Even though there are disadvantages, the observation technique offers great promise in health research, and beginning researchers should not hesitate to use it in their investigation.

TYPES

The investigator's degree of involvement in the observed events can vary.

For our purpose, we break down the observer role as follows. First is the participant within a group situation who is not interested in research but is there solely for his/her role in the event. Second is the participant-observer who gathers data but never announces his/her intentions to the group. However, he/she is a legitimate group member. The third type is the participant-observer who asks permission of the other participants to gather data. The fourth is the nonmember who observes and collects data without announcing his/her intentions, and the fifth type is the nonmember who observes and collects data after gaining permission from the group (Figs. 19-1 and 19-2).

Batten cites instances in which the participant-observer may decide not to function or may not be allowed to participate. Such instances are observation of a family, a board of directors of a large corporation, prison, prostitution, and others.[4] Certain groups might require the observer to occupy a particular niche or social status. To pretend to be a member of the subculture, the observer would have to know the appropriate cultural dialect, response, and jargon or slang used by the social unit.

The observer must remain within the group long enough to find their established routine. However, if the observer remains in the subculture too long, he/she may begin to think like the other members and lose the advantage of having an outside viewpoint.

A good example of a participant-observer situation is given by Festinger, Riecken, and Schachter in *When Prophecy Fails*.[5] These authors heard of a woman who could

[4]Batten, Thelma F.: Reasoning and research, a guide for social science methods, Boston, 1971, Little, Brown & Co., p. 131.

[5]Festinger, L., Riecken, H., and Schachter, S.: When prophecy fails, Minneapolis, 1956, University of Minnesota Press.

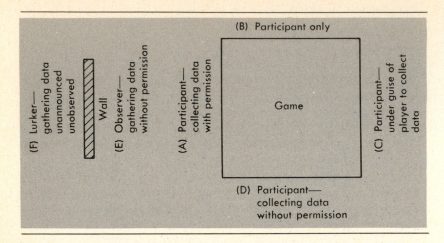

FIGURE 19-1   Observation: legitimate group (friends).

receive automatic handwriting from outer space and predict the future. The researchers, pretending to be interested members, joined the group formed by this woman. The big question is the effect the researcher team had on the other members of the group. There were only a few individuals in the organization, and the arrival of additional members who seemed dedicated may have added a new dimension to the belief of the rest of the subculture.

Consider a research study on card playing. Even though the researchers could take part in card playing, they would have to make the decision whether or not they would play if they were invited to participate. If they do not participate, how do they record

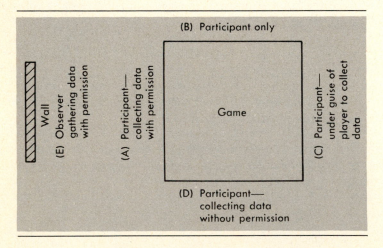

FIGURE 19-2   Observation: public group.

events? How skilled should the researchers be at card playing? Should they try to win or lose?

Batten asks: if we do enter a group as a participant-observer, what will the status of the observer be? Will it be on a lower level or a higher level than the members?[6]

The timing for the observer researcher to enter a group is not to be overlooked. He/she may already be a legitimate member before deciding to observe the behavior of the members, or he/she may have to go through the process of joining the group to do research (either announced or unannounced).

A researcher was required to observe an elementary school classroom as an assignment. Both pupils and teacher knew that a student researcher from the university was coming to observe the class. Since researchers often came to observe the class session, the pupils apparently were unconcerned. In another situation, the researcher might simply enter a classroom or other public meeting, and the group might assume that the observer is really just another one of the class. Or the participant-observer might actually join the group meeting, passing himself off as one of the group.

Kahn and Mann suggest four ways the participant-observer can enter a situation. These include (1) dual or multiple entry, (2) contingent acceptance at successive organizational levels, (3) double liaison, and (4) double access.[7]

RECORDING DATA

There are two ways to collect and record data from observations. It is possible to use a **quantitative** scale. As an example, one can check the number of times people talk. Evaluation scales use instruments for measuring precisely height, weight, time, and temperature.

Another scale is a **qualitative** one in which some variable is estimated. The following example illustrates a qualitative instrument. A student hypothesized that one section of the United States was more conservative in dress than another area. The student selected one university located in each of the two sections chosen for the study. To collect data, the student stood in the student union in each of the universities at the same hour of the day, the same time of the week, and observed the students who walked through. She had to make some kind of judgment on such characteristics as length of sideburns and hair, beards, and styles of clothing. Had there been another observer along, they might have disagreed on the measurement of each of the variables.

Checklists are frequently used to facilitate the recording of precisely defined observations. These should be prepared ahead of time in logically sequenced placement and the number of items should be limited to 10 or less, according to Morris and Fitz-Gibbon.[8] Chapter 20 provides further information concerning checklists.

[6]Batten, p. 131.
[7]Kahn, R., and Mann, F.: Developing research partnerships. In McCall, G.J., and Simmons, L.L., editors: Issues in participant observation. Reading, Mass., 1969, Addison-Wesley Publishing Co., Inc., pp. 45–52.
[8]Morris, L.L., and Fitz-Gibbon, C.T.: How to Measure Program Implementation, Beverly Hills, 1978, SAGE Publications, Inc., pp. 195–199.

OBSERVER'S TRAINING PROGRAM

If more than one person is to do the observations, there must be a training program. Again, using the illustration of dress, if the person observes students in two places, and all data were obtained from the observation of just one observer, at least the biases would all be the same. But if there was reliance on several people to do the observing, there should definitely be a training program so all the observers are in agreement (inter-rater reliability).

One method by which it is possible to train one or more assistant observers is to use a film. The observers would practice observing the film until the desired skill is developed. In case several observers are involved, training would have to be carried out until all the observers agree on a minimum of 85% to 90% of their individual observations.

It should suffice to mention again that if observers develop a bias during training, at least all the observers have the same bias and it should be identified in the report.

Selltiz and co-workers suggest that a training program begin with an explanation of the purpose and the theory involved in the study, and then move on to an explanation of the categories and rules for the study. The purpose of each category in relationship to the theory and the specific hypothesis is given. After the trainees have had an opportunity to ask questions, they would then use their observation schedule on a group that demonstrates the phenomenon they are observing. The trainees would obviously have trouble fitting certain categories in the observation schedule to actual situations. These difficulties are resolved through discussion and further practice.[9] In other words, suppose the student researcher is observing obesity in a particular community and could not decide if a given individual should be categorized as overweight. Through discussion the entire team could establish criteria to define overweight. Subjects in the field would be evaluated against the criteria and classified appropriately. The pilot study would provide an opportunity for correcting or revising borderline cases.

We suggest that tape recorders and pictures could be used to check those instances in which there has been disagreement.

Selltiz and co-workers state that in an observational study four broad questions confront the investigator. "(1) What should be observed? (2) How should observations be recorded? (3) What procedures should be used to ensure the accuracy of observation? (4) What relationship should exist between the observer and the observed, and how can such a relationship be established?"[10]

CONSIDERATIONS FOR THE OBSERVER

There are some factors that the single observer must take into consideration. It is necessary to check personal biases and selective perceptions in research. There must be objective standards against which to correct any measurements; vague impressions must

[9]Selltiz, Claire, and others: Research methods in social relations, rev. ed., New York, 1962, Holt, Rinehart & Winston, Inc., p. 232.
[10]*Ibid.*, p. 205.

be replaced by empirical measurements. Guesses must be replaced with correct and exact definitions. Hunches must be checked by counts, cross-tabulations, and other mathematical forms. As the researcher's ideas become deeper, they will be subjected to more and more controlled observations. Labovitz and Hagedorn have suggested that observers are either judges or participants. A judge is an impartial observer who should be detached from the circumstances; a participant partakes in the situation. The judge's task is to rank or put the responses in some order. The resulting data are either descriptive or inferential.[11] At best, data must be consistent, behaviors must be classified according to pre-established criteria, categories must be standardized, and rules covering every situation must be understood by all observers.

RECORDING OBSERVATIONS

Many techniques have been devised for recording observations. One is Bales Interaction Analysis, by Robert F. Bales, in which he has identified 12 interaction categories that may be checked during the observation process. Bales has made effective use of the observation method in his Interaction Analysis Checkoff (Fig. 19-3).[12]

When recording interactions, the researcher observes a group and makes a check indicating that an individual in the group exhibited one of the characteristics listed on the observation form. This instrument has gone through a number of refinements and has received favorable criticism for its reliability. Obviously, an instrument such as the Bales Interaction Analysis form would be much more valuable than a new and untested instrument.

It is possible to observe people in an experimental setup that, in actuality, is a type of field experiment. For example, we might want to observe nurses' behavior in a clinical setting. Suppose the purpose of the observation is to see how their behavior differs in the presence of a physician as compared with their behavior in the presence of another nurse. An effort would be made to hold all the variables constant. The only difference would be the presence of a physician or of another nurse. An actual experimental situation would be so artificial that subjects would not respond normally. Yet the possibility of an experimental situation is present and almost always available for research somewhere in a large hospital. All the alert researcher need do is observe. This is a circumstance that also might be observed by a nurse-researcher during the normal daily routine.

Suppose a nurse wanted to investigate the situation in the example just mentioned. After each observation, the results could be quickly recorded by the nurse while on duty rather than when acting as an outside observer. The nurse might repeat this observation for a number of days, observing as a group member rather than a participant observer.

One student hypothesized that truck drivers are more friendly than other people. The student stood on a bridge over a freeway and waved at people in cars and trucks. The percentage of responses (waved back) for car drivers and truck drivers was compared.

---

[11]Labovitz, Sanford, and Hagedorn, Robert: Introduction to social research, ed. 3, New York, 1981, McGraw-Hill, Inc., p. 72.
[12]Bales, R.F.: Interaction process analysis: a method for the study of small groups, Reading, Mass., 1950, Addison-Wesley Publishing Co., Inc.

1. Shows solidarity	Raises other's status
	Gives help
	Rewards
2. Shows tension release	Jokes
	Laughs
	Shows satisfaction
3. Agrees	Shows passive acceptance
	Understands
	Concurs
	Complies
4. Gives suggestion	Direction
	Implying autonomy for other
5. Gives opinion	Evaluation
	Analysis
	Expresses feeling
	Wish
6. Gives orientation	Information
	Repeats
	Clarifies
	Confirms
7. Asks for orientation	Information
	Repetition
	Confirmation
8. Asks for opinion	Evaluation
	Analysis
	Expression of feeling
9. Asks for suggestion	Direction
	Possible ways of action
10. Disagrees	Shows passive rejection
	Formality
	Withholds help
11. Shows tension	Asks for help
	Withdraws out of field
12. Shows antagonism	Deflates other's status
	Defends or asserts self

FIGURE 19-3   Twelve categories.

From Bales, R.F.: Interaction process analysis: a method for the study of small groups, Cambridge, Mass. 1950, Addison-Wesley Publishing Co., Inc., Copyright by R.F. Bales.

In the behavioral sciences, observation has played an important role. Freud and Durkheim collected large bodies of knowledge from their observations of natural phenomena.

Ethnography, the anthropological approach to the study of human origin based on descriptive measures, has made use of participant observation. This method of collecting data permits researching other cultures of lifestyles in their natural settings. (See Chapter 20.)

Unknown and unrevealed observers also can collect data by many creative techniques. Researchers have used one-way mirrors, hidden recording devices, or hidden cameras, all of which have been condemned as unethical. Numerous public gatherings allow observers to collect information that will contribute to the understanding of human behavior. Such instances provide opportunities for meaningful observations and ensure anonymity for the participants.

An example of this observation technique is a study called "Status of Frustrator as an Inhibitor of Horn-Honking Responses," reported by Doob and Gross.[13] The researchers placed observers and drivers in an old car and a new car. The drivers stopped at lights that had just turned red. They would sit through the red, and when the light turned green they counted the number of seconds it took the driver of the vehicle behind the experimental car to honk. The researchers hypothesized that drivers would honk sooner at the old car (with its khaki-jacketed driver) than at the new expensive model (whose driver wore a plaid sport jacket and white shirt). The results were in the direction indicated by the hypothesis: the low status car received more horn honks than the high-status car. This is an example of a creative field experiment involving strangers who were reacting to what is apparently a normal situation. Their identity was never known, and yet they contributed data by acting naturally in an experimental setting.

LURKING

Lurking is described as making observations from the periphery of a social setting in such a way that the researcher is present but is not required to interact extensively with others. The lurker does not make his/her intentions known to the group, nor does he/she make any effort to participate.

We agree with Stickland and Schlesinger that the lurker obtains a different kind of data than the participant observer. We would have to agree that the person who actually takes part in a group will influence the members. By lurking, the observer may be able to pass relatively unnoticed or perhaps completely unknown to the subject and is often able to gather a great deal of information.

People talking in public are not usually known and hence will not be identified in a study by a researcher who is lurking and listening. Usually we do not care if people overhear our normal everyday conversations in restaurants or on buses.

An example of this observation technique was devised by a student interested in seeing what percent of people's conversations were related to the opposite sex. The observer sat in a booth in a coffee shop and listened to people's conversations in nearby booths. She recorded the number of minutes devoted to the opposite sex in each conversation.

Strickland and Schlesinger say that of all modes of uninvolved observation, lurking is the most likely to become meddlesome or to introduce observer bias. There is always the risk that the observer will become involved in the group to the point of abandoning his role. Also, when the observer is not nearby, there is difficulty in hearing, which leads to misunderstanding. There is also the risk of attributing false motives, ideas, or feelings to

[13]Doob, Anthony N., and Gross, Alan E.: Status of frustrator as an inhibitor of horn-honking responses, J. Soc. Psychol. **76**:213–218, 1968.

the observed. The researcher may receive false impressions because he/she usually arrives after the start of an event and only observes a part of a situation.[14]

Erickson[15] presents a case against disguised observation, whereas Denzin argues in its defense.[16] Not only are the published results to be considered, but also what the observer did by entering into the group—how was the group action influenced? The fact than an observer is present and shows interest may be seen as hypocritical by the subjects and may somehow influence their responses. A stranger who enters a situation to observe may unknowingly produce some negative consequences, even though the written report of the situation may be harmless to the subjects.

The disguised observation may discredit other responsible professionals in the field if the method or technique becomes known and receives unfavorable criticism. Researchers using any methodology for collecting data can come under criticism. However, the overall gain in knowledge cannot be ignored, nor can research be discontinued because of negative comments.

It has been argued that since the people whom we study seldom read the findings, we need not worry about how the subjects feel. This is usually true, but in William Foote Whyte's *Street Corner Society* his subjects did read the report and were disappointed with his conclusion.[17] They felt that he had misinterpreted them.

Another ethical consideration is raised regarding the attitude of professionals toward their student researchers. Can we ask students to do research when they have reservations about the ethical integrity of the research assignment?

The final objection raised is that any masquerading disregards the intricacies of human interaction and results in faulty conclusion. It is really impossible to enter a group and be part of the group when we are only playing out a role that we do not play in real life.

On the positive side, lurking is sometimes used in a social setting to validate findings revealed by other methods. Undoubtedly, other uses for lurking may be found that do not violate ethical codes.

THE HAWTHORNE EFFECT

The problem of the Hawthorne effect, as described by Simon, is an influencing factor of unknown dimension. This effect occurs when people are aware that they are under observation and react differently.

The Hawthorne effect was discovered when a group headed by E. Mayo was doing research at the Hawthorne plant of Western Electric. They were investigating the effects of varying working hours and plant lighting on the productivity of women factory workers. Regardless of the conditions, productivity increased. They could reduce the lighting or the working hours, but the employees still increased production. It was finally

---

[14]Strickland, Donald A., and Schlesinger, Lester E.: Lurking as a research method, Hum. Organization **28**(3):248–250, Fall 1969.
[15]Erickson, Kai T.: A comment on disguised observation in sociology, Soc. Problems **14**(4):366–373, Spring 1967.
[16]Denzin, pp. 502–504.
[17]Whyte, William Foote: Street corner society, Chicago, 1955, University of Chicago Press.

concluded that the workers were aware of being observed and because of the attention were putting forth more effort.[18]

The Hawthorne effect is similar to the placebo effect. There are at least two ways to introduce the placebo into a study. One is to give the subjects a placebo without their knowledge. The researcher is informed about what is happening, but the subjects are not. Another method is a double-blind system in which neither the researcher nor subjects know who is receiving the real treatment and who is receiving the placebo. The double-blind system is valuable in medical research when a new medication is being tested. The double-blind system forces the equal treatment of the experimental and control groups and helps adjust for any bias the researcher might pass on to the experimental group. Someone outside the research project knows the placebo from the real medication, but no one working on the project knows until all the data are collected.

A similar situation could be designed for observation to avoid any Hawthorne effect. In the Hawthorne plant, the observers might have varied the amount of time they spent with the workers and their behavior toward them. The intensity of the light could have fluctuated without either worker's or researcher's knowledge, as one attempt toward a double-blind system.

RELIABLE DATA

Fox says that the independent observations of two trained observers should agree at least 85% of the time. Less agreement than this of data gathered by only one individual can only be considered tentative.[19]

The observer has a problem in using precise instruments for measuring. We recall a case in a physics class when students were required to measure small wooden blocks. Several readings were taken on each block, and then the average was computed. The blocks were difficult to measure precisely because they were irregular and the measuring instrument was finely calibrated.

Every observer has his/her own personal or cultural frame of reference or bias, which in a sense, determines how the observer perceives a situation. A person trained in music might go to a foreign country and only notice the types of musical instruments, whereas another individual interested in sports might only observe athletics.

Researchers can never assume that they know the motivation behind an act—they can never be sure that they understand what they see. Simon mentions some interesting variables concerning sequence effects. Either the first observation or the most recent stimuli will be remembered best. Investigators can try varying the order of conditions under observation rather than taking them in the same order each time. They can attempt observations at different times of the day—anything that will prevent the observation procedure from becoming routine. This, of course, takes a great deal of insight into human behavior.[20]

[18]Simon, Julian L.: Basic research methods in social science, New York, 1969, Random House, Inc., pp. 97–98.
[19]Fox, David J.: Fundamentals of research in nursing, ed. 4, New York, 1976, Appleton-Century-Crofts, p. 199.
[20]Simon, p. 95.

RECORDING

Careful measurements are mandatory. Suppose an observer wants to count the number of people who participate in a particular activity or event. A well-defined phenomenon such as the number of individuals who enter the emergency room between 10 AM and 11 AM on Monday morning is easy to calculate and record. A less well-defined act, giving good nursing care, would be more difficult to tabulate because a great deal of forethought and planning would be entailed in defining all possible acts of good nursing care.

In a study of courtesy conducted by a student, a *courteous* person was operationally defined as one saying thank you when someone held open a door. Failure to say thank you was operationally defined as being discourteous. The act was clearly delineated, and all observers could agree to categories. This is an excellent example of classifying a continuous variable into a discrete category. However, social situations are seldom well defined. It is a credit to the researchers when they are able to to operationally define an abstract variable, making it measurable in discrete units.

There are certain types of mechanical recording devices, such as tape recorders and audiovisual cameras, that may be used in the process of observation. This equipment provides possibilities for examining an incident a second time. Recorders and cameras capture details of movement, inflections and volume of voice, and gestures, which are all recorded for later interpretation or replay. If we must rely on observers to write down or record all these observations, we lose almost all environmental cues. Of course, the more precise we can make our measurements, by actually timing an event with a watch to the exact second and weighing carefully with scales and measuring with rulers, the more confidence we can have in the reliability of our data.

Some of our most commonly used mechanical measures in the social sciences, according to Labovitz and Hagedorn, are audio and visual tape recorders (video tapes), still and movie cameras, and the interaction chronograph (measured frequency and direction). Recording devices give complete records, provide the exact sequence of events, measure the length of interaction intervals, and allow for replay of events to check results when more than one observer must evaluate the event in case of error or doubt.

Physical trace evidence provides an additional method of securing data. Physical trace evidence is the result of wear, erosion, chemical remains, artifacts, and so on.[21] One of us remembers walking along on campus one day when there had been a snowfall. It had packed down, and on the surface of the hard-packed snow were imprints of high-heeled shoes. We wondered, "Why would so many women be here? Why would these women have been walking in this particular area across campus?" Suddenly, we realized that other types of shoes would not make imprints in the snow, only the spiked heels of women's shoes. Physical trace evidence can be meaningful, but it must be interpreted accurately. The interpretation of evidence can become a problem, not the evidence.

Will we ever know the truth about the assassination of John F. Kennedy in Dallas? We have testimonies, fingerprints, and bullets, but their interrelationship is still under investigation.

A few examples of physical trace evidence denoting frequency of use are (1) the amount of wear on a library book, (2) the traces of wear on certain doors of a building,

---

[21]Labovitz and Hagedorn, pp. 76–78.

and (3) the playground equipment that wears out first. These are only a few kinds of physical evidence that provide the researcher with information that may be useful.

Two other questions are involved in recording data. When should the observer make notes, and how should the notes be kept? The sooner the information is recorded after the observation, the better. In some cases, the researcher may have to wait to record the new data, but recording should be completed as soon as possible. A student once made observations on various shopping centers. The observer sat on a bench and made notations on a clipboard. People often expressed interest in her activities and offered comments and information because they were intrigued by the topic.

Notetaking may influence the quality of the observation because the observer is concentrating on writing the notes rather than on the phenomena. But how can observers remember every statement in an interaction, as well as nonverbal cues, if they must record them later? How can researchers find time to observe and record an interaction simultaneously? The danger of biased data is great unless measures are taken to minimize the amount of time the observer spends recording the data. If observers are required to take their eyes from the scene, they either fail to see the complete sequence of events or do not have time to record all the details. In an effort to help recall the events of a phenomenon, it is sometimes helpful to use associations.

When writing reports, researchers can use various techniques for recalling activities associated with the observation. They may try associating the first event with number one and the second event with number two, or a word beginning with A or B. Often it is possible or convenient to have a checkoff form for recording observations. For example, we could simply make a check in the appropriate column when the event occurs. In some situations, the time of day, the weather, and the circumstances may later prove to be important evidence.

The average number of time an event occurs each minute, hour, or week may provide a meaningful measure for interpreting data. The more precise the category is, the more accurate the judgments will be. An observer who has to place the variable in several distinct categories will be more accurate than the observer who has only two categories in which to place the data.

Counting the number of times an event occurs occasionally requires keen perceptions. If it seems likely that a single individual might not be able to count fast enough, a second observer may be needed to help record the observations. For example, a team of two nurses went from house-to-house in a refugee camp conducting a survey of families in which one member was under treatment for active tuberculosis. During each interview, one nurse recorded the answers to her questions while the other nurse observed health standards. In this instance, it took two investigators to conduct and record their observations.

In conclusions, the observation technique for data collecting is an effective tool for health research. It is hoped that the nursing profession will continue to rely on observation as a research tool for improved nursing practice.

SUMMARY

Observation is a common technique used in nursing and is one of the major means of collecting data. The same uses that general education has made of observation are also applicable to nursing education. However, there are ethical and moral questions involved when one is observing human behavior.

The advantages of the observation technique are that it is valuable for studying nursing; it is inexpensive; subjects are readily available; it lends itself to the use of recording equipment; it requires simple data-collecting instruments; it allows for the observation of a sequence of events; and it may be stopped at any time.

Disadvantages are that the time and duration of an event cannot be predicted usually; the researcher may have to wait for an event to occur; the presence of the observer may influence subjects; objectivity is subject to the bias of the observer; observations are difficult to record; extensive training is needed for observers; some situations are not open to observation; data from two or more observers may not be in agreement; observers may become personally involved in the event; and observers limit their range of observation by placing themselves in only one position.

Observation can be placed in the pure and field categories. The pure form allows for a participant observer, whereas in the field form, the observer remains an outsider.

In the observation technique, the observer always influences the group in some way. Data may be measured with a quantitative scale or a qualitative scale. Observation training may be facilitated through the use of tapes or films.

Researchers must consider their particular biases when observing. Cultural backgrounds or peculiar interests will influence their perceptions.

The Bales Interaction Analysis technique is an effective tool for observing and recording group interaction. Other observation techniques include the field experiment, lurking, and the field study. The Hawthorne effect is an influencing factor, resulting from the subjects' awareness of being observed.

There should be strong agreement between observers on what is to be observed and how before they are permitted to gather data. Mechanical devices that facilitate recording data include tape recorders, cameras, thermometers, watches, and scales.

Physical trace evidence provides clue for gathering data. An example of physical trace evidence is wear.

DISCUSSION QUESTIONS

1 How would you react if you learned that someone had used you as a subject in a research project by observing your reactions? In what way would you feel differently if the researcher were a complete stranger?

2 What would you think if you read a research report and were able to identify yourself by the statement, "One of the subjects discussed last night's party for more than three minutes before answering the patient's light?"

3 How reliable are your observations about a patient before you read his chart or file? Do you retain some of your first impressions after you read the chart? Explain.

4 If two observers are trained for a particular research project, and they reach the point of 85% agreement, are they really observing reality or have they agreed to agree on what they see? Why?

5 Suggest an hypothesis using physical trace evidence.

6 List three topics in which observation would be the most appropriate method for collecting data.

7 Relate observations and experimentation as complementary approaches to research.

8 How would you go about developing a new instrument for recording behavior in the outpatient clinic?

9 How would you go about developing an observation instrument for studying standards of cleanliness in a culture with which you were unfamiliar?

10 Would a movie camera be an ethical research recording device to use in a shopping mall if it were concealed behind a one-way mirror? Justify your answer.

CLASS ACTIVITIES

Track I

1 Class members are to go to any site they choose and observe people's behavior for 15 to 30 minutes. Observations are to be recorded afterwards and an hypothesis developed. The hypothesis and observations are then shared orally with the class.

Track II (Steps of Research Project)

1 Members of each research group or students working alone are to plan an observation experience that will provide useful data for testing the project hypothesis.

2 If possible, groups are to apply the observation technique to their hypothesis.

SUGGESTED READINGS

Baker, F.: Data sources for health care quality evaluation, Evaluation & the Health Professions 6(3):362–381, September 1983.

Batten, Thelma F.: Reasoning and research, a guide for social science methods, Boston, 1971, Little, Brown & Co., pp. 130–131.

Cassell, J.: The relationship of observer to observed in peer group research, Hum. Organization 36(4):412–416, Winter 1977.

Cooley, W.A.: Explanatory observational studies, Educ. Res. 7(9):9–15, October 1978.

Cunningham, R.: Participant observation: a research technique in public health nursing, Can. J. Public Health 69(2):101–106, March–April 1978.

Dillman, C.M.: Ethical problems in social science research peculiar to participant observation, Hum. Organization 36(4):405–407, Winter 1977.

Henerson, M.E., Morris, L.L., and Fitz-Gibbon, C.T.: How to Measure Attitudes, Beverly Hills, 1978, Sage Publications, Inc.

Herbert, J., and Attridge, C.: A guide for developers and users of observation systems and manuals, Am. Educ. Res. J. 12(1)1–20, Winter 1975.

Jackson, B.S.: An experience in participant observation, Nurs. Outlook 23(8):552–555, September 1975.

Jackson, B.S.: Participant observation in nursing research, Superv. Nurse 4(5):33, 36, May 1973.

Morris, L.L. and Fitz-Gibbon, C.T.: How to Measure Program Implementation, Beverly Hills, 1978, Sage Publications, Inc.

Robertson, C.M.: A description of participant observation of clinical teaching, Journal of Advanced Nursing 7(6):549, November 1982.

Taylor, S.J. and Bogdan, R.: Introduction to Qualitative Research Methods, The Search for Meanings, ed. 2, New York, 1984, John Wiley & Sons.

Thomson, R.W.: Participant observation in the sociological analysis of sport, Int. Rev. Sport Sociology 12(4)99–109, 1977.

CHAPTER 20

COMPUTER SIMULATION AND OTHER TECHNIQUES

Other common research methods include content analysis, systems analysis, the Q-sort, the checklist, the critical incident, ranking, rating, simulation, Delphi techniques, projective devices, clinical field trials, and use of the semantic differential. These techniques are often used, but it is hoped that other techniques will be developed as nurse-researchers increase in number. Beginning researchers should be aware of as many research techniques as possible so that they will have some choice in the methods they use in their first project.

CONTENT ANALYSIS

Content analysis is a systematic, objective analysis of a text and is frequently used in a survey of written materials or periodicals. It is usually applied to speeches, writing, or other written forms of communication. Often it involves counting how many times a particular word occurs. To be meaningful, it requires some method of measurement.

Content analysis is often used to study mass media, such as newspapers or magazines. One investigator, in studying a specific periodical over several years, counted the number of times certain words were used. She also was interested in how the usage and meaning of particular words changed. Current nursing journals were searched to determine the most commonly used term. It turned out to be *problem-solving*. The next step was to study the meanings given to the term by the authors of the different articles—they had used the term in three different ways.

An interesting type of content analysis is the study of references to nursing made by the medical profession (or any of the allied health areas), as used in medical journals, to detect how the concept of status of nursing has changed. There are a number of ways to do this. We might compare the number of times the word *nursing* was used or the intensity with which it was used in the past with the present. We might note how the concept of nursing has changed over the years and how the name itself may even have changed. We could do the same for any health profession.

Content analysis may be the method selected to identify biased treatment and prejudice against minority groups. The content of books, magazines, and newspapers can be compared to see how often the words *black* and *white* are used in reference to race. The frequency with which certain words are used may indicate a particular religious or political viewpoint. Content analysis of newspaper reports on the occurrence of various crimes would give some indication of the increase or decline of a particular crime. This technique also would be useful in studying the trends in advertising. Are magazine ads in medical and nursing journals getting smaller, larger, more wordy, or what? What changes have taken place in popular reading materials regarding the role of the nurse? Are recent nursing trends reflected in current popular fiction?

Content analysis is a precise, authoritative procedure to document, describe, and quantify a specific phenomenon. This method provides a great deal of insight into the topic under study, the communication vehicle, and societal changes all at one time.

Unfortunately, content analysis may require researchers to sift through a great deal of material. As a remedy for this, researchers may choose every n^{th} appearance of the phenomenon (perhaps in the nth journal, newspaper, or other publication) or use a random selection or other sampling technique. Another disadvantage of content analysis is that the classification systems used may be so ambiguous that an occurrence of a specific phenomenon may seem to fit into two categories.

The document or communication vehicle chosen to represent the phenomenon being studied may not best represent the phenomenon. The journal *Nursing Research*, for example, may not provide as good a representation of nurses' attitudes toward research as another journal. *Nursing Research* would be expected to discuss research, whereas another journal might better reflect the nurses' attitude toward scientific investigations.

Another disadvantage in the use of content analysis lies in the fact that some biases and prejudices in the scoring method could be detrimental to the outcome of a study. A positive or a negative attitude could easily influence the scoring process, so disinterested researchers or independent judges should be consulted to avoid biases.

To be effective, content analysis must follow a systematic classification scheme to quantify the data. Content analysis enables the researcher to quantify abstract impressions and concepts and to provide for long-term analysis of the materials under study. Moudgil and Sampson report the use of content analysis to determine the kinds of material published in the *Nursing Journal of India*. They discovered that only 3 pages out of 3,846 were related to research over a 10-year period.[1]

The instrument used for content analysis is usually a check-off list on which is recorded each occurrence of the phenomenon. Most often, content analysis is used to make a descriptive statement concerning an attitude, a word or concept frequency, a style change, a social condition, or propaganda.

Advantages

1. Through some form of random selection of every n^{th} occurrence, only a sample of the total literature must be searched to reveal a trend.
2. It is a precise, authoritative method of studying phenomena.
3. It is a convenient way to ascertain trends that are occuring and forms a basis for projection.

[1] Moudgil, A.C., and Sampson, Prema: A study in content analysis, Nurs. J. India **64**:193–194, 209, June 1973.

Disadvantages

1. The technique requires a considerable expenditure of time.
2. The classification of terms, ideas, and trends is ambiguous and an occurrence of a specific phenomenon may seem to fit into more than one category.
3. Biases and prejudice may be difficult to control.

SYSTEMS ANALYSIS

Systems analysis is a technique recently applied to research. A system is a unit composed of many interacting parts that are subject to a common purpose. For instance, our solar system is a system of planets moving about the sun in an orderly arrangement. An order is evident because the positions of the planets can be predicted precisely over years. Each planet in the system influences its neighbor. And our solar system, as a unit, operates independently of other solar systems.

Lillian Pierce traced the historical development of systems research to the pre-World War II period. Systems may be classified as conceptual when they are composed of words, symbols, or numbers, and real when they are natural or manmade. A further distinction is made between open and closed systems. Open systems exchange matter or energy with their environment, whereas closed systems do not.[2] Many disciplines recognize the usefulness of systems as a means of gaining a theoretical understanding of the world.

Biologists are and have been deeply involved with systems as related to some of their theoretical problems. Basic to the understanding of systems theory is the notion that any given system influences the environment and that the environment in turn influences the system.

Systems research techniques are similar to any other research in that they also use questionnaires, statistics, and computers. But the theoretical approach to systems analysis does differ from other theoretical approaches to research. Traditional research seems to focus on more specific, empirical questions, whereas systems analysis investigates a network of relationships and perhaps reduces the network to the most promising relationship. Results from systems analysis may suggest more specific, promising, or productive approaches.

The Minnesota Systems Research organization has undertaken projects such as the following: (1) Analyzing the nutritional results of food habits, attitudes, and food-seeking behavior of impoverished children. This study also investigates the effects of various foods and subsidy programs on the poor when they acquire food. (2) Evaluating the implementation of a computerized information system in a large general hospital. Factors such as cost-effectiveness, manpower utilization, and general performance measures are studied. (3) Undertaking a study in cooperation with state and regional planning agencies toward development of simulation models to evaluate the efforts of alternative health care delivery systems.[3]

[2]Pierce, Lillian: Usefulness of a systems approach for problem conceptualization and investigation, Nurs. Res. **21**(6):509–510, November–December 1972.
[3]State-of-the-art management methods in the fields of health, education and welfare, Minneapolis, December 1971, Minnesota Systems Research, Inc.

Lillian Pierce reported a study using the systems approach in a patient care model. This model views the patient as a communication source for various members of the health care team. Since differences exist between healthy individuals and patients, the health care team attempts to reduce the differences and to restore the patient's equilibrium (state of health).[4]

Von Bertalanffy identifies two main trends in the systems approach: mechanistic and organismic-humanistic.

A mechanistic approach is concerned with computers, cybernitics, feedback, flow charts, cost analysis—all processes which aim to solve health maintenance and nursing delivery problems.

The organismic humanistic system is concerned with the body of an organism, a live emotional, feeling creature which can be helped by the fields of science.[5]

Advantages

The possibility of finding cause-effect relationships is greatly increased with the systems approach. The understanding necessary to develop systems research demands considerable insight. Since input is high, output also should be high.

Replication research could be conducted on only the most promising findings rather than duplicating original research. The nature of systems research demands a greater depth of understanding; thus a well-conceptualized study would render reliable findings and reduce need for replication.

Numerous questions, possible solutions, and new problems can be raised, developed, and tested through systems research. Hypothesis testing, the aim of most investigations, is only part of systems research.

Disadvantages

Systems research is highly theoretical. It demands a deep understanding of the real, the practical, and the basic elements of the unit under investigation; insight into relationships, and purpose of functions; and an understanding of the effects of a multitude of border systems. In other words, it is relatively easy to study the relationship between two variables but much more difficult to study the relationship between two variables within a whole system of relationships.

Open and closed systems are not easily defined. To study the cause of a disease within the relatively closed system of germ theory would neglect the cultural, psychological, and physiological (to name only a few) aspects of disease. How far is it feasible, possible, or desirable to extend the systems in a research project?

Since vast amounts of data could be accumulated through the use of systems research, analyzing data and developing conclusions would involve considerable effort, time, and talent.

The possibilities for systems research within nursing as in other fields are vast. As the capabilities of computers are expanded and as knowledge and technology increase, it seems logical to predict that systems research may be the science of the future.

[4]Pierce, pp. 509–513.
[5]von Bertanlanffy, L., Werley, H.H., and others (ed.): The Systems Approach, New York, 1976, Springer Publishing Co., p. 9.

Q-SORT

According to Best, the Q-sort method, devised by William Stephenson for scaling statements or objects, is effective in ranking attitudes and judgments.[6] A Q-sort is similar to a questionnaire in that an answer is given by the subject; however, it has some different features, too. Statements (alternatives) are typed on cards or slips of paper and presented to the subject. The researcher usually asks the respondent to place these items in 9 to 11 piles ranging from most to least important on a relative scale. A Q-sort is especially effective when there are at least 50 items.

By way of illustration, we might decide to develop a Q-sort in which we ask the subject to sort out patient care procedures in terms of their importance. The procedures might include a backrub, hypodermic injection, personal conversation, or proper medication. All the items would be presented on cards that the subject could place in order in a predetermined number of piles according to the purpose of the investigation.

Researchers who select the Q-sort as their study method should be aware of the theoretical assumptions that are basic to the items they include and the criteria on which their Q-sort is based. Q-sorts are often used to find the attitude of a subject or to discover the ruling of a panel of judges who rearrange or evaluate each item on a specified scale. For example, a group of nurse educators could determine the attributes of a professional nurse and then compare their arrangement with the responses of a group of students.

In the Thurston type of scaling, the judges put as many statements in a pile as they want. In the Q-sort, the number going into each pile is predetermined. An advantage in having the subject place a specific number in each pile is that the rater must distribute the items evenly over the whole scale. The subject is thus forced to make a choice, and the researcher is able to measure what the subject considers average and extreme. If the number going into every pile is not specified, the subject could put all the cards in a single pile.

Sometimes individuals are instructed to compare each case with every other case. Suppose we have 7 piles and 50 statements. Theoretically we want the subject to compare each one of the 50 statements with the other 49 and, on the basis of this judgment, to place it on one of the piles.

Cummins provides a summary in the *Journal of Educational Research*.

> Q-methodology consists of a set of principles drawn from philosophy, psychology, and statistics. It is designed to set up experiments in terms of people, to evaluate qualities of performance for each person, and then to run correlations between them. It considers behavior as a whole rather than discrete phases, e.g., intelligence, emotions, readiness, etc. On the basis of a preconceived theory, it seeks particular factors operative in individual human behavior. Q is small-sample theory. It does not require data from many people. Rather its population consists of traits, characteristics, and attitudes for a single person. It is a study in depth, resting its case on the belief that a person will "give himself away" in completing the Q instrument.[7]

[6]Best, John W.: Research in education, ed. 4, Englewood Cliffs, N.J.,1981, Prentice-Hall, Inc., p. 186.
[7]Cummins, Robert E.: Some applications of "Q" methodology to teaching and educational research, Journal of Educational Research **57**(2):96–98, October 1963. Used with permission of Dembar Educational Research Services, Inc., p. 96.

Advantages

The following characteristics contribute to the strengths of the Q-sort:

1. One of the real values of the Q-sort is its provision for completeness. In the questionnaire method, the subject may skip questions or leave spaces blank, whereas the Q-sort forces the respondent to complete the entire operation. All items in the Q-sort are used; the subject is responsible for placing each item into a category.
2. The Q-sort is inexpensive to use and adaptable to many situations.
3. The Q-sort can be particularly well adapted to theory.
4. A Q-sort allows precise measurement of variables, as well as of the attitudes and beliefs of individuals.
5. The Q-sort is a powerful tool for in-depth research into human attitudes and behavior.
6. Data from the Q-sort are simple to analyze. It is possible to use statistics or to "eyeball" the results.[8]
7. Data are objective.

Disadvantages

There are several disadvantages in the use of the Q-sort method.

1. The procedure is time-consuming particularly if the Q-sort is administered to a large number of subjects.
2. There are difficulties inherent in sending a Q-sort instrument through the mail. Directions may be misinterpreted, and there can be problems in returning the selected piles of cards.
3. It is difficult to develop valid items for the instrument.
4. When subjects are forced to place a number of closely related items into distinct category piles, they sometimes make mechanical choices to get rid of the cards. The piles indicate specific differences, but the importance of the items may differ in the mind of the individual on different days. This raises the question of the instrument's reliability.
5. It is difficult to place the data into meaningful categories and to interpret the results in relation to the theory or hypothesis because it involves considerable forethought.
6. It is difficult to relate the data to an hypothesis.
7. Data analysis is a difficult procedure.

CHECKLIST

A checklist is a prepared list of items with marked columns in which the respondents indicate their participation in a certain activity. Checklists can be checked off by the observer or by the subject. The lists are usually given some hierarchical arrangement. Such lists may be of traits, habits, behaviors, or actions.

Checklists come in many types. There may be categories such as often, seldom, or never. On the other hand, checklists may provide for only yes or no responses. In certain complicated procedures for operating technical equipment, checklists are used to ensure

[8] *Ibid.*, pp. 96–97.

that no task is left undone. In carrying out nursing procedures, instructors may check off steps completed by the student for the purpose of progress, diagnosis, or grading.

The checklist as seen in Fig. 20-1 would be useful as a questionnaire or for observation of nurses skilled in establishing rapport with patients. Researchers could use the same instrument to assess nursing students' performances after an initial experience in the clinical unit. Then they could compare the data from both groups and use the results as a teaching tool when discussing the topic of rapport with inexperienced students.

A checklist is somewhat like a questionnaire in that it requires paper and pencil. The advantages are that (1) it can be completed through the mail; (2) it is a useful way to obtain a large amount of data; and (3) the resulting data are in definite categories, because the subject either does or does not engage in some acts.

The distinct disadvantages of checklists are that (1) there is no opportunity for the respondent to classify his/her judgments; (2) it is a rigid method in both the question and the response; (3) extra time must be planned for pretesting and validating the instrument; (4) the respondent is required to make a forced choice response, so each item must be carefully worded and be based on the purpose of the research; and (5) it is easy for certain important items to be omitted.

Ideally, to develop a checklist, the researcher would use the open-ended questionnaire method first. The items in Fig. 20-1 could be obtained by asking several nurses what techniques they use to establish a rapport with patients. After careful examination, the researcher could place these statements in several categories. Some statements (such as tweaking the patient's toe) might be mentioned so rarely that they would not be included in the final checklist. Only those items that receive popular support are included in the final checklist.

CRITICAL INCIDENT

Critical incidents are specific events described by individuals as having significant meaning. The incidents are categorized according to the purpose of the researcher. Subjects respond to the items in the instrument by indicating how important they believe the category or the activity to be. In other words, the critical incident technique is a process of presenting incidents or summarized events to subjects as a means of gaining insight into their beliefs, attitudes, and values.

This technique is done either in a face-to-face interview or with paper and pencil. The researcher should include a large number of episodes that have been suggested by persons experienced in the field as critical incidents. A full range of situations must be available to estimate the frequency with which each type of circumstance occurs. It is necessary, therefore, that a large sample of incidents (behaviors) that definitely led to failure or success be identified. Psychological traits are inferred from the frequently mentioned behaviors and then placed on a rating scale. Respondents later describing an event may or may not mention the behaviors identified by the experts. If these behaviors are omitted from the respondents' accounts of their experiences, these factors are omitted from the data. An estimate of the intensity of the occurrence of a specific behavior is made on the basis of the respondent's description of the event. To elicit the desired information and to be more precise in defining the critical incident, a great deal of structure has to be built

PROCEDURE USED IN GAINING RAPPORT WITH BED PATIENTS

PROCEDURE	FREQUENCY OF USE				
	ALWAYS	FREQUENTLY	OCCASIONALLY	SELDOM	NEVER
"Hello," begin conversation					
"Good morning," begin conversation					
"Hello" or "Good morning" with a gesture, conversation					
"How do you feel?" informal discussion					
"How do you feel?" formal discussion					
Formal greeting, professional discussion only					
Walk in and begin talking about generalities					
Place hand on patient, then speak					
Tweak patient's toe before speaking					
Hold patient's hand before speaking					
Smile before speaking or greeting					
Gesture before speaking or greeting					

FIGURE 20-1   Checklist.

into the situation described to the respondent. Regardless of how well the information describing the experience is structured, the researcher must depend on the respondent to define the intensity of his experience.

Flanagan used the technique as a follow-up in the longitudinal study, Project TALENT. More than 6,000 critical incidents were collected from 1,800 individuals who had a wide variety of backgrounds. The incidents were categorized into 15 aspects of the quality of life under five major groupings: physical and material well-being; relations with other people; social, community, and civic activities; personal development and fulfillment; and recreation. The 500 respondents were asked to indicate the importance and satisfaction of these 15 aspects of the quality of life. Health was indicated as the most important quality of life by both men and women, whereas political activities were least important and least satisfying.[9]

Jacobs and others conducted a study for the Council of State Boards of Nursing. American Nurses' Association, on the validity of the State Board Test Pool Examination. The purpose of the project was to develop a pool of critical incidents of nursing behavior that would be used to validate the State Board Test Pool Examination. Although they had planned to collect 2,000 incidents, the final submissions came to approximately 14,000 incidents. Respondents had been asked to write four marginal incidents (close call) and one effective and one ineffective treatment procedure.

The items were classified to facilitate application by the nursing profession. Some of the planned uses included developing nursing standards, measuring on-the-job performance, and developing certification programs and future State Board Test Pool Examinations.[10]

Advantages

1. It is a valuable tool to assess knowledge and insight.
2. It is valuable for use as a teaching tool.
3. It is a covert technique that may encourage and/or allow the subject to reveal aspects of self and knowledge that might not be possible in direct questioning.

Disadvantages

1. It requires a large number of incidents to provide valid and reliable results.
2. The types of incidents, the meaning of the responses and the evaluation of results may be subjective judgments rather than factual data.

RANKING AND RATING

There is some confusion in distinguishing between ranking and rating. *Ranking* is the placement of a series of variables in ascending or descending order or the placement of items in categories according to quantity or intensity. One individual may rank higher than another in a language examination, for example.

In *rating*, an item is given a measure of worth. When we rate a variable, we assign a value to it. Ranking and rating techniques differ in that ranking is the comparison of items against each other, whereas rating is the comparison of items against an absolute scale.

When speaking of percentile rank, we are thinking in terms of how case A compares with all other cases. We frequently hear about high school rank, college rank, and class rank. A person who ranked first in his/her class obtained the highest grades in the class. A rank is in relation to all the other units in the system being measured. Rank is meaningless

[9]Flanagan, John C.: Education's contribution to the quality of life of a national sample of 30 year-olds, Educ. Res. **4**(6):13–15, June 1975.
[10]Jacobs, A.M., and others: Critical requirements for safe/effective nursing practice, Kansas City, 1978, American Nurses' Association, ANA Pub. No. B-41.

unless it is given in relation to the total. High school rank is often considered an indicator of a student's ability to succeed in college. If the person ranked in the 50th percentile, it means that he/she excelled over 50% of his class. If the person ranked at the 75th percentile, then his/her grade point average (GPA) was higher than 75% of his/her classmates. The percentile rank is figured on the basis of the total number of individuals in a class (or group), whether there are 20, 50, or several hundred.

A person who received a raw score of 80 on a test might be in the 98th percentile, whereas someone who received a raw score of 20 might be in the 1st percentile. the differences between the percentile ranks are not the same as between the actual raw scores. It is difficult to actually determine how much difference there is between units by using percentile rank. In other words, one percentile rank may cover a few or many scores in an actual case. Percentile rank is figured by using the formula:

$$\text{Percentile rank} = 100 - \frac{(100 \times \text{rank from top} - 50)}{\text{Number (of sample)}} =$$

(rounded to nearest whole number)

For example, Barbara ranked 26th in a class of 125 students. Twenty-five students ranked above her and 99 ranked below her.

$$\text{Percentile rank} = 100 - \frac{100 \times 26 - 50}{125}$$

$$= 100 - \frac{2600 - 50}{125}$$

$$= 100 - 20 = 80$$

Let us digress to explain that there are four types of measuring scales; nominal, ordinal, interval, and ratio. A nominal scale categorizes or distinguishes between essentially two possibilities. For example, a person is either male or female. The ordinal scale is based on an ordering from more to less. This may be demonstrated with stones: one stone will scratch another so that the degree of hardness is the basis of comparison. The interval scale uses actual numbers—equal units of measurement. A thermometer is read on an interval scale. The ratio scale has the same properties as the interval scale except that it has two additional advantages: an absolute zero and the fact that the values have exact worth. A ratio scale has true numbers that can be compared. By the use of this scale. 4 is twice as much as 2, as seen in the case of money, apples, and so on (Chapter 23).

Ranking is used as an ordinal scale only. It simply says that one is higher than the other, although it does not specify how much higher. A discussion of ranking should consider what method is needed to produce equal-appearing intervals. Ranking, or scaling, of attitudes, ideas, or events is related to the idea of equal-appearing intervals. For example, some students in a class will do better academically than others. But as we attempt to discern differences between various students and their abilities, problems arise. There is considerable difference between the student who clearly earns an A grade, and the student who barely receives an A−.

If we transfer this problem into a questionnaire item, we have some idea of the problems involved in creating equal-appearing intervals. To have clear, distinct cutoffs between each category requires experimentation. If questionnaire items are written with discrete, clear-cut categories, it will be much easier for the subject to complete the instrument. As an illustration, it would be unfair to expect an individual to distinguish, by lifting, between a 14-ounce and a 14½-ounce package. Obviously the difference is too close for anyone to evaluate the weights with any degree of accuracy. The same problem exists in many questionnaires or in Q-sorts. The difference between items or intervals is so small and imperceptible that the resulting data may be questioned.

The following example is a practical problem about ranking items. A student was asked to rank violent types of weapons. He was to rank the following in order of intensity: bomb, gun, stick, stone, and fist. He had no difficulty deciding that the bomb was the most dangerous and the fist the least dangerous. Most students considered the gun to be the second most dangerous, but where along the continuum did the stick and the stone go? Students began to argue and ask questions. "How big is the stick?" "How big is the stone?" "How big is the man with the fist—is he a boxer?" Could we say that there were equal intervals between stick and stone? No. A scale has to have intervals that appear to be equal.

Rating may be done by assigning a number to an object, an attitude, or a subject. What happens when judging is done at a sports event? One judge may rate the athletes on how well they are able to execute certain figures and motions, whereas another judge may rate them on the ease and smoothness of performance. A third judge may rate participants on the degree of difficulty of their routine. Each judge gives the performer a rating of 1 to 10 and then the composite score of the three judges is calculated for a total rating. Obviously the person who rates the highest also will rank the highest, but the judges were not ranking them from best to worst. The judges, being experts, were giving the athletes a rating, not a ranking. As the scores are reported for all the participants, they form a series. Then the rank of one athlete can be seen in relation to all the others.

Rating scales are often used to poll the judgment of a number of individuals on a variable. In the nursing field we might poll the opinion of a group of nurses on which jobs in the hospital have the most prestige. We would need to consider three factors: the judges themselves, what will be rated, and the continuum or scale along which the phenomenon will be judged. The design of the study must adequately satisfy all three of these, as well as assure that the judges, the subjects, and the continuum are logically related, if the results are to be valid and reliable.

Advantages

There are major advantages in using rating systems. It is possible for the researcher to consider suggestions or ideas from several sources before making a decision, and rating scales allow data to be placed in objective categories. Such scales are easy to complete and enumerate.

Disadvantages

Rating scales are useful tools in research, but their negative features must be considered as well. There are at least four disadvantages to the use of rating scales. The halo effect is a distinct disadvantage to the use of rating systems. We tend to rate people we like higher than those we dislike or feel we are disliked by, regardless of the category. The subjectivity called for in this procedure leaves room for the expression of such bias. Also, raters tend to be too generous. They may rate at least half to three quarters of a randomized group above average in all traits. In actuality most people are average, and as many are below average as above. Another disadvantage is that the terms used for calibrations may not share the same meaning for all judges. Categories such as "superior" to "inferior" and "strongly agree" to "strongly disagree" are preferable to categories such as "good" to "poor" and "often" to "seldom." Items that imply rather than specify are difficult to translate into meaningful and specific behaviors. The subject is then likely to read in meanings that were never intended by the researcher. Other disadvantages include the difficulty of distinguishing differences between several items. The distinction between categories also may seem indiscernible or poorly defined.

RATING

Rating is the assigning of a value to a variable, whereas ranking is placing subjects in order on some variable. When alternatives are rated for the coding process, it is better to use the highest number for the most rather than the least. Hypotheses are usually worded in such an order that "the higher X is, the higher Y is." Therefore, if the alternative responses are coded so that X has a higher number than Y, it is easier to see if the hypothesis is true. If the hypothesis is worded so that the smaller number is the larger quantity, confusion is more likely to occur. Such a direction is anticipated with the hypothesis: "The higher the education, the higher the income."

In this example (Fig. 20-2), if the hypothesis were true, we expect that persons rated with high numbers such as 8 or 9 will have higher incomes than those who are rated at 2 or 4.

Types of Rating Scales

Both scaling and indexing are techniques used in research to assess the subjects' attitudes and opinions. Authors differ in their definitions of index and scale so that sometimes the words seem to be interchangeable. We will not present a discussion of indexing, since some of the same procedures apply to both techniques. Scales can be developed that produce precise, empirical data about attitudes, beliefs, and opinions.

There are several commonly used types of rating scales. In the *graphic rating scale*, the subject places a check mark along a continuum. The line may run from 1 to 5 or from 1 to 7. The number one is least, and the high number is most. The subjects are directed, for example, to check the most important reason why they considered entering nursing. They may be asked to check or rate each reason from 1 to 5. The advantage of the graphic rating scale is that it makes fine discriminations possible (Fig. 20-3).

Rating scales usually have odd numbers of choices for each item (5, 7, 9, and so on). the midposition allows the extremes to fall on either side. Even-numbered scales do not allow the respondent a middle ground, but are easier to quantify and permit all data to be used.

Another type of scale is the *itemized rating scale*. Each unit on the scale is identified and given a rating. An itemized rating scale of education is shown in Fig. 20-4.

PERSONAL INFORMATION

B. What was the highest grade attained by your mother?

		CORRECT	INCORRECT
_____	1. Some grade school, with/without business or vocational training	1	9
_____	2. Grade school education	2	8
_____	3. Some high school, with/without business or vocational training	3	7
_____	4. High school diploma	4	6
_____	5. High school diploma plus business or vocational training	5	5
_____	6. Some college	6	4
_____	7. Some college, plus business or vocational training	7	3
_____	8. College degree with/without additional schooling	8	2
_____	9. Graduate degree, with/without additional schooling	9	1
_____	10. Don't know	0	0

FIGURE 20-2   Personal information.

The *comparative scale* is the third type of scale. In the graphic and itemized scales, raters make judgments based on themselves alone, not in reference to other individuals. In a comparative rating scale, on the other hand, the rater evaluates positions in terms of relationships to other individuals or groups whose characteristics are known.

An interesting study is to have subjects rate themselves on some variable and then have another person rate the subjects on the same variable and compare the two ratings. People tend to make checks near the middle choices and to avoid extremes. Few choices or situations in real life fall at the extremes; rather, the majority fall in the middle area. A researcher has reason to be skeptical when respondents continually mark checks in one of the extreme categories. Raters must be given some training or precise directions, since they tend to judge people subjectively. Often, respondents rate individuals on a faulty definition. Many people, for example, do not know what liberal and conservative mean. If we ask the sample to rate the behavior of a group of nurses as liberal or conservative, we must provide good descriptions of what is meant by liberal and conservative—even write some examples of the terms.

Again, we want to stress that it is better for a continuum scale to have too many choices rather than too few. Responses can always be grouped together, but it is difficult to spread responses out when only a few categories are available to the subject.

Ratings can often be made by groups of judges, especially if the researcher is interested in rating a technique or a quality. Raters working in terms can cancel out biases in either direction. The more specific and the more objective the categories are made, the more likely they are to be valid. To describe some category as *good* is not enough. If *good* is defined precisely and numerically, the term becomes meaningful. One school of nursing received a recommendation for a woman who wished to enroll. The recommendation said that she would be a good nurse because she had a nice smile.

Remmers suggests that rating scales should be judged by some of the following measures:
1. Objectivity—the instrument should yield verifiable, reproducible data.
2. Reliability—if used by the same people, it should give consistent results.
3. Sensitivity—it should produce as fine a distinction between units as is normally found in the actual situation.
4. Validity—the scale should measure the variable with a high degree of accuracy. Validity is usually tested by comparing the scale with some other scale or known measure of the quality under investigation.
5. Utility—it should yield information that is relevant and easy to collect.[11]

Three commonly used scaling devices are the Guttman, Likert, and Thurston scales (Table 6). Guttman scaling technique provides for a progression of attitudes from weak to strong. The subject is required to choose some point along the continuum of provided responses, for example:

1   Have you ever been a second lieutenant?
        ☐ Yes ☐ No
2   Have you ever been a first lieutenant?
        ☐ Yes ☐ No

[11]Remmers, H.H.: Rating methods in research on teaching. In Gage, N.L., editor: Handbook of research on teaching, Chicago, 1963, Rand, McNally & Co., p. 330.

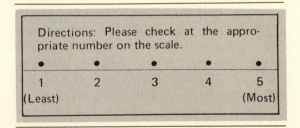

FIGURE 20-3   Graphic rating scale.

EDUCATION
(1) Some grade school
(2) Finished eighth grade
(3) Some high school
(4) Finished high school
(5) Some college

FIGURE 20-4   Itemized rating scale.

3 Have you ever been a captain?
    ☐ Yes ☐ No
4 Have you ever been a major?
    ☐ Yes ☐ No
5 Have you ever been a lieutenant colonel?
    ☐ Yes ☐ No
6 Have you ever been a colonel?
    ☐ Yes ☐ No

The items in this scale are cumulative; if the respondent checks number 6, we can assume that he also would check the other five. This structuring of items is called *scalogram analysis*. A unidimensional scale meets this objective at least 90% of the time.

The Guttman scale also may be used to measure a personality trait such as timidity.

Normally, I would (*Please check*)
1 ☐ Talk with a friend only when spoken to.
2 ☐ Initiate a conversation with a friend.
3 ☐ Talk with a stranger only when spoken to.
4 ☐ Initiate a conversation with a stranger.

These items progress from weak to strong or soft to hard. If the respondent checks number 3, the individual's behavior probably would include numbers 1 and 2.

Likert-type scales are frequently used in survey questionnaires and opinion research. Statements are submitted to the respondents who are asked to choose one of five responses that best reflect their position: strongly agree, agree, undecided, disagree, and strongly disagree. Note the progressive intensity of these items.

The range of scores is from 5 to 1, respectively. The scores from the statements are totaled to give a rating to the subject's opinion. A Likert-type scale is developed from a pool of statements that are submitted to individuals similar to those who will be in the major project. The most discriminating items are retained for use in the research project.

Likert-type items are easy to develop but are highly subjective. Therefore, the researcher must try to interpret the data objectively. Likert-type scales should have approximately equal numbers of statements that are positive and negative about the attitude under study.

Thurston developed a method of assessing attitudes in which many statements are submitted to a panel of judges. The items must meet the criteria of relevancy and clarity. Then the judges arrange them into 11 piles ranging in intensity between two extremes. When the judges agree on the inclusion of a statement, it is retained. When there is disagreement, the statement is deleted. Each of the retained items is assigned a position from 1 to 11. For example, a score of 1 is assigned to a statement that seems the least dependable and 11 is assigned to a statement that seems the most dependable. The final selection of approximately 20 items is then submitted to the subjects who indicate the statements with which they agree. Scale values for each respondent are obtained by calculating the total average value.

Scales are being developed by nurses to measure the quality of patient care and the nurse's performance in the clinical setting. Williams reports the use of three such rating scale: the Phaneuf Nursing Audit (50-item instrument); the Slater Scale (84-item scale);

TABLE 20-1 Characteristics of Guttman, Likert, and Thurston Scales

Characteristics	Gutman	Likert	Thurston
How developed How used	Researcher makes decisions Cumulative scores Subjects can be placed on a definite position in a continuum Administered before being ranked	Researcher makes decisions Summated scores Subject responds to all items on a 5-point scale Responses given a value, and individual attitude is expressed in a numerical quantity	Items selected by judges (experts) Subjects agree or disagree to a series of items and receive a quantified score
How items are retained	Through numerous applications to people	Through administration to a group of trial subjects; items correlating high with total test, retained	Ambiguous items discarded; irrelevent items avoided; high agreement items retained
Popularity	Very popular	Very popular	Less popular because of difficulty of development
Advantages	Relatively easy to develop items Cumulative items Goes farthest to test for unidimensionality	Easy to construct; takes less time Does not require judges Precise Reliable Uses actual subjects rather than a panel	Valid Equal-appearing intervals between items
Disadvantages	What is a Guttman scale for one group may not be a Guttman scale for another Results may vary from one group to another	High subjective element in interpretation of results by researcher	Need for periodic updating Arduous and time-consuming because of difficulty in judging items May be difficult to obtain judges Judges may bias Subject may not be permitted to give adequate response
Features	Permits transformation of nominal data into an ordinal scale of greater—or lesser—than properties	Assumes that specific attitude variable is being measured May or may not have ordinal or interval properties	Relatively high correlation between Thurston and Likert results

and the Quality Patient Care Scale (Qual-PaCS), a 68-item scale.[12] Volicer and Bohannon also report a rating scale on hospital stress.[13] Developing these types of instruments increases the probability of finding answers to nursing questions. The scales can be refined through extensive use.

SIMULATION

Simulation is an artificial process for the purpose of gaining knowledge without the use of the real object or situation. A simulation may be symbolic or it may be a natural model. In some cases, the two are combined. A model is an imitation of something real; it is not the real object, but it is similar to the real object. Model trains and airplanes are familiar examples. In recent years, everyone has had the opportunity to watch simulations of the astronauts' flights into outer space on television. Use of simulations can often give the researcher a great deal of insight into a subject or event. Research models are so much like the real world that they can provide information and data for the study of a process. They give researchers the opportunity to integrate and test their understanding of the theoretical basis of a phenomenon with research methods.

Models are used in building bridges or planning construction projects. Engineers can build a model of a bridge and then put it through various types of stress and strain to see how much weight it will carry or how long it will last under pressure. Likewise, they can place an airplane in a wind tunnel to simulate real conditions without risking life or property.

At least three kinds of simulation have been identified: iconic simulation (model has some basic properties of the original but with a different scale), analog model (can be manipulated to simulate another process), and symbolic simulation (a method of numerical evaluation of equations).[14]

In any given field, Jean-Paul Gremy says that the technique for the automated processing of information goes through three stages: (1) existing procedures become automated, (2) automated procedures are borrowed from other more advanced disciplines, and (3) the possibility of new procedures is made available by data processing. As an example, Hagarstrand used a geographical distribution of the economic and cultural characteristics of a farm to study the consequences of introducing a new technique in farming. The geographical characteristics of the area—fjords, lakes, and forest—were intertwined with the social characteristics of the area. The model artificially produced a communication network composed of telephone communications, migration of labor, buying and selling of land, and marriages. It was hypothesized that the social, cultural, and geographic features of an area will determine how new ideas are diffused. This

[12] Williams, Lillian B.: Evaluation of nursing care: a primary nursing project. Part I. Report of the controlled study, Superv. Nurse **6**(1):35–36, January 1975.

[13] Volicer, B.J., and Bohannon, M.W.: A hospital stress rating scale. Nurs. Res. **24**(5):352–359, September–October 1975.

[14] Ackoff, Russell L., Gupta, Shiv K., and Minas, J. Sayer: Scientific method optimizing applied research decisions, New York, 1968, John Wiley & Sons, Inc., pp. 349–350.

hypothesis could then be tested using simulation techniques by programming all these variables into a computer.[15]

One of the chief advantages of simulation research is that we can manipulate the independent variables. If one of the independent variables causes effect X, we can substitute another independent variable to observe what effect it will have. Another advantage is that the techniques are suited to long-term studies. In this instance, simulation may be combined with other research techniques such as observation and interviews.

In the study of human behavior, simulation has the disadvantage that theory as a whole is not being tested in experiments where there is a high degree of control. Neither is theory being used to its maximum for the purpose of understanding and controlling the process taking place in experimental situations. We should try to apply theory to the greatest extent possible in our attempt to understand the real world.

Simulation can be carried out with human beings in a number of ways: in games, with films, and in role-playing. Some simulation can be done with animals. Often, simulation is done by programming variables into a computer and allowing the computer to respond to the variables. In a short time the computer can arrive at answers that might take months or years to find in real life. The computer could be programmed to cover longer periods of time than could actually be studied.

Simulation Game

Simulation has often been used in the field of game theory. In game theory the researcher allows a group of people to play games and then observes and records their interactions. The game is a simulation or a model of what happens in actual life. Simulation incorporates a high degree of abstraction, although important characteristics from real-life circumstances are selected for study. It is important, of course, that all the intricacies of behavior in the natural situation be included in the simulation.

Van Dyne reports on Goodman's game designed to simulate growing old. Loss of physical mobility is simulated by attaching players to furniture with ropes that are shortened as the players "get older."[16]

Once, when using an urban redevelopment game, students were allowed the choice of being a real estate broker, an urban developer, or a community planner. As the game progressed, natural leaders evolved in each of the groups and a spirited dialogue developed. Buying and selling continued until the players reached a stalemate and refused to cooperate anymore. A discussion revealed that insights had been gained into the psychology of human behavior, the patterns of leadership, the diplomacy of bargaining, and the need for cooperation within and among organizations. The students agreed that the game produced more interest and insight than the same amount of time spent on a lecture on the topic.

A game is often though of as a fun way to find out how decisions are made, what resources are used in making decisions, how decisions affect relationships, and how relationships affect decisions. One professor used a game with a group of students to help

[15]Gremy, Jean-Paul: The use of computer simulation techniques in sociology. International Social Science Journal 23(2):204–211, 1971.
[16]Van Dyne, L.: Teaching with games? Chronicle of Higher Education 9(1):7, September 23, 1974.

simulate what it is like to be female in a male-dominant society. The players threw dice and moved their markers along a board. The underlying theme was that women are at a disadvantage when dealing with men in the business world. The game was intended to help the students propose hypotheses related to human behavior while they tried to win. At the end of the session, each student suggested three hypotheses. Some interesting observations were that winners enjoy that game, women are expected to lose, and losers blame their losing on bad luck while winners attribute their success to skill.

Such a game could be designed to simulate the interaction of nurses, physicians, and patients in a health care facility. Part of the game might hinge on making decisions regarding appropriate methods of patient care. As a penalty players could be required to answer questions related to understanding nursing intervention. Such a simulation game would be used to develop insight into relationships among team members, to teach appropriate procedures in health care, and to suggest or develop hypotheses for testing.

Advantages

1. It is an interesting and entertaining way to learn about real life in a closed environment.
2. Because games focus on competition, subjects become involved and react naturally.
3. Results are often obtained much faster and easier than in real-life situations.

Disadvantages

1. Subjects or researchers may become involved in the game or social interaction to a degree that reality is lost.
2. Results and values of simulation games are subjective and require skill and expertise in interpretation.
3. This technique requires time and subjects who are willing to participate.

COMPUTER SIMULATION

In computer simulation, mathematics or other logical formulations are entered into the computer in the same order and with the same types of decisions that people might make in real life or in a game. For example, we might have people play a game, and then the choices they made while playing the game are put into the computer. Whereas it might take the participants hours to play the game, after the data are put into the computer and properly programmed the results come back in a short time—from a fraction of a second to a few seconds.

A computer simulation could be built around the theme of nutrition and its effect on health. A simulation package could be developed with a formula that computes the effect of variables such as calories, exercise, metabolism, diet, and sleep on health. The researchers could put quantities into the computer and retrieve information on the correct diet for good health that includes weight control, adequate caloric intake, an exercise program, sufficient vitamins, and adequate rest.

Another advantage of computer simulation is that once information is obtained, it can be placed into the computer again for a more elaborate and detailed simulation study. The researcher can continue to refine his/her theoretical basis and reconstruct various aspects of the study until he/she can develop a simulated situation entirely by computer.

One must remember that data coming from a computer simulation are no better than the information that was fed into the machine. Not only must all details be put into the computer, but they must be entered in the correct order. Only well-programmed data can return meaningful information. The results cannot be greater than the sum of the parts; no one can expect the computer to bring out more than has been put in by the researcher.

DELPHI TECHNIQUE

The Delphi technique is a useful method for long-range forecasting, quantifying expert judgments, or determining priorities. First, a panel of experts on a particular subject is invited to participate in a study. Those who accept, whether they are educators, practitioners, specialists, scholars, or others, are asked to complete a questionnaire. The instrument may gather opinions, estimates, or future predictions on some special topic. The responses are collected, and the results are summarized and returned to the experts. Using the combined information of all the experts, a new questionnaire is made up. Each individual then responds to the information in the new questionnaire. This process is usually repeated four times until the resulting data are a consensus of the opinions, predictions, or beliefs of all the experts. Such information is useful for planning courses of action, finding a consensus of opinion, or for predicting future conditions. This useful technique can be modified or adapted to fit many situations.

A creative example of the Delphi technique applied to nursing was conducted by WICHE and reported by Carol Lindeman. In this project, 433 participating members were asked to identify five burning issues in nursing practice. Three hundred forty-one individuals from a number of states, representing a broad educational and experiential base, completed all four questionnaires. Results from the survey were helpful to the advisory committee for the WICHE Regional Programs for Nursing Research Development. This committee decided in September 1974 that the target of research would be to "determine valid and reliable indicators of quality nursing care.[17]

Certainly, the concentrated effort and talent of a group of this magnitude represent a significant consensus—possibly the best judgment available concerning what should be done in nursing research.

Advantages

Advantages of the Delphi technique include the following:
1. Experts (respondents) need not attend a meeting, be intimidated by individuals of a higher status than themselves, or be influenced by other experts. All opinions or statements receive the same priority (equal treatment). Expert opinions are obtained without great demands on time.
2. Each expert can review the other judges' responses and can compare and evaluate their own opinions with those of the other respondents.
3. The response rate is reasonably consistent and known in advance, since each of the experts has previously committed himself/herself to the study. If desired, members of the expert panel may remain anonymous.

[17]Lindeman, Carol: Priorities in clinical nursing research, Nurs. Outlook **23**(11):693–698, November 1975.

4. The four-step time cycle is conducive to a precise, clearly defined conceptual under-standing of many individuals' opinions condensed into a few statements or only one statement.
5. The results should be extremely useful because they represent a form of accumulated knowledge that would be difficult to obtain otherwise.

Disadvantages

The disadvantages of the Delphi technique include the following:

1. It is a costly and time-consuming procedure for the researcher. Each expert must be contacted, and some of them will probably refuse or fail to respond. The results of each questionnaire must be tabulated for the next questionnaire. The postage, tabulat-ing, and printing of the different questionnaires are expensive.
2. The operation is dependent on the cooperation and speedy response of each partici-pating expert. Second, third, and fourth questionnaires can be distributed no sooner than the receipt of the last respondent's instrument.
3. A number of biases may be introduced, including an overabundance of particular personalities; only certain types of individuals or disciplines may be invited to participate or may accept the invitation. The instrument may or may not be reliable or valid; interpretation of results from the first wave of questionnaires may influence second questionnaires, and so on.
4. The results are the opinions of experts, and experts' opinions may or may not represent reality.

SEMANTIC DIFFERENTIAL

The semantic differential measuring scale requires the subject to select a point along a continuum between two extremes. Osgood designed the scale to investigate the perceptions, the attitudes, and the feelings of respondents. However, it has sometimes been used with psychological overtones to study *how* the subjects scored the scales.

Fig. 20-5 is an example of the semantic differential scale used to evaluate a learning resource center. In this illustration, the positive elements are on the left and the negative on the right. Sometimes positive and negative elements are switched from left to right, respectively.

It is assumed that the same sets of words can be used to measure an attitude toward any object or person. Osgood sees another dimension to this scale; the subject's subtle feelings toward the object can be represented by a word.[18] Evaluation, activity, and potency are connoted in people's responses to many polar pairs of adjectives. For that reason the three polar pairs of words—hard-soft, clean-dirty, valuable-worthless—could function as a universal scale on which to evaluate many objects, words, or ideas.

In actual use, the researcher selects the subject, object, or attitude for study. A list of opposing word-adjectives is developed which appear to cover the area of research. The following word combinations could be useful for a variety of situations: active-passive, complacent-assertive, definitive-rambling, sharing-closed, and bold-timid. Such combi-

---

[18]Kerlinger, Fred n.: Foundations of behavioral research, New York, 1973, Holt, Rinehart & Winston, p. 568.

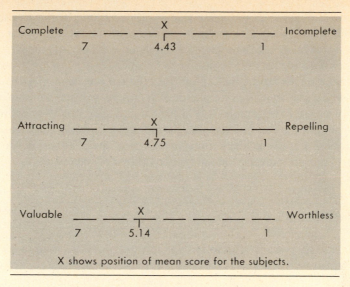

Complete	___	___	X ⌐	___	___	___	___	Incomplete
	7		4.43			1		

Attracting	___	___	X ⌐	___	___	___	___	Repelling
	7		4.75			1		

Valuable	___	___	X ⌐	___	___	___	___	Worthless
	7		5.14			1		

X shows position of mean score for the subjects.

FIGURE 20-5   Semantic differential scale.

nations could well describe individuals, groups, and organizations. The sharing-closed set could be used in a creative fashion to evaluate a particular unit in a hospital, clinic, medical center, or client-family. The semantic differential is adaptable to many purposes and its effectiveness can be increased by the use of insightful word pairs.

Advantages

The advantages of the semantic differential include the following:
1. It is an indirect approach.
2. It tends to arouse the subject's interest.
3. It provides data that can be placed in objective categories.
4. It is more difficult for the subject to disguise his feelings.

Disadvantages

The disadvantages of the semantic differential are as follows:
1. The researcher must be well trained in psychological interpretations.
2. It is difficult to determine the appropriate balance of pairs representing the polar extremes.
3. It is difficult to test the reliability and validity of the device.

PROJECTIVE DEVICES

A projective device is a method designed to reveal the underlying attitudes, feelings, and motivations of respondents as demonstrated by their responses to a testing tool. Unfortunately, the administrator's interpretation of the response is difficult to validate. One of the best known examples of a projective technique is the Rorschach test in which subjects interpret ink blots.

Enthusiasts of this technique believe that a given response has a specific underlying meaning. This meaning or attitude may be unknown to the respondent or may be subconsciously rejected or feared. It is assumed that the easiest way to learn the subject's hidden feelings is by the indirect projective technique.

In the case of the Thematic Apperception Test, the subject tells stories about individual pictures in a series. The Sentence Completion Test requires subjects to complete sentences with their own words. For example, "My father was _____" or "Nurses are _____."

Another projection technique is to question the subject about a particular topic. The response demonstrates the subject's frame of reference. In all fairness it also may be said that the interpretation indicates the interpreter's frame of reference.

QUALITATIVE RESEARCH

For the benefit of individuals who want to gain beginning skills in both qualitative and quantitative research, this chapter provides an introduction to qualitative research. There has been a growing realization among nurse researchers that quantitative methodology does not answer all questions. Learning the frequency of events, although informative, does not provide a holistic, natural world view of the phenomenon that qualitative research can produce. Although criticized by some researchers as unscientific, qualitative investigation is considered productive and beneficial by many who believe that the *what* needs to be known as much as the *amount*.

Gortner calls for greater explanatory power in nursing research as a means of influencing policy formation.[19] Such explanatory power also gains the respect of researchers in other disciplines as they recognize the contribution that nursing qualitative research makes to new knowledge. The expansion in understanding of the human being—the focus of all nursing—cannot be comprehended at the present status of nursing research. But as nursing investigators develop new modes of inquiry through description and induction as well as prescription and deduction, the answers to why and the meaning will result.

Techniques Used

The most common techniques used in qualitative research are observation, content analysis, and interviewing. Other popular techniques include unobtrusive measures, historical analysis, ethnography, self-reports, and case studies. In contrast to quantitative research, a diversity of data sources is preferred in qualitative research.

1. *Observation* has been identified as the core of qualitative research methdology. It generally falls into two categories; complete observer and participant-observer. By knowing what to look for and recognizing it when it occurs, the complete observer can gain an understanding of a phenomenon that cannot be acquired any other way. Social interaction, timing of events, and documentation of various kinds can accurately

[19]Gortner, S.R.: Knowledge in a practice discipline: philosophy and pragmatics. In Williams, C., editor: Nursing research and policy formation: the case of prospective payment, American Academy of Nursing papers of the 1983 scientific session, Kansas City, 1984, American Nurses' Association, p. 5.

be recorded and described. The participant-observer, on the other hand, becomes involved in social interaction with informants and the context of their behavior. He/she collects data systematically and unobtrusively and interprets it in language that reveals a full and rich analysis.

2. *Ethnography* refers to a qualitative methodology that has long been used by anthropologists in its various styles, and that results in purely descriptive studies of the culture. Extensive fieldwork is conducted using such techniques as participant-observation, filming, formal and informal interviewing, collecting documents, and recording.

3. *Content analysis* of documents is effective in evaluating programs. The technique includes analyzing the conceptualization, implementation, and ongoing processes. Insight can be gained into the philosophy, factors that affected change over time, the key individuals, and circumstances that influenced the program.

4. *Interviewing* may be formal or informal. In some cases, the data may be collected during informal conversations. At other times, interview guides may be used. The researcher must determine if the response is to be limited or open-ended. When an interview guide is used, the researcher must be sure that assistants are well-trained and skillful in probing for the information sought.

5. *Unobtrusive measures* to collect data for qualitative research are those that do not "interfere" by not concentrating on the average but rather on the variance. Concentration is on things under study without the researcher influences on the persons and setting, according to Taylor and Bogdan.[20]

6. *Historical analysis* may be conducted in order to enlarge the researcher's perspective on a given situation. Public documents, newspapers, files of historical societies, and various archives provide a wealth of material for the investigator.

7. *Self-reports* make it possible for the researcher to gain a glimpse of the indigenous person's point-of-view concerning the phenomenon. Self-reports are closely associated with ethnography; they are at the core of gaining access to the conceptual world of those living in the culture under study.

8. *Case studies* may be conducted as a one-shot investigation in which the researcher observes one sample or population at only one point in time. The study might involve one person, a community, organization, or institution. The intent is to describe rather than to test an hypothesis. Case studies provide a holistic approach to a field of study. They may be singular or multiple in number. Case clusters call for limiting the parameters for the units to be analyzed.

Triangulation

Researchers may choose to complement their quantitative research project with a qualitative one. Combining the two types is called triangulation. Jick believes that triangulation can uncover a unique variance that might not have appeared in a single method of investigation.[21] He suggests that it increases confidence in results and allows

[20]Taylor, S.J., and Bogdan, R.: Introduction to qualitative research methods, the search for meanings, ed. 2, New York, 1984, John Wiley & Sons, pp. 117–118.
[21]Jick, T.D.: Mixing Qualitative and quantitative methods: triangulation in action. In Van Maanen, J., editor: qualitative methodology, Beverly Hills, 1983, SAGE Publications, Inc. p. 138.

for creative methods. At the same time, new ways of seeing a problem that may have been overlooked before may be balanced with the common methodologies, and a new dimension of the problem may be uncovered.

COMPARISON OF QUALITATIVE AND QUANTITATIVE CHARACTERISTICS

Qualitative research is concerned with meaning and multiple sources; quantitative research assumes the meaning and more frequently uses one source. Qualitative research is concerned with the nature of something rather than with the amount. It is process-oriented rather than product-oriented. Qualitative research investigates components that are unevenly distributed rather than those that are just existing. Phenomena are studied in their settings.

It is widely recognized that differences in qualitative and quantitative research exist, but there can be overlap at times. Observation can be quantified as can interviews, but qualitative researchers are more likely to describe what has occurred as a process than to report it as a social structure.

Qualitative research does not begin with the identification of a problem and literature review; rather, the investigator enters the arena and observes the natural world as it exists. Although there is no hypothesis to be tested, discovery can be the result. Symbolism has a place in qualitative research as does exploration for theory. The qualitative researcher is intent on capturing new insights and uses himself/herself as the tool.

SUMMARY

Investigators often become attached to a few favorite approaches for their research studies. When there is a variety of methods from which to choose, research is made more effective.

Content analysis is a systematic enumeration of the occurrence of specified words or concepts in written and verbal material. This analysis is usually done on every n^{th} publication over an extended period of time.

Systems analysis is a research technique that concentrates on all the interacting units in the whole system. Rather than consider the physiological cause of illness, the systems approach may evaluate the relationship of social, economic, and psychological factors.

The Q-sort is made up of a series of statements reviewed by professionals and submitted to the subjects in the sample. The subjects place the statements in order or in a designated number of piles, either from one extreme category to the other or on a specified scale. The Q-sort is characterized by its facility of theoretical orientation, its provision for completeness, its economy, its interpretation, its depth, and its precision. It is equally adaptable for attitudes, beliefs, and values.

Checklists are prepared lists of items with appropriate columns whereby the respondent may indicate preference or indulgence in certain traits, habits, behaviors, or attitudes. Open-end questions are used to develop items on a checklist.

Critical incidents are described situations presented to subjects to elicit recall of similar phenomena. On the basis of psychological inferences, subjects are judged acceptable for some occupation or some other value.

Ranking and rating are similar techniques whereby individuals or circumstances are evaluated. Ranking and rating differ in that ranking requires the judges to make decisions by comparing one item against another rather than against an absolute scale. High school percentile rank is an example of the use of rank. It is difficult to determine the actual difference between two units by their percentile ranks. Since ranking is a type of ordinal scaling, some consideration should be given to equal-appearing intervals. When categories in a questionnaire or other instrument are not distinct and clear-cut, then responses are also vague, and the validity of the instrument may be questioned. Rating may be used for obtaining subjects' responses, or judges' opinions, or for assigning values to a variable for measurements. Individuals often rate their friends above average on any measuring scale, in spite of the fact that half the population is below average.

Three of the common scaling devices are the Guttman, Likert, and Thurston scales. Nurses are beginning to develop scales in clinical nursing to measure the quality of nursing care and nurse performance.

Simulation is an artificial process for the purpose of gaining knowledge without the use of real subjects. Simulation has the distinct advantages of manipulating the independent variable and providing immediate results that can be reprogrammed. Simulation is often accomplished by use of computers, games, and films. The results of computer simulations are only as good as the data programmed into the machine.

The Delphi technique uses questionnaires that are sent to experts. These are summarized, and the results are sent to the sample along with the next questionnaire. This four-time procedure is useful for predicting and obtaining a consensus.

Semantic differentials are scales used to measure subjects' perceptions. Projective devices are designed to measure underlying attitudes and feelings.

Qualitative research answers *what*, quantitative research is concerned with *amount*. Some common types of qualitative research are observation, ethnography, content analysis, interviewing, unobtrusive measures, historical analysis, self-reports, and case studies. Triangulation is the combining of qualitative and quantitative methods. Qualitative research does not test hypotheses, but specializes in rich insights.

DISCUSSION QUESTIONS

1 Why do you think the authors titled this chapter "Other techniques" since the techniques in this chapter still involve questionnaires, interviews, records, observations, and experiments?
2 Suggest a way to use content analysis other than with published material.
3 Comment on the following statement, "The future of research will probably revolve around the systems analysis approach."
4 How could you combine simulation and the Delphi technique to study the future of nursing?
5 Defend the position that researchers could learn by developing their skills and by concentrating on one research technique than by using a variety of approaches.
6 Which technique presented in the chapter would you like to try? Why?
7 Suggest a questionnaire item using the semantic differential technique to gather data from a sample of patients who only recently arrived from a nonEnglish-speaking country.

8 Develop five items for a Q-sort, two for each extreme and one for the midpoint.
9 In what way are the critical incident and Q-sort techniques similar?
10 Defend the position that rating is a better way of assigning course grades than ranking.

CLASS ACTIVITIES

Track I

1 The class is divided into groups. Each group is to suggest ideas that could be considered for a computer simulation program dealing with doubling the size of a selected health care facility.
2 The class is divided into groups. Each group is to plan a short questionnaire concerning nutrition in an educational institution using the Delphi technique.
3 Each group is to design a checklist or semantic differential scale for a project suggested by the instructor.

Track II (Steps in Research Project)

1 The class is divided into the project groups.
   a Each group or student working alone is to complete the instrument it intends to use in the investigation and to prepare to pretest it.
   b Prepare enough copies of the instrument to pretest it using the pilot study sample.

SUGGESTED READINGS

Abraham, I.L.: Univariate statistical models for meta-analysis, Nursing Research 32(5):312, September–October 1983.
Ackoff, Russell, L., Gupta, Shiv K., and Minas, J. Sayer: Scientific method optimizing applied research decisions, New York, 1968, John Wiley & Sons, Inc., p. 210.
Best, John W.; Research in education, ed. 4, Englewood Cliffs, N.J., 1981, Prentice-Hall, Inc., Chapter 7.
Bond, S.: A Delphi survey of clinical nursing research priorities, Journal of Advanced Nursing 7(6):565, November 1982.
Brower, H.R., and Crist, M.A.: Research priorities in gerontologic nursing for long-term care, Image XVII(1):22–27, Winter 1985.
Carlberg, C.G., and others: Meta-analysis in education: a reply to Slavin, Educational Researcher 13(8):16–23, October 1984.
Case studies, Nursing Research, 135–136, November–December 1977.
Clark, M.J., and Clark, P.E.: Personal computers and database access, Image XVII(1):21, Winter 1985.
Cohen P.A.: Student ratings of instruction and student achievement: a meta-analysis of multisection validity studies, Review of Educational Research, 51(3):281–309, Fall 1981.
Coleman, James S., and others: The Hopkins games program: conclusions from seven years of research, Educ. Res. 2(8):6, August 1973.
Cooper, H.M.: The integrative research review, a systematic approach, Applied Social Research Methods Series, Vol. 2, Beverly Hills, 1984, Sage Publications, Inc.
Conners, C.K. and Wells, K.C.: Single-case designs in psychopharmacology, New Directions for Methodology of Social and Behavioral Sciences: Single-Case Research Designs, no. 13, San Francisco, 1982, Jossey-Bass.
Cook, T. and Leviton, L.: Reviewing the literature: a comparison of traditional methods with meta-analysis, J. of Personality 48(4):449–472, December 1980.

Cornell, S.A.: Development of an instrument for measuring the quality of nursing care, Nurs. Res. 23(2):117, 1974.

Denenberg, V.H.: Comparative psychology and single-subject research, New Directions for Social and Behavioral Sciences: Single-Case Research Designs, no. 13, San Francisco, 1982, Jossey-Bass.

Downey, H.K. and Ireland, R.D.: Quantitative versus qualitative: environmental assessment in organizational studies, Qualitative Methodology, Beverly Hills, 1983, Sage Publications, Inc.

Fawcett, J.: The family as a living open system: an emerging conceptual framework for nursing, Int. Nurs. Rev. 22(4):113–116, July–August 1975.

Field, P.A.: An ethnography: four public health nurses' perspectives of nursing: an approach for clinical nursing research, Journal of Advanced Nursing 8(1):3–12, January 1983.

Flanagan, J.C.: Education's contribution to the quality of life of a national sample of 30-year-olds, Educ. Res. 4(6):13, June 1975.

Garmezy, N.: The case for the single case in research, New Directions for Social and Behavioral Sciences: Single-Case Research Designs, no. 13, San Francisco, 1982, Jossey-Bass.

Glass, G.V.: Primary, secondary, and meta-analysis of research, Educational Researcher 5(10):3–8, November 1976.

Glass, G.V.: Integrating findings: the meta-analysis of research, review of research in education, Review of Research in Education, vol. 5, 1977, American Educational Research Association.

Gorden, R.L.: Unidimensional scaling of social variables, concepts and procedures, New York, 1977, The Free Press.

Hall, J.E., and Weaver, B.R.: A Systems approach to community health, ed. 2, Philadelphia, 1985, J.B. Lippincott Company.

Hambleton, R.K.: Testing and decision-making procedures for selected individualized instructional programs, Review of Educational Research 44(4):373, Fall 1974.

Hedges, L.V. and Olkin, I.: Analyses, reanalyses, and meta-analysis, Contemporary Education Review 1:157–165, Fall 1982.

Helmer, O.: Analysis of the future: the Delphi method, Santa Monica, CA., 1967, RAND Corporation.

Herriott, R.E., and Firestone, W.A.: Multisite qualitative policy research: optimizing description and generalizability, Education Researcher 12:14, Fall 1983.

Hildebrand, D.K., Laing, J.D., and Rosenthal, H.: In Uslaner, E.M., editor, Series: quantitative applications in the social sciences, no. 07-008, Beverly Hills, 1977, Sage Publications, Inc.

How to use qualitative evaluation methods, how to: evaluate education programs: a monthly guide to methods and ideas that work, pp. 1–6, January 1985.

How to: evaluate education programs, Arlington, VA, January 1985, Capitol Publications, Inc.

Jacobs, A.M., and others: Critical requirements for safe/effective nursing practice, ANA Pub. no. B-41, Kansas City, 1978, American Nurses' Association.

Jick, T.D.: Mixing qualitative and quantitative methods: triangulation in action. In Van Maanen, J., editor: Qualitative methodology, Beverly Hills, 1983, Sage Publications, Inc.

Johnson, D.W., Johnson, R.T., and Maruyama, G.: Interdependence and interpersonal attraction among heterogeneous and homogeneous individuals: a theoretical formulation and a meta-analysis of the research, Review of Educational Research 53(1):5–54, Spring 1983.

Kerlinger, F.N.: Foundations of behavioral research, New York, 1973, Holt, Rinehart & Winston.

Krieger, D.: Therapeutic touch: the imprimatur of nursing, Am. J. Nurs. 75(5):784–787, May 1975.

LeCompte, M.D., and Goetz, J.P.: Problems of reliability and validity in ethnographic research, Rev. of Educational Research 52(1):31–60, Spring 1982.

Lindeman, C.: Priorities in clinical nursing research, Nurs. Outlook 23(11):693–698, November 1975.

Linstone, H.A., and Turoff, M.: The Delphi method, techniques, and applications, Reading, MA, 1975, Addison-Wesley, Publishing Co., Inc. p. 10.

McClintock, C.C., Brannon, D., and Maynard-Moody, S.: Applying the logic of sample surveys to qualitative case studies: the case cluster method. In Van Maanen, J., editor: qualitative methodology, Beverly Hills, 1983, Sage Publications, Inc.

McIver, J.P., and Carmines, E.G.: Unidimensional scaling, series no. 07-024, Beverly Hills, 1981, Sage Publications, Inc.

Melia, K.M.: Tell it as it is—qualitative methodology and nursing research: understanding the student nurse's world, Journal of Advanced Nursing 7:327, July 1982.

Miles, M.B., and Huberman, A.M.: Drawing valid meaning from qualitative data: toward a shared craft, Ed. Researcher 13(5):29–30, May 1984.

Mintz, J.: Integrating research evidence: a commentary on meta-analysis, Journal of Consulting and Clinical Psychology 51:71–75, 1983.

Mintzberg, H.: An emerging strategy of "direct" research. In Van Maanen, J.: editor: Qualitative methodology, Beverly Hills, 1983, Sage Publications, Inc.

Mullen, P.D., and others: Qualitative methods for evaluation research in health education programs, Health Education 13:11–18, May–June 1982.

Murphy, J.R.: Preparing research data for computerization, Am. J. Nurs. 79(5):954–956, May 1979.

Newman, M.A., and others: Experiencing the research process via computer simulation, Image 10:5–9, February 1978.

Oiler, C.: The phenomenological approach to nursing research, Nursing Research 31:178, May–June 1982.

Omery, A.: Phenomenology: a method for nursing research, Advances in Nursing Science 5(2):49–63, January 1983.

Pearson, B.D.: Simulation techniques for nursing education, Int. Nurs. Rev. 22(5):144–146, September–October 1975.

Phaneuf, M.C.: The nursing audit: profile for excellence, New York, 1972, Appleton-Century-Crofts.

Quantitative and qualitative methods: a choice or a combination? Epidemiological Bulletin 4(6):12–13, 1983, Pan American Health Organization.

Redfield, D.L., and Rousseau, E.W.: A meta-analysis of experimental research on teacher questioning behavior, Rev. of Educational Res. 51(2):237–245, Summer 1981.

Rees, R.L.: Understanding computers, J. Nurs. Admin. 8(2):4–7, February 1978.

Robertson, M.H.B., and Boyle, J.S.: Ethnography: contributions to nursing research, Journal of Advanced Nursing 9(1):43, January 1984.

Rosenshine, B.: Evaluation of classroom instruction, Review of Educational Research 40(2):279–300, April 1970.

Rosenthal, R.: Meta-analytic procedures for social research, Applied social research methods series, Vol. 6, Beverly Hills, 1984, Sage Publications, Inc.

Sanday, P.R.: The ethnographic paradigm(s). In Van Maanen, J., editor: Qualitative methodology, Beverly Hills, 1983, Sage Publications, Inc. pp. 19–36.

Slavin, R.E.: Meta-analysis in education: How has it been used? Educational Researcher 13(8):6–15, October 1984.

Slavin, R.E.: A rejoinder to Carlberg, et al, Educational researcher 13(8):24–27, October 1984.

Smith, M.L., and Glass, G.V.: Meta-analysis of psycho-therapy outcome studies, American Psychologist 32:752–760, September 1977.

Swanson, J.M., and others: Why qualitative research in nursing? Nursing Outlook 30:241, April 1982.

Thomas, B.: Using nominal group techniques to identify researchable problems...research preparation in nursing, Journal of Nursing Education 22(8):335, October 1983.

Touching, Nurs. Care 8(2):33, February 1975.

Van Maanen, J., editor: Qualitative methodology, Beverly Hills, 1983, Sage Publications, Inc.

Van Maanen, J.: The fact of fiction in organizational ethnography. In Van Maanen, J., editor: Qualitative methodology, Beverly Hills, 1983, Sage Publications, Inc.

Van Maanen, J., Dabbs, J.M., Jr., and Faulkner, R.R.: Varieties of qualitative research, Studying organizations: innovations in methodology, 5, Beverly Hills, 1982, Sage Publications, Inc. Published in cooperation with Division 14 of the American Psychological Association.

Volicer, B.J., and Bohannon, M.W.: A hospital stress rating scale, Nurs. Res. 24(5):352–357, 1975.

Wainer, H., and Thissen, D.: Graphical data analysis, Ann. Rev. Psychol. 32:191–241, 1981.

Walberg, H.J.: Quantification reconsidered, In W. Gordon, editor: Review of research in education, 11, Washington, D.C., 1984, American Educational Research Association.

Waltz, C., and Bausell, R.B.: Nursing research: design, statistics and computer analysis, Philadelphia, 1981, F.A. Davis Company.

Wandelt, M.A., and Stewart, D.S.: Slater nursing competencies rating scale, New York, 1975, Appleton-Century-Crofts.

Webb, E., and Weick, K.E.: Unobtrusive measure in organizational theory: a reminder. In Van Maanen, J., editor: Qualitative methodology, Beverly Hills, 1983, Sage Publications, Inc.

Werley, H.H., Zuzich, A., Zajkowski, M., and Zagornik, A.D.: Health research: the systems approach, New York, 1976, Springer Publishing Company.

Williams, C.A., editor: Nursing research and poligy formation: the case of prospective payment, Papers of the 1983 Scientific Session, American Academy of Nursing, Kansas, 1984, ANA.

Willson, V.L.: Research techniques in AERJ articles: 1969 to 1978, Educ. Res. 9(6):5–10, June 1980.

Wilson, S.: The use of ethnographic techniques in educational research, Review of Educational Research 47(2):245–265, Spring 1977.

CHAPTER 21

THE PILOT STUDY AND PRETESTING THE INSTRUMENT

Pretesting the research instrument and conducting the pilot study are important to the success of an investigation. Pretesting the research instrument and the entire pilot study precede the gathering of data for the actual research project. For our purpose, pretesting is the process of measuring the effectiveness of the instrument (vehicle or tool used to gather data), and the pilot study is the preliminary small-scale trial run of the research study.

By way of review, we have discussed the research approach with an emphasis on nursing and on the basic aspects of investigative theory and methodology. Knowledge of the scientific method and an understanding of the terms commonly used in the research process provide a basis for insight into the relationship between theory and method.

By the time the pilot study is ready to be conducted, the investigator has completed all of the preliminary steps of the research process. The researcher has conceptualized the problem, thought through the ethical implications, completed the library search, stated the hypothesis or question, determined the sample, and developed the instrument.

The need for a library search cannot be stressed too strongly. If the library has been developed into a learned resource center, there may be additional learning aids available that are useful for selected topics. Especially valuable and stimulating are professional journals, abstracts, and dissertation abstracts. All of them are useful for introducing new methods and new topics. Library materials can help the investigator to gain additional information, review old facts, and develop different perspectives.

Before testing the hypothesis, the researcher must carefully work out the research design. He decides on the sampling technique, as well as the method for testing the hypothesis.

Along with developing a conceptual or theoretical framework for his research, the investigator must plan on testing his data-collecting methods. Pretesting the instrument and conducting the pilot study are somewhat similar to the driver getting his automobile ready for the main race. He makes a trial run around the track before the main event begins. Researchers make a trial run to "get the bugs out" of their instruments and study designs.

This chapter includes a section on the development of tables because the researcher needs to know if the sample data will "fit" into the tables. If they do, the researcher has assurance that the items provide the variety of data needed in the study. If they do not, a revision of the tables must be made before the data for the major study are collected. In case it becomes apparent that the instrument does not provide a sufficient variety of items, the instrument will need further revision and pretesting before the researcher engages in the collection of study data.

PRETESTING THE INSTRUMENT

The word *pretest* has at least two meanings; however, for our purpose the word *pretest* refers to the trial test of the instrument developed for testing the hypothesis. The pretest is a time for checking the reliability and validity of the instrument developed for the study. Other researchers may think of using the pretest for comparison with the posttest that follows the experiment. Other authors and researchers speak of the pretest as a process for finding out something about the subject at a given time for comparison with a later time. In this chapter we use the term *pretesting* as a process (verb). The pretest is a check on the instrument to evaluate such factors as its length, wording, and validity.

Instrumentation is closely linked to pretesting in that the focus is on the measuring instrument. If a mechanical device is used, changes might occur in it during the measuring process. If the change is in the observer or the scorer of the subject's product, then a threat to internal validity exists. Changes in the variable being measured might be the result of practice, boredom, attitude, or fatigue.

The Process

There are two types of activities relative to instrument development. The first is the information-gathering procedure, a kind of probing in which open-ended questions are asked, and the responses are used in the development of the research instrument. After the tool is completed, it must be tested on subjects who meet the criteria for the study sample, but who will not participate in the major project.

The purpose of a pretest is to reveal problems relating to answering, completing, and returning the instrument and tabulating the data. It also will point out weaknesses in the administration, organization, and distribution of the instrument.

The pretest may be in any form that contributes to the testing of the instrument. It is sometimes necessary to interview or by other means find out the opinions of people differing in education, temperament, and viewpoints to see if they understand the questions and are able to give complete and pertinent answers. During the pretest, the researchers must keep in mind the purpose of the study and at the same time must be aware of the aim and specific intent of each question. Is the question understood and answered by the respondents in the manner intended (that is, does the question ask what it was meant to ask)? The investigator must be alert to the respondent's every reaction, comment, and nonverbal cue and should carefully record them. Alternative wording of questions should replace those that are not clear.

Respondents may be asked what the question meant to them, what difficulties they experienced in answering, and what ideas were not brought out by the questions. Often in asking questions, the respondent does not have enough choices or is forced to choose between two categories, neither of which is acceptable to him/her.

When subjects answer questions by saying, "I don't know," or fail to respond altogether, they should be questioned further to elicit the reason why they cannot answer. What was the reason their opinion could not be or was not tapped?

Interviewers should record their own observations, criticisms, and suggestions for improving the instrument as suggested by the difficulties in locating or interviewing respondents, questions causing embarrassment or resistance, problems of maintaining rapport, and respondents who were bored or impatient. Likewise, they should note which questions needed further information or clarification, if sufficient space was allowed for recording answers, and if the instrument was too long.

The researcher cannot assume that the subjects have as much knowledge or interest in a topic as the researcher. Nor can he/she assume that respondents always know what is meant by the wording of a question. A sweet little lady who did not know very much about cars observed that her next door neighbor, a dealer for American Motors, frequently came home driving a different car. One evening it might be a sedan, and the next day a sports car or station wagon. On this particular day, while admiring his new car, she asked, "What kind of a car is a Rambler? Is it a Chevy or a Ford?" We could have asked her in a questionnaire or interview if she preferred a Rambler or a Ford, but her response would have been meaningless, because she knew so little about car makes and models.

An example of how testing is undertaken is a short questionnaire, which was developed by a researcher and given to a professional colleague to criticize. His suggestions were incorporated into the instrument. The questionnaire was then given to six people who were asked if there were any questions they did not understand, and why they answered the items the way they did. It was discovered that some questions gave rise to misunderstandings, so the questionnaire was rewritten and given to the professional researcher to review again. His corrections were considered, and the questionnaire was once again submitted to another group of six people. Shortcomings, weaknesses, and strengths of the instrument were discussed; more changes were made and approved by the expert. At this point tests of the instrument's reliability and validity were conducted. Finally the instrument was administered as the tool for the research project.

If it is possible to locate someone who is experienced in the formulation of questionnaires or who can criticize the instrument, the result will be an improvement of its quality and a reduction in its errors.

When the research hypothesis is based on theory, interview questions or data-collecting instruments must be formulated to comply with the theory. It is also quite possible that the theorist or other researchers in the field will have developed a questionnaire that can be useful. In addition, there are books that provide scales and types of instruments that have been tested in the field. If we can locate instruments that have been found effective, then we should by all means make use of them.

Both the pretest and the pilot studies should be set up according to the study design. It should be clear that no amount of thinking, and careful, logical, or brilliant planning can compare with a careful pilot study out in the field.

The concept of pretesting is based on the idea that experience is the best teacher. This does not mean, however, that either the pretesting of an instrument or the use of a pilot study will eliminate all flaws, because there will be some mistakes that will not be noticed in a small study but will be evident later in the larger study, which involves more subjects.

For example, a student attempted to formulate a questionnaire concerning athletics. The respondents were to check off their attendance at sporting events. Later, the instructor happened to be sitting beside a student who was filling out one of the questionnaires. The student suddenly threw down the paper in disgust and said, "This is a stupid questionnaire." When asked why, he responded, "Well, look at this question. They shouldn't have asked us to give a scaled answer here. They should have simply asked for a 'yes' or 'no' answer. 'Yes, we do' or 'No, we don't' would have been sufficient. I don't know how to answer when we have to scale all these percentages." The designer of the questionnaire had pretested the instrument, but no one had pointed out that particular flaw; and yet, on close examination of the item, the disgruntled student was clearly right. It was a very poor question and should have been noticed earlier. Some misunderstandings had been detected in the pretest but not this particular one.

Concerning the pretest, Goode and Hatt have said:

> The pretest accepts the fact...that no amount of intuition, native talent, or systematic thought will substitute for the careful recording, tabulating, and analysis of the research facts. These facts must be obtained before the final investment of much time, money, and energy in a full-scale project. It is quite likely that the undergraduate student, carrying out his first project, will be unable to divert so much energy to each phase of the study as is desirable. On the other hand, he must keep in mind that the project will, as a consequence, be deficient in many regards. Furthermore, if undergraduates form research teams for such projects, it is likely that each of these steps can be covered with a small sample.[1]

So far, we have discussed the pretesting process in terms of its relationship to a questionnaire. Pretesting should be conducted on all instruments regardless of the method used for collecting data. If a check-off sheet is used in conjunction with observation, it should be pretested on a series of subjects similar to those who will participate in the major study.

When records are selected as a source of data, some kind of check-off list or compilation sheet may serve as the instrument. This instrument ought to be developed and then evaluated after actual use. The alert researcher would no more collect data using an untested instrument than a basketball team would enter a contest without practice. Suppose patients' charts are used to obtain data for a particular project. After a compilation form is developed, data from a number of charts are recorded into the prepared spaces and summarized. In this way, actual experience is used to discover strengths and weaknesses of the instrument that was developed specifically to elicit information from patients' charts.

If data are obtained through experimentation, some form of recording device or test is necessary. The instrument should be pretested in a miniature study to evaluate its validity and reliability (Fig. 21-1).

Instruments used in case study research should be pretested. Experts may be asked for recommendations to improve the tool. Standardized instruments that have been published need not be pretested, but the administration of the standardized form should be tried out to detect any problems. Such forms have already been pretested, and reports of their reliability are available from the publisher.

---

[1]Goode, William J., and Hatt, Paul K.: Methods in social research, New York, Copyright 1952, McGraw-Hill, Inc., p. 147. Used with permission of McGraw-Hill, Inc.

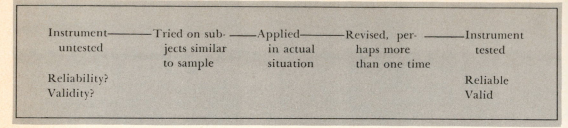

FIGURE 21-1   Process of pretesting an instrument.

THE PILOT STUDY

A pilot study is a small preliminary investigation of the same general character as the major study. It is designed to acquaint the researcher with the problems to be corrected in preparation for the larger research project. It also provides the researcher with an opportunity to try out the procedures for collecting data. During the pilot study, the instrument is going through a pretest, although the instrument content is expected to be in final form by this stage.

The pilot study, then, is a miniature trial run of the methodology planned for the major project. It is a time for detecting errors and flaws in the instrument for gathering data. When the actual study is carried out, the researcher can profit by the mistakes made in the pilot study. Thus the purpose of the pilot study is twofold: (1) to make improvements in the research project and (2) to detect problems that must be solved before the major study is attempted. Sometimes a rather limited but significant initial study later serves as a pilot study for an even more complete investigation with a larger sample.

It is important that all steps in a pilot study be carried through, because it is only by completing the full procedure that weaknesses can be identified. A thorough methodologist will tabulate the data to detect problem areas that are hidden. Perhaps the subjects do not give the responses expected. Poorly worded items, ambiguous answers, and a rather high proportion of respondents who refuse to be interviewed or who refuse to return questionnaires and marginal comments all point to corrections that should be made before the research tool is used in the major study.

One of the benefits of going into the field to carry out the interviewing procedure is that it gives respondents the opportunity to explain their answers. Responses that appear most frequently should be retained for future reference. Only those items that have the most popular responses are included as items in the final draft of the instrument.

When examining the results of the pilot study, researchers may discover that major changes must be made. They may notice that some objects do not meet the criteria for the sample, the subjects do not understand the items, a given question is not eliciting the desired information or is irrelevant, important items have been omitted, or there is a gap between some of the questions. Reformulation of items may be necessary, or additional questions may be required.

Checklist for Use in Pretesting an Instrument
1. Administration (researcher and assistants)
   a. Make sure assistants understand the purpose of the study
   b. Brief assistants thoroughly before going out to pretest the instrument
   c. Note difficulties in locating respondents
   d. Note difficulties encountered when interviewing respondents
   e. Note any problems in establishing rapport with respondents
2. The interviewer (researcher and assistants)
   a. Note whether the questions were understood
   b. Note if the respondents had difficulty answering any question
   c. Record verbatim the respondents' comments
   d. Note nonverbal reactions
   e. Write own criticisms and comments regarding the tool
      (1) Was the instrument too long? (Perception of time differs from culture to culture.)
      (2) Was there a problem with the sequence of items? Do the questions flow smoothly from one to the next?
      (3) Was there enough space for recording answers?
      (4) Were the respondents offered enough choices in a question?
3. The instrument items (researcher and assistants)
   a. Note questions where respondents needed further information
   b. Note points where respondents showed impatience
   c. Note words that needed to be simplified
   d. Note vague phrases that needed to be clarified
   e. Note any questions that seemed to embarrass respondents

---

Pilot Study Size

How large should the pilot study be? It should include enough subjects to reveal any misunderstandings that might arise from the wording of items. In addition, it must provide a fairly accurate measure of the amount of time required by each subject to complete the instrument or experiment.

If we were to carry out a project using 100 people as the sample, a pilot study participation of 10 subjects should be a reasonable number. A sample of this size would give some indication of the major problems that will arise in the research study.

However, time and cost may limit the pilot study size. Size is partially determined by the amount of time available to the researcher to conduct the total research project. Only a fraction of the total time can reasonably be devoted to the pilot study, and the investigator must arbitrarily determine that fraction. To help minimize the cost of the pilot study, the instrument need not be in a finished form (for example, mimeographed copies rather than offset printed forms may be used). If the number of subjects or objects is sufficient to test the usefulness of the instrument, then the size of the pilot study is adequate.

Confidentiality

It is very important that information discussed during the pilot study or pretest be kept confidential. Subjects in the major study should not be contacted ahead of time, since neither the procedure nor the items should be discussed with them. The purpose and hypothesis of the study should be kept confidential until the appropriate time for announcement.

Confidentiality is especially important in experimental research. Experiments are difficult to duplicate in another setting where individuals are likely to discuss the procedure with other potential subjects. This is true of almost any research. Therefore, the investigator must stress that the subject maintain silence until a specified time.

Pilot Study Results

Pilot studies are always under the influence of the serendipity principle. The possibility that serendipity can occur makes the pilot study valuable. Not only does this preliminary study reveal weaknesses and flaws, but it can also open up unexpected and exciting new possibilities (Fig. 21-2).

Why does the pilot study fail to point up all the flaws that are built into the research design? Two major reasons are: (1) the pilot study is an artificial situation, and (2) the sample size is not large enough. If opinions are obtained from only a few people, investigators will not encounter the variety of behavior and personalities or characteristics that are pertinent to the study. Because there are a multitude of subjects, kinds of people, and types of personalities the pilot study may not include a great enough variety to detect problems in the methods used. Larger numbers of subjects may be required to point up certain errors, inadequacies, or flaws.

Suppose that 10 mothers are interviewed in a pilot study, and only 1 of the 10 does not understand the question. Later, however, in a larger study of 1,000 subjects, if 10% or more have difficulty with the wording the problem becomes serious. The sample in the

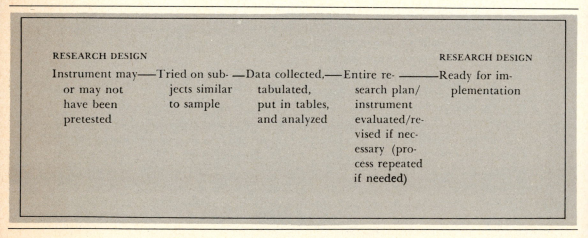

RESEARCH DESIGN   RESEARCH DESIGN

Instrument may——Tried on sub- —Data collected,——Entire re- ———————Ready for im-
   or may not   jects similar   tabulated,   search plan/   plementation
   have been   to sample   put in tables,   instrument
   pretested   and analyzed   evaluated/re-
                                                           vised if nec-
                                                           essary (pro-
                                                           cess repeated
                                                           if needed)

FIGURE 21-2   Process of conducting a pilot study.

first case was not large enough to show the problem. Even though all the difficulties are not revealed in the pilot study, this does not mean that the trial run should be omitted. This aspect of the research process should definitely be undertaken for the very reason that it does fail. The fear of failure sends the conscientious researcher to the library beforehand to review research material, since it contains a description of problems and solutions reported by other investigators. Beginning researchers, likewise, are obliged to write up the results of their studies, pointing out their difficulties so that other researchers, reading the findings, can benefit from the first researchers' experiences, failures, and successes.

Every detail of the major study should be undertaken in the pilot study—from administering the instrument, tabulating data, and placing them in tables, to analyzing the data and noting any trends in the findings. If the data do not fulfill methodological requirements, a deficiency exists. In conceptualizing the research plan, the researcher must decide if the methodology meets the requirements for testing the hypothesis.

The purpose of developing tables prior to collecting data for the pilot study is to give the researcher an idea of what the data will look like when collected. It is also an aid to conceptualizing the results of the major study. Unless the researcher knows what is being trapped, he/she does not know what kind of trap to build. In this case the *trap* is the tables. By looking at the table content, it should be possible for the researcher to tell whether the hypothesis is accepted or rejected. During the planning stages, the researcher should ask, "If the hypothesis is accepted, what will the tables look like?"

As part of the research strategy, the investigator should have made a decision as to the type of statistics to be used. The format of the tables is dictated by the statistical measures that are selected. If percentages are used, predesigned tables are still necessary. A research design without considering tables is incomplete.

TABLES

Tables are an important aspect of the interpretation of data. Unless tables are set up correctly, are identified fully, and contain appropriate information, they are meaningless to the reader and hinder the interpretation of the collected information. A table heading must be so well defined that the table can stand alone without additional explanation in the text.

A well-qualified researcher once said, "I like to read the tables first and see what conclusions I arrive at. Later, I like to read what the author of the article had to say and see what his conclusions are. If I cannot understand his tables until I have read the text, then the tables are poorly constructed and poorly labeled."

Cross-tabulation, presenting data in tables, is a valuable technique in which one variable is broken down categorically for comparison with another variable (Table 21-1). For example, we might analyze age categories as they relate to an illness or common disease. As a hypothetical example, if patients with gout are studied, we might make a comparison between them regarding age, income, education, occupation, and marital status. We might notice that men who have a high income tend to have a higher of gout attacks than men with low incomes. This would be an important discovery, and one that would not have been found by simply glancing at a table of incidents. Only after the process of cross-tabulation, in which the number of gout attacks was compared with income, did we notice the relationship.

Tables are a help; however, they are not an end in themselves. A table can show relationships that are easily seen but difficult to explain in words. An effective table, along with a simple, concise explanation, gives the reader two opportunities to grasp the meaning of the research data.

Tables should be simple in format and should not present more than three variables at a time. In Table 21-1, the two variables being categorized are sex and school. If a table showing number and percentage is provided in the appendix, then the table, as presented in the body of the research report, may show only the percentages (Table 21-2).

Tables should be organized so as to focus attention on the data as it clarifies the meaning and significance of the information presented. If the table is difficult to understand, the reader's attention will be turned to the details of the presentation rather than to the data. Readers sometimes find the tables so difficult to comprehend that they do not bother to read the report. Pertinent studies are sometimes omitted from the review of literature section of a report because the investigator was unable to comprehend the tables.

Each researcher has a particular style of writing, and the table and graphic presentations may reflect the researcher's particular style as well. The format of the table should facilitate the reader's understanding. As the table style begins to develop, giving uniformity to the details, the reader learns to expect the researcher to present data in a consistent manner. The reader is thus able to concentrate his/her attention on the content rather than on trying to decipher distracting elements in the table. The type of material being presented frequently dictates the nature of the visual aid.

A typewritten report imposes certain restrictions on the writer, whereas the commercial printing process is more versatile. Any kind of drawing, statistical formula, or vertical line is possible through printing. In the report the researcher should have all tables typewritten, with vertical lines and statistical formulas neatly lettered in a black ink that matches the typewriter ribbon as closely as possible.

Types of tables.   There are two types of tables: general purpose and special purpose. The reference table that presents a broad scope or arrangement of data is an example of the general purpose table. A special purpose table demonstrates an analytical point or an

TABLE 21-1   Number and Percentage of Freshmen Enrolled in Five Schools, Classified by Sex and School

| | Sex | | | |
| | Male | | Female | |
School	Number	Percent	Number	Percent
A	72	20.3	71	18.0
B	54	15.2	52	13.1
C	56	15.7	67	17.0
D	116	32.7	119	30.1
E	57	16.1	86	21.8
TOTAL	355	100.0	395	100.0

TABLE 21-2 Percentage of Freshmen
Enrolled in Five Schools,
Classified by Sex and School

School	Sex	
	Male (%)	Female (%)
A	20.3	18.0
B	15.2	13.2
C	15.7	17.0
D	32.7	30.1
E	16.1	21.7
TOTAL	100.0	100.0

answer to a specific question. Tables can help the researcher arrange data in columns and rows. This type of visual aid serves the purposes of (1) reference, (2) relationship, (3) comparison, and (4) continuity.

A *reference table* can be simple or complex. Usually, reference tables are found in the appendix of a report or a book. They provide detailed information for the reader's use. Conversion tables and degrees of freedom tables are examples of reference tables. Table 21-3 illustrates a reference table commonly found in texts.

Note that Table 21-3 is a general purpose table, whereas the other tables in this chapter illustrate or demonstrate particular ideas. They are single-use tables, since the data would change if the study were repeated in another setting or at a later date.

A *table of relationships* may be used to show the interpretation of data, as well as relationships between two variables, events, quantities, and so on. An example of such a

TABLE 21-3 Square Roots of Numbers 1 to 60

Number	Square Root	Number	Square Root	Number	Square Root
1	1.0000	21	4.5826	41	6.4031
2	1.4142	22	4.6094	42	6.4807
3	1.7321	23	4.7958	43	6.5574
4	2.0000	24	4.8990	44	6.6332
5	2.2361	25	5.0000	45	6.7082
6	2.4495	26	5.0990	46	6.7823
7	2.6458	27	5.1962	47	6.8557
8	2.8284	28	5.2915	48	6.9282
9	3.0000	29	5.3852	49	7.0000
10	3.1623	30	5.4772	50	7.0711
11	3.3166	31	5.5678	51	7.1414
12	3.4641	32	5.6569	52	7.2111
13	3.6056	33	5.7446	53	7.2081
14	3.7417	34	5.8310	54	7.3485
15	3.8730	35	5.9161	55	7.4162
16	4.0000	36	6.0000	56	7.4833
17	4.1231	37	6.0828	57	7.5498
18	4.2426	38	6.1644	58	7.6158
19	4.3589	39	6.2450	59	7.6811
20	4.4721	40	6.3246	60	7.7460

table is Table 21-4. Senior students in this case were rated before and after a special experience (experience T) in which they assumed the responsibilities of beginning staff nurses, under the guidance of a nursing faculty member. They were rated on a five-point scale before and after this experiment. The relationship of the second rating to the first was reported as the degree of change. The amount of change was not identified, only the fact that there was change.

A *comparison table* shows one or more variables being held constant or running in series and another event or variable being compared with the first variable. In Table 21-5 there is a comparison of men and women participants by age categories. In this particular study, the patients were interviewed, and the investigator's recognition of their felt need was assessed.

A *continuity table* shows a continuous increase or decrease from one cell to the next. In Table 21-6 we see the results of a study done to test the hypothesis, "The more Bible-oriented the curriculum of a college, the greater the ratio of females to males enrolled." Note that the data show a steady progression from the most Bible-oriented institution to the least Bible-oriented institution. The proportion of women is from 6.66% at one extreme to 33.33% at the other extreme (Table 21-6).

The researcher should include formal tables in the report. A *formal table* observes all the rules of table construction and includes headnote, footnotes, stub and box head, title, and number (Figs. 21-3 and 21-4). A leader table (simple two-column table without title) and a text tabulation table (ruled tables that must be explained) are not suitable for a professional research report.

The parts of a formal table (Figs. 21-3 and 21-4) are as follows:

heading: The table heading is its title, headnote (if any), column heads, stub head, spanner head, and table number.

Table 21-4   Changes in Student Behaviors Observed after Experience T. Classified by Change in Ratings*

Behaviors	Change in Ratings			
	Lower Percent	Same Percent	Higher Percent	Not Observed Percent
N = 70				
Determining priority of needs	8.6	45.7	45.7	0.0
Planning patient care	7.1	54.3	38.6	0.0
Performance of nursing techniques	11.4	40.0	44.3	4.3
Function as team leader	7.1	45.7	42.9	4.3
Communication skills	10.0	54.3	32.9	2.9
Personal responsibility	4.3	57.1	37.1	1.4

*Students were rated on a five-point scale prior to and at the end of experience T. The relationship of the second rating to the first is reported as the degree of change. The highest rating was 1; the lowest 5. Amount of change was not identified, only the fact that there was change.

TABLE 21-5 Number of Patients Interviewed, Classified by Age Group and Sex*

Sex	Years of Age					
	20-29	30-39	40-49	50-59	60-69	70-79
N = 22						
Male (N = 11)	4	2	0	1	2	2
Female (N = 11)	1	2	2	2	2	2
TOTAL	5	4	2	3	4	4

*This does not include two patients interviewed in the trial run.

spanner head: The spanner head is the descriptive title that applies to the columns it heads. These columns all contain the same type of information.

column heads: The column heads are the descriptive titles for the verticle display of the data that they head.

stub head: The stub head is the descriptive title given to the stub listing.

stub: The stub is the lefthand column that contains the data classifications.

line caption: This descriptive title applies to the type of data appearing in a row. In this case, the terms *line* and *row* are used synonymously to describe a horizontal display of data.

subhead: The subhead is the title of the heading for two or more line captions.

block: The block is a section of the stub and is composed of related line captions and subheads.

field: The field is located to the right of the stub and below the heading. All tabulated data are found in this portion of the table.

grand total: The term *total* applies to the sum of the column entries. If the summary provides information that is not obtained by adding up the columns, then a descriptive phrase is used to identify the fact that this information applies to a specified group, such as all nurses or all patients.

cell: A cell is the space allotted for a single numerical entry of data.

footnote: The footnote is placed directly beneath the table and contains information necessary to interpret the table. This special table footnote is not part of the footnoting system used for the report or the manuscript.

source: The source of a table must be identified when the table is taken from someone else's work (Table 21-6).

TABLE 21-6 Percentages of Freshman Students Enrolled in Colleges, Classified by Sex and Degree of Bible-Oriented Curriculum*

Institution	Sex	
	Male (%)	Female (%)
College A (all Bible-related classes)	33.33	66.66
College B (Bible college with some liberal arts)	40.00	60.00
College C (church-related liberal arts college)	50.00	50.00
College D (university)	66.66	33.33

*Source: This table was included in the report of a class project (J.T.).

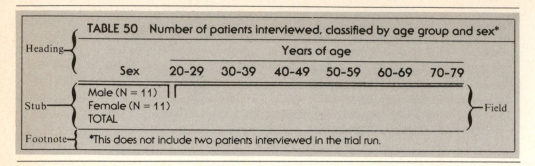

FIGURE 21-3   Major parts of a table.

The table plays an important role in the analysis and interpretation of data. The visual presentation demands skill and creativity. Like a picture, a good table is probably worth a thousand words. Tables may need several modifications and changes before they are incorporated into the report. Simple tables are easier to construct than complex ones and increase the reader's understanding.

Guidelines for Table Construction

General guidelines for table construction, which aid in the appearance and the readability of the table, include the following:

1. Within the body of the report, a table should be complete on one page. A large table, provided in the appendix, may extend over two or more pages, but each page must show the column headings so that the reader does not need to turn pages to be reoriented.

2. A table should have good proportions. It should not be too wide or too narrow.

3. A table should have lines only when necessary. Horizontal lines are easy to make with a typewriter, but vertical lines are difficult. By grouping related sections of the study and using double or triple spacing between rows or columns, we may minimize the use of lines. In other situations, such as reference tables, which have continuous lines, columns, and figures, it may be difficult for the eye to travel across the page without assistance. A row of blank spaces, dots, or dashes may be inserted at every fifth row to help the reader.

4. A table should be able to stand alone. A written description of the table within the text is not necessary. The text is devoted to a discussion of the contents of the table, not a definition of it. For example, in discussing a table, the investigator might properly say: "Notice that in Table 21-7 the same number of men and women (N = 175) was interviewed. The one category that shows any measurable difference was the over 70 age group, which had only women subjects." It would not be acceptable for the investigator to refer to the information provided in the table by saying, "Table 21-7 shows a breakdown by sex in six age categories."

When the table has a heading, it is referred to by its table number, not by its table title. If a title is lacking, the researcher must identify the table by a description of the report.

Busy researchers often prefer to analyze tables and reach their own conclusions from the data. They may check later to see if the author's conclusions agree with their conclusions.

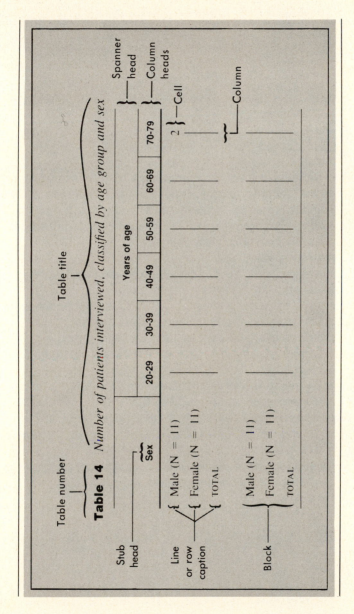

FIGURE 21-4   Parts of a table heading and a stub heading.

TABLE 21-7   Number and Percentage of Individuals Interviewed During July 1980

| | Sex | | | |
| | Women | | Men | |
Age	Number	Percent	Number	Percent
20-29	20	11.42	35	20.00
30-39	35	20.00	25	14.28
40-49	60	34.28	65	37.14
50-59	20	11.42	30	17.14
60-69	25	14.28	20	11.42
70 and over	15	08.57	0	00.00
TOTAL	175	99.97	175	99.98

5. If several tables with similar content are presented, each table should have the same format. Suppose there are four different clinical areas in our study and a table is required for each of them. The table format should be the same so the reader may quickly refer from one table to the next when comparing the same variables. The reader should be able to look in the same place on each table without having to search.

6. Similar tables call for similar titles.

7. All capitalization in a table should follow a consistent format. The period is omitted at the end of the title.

8. Box headings should be centered above the columns, except on the first and last columns where they may be set even with the margins (Fig. 21-5).

9. Reference to subject categories should be consistent (Fig. 21-6).

10. Captions should be as brief as possible. It is better to say "Men in nursing" than "Men employed in nursing."

11. All columns of figures should be aligned with the decimal point, with calculations being carried out to the same number of places (Fig. 21-7).

12. Symbols should precede only the first figure in a column (Fig. 21-8).

13. Figures of four or more digits should be separated with commas. (For example, write 4,125 instead of 4125).

14. If there is no figure for an item in column, this blank space, which can be confusing to the reader, is expressed by a row of periods, a dash or zeros (Table 21-8).

RIGHT	WRONG	RIGHT
Personnel	Number of nurses	Number of nurses
Supervisors	20	20
Head nurses	14	14
Staff nurses	35	35
Nurse assistants	10	10

FIGURE 21-5   Column placement.

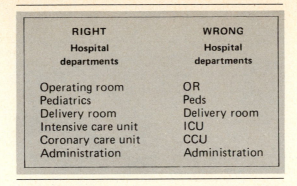

FIGURE 21-6   Consistency in subject categories.

15. Tables should be numbered consecutively throughout the entire report or within each chapter.

16. Tables in the appendix should have an identifiably different numbering system. For example, add a letter of the alphabet (B1, B2, and so on. See Fig. 21-9).

17. Tables in the appendix should have an identifiably different numbering system. For example, add a letter of the alphabet (B1, B2, and so on. See Fig. 21-9).

18. In the appendix, percentages are shown two digits beyond the decimal. When the same table appears in the text, the researcher may wish to round off the last digits to show only one digit beyond the decimal.

Steps in Developing Tables for the Pilot Study

The steps followed for developing tables for the pilot study are illustrated as follows.

1. Prepare a large (long) piece of paper to contain calculations of each item in the instrument or for each unit of data that were collected. This master sheet will serve as a ready reference for the researcher and will avoid computational errors.

2. If it will be necessary to calculate the same percentage several times in the instrument, it is better to take the time to calculate the full range of percentages to avoid computational errors. The list then serves as another reference for all similar calculations and saves time later.

RIGHT	WRONG
Percent	Percent
0.66	0.6
0.75	.750
1.06	1.06
16.75	16.75

FIGURE 21-7   Consistency in decimal placement and calculations.

3. Tally the responses to each item. Example:

	1982	1985	No reply
married	⊦⊦⊦⊦ ⊦⊦⊦⊦	⊦⊦⊦ //	//

4. Convert tally marks to numbers.

	1982	1985	No reply
married	10	7	2

5. Compute each item two digits beyond the decimal.

$$84.23$$
$$11.83$$
$$1.41$$
$$2.54$$
$$0.00$$
$$\overline{}$$
$$100.01$$

6. In most cases, round off percentages for items that appear in the text of the report or article.

$$84.2$$
$$11.8$$
$$1.4$$
$$2.5$$
$$0.0$$
$$\overline{}$$
$$99.9$$

7. Place numbers within the table that has been prepared for the item. Be sure there is a table number, informative title, column and row headings, notification of the number

RIGHT	RIGHT	WRONG
Percent		
16.23	16.23%	16.23%
7.20	7.20	7.20%
2.04	2.04	2.04%
6.75	6.75	6.75%

FIGURE 21-8   Placement of symbols.

TABLE 21-8   Percentages of
Nursing Students Participating in Nursing Home Projects

Academic Year	Students (N = 350) Percent
Seniors	49.5
Juniors	30.5
Sophomores	20.0
Freshmen	00.0
TOTAL	100.0

of respondants by N = or column total, and explanation of anything that should be brought to the reader's attention (See Fig. 21-9).

8. Tables presented in the text should be those that report the major findings of the study. After each table is analyzed separately, the researcher should cross-tabulate the variables that seem to show new information. Any new table that is constructed as a result of cross-tabulations should be presented in the text rather than in the appendix.

Even though the pilot study data fit into the tables that are prepared for them, at this stage, the pilot study is incomplete. The researcher must interpret the findings even though the sample size was limited. Does there seem to be a trend in the responses to any item, procedure, or tool? Do any threats to reliability and validity seem apparent? The analysis of findings at this stage brings an early touch of excitement. The researcher begins to suspect what might be learned from the study and anticipation heightens as collection begins for the major study.

TABLE D1* CLIENTS' CURRENT MARITAL STATUS—
      CLASSIFIED BY YEAR OF INTERVIEW

| Marital Status | Year of Interview | | | |
| | 1982 | | 1985 | |
	No.	Per cent	No.	Per cent
Married	213	85.20	299	84.23
Single	21	8.40	42	11.83
Widowed	9	3.60	5	1.41
Divorced or separated	6	2.40	9	2.54
No reply	1	.40	0	0.00
Total	250	100.00	355	100.00

*Note the use of the alphabet to eliminate confusion
in the table numbering format.

FIGURE 21-9   Table in Appendix

DATA COLLECTION

Quantifying data is an important part of data collection. The need to quantify information can be illustrated by a conversation held with a young man some time ago. The student came into the office unhappy with a grade he had received for a research paper. In his study he had asked his subjects to draw pictures under two different conditions. In one situation the students were subjected to a cold room and loud noises and were asked to draw pictures. The same students were then taken to another room where the surroundings were quiet and the temperature was comfortable. Once again they were asked to draw pictures. He experimented with the same three students in each setting and found that the drawings made in the quiet setting were of more peaceful scenes and were drawn better than those produced in the noisy setting. The student reported that he was satisfied beyond the shadow of a doubt that if people drew pictures in certain types of situations, their drawings were more skillful. There was no set standard for judging the drawings, only his opinion. Although various possible methods were suggested to him for measuring the quality of the drawings, his response was, "That is impossible to measure."

This young man had not collected any quantitative data. He had not defined levels of skills in drawing, had not used judges to supplement his personal opinion, and had accepted personal preference for fact. He had substituted private interpretation for the steps of the scientific method. Likewise, in nursing research, it is necessary to base conclusions on an adequate sample and quantities of data rather than on the private interpretation of one individual.

Historically, it was not common practice to base conclusions and judgments on information collected systematically. During the 19th century, however, the social sciences made a major contribution to society by demonstrating the need for quantified data. We should add that it was Galileo who said, "Count what is countable, measure what is measurable. What is not measurable, make measurable." Before the mid-19th century, people made statements without systematically investigating their validity. Apparently no one actually took the time to question individuals and record their opinions to arrive at a quantitative analysis.

We cannot determine an *average* opinion by interviewing only one person. Instead, we must question a large number of people to discover how the majority respond. This compilation of responses is known as data collection.

As mentioned previously, there are five basic approaches to collecting data: question-naires, interviews, records, observations, and experimentation. Each of these approaches contains numerous and ever expanding types of instruments that can be as innovative as the capabilities of the researcher allow.

Measurable Data

It is a difficult task to take one form of human behavior and transform it into a numerical quantity or quality. We can compare the numbers 2 and 4, but we cannot make a comparison between the hazy areas of "often" and "seldom." Nor can we make a comparison between "good" and "bad," or "old" and "young." Some type of numerical form must be used if we are to discover similarities or differences. Therefore, the collected data must be put into numerical form for comparison.

Numerical data can be classified into continuous and discrete categories. *Continuous data* are those that can be found at any point along a continuum or linear scale. The items may be so closely related that they cannot be separated into specific categories. *Discrete measures*, expressed in whole numbers, are distinct units. They fall into definite categories and the values cannot be interchanged.

Data collected in a nursing research study may be classified as continuous or discrete. Continuous data cannot easily be measured accurately. For example, can we measure the characteristics of students to see if they will make good nurses? Can we measure a good nurse? Since the concept of good is so indefinite, it would be difficult to measure. However, we can measure how many patient contacts a nurse makes. This is a discrete variable, because patient contacts can be translated into distinct units. How good a nurse is, on the other hand, is a continuous variable and difficult to define. Good is subjective interpretation of human behavior.

Let us consider another example of continuous and discrete measurement. A concept such as *wellness* is impossible to measure accurately. Imagine asking a subject, "How well are you today?" Wellness is a continuous variable because there is no point along the continuum that can be called well or not well. Some variables such as blood pressure, temperature, and pulse can be measured and defined as normal or abnormal. However, an individual could have a normal temperature and still not feel well. Because there is no definition of absolute wellness, the concept can be classified as a continuous variable.

On the other hand, the number of syringes on a tray is a discrete entity. Since there are only whole numbers with which to deal, we learn the exact number of syringes on the tray by counting them. Everyone would agree with the number.

In dealing with human behavior and relationships, researchers find it extremely difficult to work with continuous data, so they must make an effort to collect information and place it in a discrete form. Therefore, the researcher attempts to define variables so that they fall into discrete categories. Examples of discrete categories are sex, marital status, and number of children.

Confidentiality

Just as confidentiality is necessary for pretesting the instrument and conducting the pilot study, it is also necessary during the data-collecting stage. Quite often, when searching for information, interviewing, or mailing questionnaires, the investigator must guarantee the respondents or people who supply data, such as records, that the information gathered will not be publicized indiscreetly and that no individual names will be reported. Any promises of anonymity must be scrupulously honored. Frequently, before outsiders are allowed to use records, they must assure the administration that they will not discuss the record content inadvisedly. For example, if we wanted to gather data from records in a health care agency, the personnel there might allow us to use the records if we held a responsible job or had a meaningful use for the information. Sometimes students are allowed access to records or are given permission to administer questionnaires and other forms to be filled out, providing they agree not to reveal the names of individuals, or in some cases, even the names of institutions. In the study *Street Corner Society* by William Foote Whyte, the name of the town was never mentioned.[2] Some individuals were aware of the town being studied, but the name was never divulged in the book itself. Anonymity is frequently required in research projects before cooperation is granted by organizations or institutions.

Confidentiality is a matter of ethics. The investigator must have the subjects' permission to use their responses for research purposes, and must inform them of the use that will be made of the data.

Sponsorship of Research

Quite often, data are more easily obtained if the study is sponsored or has the approval of certain associations. For example, if we were doing a study of nurses with the approval of the State Board of Nursing, and the board's cover letter requesting cooperation accompanied the instrument, this display of support would be helpful in obtaining participants for the study. The fact that a major organization is willing to sponsor or back such a study helps in gaining the approval and participation of respondents. Any research projects, regardless of size, should state somewhere its purpose and the sponsoring organization, as well as the researcher's name and address.

SUMMARY

We have considered pretesting and pilot studies under their own definitions. For the purpose of this book, these terms have been defined as follows: *pretesting* is the process of measuring the effectiveness of the instrument used to gather data; the *pilot study* is the preliminary small-scale trial run of the research study.

After the research tool is completed, it must be tested on subjects who meet the criteria for the study sample. This is called pretesting. The pretesting of an instrument is more valuable than any other process in developing a good research tool.

Several different methods may be used in pretesting the instrument. In the initial phase of testing, after the instrument is administered. its effectiveness is discussed, checked for weaknesses, and criticized. The pretest is expected to reveal problems in the organization, administration, completion, and return of the instruments. After the instrument has been pretested, strengths and weaknesses are noted and improvements made. If possible, the research tool should be reviewed by an experienced researcher.

The pilot study is designed to help the researcher plan the major study. All the variables encountered in the major study will conceivably have been encountered in the pilot study, and mistakes that were found should be corrected before the actual study begins.

The purpose of the pilot study is twofold: (1) to improve the research process and (2) to detect problem areas. In actuality, every research project should serve as a pilot study in anticipation of an even larger project. The pilot study should only be large enough to be representative of the sample, which in some cases might be 10% of the anticipated sample size.

---

[2]Whyte, William Foote: Street corner society, Chicago, 1955, University of Chicago Press.

Pilot study participants should not discuss the study with potential subjects because this may bias the results of the study.

The fear of failure should force conscientious researchers to return to the library, to pretest their instruments, and to conduct pilot studies in the field until they have an effective tool.

A table should be labeled and its contents identified so that it is able to stand alone. Cross-tabulation tables are a breakdown of at least one variable with one or two other variables. In any analysis of data, the findings in relationship to the hypothesis should be stated (that is, the hypothesis is either accepted or rejected.)

Proper presentation of tables is based on simplicity and descriptive headings. Two or three variables are sufficient for one table. The types of tables are reference, relationship, comparison, and continuity. The major parts of a table are the heading, stub, and field. Each part is broken down into subunits with appropriate titles. With regard to its appearance and readability, a table should be complete on one page, exhibit good proportions and good composition, be able to stand alone, have a format similar to its content, and be consistent in reference to subject categories.

DISCUSSION QUESTIONS

1 When is an instrument adequately pretested?
2 Suggest a method for selecting subjects in a hypothetical pilot study.
3 Is it or is it not appropriate to use the pilot study as a time to pretest the instrument developed for a research project? Support your response.
4 If there is a target population of 1,000 people and the sample is 100, how large should the pilot study sample be?
5 What are some disadvantages of the pilot study that might be detrimental to the research results?
6 What could be learned by comparing the pilot study results with the research results?
7 Your questionnaire has already been printed, and now you conduct the pilot study. Suppose you find that your instrument has five questions that were left blank by the pilot study sample approximately 40% of the time. What do you suggest doing?
8 Why should the pilot study be tabulated, analyzed, and placed in tables?
9 Why might a research project serve as a pilot study for an even larger study?
10 To pretest an observation check-off sheet you observe five nurses talking together in the hallway. What is wrong with this method of pretesting the instrument, if anything? Support your response.

CLASS ACTIVITIES

Track I

1 The students are to revise or reorganize an instrument distributed by the instructor.
2 The students are to shorten an instrument selected by the instructor.

Track II (Steps in Research Project)

1 Project developers are to (a) pretest the instrument and revise it as necessary, (b) prepare all tables with titles for the data collected, and (c) insert the data and note if it all "fits" into each table as expected.

2 Make any revisions in the instrument and plans for its administration before proceeding with the major study.

SUGGESTED READINGS

Diers, C.: Research in Nursing Practice, Philadelphia, 1979, J.B. Lippincott Co., Chapter 10.

Doak, C., Doak, L. and Root, J.: Teaching Patients with Low Literacy Skills, Philadelphia, 1985, J.B. Lippincott Co.

Fleming, J.W., and Hayter, J.: Reading research reports critically, Nurs. Outlook 22(3):174, March 1974.

Lee, J.J.: Methods of collecting data, Physiotherapy 68(11):361, November 1982.

Marin, J., and Howe, H.L.: Physicians' attitudes toward breast self-examination, a pilot study, Evaluation and the Health Professions 7(2):193–204, June 1984.

Notter, L.: Essentials of Nursing Research, ed. 3, New York, 1983, Springer Publishing Co., Inc.

Riley, M.W.: Sociological Research, a Case Approach, New York, 1963, Harcourt Brace Jovanovich, Inc., p. 182.

Vredevoe, D.L.: Nursing research involving physiological mechanisms: definition of the variables, Nurs. Res. 21(1):68–72, January–February 1972.

PART FIVE

ANALYZING DATA

The analysis of data is the theme of Chapters 22 through 24. Following an introduction to the topic, Chapter 22 provides information concerning raw data, interpretation of data, scaling, scales, and the use of the computer. The topics in Chapter 23 include descriptive measures used in quantitative research, frequency distribution, measures of central tendency, normal distribution, and measures of dispersion. Statistical inference, analysis of variance, chi-square, steps in hypothesis testing, and power are among the topics covered. Part Five closes with Chapter 24 emphasizing the evaluation process and generalizability of the study results. The single case and qualitative research are discussed as they relate to generalizations. Other topics covered are conclusions, implications, and recommendations for further study.

CHAPTER 22

THE ANALYZING PROCESS AND USE OF COMPUTERS

WHAT TO DO WITH RAW DATA

Raw data must be presented in an orderly fashion to show relationships. If the research data confirm the hypothesis, researchers must show this confirmation in a meaningful presentation. Ideally, they should express what was found not only in words but also in a graphic presentation of the data in the form of tables or diagrams. In fact, data are meaningful only when they relate to the hypothesis being tested.

Suppose the researcher had gathered from a large number of people data that included their ages, occupations, and incomes. The researcher then listed the individuals separately with their characteristics. Such data would be worthless for any comparison or demonstration of relationships. Only when data are combined so that averages and categories can be identified do the data become meaningful. The researcher must usually carry out some type of grouping, such as placing the data in common categories and computing the number or percentage of each kind of division.

The manner of analyzing data is frequently related to the complexity of the data or the complexity of the hypothesis or hypotheses. It is usually the consensus of opinion among researchers that if tables are designed before data are gathered, analysis is simplified.

For example, suppose we are testing an hypothesis by using the classical experimental design. First, we would want to provide for the four cells; that is, the control and experimental groups' scores on the pretest and posttest. Having prepared the four cells, we simply conduct the experiment and insert the results or scores in each of the cells. If we had prepared a table beforehand, we could easily collect information, as well as provide a guide for the appropriate kinds of data needed for the tables. Well-designed tables serve the same function as blueprints in building construction.

We must make certain considerations when preparing the instrument depending on whether we are analyzing data by machine or by hand. For example, questionnaires should have spaces in the righthand margin where response identification numbers can be written. It is difficult to say where the cutoff point should be, but if there are more than 100 questionnaires or observations to be analyzed, the data should be placed on cards for use with the computer. If the data must be studied by hand, they should be extended to the right side as in Fig. 22-1 for later transfer to a larger form or to a work sheet. It is advisable that the worksheet contain the total number of responses for each alternative of each item.

Suppose we are testing an hypothesis concerning the care of the patient. The sample is made up of nurses who have checked categories that relate to the most important aspects of patient care. After we collect the questionnaires containing the responses, we transfer each response to the worksheet prepared earlier. After all the responses have been transferred to this large sheet, we then arrange the information into an orderly form. For example, we might be able to say that 25 of the 100 respondents preferred bedside nursing. Meaning is given to data when responses are tallied.

PERCENTAGES

An excellent researcher once commented that most research could probably be presented with simple percentages, and that most research, in fact, would be better off if only percentages were used in reporting findings.

Figuring percentages is done by dividing the smaller number by the total number. If there are 142 subjects in the sample and 79 are male, $79/142 = 55.6\%$. If the researcher does not have a prepared table of percentages for reference, it is helpful to make a table for the particular study. For example, if the sample has 151 respondents, calculate all the possible percentages for the number of responses from 1 to 151 or within the possible range. This will eliminate errors during data description and the need for recalculation later.

The percentage is commonly used for comparing the results of two different groups of unequal size or the proportions of the subjects within each category of a population or sample. The actual value of using percentages is seen when groups or subgroups of unequal size make up the sample, and when a comparison with the whole group is desired. If the researcher wishes to compare a group of 104 subjects with 87 subjects, it is possible to do so. Often in medicine the frequency of certain illnesses or diseases is reported by the number of persons per 1,000, per 10,000, or per 100,000. To make a percentage comparison would require more computations, and the resulting figure would be difficult to interpret.

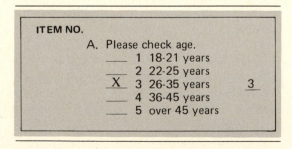

FIGURE 22-1   Coding space.

ITEM NO.

7. Do you think males should become nurses?   N = 40

   25 Yes

   5 No

   7 Undecided

   3 No response

FIGURE 22-2   Number of responses to questionnaire items.

The frequency should be reasonably large if percentages are used to describe the data. Obviously if the researcher has less than 100 cases when making a percentage comparison, every subject accounts for what seems a rather large proportion. This is especially true if there are only 6 or 8 persons in the sample. In such a case, a percentage comparison is rather misleading. The researcher must show that the independent variable under study is, in fact, the one that seems to be causing the dependent variable.

The base from which percentages are computed may cause a problem. For example, suppose that 40 questionnaires were distributed to female nurses employed at a health agency, and only 30 of the nurses gave a definite response to the question, "Do you think males should become nurses?" Should we include those 10 who were undecided, or who omitted the item in the base from which percentages are computed (Fig. 22-2)? Do we use 40 as the base, or 30, which is the number of nurses who responded yes or no to item 7? We really do not know how the 7 who were undecided or the 3 who did not answer the item would have responded if they had been pressed for a definite answer. Perhaps the question is not which base the researcher *should* use but what base *is* used.

RATIO

In addition to making a percentage comparison, the investigator also can make a ratio comparison. Ratios may be reported in a study, for example, where the number of male nurses versus female nurses is reported. The researcher may find that for every 100 female nurses in the state there are on the average 3 male nurses. The resulting ratio is 3/100, or 3 per 100. In a population where there is a comparison of men and women the concept of sex ratio is used. Sex ratio here means the number of men per 100 women. If we report a sex ratio of 95, it means that there are 95 men for every 100 women. A ratio may be reported as a pair of numbers (20/2 + 10), or it may be completed (20/2 + 10/1). A single-number ratio (for instance, 10) is a ratio to one. The researcher might ask, "What is the ratio of nurses to physicians in Latin America, in Africa, and in the Caribbean?" In some areas of the world physicians outnumber nurses. A statement of ratio would thus constitute an important factor in patient teaching by the nurse, for instance.

PROPORTION

Another useful procedure is the proportion, which is one kind of ratio. By definition, a proportion is the ratio of the frequency in a given category to the total frequency. That is, the frequency in which something (score, response, or question) occurs is divided by the total number. In our example of number of men compared with women, the proportion would be 3/100 + .030. Because the reporting of such a situation in words is unwieldy, the proportion is multiplied by the constant 100 and reported as a percentage (3% men). Thus the rule is to multiply the proportion by 100 to obtain the percentage. The procedure could be used to determine the proportion of patients who came to General Hospital last year from the suburbs as opposed to those from the inner city.

INTERPRETATION OF DATA

Quantifying data is accomplished by classifying them according to classes, units, or characteristics. Some common categories for classifying individuals are age, sex, and education. The major concern is how to present the data so that the results can be interpreted. The army sergeant confronted with a platoon of new recruits has to make some order out of all the men. He may place them in groups of 12 arranged by height. The same thing applies to researchers; they must place their findings in an orderly arrangement.

After all the data are collected, they must be quantified for calculation and placed in previously designed tables. The data must be put into forms that are understandable. Measures of central tendency (mean, median, and mode) and standard scores are mathematical terms commonly used to describe the data. These are discussed in Chapter 23.

SCALING

Since each variable in the research study must be defined in operational terms, the researcher must describe the characteristics being studied, as well as the categories that make up the variables. The descriptions that result from defining the variables in operational terms are called *scales*. The process used in developing scales is called *scaling*.

Nominal Scales

The simplest type of scale is the nominal scale. The categories into which a variable is divided are identified, and each observation is classified by its appropriate category. Two requirements for the use of the nominal scale are that (1) the categories must be mutually exclusive; that is, it is possible for the observation to be placed in only one of the categories; and (2) they must be collectively exhaustive, meaning that there are sufficient categories to accommodate all the observations. In our illustration of male and female nurses, the variable, sex, would be a nominal scale, since all people can be placed into one of the categories and no one can be classified as both. Other examples of nominal scales are the number of children in a family and marital status (married, single, divorced, or widowed). Notice that each example illustrates a condition that is so exclusive that an individual can be included in only one category (Fig. 22-3).

Ordinal Scales

Ordinal scales go a step beyond nominal scales; that is, in addition to being composed of mutually exclusive classes, each class fits into a specific order. Ordinal scales break down the either-or choice in nominal scales. In other words, the researcher has the opportunity to categorize an observation a little above or a little below the other observations. *Good, better, best* is an illustration of the ordinal scale; there is order in the sequence, with some leeway within each category. There is no indication of how good is good, although it is recognized as a category. As another example, the degree of hardness of various woods could be arranged in order from the hardest to the softest. The contestants in a race could be arranged by order of finishing. The fastest runner finishes first; the second fastest runner finishes after the first but ahead of all the others. There is an order to the position of contestants, in relationship to their speed. However, ordinal scaling does not indicate how much faster, larger, or better one category or item is over another. A patient's condition is an ordinal class that could be used by nurses to categorize health status. Comparisons can be made even when an accurate judgment is not possible. (Fig. 22-4).

Interval Scales

Interval scales extend one step beyond ordinal scales in that measurement between each class is involved. Classes are not only ordered, but ordered with equal measurement between each class. Two pieces of equipment that nurses frequently encounter make use of the interval scale: the thermometer and sphygmomanometer. The scale is ordered with equal distance between the units of measurement. The units are determined arbitrarily.

Ratio Scales

Ratios, cited earlier, are considered a part of the continuing series of scales. They have all the properties of the former scales and, in addition have the property of an absolute zero point, which makes multiplication and division possible. Money is an example of a ratio scale. Two dollars is exactly twice as much as one dollar. Other ratio scales include units that measure liquids, land, and grains. For instance, two liters are twice as much as one liter. Mathematical operations are possible because each number is in a relationship to any other number and any specific value on a ratio scale can be reported as a multiple of any other. Nominal, ordinal, and interval scales do not have absolute mathematical

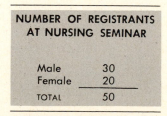

NUMBER OF REGISTRANTS AT NURSING SEMINAR	
Male	30
Female	20
TOTAL	50

FIGURE 22-3   Nominal scale.

CONDITION OF PATIENTS IN
A UNIT

Good	12
Fair	3
Stable	1
Poor	1
Critical	0
TOTAL	17

FIGURE 22-4   Ordinal scale.

values. We cannot say that the interval scale of 10° F below zero is twice as cold as 5° F below.

CROSS-TABULATION

Cross-tabulation, a technique of comparing two or more variables at the same time, is useful in testing relationships, and in finding the correlation between two variables from data that have been collected.

Cross-tabulation is sometimes referred to as multivariate analysis, which means that we are analyzing three or more variables simultaneously. This is in contrast to univariate analysis in which there is analysis of a single variable such as age, and bivariate analysis in which there is analysis of two variables.

An example of univariate analysis can be seen in the columns of Table 22-1. Ten of the respondents are under 10 years of age, eight are from 10 to 13 years of age, and so on. Cross-tabulation is evident when comparing age with types of nursing preference.

Bivariate analysis can compare the variables of age with one type of nursing, such as research. One person was 18 to 22 years of age and another person was over 23 years of age when each first thought of nursing. Table 22-1, as a whole, provides data for a multivariate analysis. Not only is age a categorized variable, but the various types of nursing provide nine other variables for study.

Suppose we designed a simple study in which we wanted to learn the sex differences of persons who go to a clinic in the local community. We distribute a questionnaire to the 116 people in a three-block radius. Table 22-2 shows the results of our hypothetical example.

The data indicate that 70 people (60%) go to City Clinic for health care. This information is not very meaningful until it is cross tabulated on the basis of sex. A percentage breakdown shows that a much larger proportion of women than men go to the clinic (81% versus 37%). If we classify the data as in Table 22-3, the results are much different. Note that there are 54 men and 62 women in the sample before proceeding to analyze the table.

In table 22-2 we observe the percentage of men and women who go to City Clinic, whereas in Table 22-3 we have computed the percentage of those who go to City Clinic,

TABLE 22-1   Cross Tabulation of Age When Senior Nursing Students First Thought of Nursing, with Types of Nursing Preference (Hypothetical)

Type of Nursing	Under 10	10 to 13	At 14 or 15	At 16 or 17	18 to 22	23 or over
Research					/	/
Teaching and administration					//	//
Maternity nursing			/	//	/	
Mental health		/	//	/	//	/
Children	///	//	/	//		/
Medical-surgical nursing	///	/	/	//	//	
Community nursing	/	/	/	/		
Operation room	//	/	/			
Medical-surgical specialties	/	//				

classified by sex. the numbers of men and women in the first table are summed at the bottom of the columns, whereas they are placed at the beginning of the row (N) in the second table.

Table 22-2 classifies the data on the basis of sex, whereas Table 22-3 classifies the data on the basis of going to the clinic. We can correctly analyze our data through Table 22-2 because we are interested in sex differences, not in attendance differences. When the emphasis is on sex differences, using Table 22-3, an additional calculation must be done using the N at the beginning of each row.

We may wish to proceed and learn why more women than men go to the clinic.

Men and women might be compared simultaneously in other categories of the research study. Obviously, as the number of variables increase in the data, or as the number of questions increase in a questionnaire or interview, the number of combinations becomes larger and larger. In our illustration, we could break down the variables and look at the educational background of the parents of men and women who go to community clinics. Suppose we find a significant difference between the number of women who go to clinics and the number of men who go to clinics, with the difference depending on the amount of education of one of the parents. The number of possibilities for cross-tabulation is limited only by the amount of data on hand, which is one of the reasons why the more items there are in an instrument, the more chances there are of finding factors that contribute to causal relationships.

Normally, if there is excessive tabulation to be done, it is appropriate to program the data into a computer. Card sorters also may be used to separate data (variables such as sex and occupation) and to sort them into piles. Then each pile can be run through again, setting the sorter to separate cards by another variable such as education. By having several variables punched separately on a computer card, almost endless tests of variable relationships can be cross-checked.

TABLE 22-2 Number and Percentages of Men and Women Living in Midtown Neighborhood Who Go to City Clinic for Health Care, Classified by Sex

| | Sex | | | |
| | Men | | Women | |
Attendance at Clinic	Number	Percent	Number	Percent
Attend	20	37.0	50	81.0
Do not attend	34	63.0	12	19.0
TOTAL	54	100.0	62	100.0

Cross-tabulation can be done by hand through the use of cards that are punched for appropriate data along the outside border. By running a wire wand through the pile of cards, those cards on subjects who exhibit the characteristic under study can be extricated from the stack. However, we do not suggest this system if there is a large number of cards.

We can show a cross-tabulation by writing tally marks in a two-way table (Table 22-1). Each tally mark is inserted in the cell that agrees with both the column head and the line caption.

Another technique for hand sorting cards in the use of drawn lines and symbols on 3 × 5 cards or regular, punched IBM-like cards. Using crayons or colored pencils on the cards, identification code marks can be made so that it becomes quite easy to sort the cards into piles. If, for example, we wanted to put a small green **x** on a specific corner of every women's card in one group, it would be easy to flip through the cards and count the number of women (green **x**'s). Then we would automatically know that the remainder of the cards represent men.

To identify a certain variable, instead of using lines and symbols the investigator can clip off the corner of one card belonging to data of predetermined identification. Even an unskilled assistant can soon learn to count hundreds of cards within a few minutes.

USE OF THE COMPUTER

We mentioned earlier that the computer can save the researcher a great deal of work. Not only can it tabulate and analyze data, it can compute the statistics. The computer also can be used for researching libraries. There are many operations that the computer can carry

TABLE 22-3 Number and Percentages of Persons Living in Midtown Neighborhood Who Go to City Clinic for Health Care, Classified by Sex

| | Attend | | Do Not Attend | |
Sex	Number	Percent	Number	Percent
Men (N = 54)	20	29.0	34	74.0
Women (N = 62)	50	71.0	12	26.0
TOTAL	70	100.0	46	100.0

out, thus making it a useful tool for the researcher. It is not only thorough and complete in its operations, but the computer can calculate with infinitely greater rapidity and accuracy than human mathematicians.

However, a computer cannot think for itself; everything must be planned. If the computer is correctly programmed, it will follow all requests. Often the researcher will find it more difficult to develop a large, complex program than to do some calculations with smaller, less complex machines.

Before the research data are entered into a computer file by teletype, key-disc, magnetic tape, key-tape, or card, the data must be prepared for entry.

Computers are classified as either digital or analog. Digital computers count data digit by digit; they perform by adding, subtracting, and multiplying. Analog computers are used for simulation. They represent continuous data such as distance and angles. The machine and its tangible components are called the hardware; the information, which includes the data and the computer program, is called the software.

The process of tabulating by hand is definitely less efficient and more time consuming than using a computer. However, when a computer is available, there is the danger that the investigator will try to find relationships just for the sake of finding relationships. Then he/she may report only those findings that were statistically significant rather than those that demonstrated insignificance, thus resulting in misconceptions and erroneous conclusions.

Computers allow for long-term storage of data on magnetic tapes that travel at a high speed over a magnetic head for rapid retrieval. Memory units provide storage for a large number of words and allow split-second access to information. Magnetic tapes provide convenient, low-cost storage of great quantities of data, whereas memory units allow easy access and swift retrieval of data. Names and addresses can be conveniently and quickly retrieved from a memory unit, but the magnetic tape would have to be run over the head until the data were found, which would take longer.

Computers are a binary system (based on 2) rather than a decimal system based on 10. This means that the binary digit has a possible value of 0 or 1. *On* represents 1 and *off* represents 0.

An IBM or data-processing card is the most common means used to enter data into a computer (Fig. 22-5). These cards are punched with a key punch, which looks like a typewriter. A person places the card in the machine and punches in the material to be programmed. Data are transferred from the code space on a questionnaire, for example, to an appropriate column on the cards that is reserved for each variable being studied. Notice that up to 80 pieces of information with at least 9 responses for each variable are possible. We might think in terms of having columns 1 and 2 for some type of special identification, column 3 for the institution's code number, column 4 for the respondent's sex, column 5 for his age group, and so on. Beginning with column 6 or 7, the coded responses to variable 1 may be punched. As suggested previously, each questionnaire is coded so that all the keypunch operator must do is punch the coded number on the righthand side of each page. After one card is made for each of the questionnaires, the data are ready to be put into the computer or the card sorter.

Many kinds of information can be obtained through the use of the card sorter. A card-sorting machine is used to sort the punched cards on any given line (entry). We might designate sex as male (1) and female (2), and then place the cards in the sorter, set

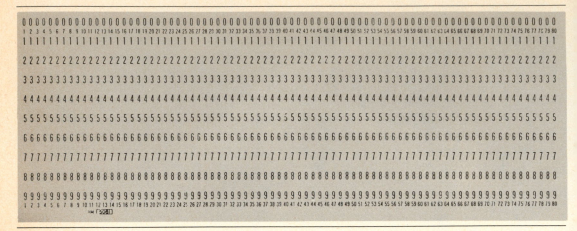

FIGURE 22-5   IBM card.

the indicator on column 4 (the column for "sex"), and press the start button. The card sorter will separate the cards of men into one stack and women into another. Some card sorters also have a counter that counts the number of male and female respondents, thus saving the researcher from counting the cards in each stack by hand.

A cross-tabulation is possible as a second step. We might take the female respondents' cards, set the card sorter on the column for age, and separate those cards accordingly. Again, if we want a run on another variable, say occupation, we could find how many respondents between 20 and 40 years of age are nurses. The operation just described is a cross-tabulation with the card-sorter—a valuable technique for studying collected data.

If we have a large number of cards (500 or more), the computer can be used for all computation. First, however, we will have to write a program for the cards if there is not a canned program available. We might find it possible to do several procedures such as chi-square, analysis of variance, or other statistical techniques with the data simply by using a canned program and a few preliminary cards. Canned programs have all the preliminary cards written for basic procedures, and the researcher needs only to add his/her specific data.

The researcher may have access to a card sorter and computer or may request that the various procedures mentioned be done by someone who does have access. In that case, the researcher will probably have to be taught how to read the printout of the data or how to carry out some of the procedures personally.

In addition to large computers, technology has provided small computers that are changing so fast that it does not seem wise to describe their use at length. Some are small desk-type machines that can calculate mathematical problems, whereas others are desk-type machines that accept a plastic card or a paper tape program plus the data for the individual research study. Some small ateletypes and terminals are hooked up to larger computers. Since most researchers are not skilled in doing complicated procedures with computers, they will need the assistance of a specialist who works with computers full time. *Be sure to use the services of an expert when necessary.*

It no doubt seems obvious that researchers are forced to translate human behavior into numbers. A machine can utilize 1, 2, 3, 4, and 5, but it can do nothing with terms such as old, sick, well, good, bad, or deviant. A computer cannot work with abstract concepts. Instead, the machine must work with concrete, discrete variables of behavior categorized by numbers.

An important tip to remember is to make a duplicate set of cards if they are to be run through the computer. If one card is lost or damaged, it becomes very difficult to find out which card is missing. sometimes a card is damaged so badly that it cannot be put through the duplicator for replacement. After several runs through a card sorter, cards become dog-eared and jam the machine. It is good and cheap insurance, therefore, to have an extra, complete deck of cards made before sorting or calculations are begun. It is also wise to number each questionnaire and to keypunch this identifying number on each card. If there is an error on a card, it is easy to refer back to the questionnaire. Many reject cards are the result of incorrect keypunching. By correcting the rejected cards, a conscientious researcher can have a virtually error-free deck.

Programming a computer is extremely complex since the machine has no reasoning ability. Every consideration for decision must be entered in the program. As a simple illustration, the program must be directed that April has only 30 days, not 31. A year has 12 months, and so. Once it has been programmed for dates, a transposed day and month (April 14) entered as 14-4 would be rejected as "error." Even misplaced commas will be indicated as error.

Programming a computer to calculate standard deviation requires many hours. the programmer must understand the basic theory of the statistics, how to calculate the statistic by hand, how to write the program to perform the mathematics correctly, and anticipate any user errors so that the program will not run if given wrong data. After the program is developed, the user must be computer literate and understand the program. Even if the user can calculate the formula by hand, he/she may not be able to enter the data in the correct form for the computer to run. It is not entirely incorrect to say that more knowledge is needed to get data into appropriate form for a computer than to calculate by hand. The great advantage of the computer is accuracy and speed.

Some terms used in computer technology include:

input: entering data into the computer with cards, tapes, and optical scanners.

output: the computer's response to a request for information. The response, called a printout, is in the form of a printed page, display on a screen, or tape.

storage: a system of retaining large quantities of information, which might include the results of a survey or scores from thousands of persons in an experiment, and so on. The storage containers include tapes, disks, or magnetic cores.

controls: the direction part of computers is known as the program. This is a series of instructions written in computer language such as FORTRAN, COBOL, ALGOL, or BASIC.

software: includes programs and other instructions to perform functions or solve problems.

hardware: mechanical parts, physical, and electronic components of the computer.

CPU (Central Processing Unit): makes and performs mathematical calculations.

time sharing: a computer is shared on a short-term basis by several programs.

delay: turnaround time between input and output.

The following is an example of computer usage in clinical research. The microcomputer can be used to evaluate biomedical profiles of patients using multivariate techniques.

Analyzing several profiles provides more valuable information than a single analysis. Comparisons are made on the basis of confidence levels. Patients diagnosed as normal are within the confidence level while the more severe cases are outside the confidence level. Evaluation profiles can be performed by SIMCA with FORTRAN or SPSS (Statistical Package for the Social Sciences). In addition, several programs are especially adapted for the computer for statistical analysis such as BMD (Biomedical Computer Program) and SPSS.

WRITING THE ANALYSIS OF DATA

Analysis of data tends to be the longest section in most research studies. The researcher reports how the data were classified scientifically by placing items that have similar attributes together in one class and how data were ordered, manipulated, and then summarized in order to answer the question under study. The analysis sets the stage for the interpretation and conclusions that are drawn.

Lengthy narrative descriptions of the data are not appropriate. Instead, the researcher should present some of the data in tables, include some of the highlights, and if need be, explain the findings. The usual procedure for presenting findings is for the researcher to explain why the results shown in the report text came out as they did. Other studies may be mentioned in which the results were the same or different. The researcher also should attempt to explain why any discrepancies occurred in the findings. Why are the results different from what was expected? Some of the tables in the body of the report may show the results of a single instrument item, whereas a few tables may be developed to combine the findings of two or more items. In addition, a graphic design may present combined findings. It is important that several complex ideas not be included in one table or visual presentation.

It is permissible for the researcher to discuss findings other than those related to the hypothesis or question but the central theme should not be neglected. The instrument specifically designed or selected to test the hypothesis should receive the focus of attention.

Readers of the research report will want to know something about the sample and the study setting. Data based on personal information about the sample should be discussed.

SUMMARY

A research study is no better than the quality of the analysis. Plans for the interpretation of data must be made prior to the collection process and should include the formats to be used in presentation of the data. The method used in analyzing the data is a prime factor in the interpretive process. Meaningful interpretation of research findings hinges on correct analysis of data.

Beginning researchers ask the question, "Now that I have my data, what do I do with it?" This chapter describes possible ways of analyzing data. Prose descriptions should always be reinforced with visual arrangements of the data in tables, graphs, or charts. It is the consensus of many researchers that tables should be developed, and then the data collected to fill the tables. This procedure is preferable to designing tables after the data are collected.

We recommend that space and time be made available for coding answers. This will facilitate transfer of the information to IBM-like cards. We recommend the use of a large worksheet to compile responses given to each item.

Percentages are especially valuable for comparing two quantities. Ratios also are useful in numerical comparisons. To be meaningful, data must be placed in some sort of order. The measures of central tendency (mean, median, and mode) and standard scores all provide valuable arrangements. Other techniques for descriptive data are scales. *Nominal scales* place data in mutually exclusive categories, such as male and female. *Ordinal scales* are an ordering of categories. *Interval scales* make use of measurement between classes. *Ratio scales* have an absolute zero point and are mathematically manipulatable.

Cross-tabulation tables are a breakdown of at least one variable with one or two other variables. In any analysis of data, the findings in relationship to the hypothesis should be stated (that is, the hypothesis is either accepted or rejected).

The computer and card sorter are especially useful machines for counting and sorting data cards. Working with computers may require the use of a professional programmer or special training to learn their operation. Canned programs may be obtained for many statistical procedures. A duplicate deck of data cards is essential.

DISCUSSION QUESTIONS

1 Why is it important to analyze the data collected by the research instrument?
2 What is meant by quantifying data?
3 How is quantifying data part of the analysis process?
4 How does coding help organize the instrument?
5 Defend the statement, "Percentages are the most meaningful statements about the research findings."
6 Why would a researcher be interested in whether the data could be placed in nominal, ordinal, interval, and ratio scales?
7 If a researcher ignored the possibility of type I and type II errors, how would it affect research results?
8 Why is the level of significance important?
9 Why is the program the most important part of computer analysis?
10 Why would the preparation of data for computerization be an important component of the research design?

CLASS ACTIVITIES

Track I

1 The instructor is to provide raw data for the class. Data are quantified, put into percentages, placed into a selected scale, and analyzed.
2 Using raw data from previous class projects, a demonstration is given to show what can be learned through computer analysis.

Track II (Steps in Research Project)

1 Each group or single researcher uses the revised instrument to collect data for the research project.
2 The data are collected, tallied, and placed in tables.
3 Data from each item or question are analyzed.

SUGGESTED READINGS

Burnstein, L.: Secondary analysis: an important research for educational research and evaluation, Educ. Res. 7(5):9–12, May 1978.

Computer technology and nursing education, Southern Council on Collegiate Education for Nursing, Atlanta, GA, 1984.

Daniel, W.W., and Longest, B.B., Jr.: Statistical sampling and the nurse-researcher, Nurs. Forum 16(1):36–55, 1977.

Davitz, J.R., and Davitz, L.L.: Evaluating research proposals in the behavioral sciences: a guide, ed. 2, New York, 1977, Teachers College Press.

Fleming, Juanita W., and Hayter, Jean: Reading research reports critically, Nurs. Outlook 22(3):175, March 1974.

Gardner, Paul Leslie: Scales and statistics, Review of Educational Research 45(1):43, 45, Winter 1975.

Gorden, R.L.: Unidimensional scaling concepts and procedures, New York, 1977, Macmillan, Inc.

Henkel, R.E.: Tests of significance. In Uslaner, Eric M., editor: Series: quantitative applications in the social sciences, Beverly Hills, Calif., 1976, Sage Publications, Inc.

Hildebrand, D.K., and others: Analysis of ordinal data. In Uslaner, Eric M., editor: Social sciences, Beverly Hills, 1977, Sage Publications, Inc.

How to use a statistical consultant, Am. J. Nurs. 79(5):956, May 1979.

Kibrick, A.K.: Data analysis and interpretation of results. In Wechsler, H., and Kibrick, A., editors: Explorations in nursing research, New York, 1979, Human Sciences Press, Inc. pp. 309–315.

Marciniak, S.P., and Guttman, L.: Data analysis and statistics, AORN J. 33(2):289–297, February 1981.

Murphy, J.R.: Preparing research data for computerization. Am. J. Nurs. 79(5):954–956, May 1979.

Rees, R.L.: Understanding computers, J. Nurs. Adm. 8(2):4–7, February 1978.

Reynolds, H.T.: Analysis of nominal data. In Uslaner, Eric M., editor: Series: quantitative applications in the social sciences, Beverly Hills, Calif., 1977, Sage Publications, Inc.

Skiba, D.J., and Slichter, M.: of bits and bytes, Am. J. Nurs. 84(1):102–83, January 1984.

Suen, H.K.: A Bayesian aggregate meta-analytic evaluation approach, Evaluation and the Health Professions 7(4):461–470, December 1984.

Zeisel, Hans: Say it with figures, ed. 5, New York 1968, Harper & Row Publishers.

CHAPTER 23

DESCRIPTIVE AND STATISTICAL DATA ANALYSIS

Descriptive measures and data analysis are used to present the results of each of the research approaches. The ultimate aim of the researcher is to make generalizations about what has been observed in a single study. It is through description that both the researcher and reader gain insight into the total impact of the data. It is required, therefore, that the descriptive presentation be both systematic and objective if generalizations are to be accurate and consistent.

In this chapter we explain how data are prepared for reporting simple collective characteristics by means of the arrangement of measurement values into selected descriptive indexes. Since the distribution of measurements is the basis for descriptions and descriptive measures, the frequency and shapes of distributions are considered first. The three measures of central tendency show how scores tend to cluster on an ordered scale, and the measures of dispersion show the degree of spread or dispersion around the central position.

FREQUENCY DISTRIBUTION

When data consist of a long series of measurements in which it is impossible for a subject to belong to more than one class, these classes are mutually exclusive. It is inconvenient to handle each subject individually, so we generally look at the lowest and highest measurements to determine the range of our observations. On a scale of 0 to 100, if the lowest score is 75 and the highest is 92, the range is 17 points (75 to 92).

Next, we divide the range into steps or intervals and tabulate the number of units falling into each interval. These steps and the frequency of units or subjects belonging to each step constitute what is known as a frequency distribution. To make a frequency distribution, we list the appropriate categories and then tabulate the frequency of each occurrence. If we listed the ages of students in a clinical class, they might appear as in the list on the following page.

The simplest form of presenting research data is the frequency distribution table. A frequency distribution table has two columns. The lefthand column shows different qualities or attributes of a variable, and the righthand column lists the frequency with which the attribute or quality occurs. Note in Table 23-1 that the frequency column

Age	Tally marks	Frequency
24	/	1
23	/	1
22	//	2
21	///	3
20	//// ///	8
19	/	1

reports the number of registered nurses employed on February 1 each of the years under study (1970 to 1975).

There are several important rules to consider when using a frequency distribution table. First, the units entered in the lefthand column describe the qualities or values, and when grouped must be mutually exclusive as well as exhaustive. Overlapping values lead to a great deal of confusion. In other words, a response must be so clearly defined that it cannot be placed into two categories, and there must be sufficient numbers of categories available to record all responses.

Second, to be the most useful, the tabulation must have internal logic, be consistent, and be ordered. For example, if we are tabulating the incomes of the members of our sample, we should record them systematically, either from highest to lowest or from lowest to highest. They should not be listed randomly. Note that in Table 23-1 the years are listed in chronological order.

The third requirement for the lefthand column of a tabulation is that it be in a quantitative variable carefully and reasonably chosen. Intervals should be of uniform size when we are dealing with scores or whole units. However, as in Table 23-2, the ages of senior students are grouped according to the periods of time young people are most likely to make vocational and career choices.

Intervals should not be so small that they cannot be summarized or so large that they conceal the most important characteristics of the distribution. If we were selecting certain age categories, we would not want to use every age separately (such as 1 to 100 years); but we might make logical intervals such as up to 5 years, 5 to 10 years, 10 to 15...90 to 95 years, and 95 and over. The more we know about the subject, the better prepared we are to know how to divide the variable into subunits. If every year is included in a column, the table becomes too long; if the subunit is too inclusive, an important variable may be lost. For example, if we were to use only three categories of age (1 through 15 years, 16 through 30 years, and above 30 years), we could overlook some characteristics of the

TABLE 23-1   Number of Registered Nurses Employed at Midwest Memorial Hospital, 1970 to 1975 (Hypothetical)

Year	Number Employed*
1970	147
1971	155
1972	157
1973	200
1974	205
1975	208

*Number employed as of February 1, each year.

TABLE 23-2 Ages of Seniors at First Thought of Nursing and Decision to Enroll in a Baccalaureate Nursing Program (Hypothetical)

	Vocational Choice	
Age	First Thought of Becoming Nurse (N = 100) Percent	Decide to Enroll in Baccalaureate Nursing Program (N = 100) Percent
Before 10	20.2	2.0
Between 10 and 13	16.1	8.1
At 14 or 15	18.3	25.0
At 16 or 17	40.2	59.4
Between 18 and 22	4.2	3.1
Since 23	1.0	2.4
TOTAL	100.0	100.0

variable we are trying to study. A class interval, likewise, should preferably be of a length that makes for ease of calculation, such as 5 or 10 rather than odd numerical divisions that require excessive effort to compute.

After interval size has been determined, it is important that the size be clearly designated in the frequency table. For example, in a discussion concerning income, categories should be clearly specified with no overlap allowed. It should be noted that if an interval includes from $5,000 to $10,000, the next higher category begins at $10,000.01 or perhaps $10,001. The categories should continue in this manner to the top of the scale. If for some reason the intervals are of unequal size, they still should not overlap.

MEASURES OF CENTRAL TENDENCY

Measures of central tendency are commonly called averages. They are characteristic representations of a group and allow comparison between groups. The common trait of a group provides a general description of that group that is superior to defining each object individually. A term for this common characteristic is *central tendency*. It tells us something about the trait being measured.

The following example illustrates the use of a measure of central tendency. Suppose we want to compare a group of athletes with nonathletes in their ability to run the 100-yard dash. We can record each runner's time on the 100-yard dash and then compare the average time for the athletes versus the nonathletes.

Three measures of central tendency are the mean, the median, and the mode. Each measure requires a different procedure for calculation, and each measure has a different interpretation. These three measures, as well as the distribution curve, standard score, and standard deviation, are discussed later in the chapter.

Mode

The mode (usually abbreviated Mo.) is often identified as the most frequently appearing value. It also can be defined as the most common characteristic of a group of observations. Notice in Fig. 23-1 that the most frequent score is 95. Although we usually think of an average as falling in the middle of a group of scores or observations, the mode may fall at any point.

Consider another situation in which seven students' test scores run from 78 to 93. Note that two students in Fig. 23-2 receive the same score. In this case the score of 88 would be the mode, since no other score appears twice. When measuring the height of several hundred men, the mode would probably cluster around an average of 5 feet 8 inches to 5 feet 10 inches. The height found most often would be the mode.

The mode may be determined quickly. It is not affected by extreme scores; however, it is affected by changes in the grouping of data. Other disadvantages are that it is a poor measure of central tendency, especially in small samples, and it cannot be used for algebraic manipulation. The mode from one sample cannot be averaged with the mode from another sample to find the mode of the combined frequency distributions. Of course it is possible that there will be no mode within a given distribution if all scores have an equal number of observations.

Bimodal distribution.   When a distribution has one modal class it is unimodal, but when there are two modal classes, it is bimodal. Bimodal means that there are two modes or two values where there are clusters of observations. For example, if there are two points along a baseline where large clusters of scores appear, this is called a bimodal distribution. The bimodal effect may be seen in the number of tally marks in Fig. 23-3 and in the graph in Fig. 23-4.

Tate points out that if the data demonstrate a bimodal effect, then the researcher may question if the data are homogeneous. The researcher should look closely at his research design to determine if he is combining two different qualities within one measure. It is important that the researcher point out the presence of two modes, but these should not be combined to report a single average.[1]

Median

Another measure of central tendency is the median (Md. or Mdn.). The median is the score that has half the number of values above it and half below it on a scale; that is, half the scores or values are larger and half are smaller. It is the middle or halfway point in a median distribution.

[1] Tate, Merle W.: Statistics in education and psychology, a first course, New York, 1965, Macmillan, Inc., p. 47.

SCORE	FREQUENCY
95	/̶N̶/ /̶N̶/ (mode)
90	/̶N̶/
85	/̶N̶/ //
80	/̶N̶/
75	//
70	/

FIGURE 23-1   Mode: frequency distribution table.

STUDENT	SCORE
Carol	93
Jane	92
Sally	91
Nancy	88——
Naomi	88——
Karen	86
Diane	78

FIGURE 23-2   Mode: two scores identical.

If data are ungrouped, then the researcher simply counts up from the bottom score or value to the middle one to report the median. If a series of scores was 78, 81, 85, 92, and 96, the median score would be 85. Needless to say, all values must be in numerical order before they are counted. If there are an even number of scores, the median is usually defined as a point halfway between the two middle scores. For example, if we had scores 93, 92, 91, 88, then the median would be at a point between 92 and 91.

It is necessary to use a formula when computing the median for grouped data. Fig. 23-5 illustrates the use of the formula. An advantage to using the median is that it is less affected by extreme scores. A disadvantage is that it cannot be combined with other medians to give a combined median from other distributions. Like the mode, it is a nonalgebraic measure.

Franzblau says:

> While the median, because of its ease of calculation, is a useful approximate measure of central tendency, it is not satisfactory when more exact information is desired. The reason for this is that it does not give proper weight to variations which may occur within the group of measures. In counting to the middle of the group, it disregards completely the measurements of all who are passed by.[2]

Because the median is a measure that divides a group into equal halves, it may be possible to determine it without calculation. By lining up a group of children according to

[2] Franzblau, Abraham N.: A primer of statistics for non-statisticians, New York, copyright 1958, Harcourt Brace Jovanovich, Inc., p. 25.

SCORE	FREQUENCY
95	/X/ /X/ (mode)
90	/X/
85	/
80	//
75	/X/ /X/ (mode)

FIGURE 23-3   Bimodal distribution: frequency distribution table.

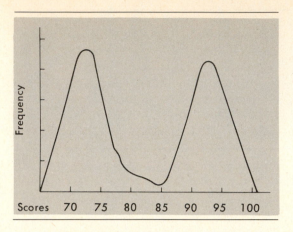

FIGURE 23-4   Bimodal distribution: graph.

height, we can see that the middle child is the crucial subject. If there were 15 children in the group, the height of the eighth child would be the median height.

The median and the mode may have different values within a given distribution. We note in Fig. 23-6 that the mode is 95, whereas the median score is 90. Different values also occur in Fig. 23-9.

Mean

The third measure of central tendency is the arithmetic mean, usually referred to by the shortened form, mean. The mean is best described as the average. It is computed by adding all the scores and dividing the sum by the total number of scores. We notice that the test scores of the 7 students total 616 in example 1 (Fig. 23-7). By dividing 616 by 7 (the number of students), the mean score is 88.

The mean has two advantages: it is the most reliable and accurate of the three measures of central tendency, and it is suitable for mathematical calculations. However, the mean has a disadvantage in that it is influenced by highly unusual scores. Suppose the salaries listed in Fig. 23-8 were paid to employees in one department during one month. Note the mean, median, and mode.

Notice that it is possible to bias a report by saying average without explaining if it is the mode, median, or mean. In this case if the researcher wanted it to appear that high salaries were being paid, he could say that the average wage was $560.00 per month, or if he wanted it to appear that salaries were low, he could say that the average wage was $500.00 per month.

Notice what happens to the mean when Diane's score is changed in Fig. 23-7 from 78 to 64. The scores of the other students remain the same. This one low score brings the mean down so that the average is no longer in the middle of the median distribution.

In comparing example 1 with example 2, there is only one score that is the same as the mean (86), and one score (64) below the mean. Five remaining scores are above the mean; therefore, in example 2, because of one extreme score, the average is influenced and does not present a true picture of the distribution. The term *average* has the connotation of

**AGE OF SAMPLE ENROLLED
IN WORKSHOP 3**

Age (years)	f	cf
30-32	5	27
27-29	4	22
24-26	9	18
21-23	3	9
18-20	6	6
N =	27	

FORMULA

$$Mdn = L + \left(\frac{N/2 - F}{f}\right)i$$

L = Lower limit of class
in which median is believed
to lie

f = Frequency of the class

F = Total frequency of all
frequencies below that
class

i = Size of the class interval

N = Total cases in the distribution

cf = Cumulative frequency

N = 27
N/2 = 13.5
L = 23.5
F = 9
f = 9
i = 3

$$Mdn = 23.5 + \left(\frac{13.5 - 9}{9}\right)3$$

$$Mdn = 23.5 + \left(\frac{4.5}{9}\right)3$$

$$Mdn = 23.5 + 1.5$$

$$Mdn = 25$$

Median age of participants
enrolled in workshop 3 is 25
years (using grouped data).

FIGURE 23-5   Figuring median with grouped data.

being in the middle, whereas if the mean is considered as average, it appears at a point on the bottom of the scale.

The formula for calculating the mean for ungrouped data is

$$M = \frac{\Sigma X}{N}$$

in which ΣX is the sum of the scores and N is the number of items. Computing the mean is a simple task if the list of items is short; however, a calculating machine may be necessary for a longer list. If data are grouped, then another formula is used.

SCORE	FREQUENCY
100	/
95	//// (mode)
90	/ (median)
85	//
80	//
75	/

FIGURE 23-6   Measures of central tendency (median and mode).

By looking at the data in Fig. 23-9, the researcher can quickly see that the mean is 25. Some accuracy is sacrificed when data are grouped; the mean is actually 24.9.

The arithmetic mean is the most commonly used measure of central tendency; it is more difficult to compute than either the mode or median. But the fact that it is an algebraic quantity is a major reason for its popularity.

An example in which the mean is not seen as a useful average is the case of national income. Suppose we average the income of everyone in America. Because some people make very large salaries, whereas others earn very little, the mean wage is different from the median because the large salaries are so much more extreme. Individuals with high incomes may make many times the salary the majority of people make in a given year. The mode or the median would probably be a better indicator of the average income of most people.

THE NORMAL DISTRIBUTION

The normal distribution is a theoretical distribution, often assumed for measurements, that enables one to make useful probability statements. The idea that naturally occurring

STUDENT	SCORE Example 1	Example 2
Carol	93	93
Jane	92	92
Sally	91	91
Nancy	88	88
Naomi	88	88
Karen	86	86
Diane	78	64
Total	616	602
	Mean 88	Mean 86

FIGURE 23-7   Mean when one score is changed.

EMPLOYEES	SALARIES		
A	$1,000.00		
B	500.00	Mode	$500.00
C	500.00	Median	$500.00
D	450.00	Mean	$560.00
E	350.00		
Total	$2,800.00		

FIGURE 23-8   "Average" wages paid per month.

observations are approximately normally distributed is a useful concept. For a large number of observations we could make a frequency distribution or plot a histogram that would have properties that make it appear as though there is a normal distribution. One example is height. Suppose we were to measure the height of all the men in the United States. If we plotted these measurements on a graph, we would probably see a somewhat bell-shaped distribution. The distribution would rise in the center, reflecting a pile up of frequencies. The distribution of heights begins at a low number because very few people

AGE OF SAMPLE ENROLLED IN WORKSHOP 3

Age (years)	f	Midvalue of interval X^1	fX^1
30-32	5	31	155
27-29	4	28	112
24-26	9	25	225
21-23	3	22	66
18-20	6	19	114
	N = 27		ΣfX^1 = 672

FORMULA

$$M = \frac{\Sigma fX^1}{N}$$

$$M = \frac{672}{27}$$

$$M = 24.9 \text{ years}$$

Σ = Sum of

f = Frequency in a class

X^1 = Class midpoints

Mean age of participants enrolled in workshop 3 is 24.9 years (using grouped data).

FIGURE 23-9   Figuring mean with grouped data.

(in our illustration) would be less than 3 feet tall. It rises until many people would be included in the middle around 5 feet 9 inches tall. It slackens off at the other extreme because there are very few people 7 feet 9 1/4 inches tall.

Notice the normal curve in Fig. 23-10. We can see that 68.2% of the area is included in the area from -1σ to $+1\sigma$. Next, notice that 95.4% of the area is in the interval -2σ to $+2\sigma$, which means that 95.4% of the cases in a normal distribution lie between -2σ to $+2\sigma$ standard deviations from the mean (center line). This is true in most situations in which the normal distribution is used to approximate the distribution of observations; only a few cases will be found in the extremes.

The essential normality of a set of observations can be exemplified by plotting a graph known as a histogram. Basically, the histogram is a vertical bar graph of the frequency distribution of a group of people, things, or objects (Figs. 23-11 and 23-12). The frequency of occurrence is represented on the ordinate or vertical axis, and the value of each variable is represented on the abscissa or horizontal axis. A histogram is prepared by marking off increasing values on the abscissa from left to right. Beginning with the zero point, the ordinate scale is marked off with equal intervals to include the highest possible frequency.

If we run a line through each of the midpoints on the bars of the histogram, which represents frequency of scores or variable being measured, we have the likeness of a normal distribution. The normal distribution is symmetrical and has as many spaces on the extreme left of the mean as on the extreme right.

Skewness

The form of a frequency distribution may be called a negative skew or positive skew when the frequencies are piled up on either end. The terms *skewed to the right* and *skewed to the left* are sometimes used but are ambiguous and should be avoided. Note the five curves of Fig. 23-13. Curve A has a bell shape, or normal distribution. Curve B is peaked; it reaches a high point and then tapers off very suddenly. Curve C is flat, or has a plateau. Curve D is negatively skewed. Curve E is positively skewed.

Curve D illustrates the situation that occurs when the majority of scores tend to appear on the positive side. We might think that it should be called a positive skew, but the skew is defined by the direction toward which the distribution is pointing. The mean of a negatively skewed distribution is located left of the median; likewise, the mean of a positively skewed distribution is located to the right of the median since it is pulled toward the pointed end of the curve. In this case Curve D falls off toward the left side, so its curve is negatively skewed. Curve E is just the opposite. The pointed (lesser area) falls off toward the positive side of the scale, illustrating a positively skewed curve.

Fig. 23-13 serves as a hypothetical illustration of a census of patient's ages in a hospital. The abscissa shows the age range of patients from newborn on the left to the elderly on the right. The ordinate shows the frequency of a patient's census.

A is an example of a patient census when the majority of patients are in their 40s with equal numbers of individuals in the earlier and later years of life. B, which is a peaked curve, demonstrates a situation in which even more patients are in their mid-40s than at the extremes. Curve C shows that approximately the same number of patients are in the categories ranging from the mid-teens to 60 years of age. Curve D might occur when there

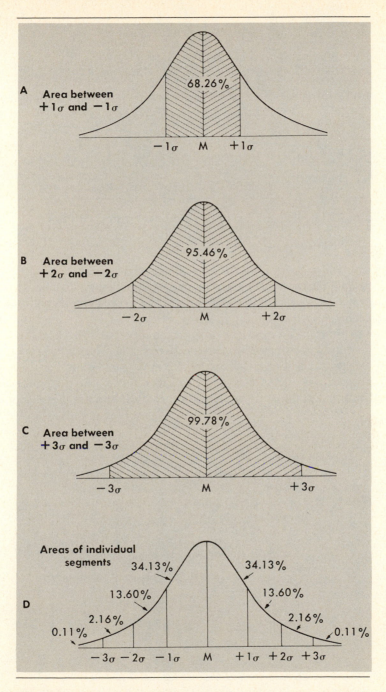

A Area between
   $+1\sigma$ and -1σ

68.26%

-1σ M $+1\sigma$

B Area between
   $+2\sigma$ and -2σ

95.46%

-2σ M $+2\sigma$

C Area between
   $+3\sigma$ and -3σ

99.78%

-3σ M $+3\sigma$

Areas of individual
segments

34.13% 34.13%

13.60% 13.60%

D

2.16% 2.16%

0.11% 0.11%

-3σ -2σ -1σ M $+1\sigma$ $+2\sigma$ $+3\sigma$

FIGURE 23-10 Areas of various segments of the normal distribution curve.

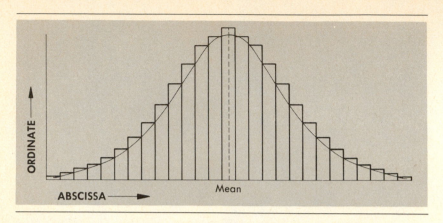

FIGURE 23-11   Histogram with a superimposed normal distribution.

is an increase in patients from 55 to 65 years of age during the late winter when the number of patients in the pediatric department happens to be especially low. The reverse situation is seen in curve E when the census of infants and young people is high because of a regional epidemic.

In a normal distribution, the mean, the median, and the mode all occur at the center of the curve or at the midway point that divides the curve in half. The curve is symmetrical, so the mean, the median, and the mode are located at the same point.

The term *construct* was discussed in Chapter 15. The normal curve is a mathematical construct that was first derived as a mathematical exercise and not based on concrete

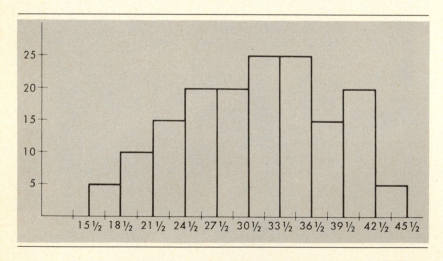

FIGURE 23-12   Histogram: distribution.

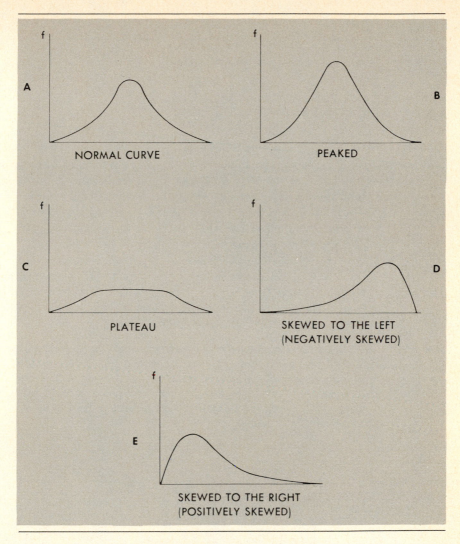

FIGURE 23-13   Frequency curves.

data. Theoretically, the curve never touches the baseline, since its range is unlimited. But it comes closer and closer to the baseline as it extends in either direction.

The question may be asked, "Of what importance is the fact that some variables seem to be normally distributed?" Perhaps the most valuable application of this fact is that we can generalize from limited observations of a limited sample to a population that has not been observed. If it seems reasonable that a variable has a normal distribution, then measures of it can be scaled to produce a normal distribution. Also, in the case of some physical measurements whose distributions are closely approximated by a normal distribution, use of the normal distribution assists in analysis.

STANDARD DEVIATION

Standard deviation (S.D.) is an index of dispersion, found by the formula:

$$S.D. = \sqrt{\frac{\Sigma x^2}{N}}$$

Standard deviation is equal to the square root of the sum of the squares of scores divided by the number, or the square root of the variance. Using this formula we can now figure the standard deviation of scores (Fig. 23-14). By computation the standard deviation is 7.48. This means that approximately 68% of the scores will fall between 7.48 points above the mean score to 7.48 points below. We will not compute a standard deviation from a large group of data; however, the formula for use with a large group of data can be readily obtained from a statistics book.

It is important that beginning researchers become familiar with measures of dispersion so these measures may be used when appropriate. Standard deviations, which are algebraic in nature, can be combined. Once computed, they can be used for a comparison of a variety of subjects or variables. The researcher might wish to compare the spread of scores of graduates from two institutions on a placement examination. Tate states:

> The methods of finding the mean and standard deviation of a total group from those of subgroups are useful chiefly in two situations: (1) when it is desired to determine the total mean and standard deviation when all that remains of the original data are the numbers, means, and standard deviations of subgroups, and (2) when it is desired to determine the effect of new groups upon old means and standard deviations without making up new distributions; for example, when it is desired to revise test norms.[3]

[3] Tate, p. 78.

SCORE X	DEVIATION FROM MEAN $(X - \overline{X}) = x$	DEVIATION FROM MEAN SQUARED x^2
24	12	144
18	6	36
14	2	4
8	−4	16
6	−6	36
2	−10	100
$\Sigma X = 72$	$\Sigma x = 0$	$\Sigma x^2 = 336$

Mean $(\overline{X}) = 12$

Then,

$$S.D. = \sqrt{\frac{336}{6}} = \sqrt{56} = 7.48$$

FIGURE 23-14   Computation of standard deviation.

Generally, the abbreviation S.D. or s stands for the standard deviation of the sample of the population, whereas the symbol σ (sigma) refers to the standard deviation of the population (Figs. 23-15 and 23-16). Tate says that "the standard deviation, as an algebraic quantity has many uses denied other measures of variability...we shall find that it deserves its place as the 'master' measure of variability."[4]

STANDARD SCORE

Standard score is closely tied to standard deviation, since standard score is expressed in units of standard deviation. Freeman says "the standard score...is the distance of any

[4] *Ibid.*, p. 79.

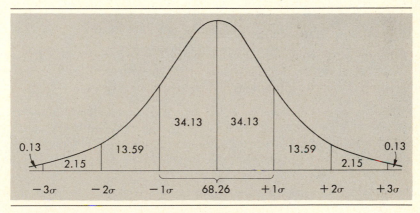

FIGURE 23-15   Normal curves.

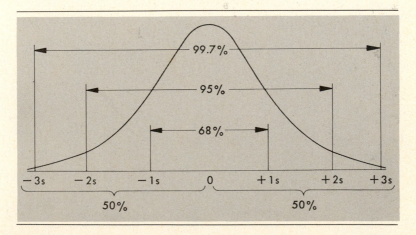

FIGURE 23-16   Percentage of cases included in segments of a normal distribution.

score from the mean of the distribution *expressed in standard deviation units;* it is the number of standard deviations from the mean of any specified score."[5]

By using standard scores, the researcher can make comparisons between one group and another. Percentile ranks are not necessarily a good means for comparison of one group with another. Someone might have one percentile rank in biology and another percentile rank in history, but this really does not tell us very much. If, on the other hand, percentile ranks are converted to standard scores, which have a constant relationship to raw scores, a comparison can be made.

When we know a standard score, we know how many standard deviations the score is above or below the mean. If we know that a score is 1 standard deviation above the mean, then it has a standard score of +1; a score of 2 standard deviations below the mean would have a standard score of −2. The unit of measure used to express standard scores is called a *z* score. Remember that a *z* score is based on the normal distribution; if the distribution is not normal, problems arise in interpreting the results. The formula for computing the *z* score is:

$$z = \frac{\text{Score obtained} - \text{Mean of distribution of scores}}{\text{Standard deviation of distribution}}$$

$$z = \frac{X - \overline{X}}{\text{S.D.}}$$

The proportion of scores above or below a certain *z* score can be figured, since approximately 34% of the area of the normal distribution lies between the mean and $+1\sigma$. Then by adding the 50% of the cases lying below the mean and the 34% that lie between the mean and $+1\sigma$, we know that 84% of the cases lie below $+1\sigma$ (Fig. 23-17). Since *z*

[5] Freeman, Linton C.: Elementary applied statistics: for students in behavioral science, New York, copyright © 1965, John Wiley & Sons, Inc., p. 63. By permission of John Wiley & Sons, Inc.

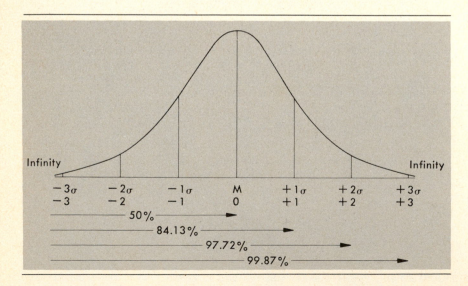

FIGURE 23-17   Percentages of area under the normal curve.

scores are usually not found as whole numbers, we must look at a special reference table located in the back of most statistical methods texts to complete the problems. If the raw score is below the mean, the standard score is negative.

Using the example of Fig. 23-14, suppose a nursing student answered 18 out of 24 questions correctly, and suppose we found by computation that the mean for the six students was 12, and the standard deviation was 7.48. The z score for this problem is

$$z = \frac{18 - 12}{7.48} = \frac{6}{7.48} = .8$$

A special table shows the proportion of the total area under the curve between the mean ordinate and the ordinate at the z distance from the mean to be .2881. Adding .50, which represents the 50% of the cases below the mean, .2881 + .50 = .7881 or .79. So 79% of the scores fall below those of this nursing student.

CORRELATION

By way of review, the measures of central tendency include three types of averages: mean, median, and mode. The measures of the spread or dispersion include deviations, standard deviations, and the spread of the distribution of scores around the mean (variance). Percentile rank, percentile scores, and standard scores indicate the position of a person or object relative to the whole group. The coefficient of correlation is a measure of the relationship between variables.

Correlation is the relationship between two variables. An investigator could say that he found a high correlation between overweight adults and coronary heart disease. This means that when an adult is overweight, he/she is more likely to develop coronary problems. Conversely, if the subject is at a normal weight, there is less tendency for heart disease to develop (low correlation between weight and heart disease).

Rank-order correlation is used as a test of association. In Table 23-3, we deal with a hypothetical case for which the formula is as follows:

$$r = 1 - \frac{6 \Sigma D^2}{N(N^2 - 1)}$$

r = Rank-order correlation
Σ = The sum of
D = Difference between ranks
N = Number of paired ranks

The formula is read: r equals one minus six times the sum of the difference squared, divided by the number of paired ranks in the sample times the number squared minus one.

We see by this formula what kind of relationship there is between the rankings given by two judges as they ranked 10 booths at a student bazaar. Is there any correlation between the rankings given by Judge Smith and by Judge Anderson? In Table 23-3, notice that the judges agreed on the order of all the booths; they placed every booth in the same order. Thus, we would say that there is a perfect correlation, or 1 (numerically

TABLE 23-3   Ranking of 10 Booths in a Student Bazaar by Judges Smith and Anderson

Booth	Smith Rank	Anderson Rank	D	D²
A	1	1	0	0
B	2	2	0	0
C	3	3	0	0
D	4	4	0	0
E	5	5	0	0
F	6	6	0	0
G	7	7	0	0
H	8	8	0	0
I	9	9	0	0
J	10	10	0	0
N = 10				$0 = \Sigma D^2$

speaking). Anything less than perfect correlation would be less than 1. When there is complete disagreement, the rank-order coefficient is −1.

$$r = 1 - \frac{6\ (0)}{10\ (100 - 1)}$$

$$r = 1 - \frac{0}{990}$$

$$r = 1$$

But suppose the judges did not rank the booths in identical order. In our second example of this hypothetical case (Table 23-4), Judge Smith ranked booth A first, but Judge Anderson ranked it second. At the same time, Smith ranked booth B second, whereas Anderson ranked it first, and so on down the line. Notice that they both agreed on the final two booths in the list as being next to the poorest and poorest in appearance.

TABLE 23-4   Ranking of 10 Booths in a Student Bazaar by Judges Smith and Anderson

Booth	Smith Rank	Anderson Rank	D	D²
A	1	2	-1	1
B	2	1	+1	1
C	3	4	-1	1
D	4	5	-1	1
E	5	6	-1	1
F	6	3	+3	9
G	7	8	-1	1
H	8	7	+1	1
I	9	9	0	0
J	10	10	0	0
N = 10				$16 = \Sigma D$

Now, what is the correlation between the rankings of the two judges? It can be seen that the relationship is less than perfect.

First, find the sum of the squared differences. The differences are found by subtracting each second rank from the corresponding one in the first column. The sum of the squared differences is 16. Now, place this sum in the formula.

$$r = 1 - \frac{6\,(16)}{10\,(100 - 1)}$$

$$r = 1 - \frac{96}{990}$$

$$r = .91$$

Notice that there is a high correlation between the opinions of the two judges regarding the rank of the booths. Such a method could be used to find the correlation between nurses' and physicians' perceptions of patients' progress.

When large numbers of pairing are involved in a study, a desk calculator is more appropriate to use. A different formula is applied in that case.

CHI-SQUARE

Nonparametric tests are used when variables are expressed in nominal or ordinal forms and when the nature of the population from which the sample is drawn is unknown. A *parameter,* by definition, is a characteristic of a population. A *statistic* serves as part of the basis for estimating the parameter. The relationship between the statistic and the parameter is described in the process of statistical inference.[6]

Chi-square (χ^2) is one of the important nonparametric tests of significance. It has many diverse applications. Chi-square is commonly used in connection with data that are in the form of frequencies or with data that can be reduced to frequencies. As a test of significance it tells us how significant the difference is between the frequencies we observed and the frequencies we expected to find.

One of the important advantages of chi-square is that it has certain additive properties that enable us to combine it with several other statistics and values in the same test.[7]

Chi-square, by definition, is the sum of the ratios or, to put it another way, it is equal to the sum of the squares of all differences, each divided by its corresponding expected frequency.[8,9] A ratio in this instance is between a squared discrepancy and an expected frequency (between those frequencies observed and those expected).

The chi-square formula may appear differently in various books because of the symbols used, but the meaning is the same: chi-square equals the sum of all the cases of

[6] Williams, F.: Reasoning with statistics, ed. 2, New York, 1979, Holt, Rinehart & Winston, pp. 38–39.
[7] Guilford, J.P.: Fundamental statistics in psychology and education, ed. 3, New York, 1956, McGraw-Hill, Inc., p. 228.
[8] Guilford, p. 228.
[9] Freeman, p. 218.

observed frequencies minus expected frequencies, squared, divided by the expected frequencies.

$$\chi^2 = \Sigma \ \frac{(f_o - f_e)^2}{f_e}$$

f_o = Observed frequency
f_e = Corresponding expected frequency

Chi-square is useful for testing hypotheses in which data are reported in the form of nominal scales. This statistic is applied in problems concerning the discrepancy between observed and expected frequencies and problems in which data are ranked.

Table 23-5, on chapel attendance, is an example of the use of chi-square. This was a study in which a sample of 157 students in a college was divided according to sex; the students were then asked how often they attended chapel. Chapel services were held daily, so it was possible for the students to attend each morning. Their responses were put into four categories: never or only once, twice a week, three times a week, and four times a week or every day.

From looking at the data, it is evident that women attended chapel more often than men did. But is it significant beyond chance that the difference would be this great? Chi-square will provide the answer.

First, let us discuss how the expected frequencies (shown in parentheses in Table 23-5) were determined. With the formula for chi-square, we find the sum of the observed frequencies minus the expected frequencies, squared, divided by the expected frequencies. There were 81 men in the group and a total of 38 people who never attended chapel or attended only once. To find the expected frequency of men attending chapel never or once, we multiply 38 × 81; then, we divide by 157 (total number of people in the sample). The result is 20 (expected frequency for men attending never or once). The remaining 18 are the expected frequencies for women attending never or once. We continue in this same manner for the remaining categories of men and women until all expected frequencies have been figured.

Notice in Table 23-6 that we have more values for our example. We complete the calculations in each column before we go on to the next column. The total is 19.63 in this case. Chi-square becomes a larger number when differences increase.

Our next step is to evaluate the significance of the value of χ^2 in our example. Since our observed frequencies differ from the expected frequencies, χ^2 differs from zero. Next, we must determine the sampling distribution of χ^2 when χ^2 is zero. Before we can turn to a

TABLE 23-5   Comparison of Chapel Attendance, Classified by Sex

Chapel Attendance	Men		Women		Total
Never or once	23	(20)	15	(18)	38
Twice per week	19	(12)	5	(12)	24
Three per week	22	(20)	16	(18)	38
Four times per week or every day	17	(29)	40	(28)	57
TOTAL	81		76		157

chi-square table, which is found in the appendix of most statistics books, we will have to determine the number of degrees of freedom for our table, since chi-square tables are set up according to degrees of freedom. The formula for degrees of freedom (d.f.) is $(c-1)(r-1)$; that is, the number of columns minus one, times the number of rows minus one. For our problem there are two columns and four rows: d.f. $= 1 \times 3 = 3$.

Consult the table of chi-square values in a statistics book, and go down the margin lines to find 3 degrees of freedom. Then read across the level to the figure you have obtained for χ^2 (in our example it is 19.63). You will find the chi-square values arranged in columns with probability headings of .05, .02, .01, and so on. If the chi-square value is closest to the probability heading .01, then we may say that the odds are about one in one hundred that chance alone could have produced the relationship found in our study. Even at the probability heading .005, χ^2 is still only 12.8 as compared with our 19.63. The relationship found in our study produced a difference so great that it could happen by chance only 5 times in 1,000. Thus, we can say that women are probably more religious than men in the situation we studied.

As we look at our data we can see that it appears unusual; out of the 38 people who attended chapel only once or never, 23 were men and 15 were women. Percentagewise they were nearly equal (20% versus 18%), although there were fewer females in the total sample. As you can see, the trend reverses at the other extreme.

Table 23-7 is an example of chi-square applied to graduates' attitudes toward their present salary. In this case there was no significant difference between the percentage of graduates who indicated satisfaction with their salary whether they planned to remain with the employer or not.

t Test

A t test is a test of differences between means, a method to determine if the differences are significant, and the probability such a difference could have occurred by chance.

TABLE 23-6   Computation of Chi-Square (Based on Table 23-5)

Cell	f_o	f_e	$f_o - f_e$	$(f_o - f_e)^2$	$\dfrac{(f_o - f_e)^2}{f_e}$
Men attending never or once	23	20	3	9	.45
Men attending twice weekly	19	12	7	49	4.08
Men attending three times per week	22	20	2	4	.20
Men attending four times or daily	17	29	−12	144	4.96
Women attending never or once	15	18	−3	9	.50
Women attending twice weekly	5	12	−7	49	4.08
Women attending three times per week	16	18	−2	4	.22
Women attending four times per week or daily	40	28	12	144	5.14
TOTAL					19.63
					$\chi^2 = 19.63$

TABLE 23-7   Attitudes of Graduates Toward Present Salary—Classified by Job
Satisfaction*

Attitude Toward Salary	Graduates Currently Employed	
	Planning to Stay† (N = 265) Percent	Planning to Resign‡ (N = 335) Percent
Very satisfied/ satisfied	61.1	54.2
Very dissatisfied/ dissatisfied	38.9	45.8
TOTAL	100.0	100.0

*X = 2.5286; d.f. = 1; $p > .05$.
†Currently working as an RN and plan to remain with employer for next two years.
‡Currently working as an RN and plan to leave employer within
next two years.

Usually, the researcher sets some probability limits, often the magical .05. If the results
are such that probability is .05 or .01, the null hypothesis of no difference is rejected.

The t test formula is:

$$t = \frac{\bar{X}_1 - \bar{X}_2}{\sqrt{\left(\dfrac{SS_1 + SS_2}{n_1 + n_2 - 2}\right)\left(\dfrac{1}{n_1} + \dfrac{1}{n_2}\right)}}$$

$\bar{X}_1$ = mean of control group
$\bar{X}_2$ = mean of experimental group
SS = sum of squares

As a hypothetical example in order to have some data, suppose a nursing intervention
plan is tried on 10 patients. Five clients are randomly assigned to a control group and 5 to
a treatment group. The experimental group receives medioswirl stimulation before
bedtime while the control group does not receive the treatment. The hours of sleep are
recorded. The data in Fig. 23-18 were collected for the study.
Degrees of freedom is found by the formula:

$$n_1 + n_2 - 2 = 5 + 5 - 2 = 8$$

Refer to a t distribution table and find 8 degrees of freedom. Since 8.57 is larger than
any of the values shown (.10, .05, .01, or .001), then 8.57 is significant beyond .001. Such a
difference could be found by chance less than 1 time in 1,000. The results are significant
and the treatment is quite likely the cause of the patients sleeping longer. It is necessary to
remember that these are only hypothetical data which were constructed in such a manner
to make calculations simple.

Analysis of Variance

ANOVA, the abbreviation for analysis of variance, is a procedure to test the significant
difference between three or more sets of data or three or more groups. ANOVA could be
used in finding the significant differences in many of the experimental designs of

Control Group		Experimental Group	
X_1	X_1^2	X_2	X_2^2
6	36	9	81
8	64	8	64
6	36	8	64
6	36	7	49
4	16	8	64
$\Sigma X_1 = 30 \quad \Sigma X_1^2 = 188$		$\Sigma X_1 = 40 \quad \Sigma X_2^2 = 322$	

$$\bar{X} = \frac{30}{5} = 6 \qquad\qquad \bar{X} = \frac{40}{5} = 8$$

$$SS_1 = \Sigma X_1^2 - \frac{(\Sigma X_1)^2}{n_1} = 188 - \frac{(30)^2}{5}$$

$$= 188 - \frac{900}{5} = 188 - 180 = 8$$

$$SS_2 = \Sigma X_2^2 - \frac{(\Sigma X_2)^2}{n_2} = 322 - \frac{(40)^2}{5}$$

$$= 322 - \frac{1600}{5} = 322 - 320 = 2$$

$$t = \frac{\bar{X}_1 - \bar{X}_2}{\sqrt{\left(\frac{SS_1 + SS_2}{n_1 + n_2 - 2}\right)\left(\frac{1}{n_1} + \frac{1}{n_1}\right)}} = \frac{8 - 2}{\sqrt{\left(\frac{8 + 2}{5 + 5 - 2}\right)\left(\frac{1}{5} + \frac{1}{5}\right)}}$$

$$= \frac{6}{\sqrt{\left(\frac{10}{8}\right)\left(\frac{2}{5}\right)}} = \frac{6}{\sqrt{(1.25)(.4)}} = \frac{6}{\sqrt{.5}} = \frac{6}{\sqrt{.70}} = 8.57$$

FIGURE 23-18   Example of a t test.

Campbell and Stanley. Remember, ANOVA is for more than two groups. The general formula is

$$SS \text{ total} = \Sigma X^2 - \frac{(\Sigma\ X)^2}{N}$$

or

Total Sum of Squares = difference between sum of
squares + within sum of squares

To state the formula another way:

SS total = SS between + SS within
SS total = total sum of squares
Σ = sum of squares
X^2 = mean of all scores squared
N = number of total groups

It is possible to say that the total sum of squares is equal to the between sum of squares + within sum of squares.

As a hypothetical example, suppose we have a control group and two experimental groups of 5 clients each for a total of 15 clients. The nurse has decided that two 15-minute teaching sessions for the patient's spouse are superior to one 30-minute session. No new material is added in the second 15-minute session, the original information is simply reinforced. Each group answers an 8-item questionnaire. The scores of each 5-client group are presented in Fig. 23-19.

Regression

The term regression refers to moving back toward a former position. In statistics, reference is often made to regression toward the mean. A personal observation is that if a teacher has one measure of student ability—for example, an exam—quite a large spread of scores will probably occur. If a single exam is the only measure of learning, it would be easy to calculate grades. But if exams, papers, verbal questions, and applications of knowledge are used, the final grades are much closer together. In other words, the students regress toward the mean. Some students are always better or worse in some form of assessment than others. If enough variety of assessment is used, the students will all have opportunity to demonstrate their abilities. Statistically, regression is concerned with relationships between variables. Further, regression is finding a measure of relationship of the independent variable on the dependent variable.

The general regression formula is:

$$Y = a + bX$$

It is necessary to discuss linear regression before explaining the formula. Scores or data begin to assume a pattern when they are placed on a scatter plot. If a line is drawn through the center of these scores, the line passes through the point that is closest to the most scores, or as the formula $Y = a + bX$ states, this line is determined at the point where the sum of squares is at a minimum. The line represents the central tendency of the data. Another way to describe regression is to say that it is a line correlation which represents the mean values of the correlation between two variables plotted on a scatter diagram (see Fig. 23-20).

Figure I is the line of best fit which illustrates the formula $Y = a + bX$. If the value of X is known, we can use the formula to calculate Y. For every X value there is a corresponding Y value. The letter a is the intercept value and b is the slope of the line (slope describes the nature of the line which varies from almost horizontal to almost vertical). The symbols a and b are known as regression coefficients. If there was a perfect correlation between X and Y (for every unit of X there was an increase of 1 unit of Y), we would have a straight line. We could then predict where any Y values would occur if we had an X value. However, if the correlations are not perfect, the line will not pass through the point where every X and Y intercept. The linear regression line will pass at a point closest to the most intercept points. The regression line also is known as the line of best fit. The formula $Y = a + bX$ will allow us to calculate the best estimate of Y if we know X along the line of best fit. The more the values of X and Y vary along the regression line, the greater the probability of error in predicting other values along the line. The SEE (standard error of estimate) will provide a statistical measure of the accuracy with which we can predict values.

	Group I Control Group		Group II 30-Minute Teaching		Group III 15-Minute Teaching X 2
Score	Score Squared	Score	Score Squared	Score	Score Squared
4	16	5	25	5	25
3	9	4	16	5	25
5	25	3	9	7	49
2	4	7	49	6	36
4	16	5	25	7	49
18	70	24	124	30	184

$$\Sigma X = 18 + 24 + 30 = 72$$
$$\Sigma X^2 = 70 + 124 + 184 = 378$$
$$N = 5 + 5 + 5 = 15$$

$$\text{SS total} = \Sigma X^2 - \frac{(\Sigma X)^2}{N} = 378 - \frac{(72)^2}{15} = 378 - \frac{5184}{15} = 378 - 345.6 = 32.4$$

Now it is necessary to find SS between

$$\text{SS between} = \frac{(\Sigma X_1)^2}{n_1} + \frac{(\Sigma X_2)^2}{n_2} + \frac{(\Sigma X_3)^2}{n_3} - \frac{(\Sigma X)^2}{N}$$

$$= \frac{18^2}{5} + \frac{24^2}{5} + \frac{30^2}{5} - 345.6$$

$$= \frac{324}{5} + \frac{576}{5} + \frac{900}{5} - 345.6 = 64.8 + 115.2 + 180 - 345.6$$

$$= 360 - 345.6 = 14.4$$

$$\text{SS total} = 32.4$$
$$\text{SS between} = \frac{14.4}{18.0}$$

Source of Variation	Sum of Squares	df*	Mean Square	F
Between	14.4 (K − 1)	2	7.2	4.8
Within	18.0 (N − K)	12	1.5	
Total	32.4 (N − 1)	14		

*df is calculated for each individual group: K = Number of groups, 3 − 1 = 2; N = Number of sample, 15 − 3 = 12; N − 1 = 15 − 1 = 14.

$$\text{Mean square} = \frac{\text{sum of squares}}{\text{degrees of freedom}} \text{ or MS} = \frac{\text{SS}}{\text{df}}$$

$$MS_B = \frac{SS_B}{\text{df}} = \frac{14.4}{2} = 7.2 \quad MS_w = \frac{SS_w}{\text{df}} = \frac{18}{12} = 1.5 \quad F \text{ ratio} = \frac{MS_B}{MS_w} = 4.8$$

Need 3.88 to exceed .05 since 4.8 is larger. There is a significant difference among the group means.

FIGURE 23-19 Example of ANOVA.

Meta-analysis

Meta-analysis is the process of summarizing the findings of several studies to find an average. Meta-analysis is not the latest research technique although it is currently receiving a great deal of attention.

Psychologist Robert Rosenthal has worked with procedures in research methods for about 20 years. Although they were not identified by the title of meta-analysis, these procedures involved meta-analysis techniques. According to Rosenthal, defining research results using meta-analysis is the attempt to explain the relationship between any two variables.[10] Since meta-analysis is used to obtain some measure of average results from several studies, it is necessary for the investigator to conduct a literature search for research studies in the particular area of interest. Books, journals, theses, dissertations, and unpublished works are sources for studies which discriminate research findings.

It is important to note that meta-analysis is used with experimental research studies that have an experimental and a control group.

Some of the uses of meta-analysis are:

1. To summarize the relationship of two variables (the same two variables) as found in several studies.
2. To find the average or median of the results of several experimental studies.
3. To find the overall average relationship between the independent and the dependent variables from several individual research projects.
4. To form an average probability by combining probabilities from several cases.
5. To establish the magnitude of the factors associated with the relationship between two variables.
6. To make a precise mathematical statement about results, which is difficult by the usual perusal method of reading the literature and summarizing the findings.

Glass differentiates between primary analysis which the researcher does with his/her original data and secondary analysis which is done by a second researcher or is re-analyzed

---

[10] Glass, G.V.: Primary, secondary and meta-analysis of research, Educational Research 5(10):3–8, November 1976.

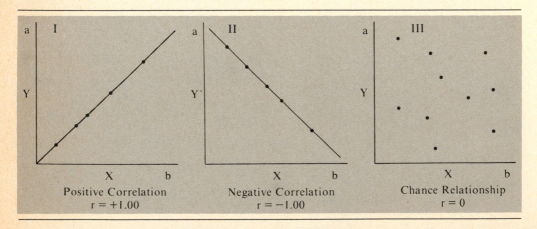

FIGURE 23-20   Scatter diagrams.

by the original researcher using different statistical measures or analyzed to test a new hypothesis. Finally, meta-analysis is the analysis of the results from several (4 to hundreds) of individual studies to integrate results into a simple dimension. As a hypothetical example, a meta-analysis of 50 studies of treatment X found that on the average clients recovered 2 days earlier with treatment X than without it. Glass believes that one of the great values of meta-analysis is the drawing together or consensus of findings into a meaningful piece of knowledge.[11]

Effect size is an important concept in meta-analysis.

$$ES = \frac{\overline{X}t - \overline{X}c}{SDc}$$

ES = effect size
$\overline{X}t$ = treatment group mean
$\overline{X}c$ = control group mean
SDc = standard deviation of the control group

The effect size is the difference between the treatment group (experimental group receiving some manipulation) and the control group which did not receive the treatment (manipulation). The effect size is the result of the statistical manipulation with the ES formula. Effect sizes can be added together to produce a mean of several experiments: Occasionally the effect size mean is computed for certain categories of studies and compared with the effect size mean of a second series of studies. Perhaps studies with 20 subjects in the treatment group would produce an effect size which could be compared with 19 or fewer subjects in the treatment group.

Other researchers might find the means of effect size from studies judged sufficiently valid with those judged invalid. An interesting phenomenon which often merges in a comparison of valid versus invalid studies is that the valid studies control for more variables but the resulting effect size is only slightly higher.

In studying the effect of teaching using higher cognitive questions, Redfield and Rousseau found effect size in all of 14 studies as +.7292. Seven studies judged valid had an ES of +.7631 while seven studies judged less valid had an ES of +.7148; thus the average student taught by a teacher using higher level questions could be expected to score at the 77th percentile whereas the untreated student would score at the 50th percentile.[12]

Glass reported analyzing 375 studies of psychotherapy which involved 40,000 subjects with more than 19 hours of treatment or no treatment. Therapists had 2 1/2 years of experience and the measurements of outcome were conducted 4 months later. The conclusion reached was that any type of therapy will move a client from the 50th to the 75th percentile as compared with those clients who were untreated.[13]

Dr. Mary Turley used meta-analysis to integrate the findings of 20 experimental studies. She found that maternal-infant interaction is increased when mothers receive information about sensory and perceptual capacities of their children.[14]

[11] *Ibid.*, p. 4.
[12] Redfield, D.L., and Rousseau, E.W.: A meta-analysis of experimental research on teacher questioning behavior, Rev. of Educational Res. **51**(2):237–245, Summer 1981.
[13] From Glass, *op. cit.*, p. 3–8.
[14] Turley, Dr. M.: Meta-analysis of informing mothers concerning the sensory perceptual capabilities of their infants: the effects on maternal-infant interaction. Unpublished dissertation presented to University of Texas at Austin.

Advantages

1. Meta-analysis is much more precise than some traditional techniques of reviewing a number of studies and defining the results in prose.
2. Meta-analysis provides a mathematical conclusion in the form of a precise quantity rather than a subjective statement.
3. Meta-analysis' strength is that it reduces each study to a standard measure of equivalency through effect size as the common denominator.
4. Since few studies are exact replications of another study, meta-analysis is a logical method of comparing studies which have at least control and experimental groups.
5. Some studies that are included in a meta-analysis research may have flaws and biases, but research of the meta-analysis results has found that "poor" studies yield effect size very similar to "good" studies.

Disadvantages

1. The combining of effect sizes can mean that poorly designed, invalid, and biased research studies are often included in the meta-analysis.
2. Combining several studies which may have been concluded under questionable controls can often result in a muddle of bewildering grey.
3. Some critics feel that combining many different types of studies is like comparing apples with oranges.
4. Possible procedural invalidity of some meta-analysis studies include such areas as retrieval, estimates of differences, difference among methods of analysis, and differences in the meaning of terms and sample sizes.

Figs. 23-21 to 23-24 present a breakdown of the most commonly used statistical terms with examples and use in research. The measures presented are not intended to be all inclusive but offer some indications of possible statistical applications.

ACCEPTANCE OR REJECTION OF THE HYPOTHESIS

When looking at our data, we should be able to say if our hypothesis was accepted or rejected. If statistics are used, we should say at what level the hypothesis was accepted or rejected and what the correlations were. Testing the hypothesis is the whole point of research, so it is extremely important that the investigator be able to report, in definite terms, just what the test revealed.

Suppose we are using a null hypothesis stating that there is no difference; if we reject the null hypothesis, this means that there was a difference. In reporting the fact that there was a difference, we should say what that difference was. On the other hand, if we are using a scientific hypothesis that states a direction, then we should report that it was accepted or rejected.

If, for example, we were using the hypothesis that the taller a person is, the more he/she will weigh, we could say that, if we found this to be true, the hypothesis was accepted. However, if the hypothesis was not accepted, then we would state that it was rejected.

Suppose we had used the null hypothesis, "there is no relationship between height and weight," and we found this to be true; then we would say that the null hypothesis was

MEASURING SCALES

	Purpose	Example	Use in Research
NOMINAL	Classifies into either-or.	Male or female.	Yes and no answers.
ORDINAL	Ordering from high to low.	Order of finish of race.	Ranking quantified answers.
INTERVAL	Equal intervals between units.	Degrees on a thermometer.	Likert scaling.
RATIO	Unit has a precise value and absolute zero.	Money from none to infinity— 2 dollars twice as much as one.	Rarely used.

DESCRIPTIVE STATISTICS

	Purpose	Example	Use in Research
MEAN	Measures	Arithmetic average, average IQ is 100.	Basis for most statistical calculation.
MEDIAN	of central	Point of score in the middle of the group.	Not influenced by extreme scores. May be a statistical requirement.
MODE	tendency	Most frequent score.	Rarely useful.
RANGE	Measure of variability.	Difference between highest or lowest score.	Useful in finding differences.

FIGURE 23-21 Methods to measure and describe data.

accepted; there is no difference. If we found, when using the null hypothesis, that there was a difference, we would report that we rejected the null hypothesis of no difference.

Errors

Concerning the hypothesis, there are two types of errors the researcher may commit. Type I error occurs when the researcher rejects a null hypothesis that is actually true, and type II error occurs when he/she fails to reject a false null hypothesis. Freeman explains:

	Purpose	Example	Use in Research
QUARTILE DEVIATION	Measure	Scores divided into 4 equal parts. Half of lower median is 25 quartile.	Useful in education and scoring.
PERCENTILE RANK	of	Score of value calculated to parts of a hundred.	
STANDARD DEVIATION	variability	Measure of difference of each value from the mean.	Extremely useful in comparison with normal curve.
NORMAL CURVE	A device to locate scores in relationship to each other.	A curve which included all possible scores from lowest to highest with 3 measures of central tendency in exact center.	Scores can be used as a measure of comparison between groups.
STANDARD SCORES	Represents distance from the mean as measured by standard deviation.		

FIGURE 23-22   Measures of variability.

Errors of the first kind, or *type I errors,* occur when we reject a null hypothesis which is true: they are determined by the level of α. It is customary, you will remember, to set $\alpha = .05$ or .01. Then, if a given result falls in the area (5% or 1%) specified by α, we reject the null hypothesis. If the null hypothesis is true, a result falling in the region of rejection is an extremely unlikely event; but it is not impossible! At $\alpha = .05$, 5% of the observed results will fall into the region of rejection just by chance. So if we consistently use $\alpha = .05$, we shall reject 5 out of every 100 true null hypotheses. At $\alpha = .01$ we shall commit this Type I error once in every 100 tests. In the general case, the probability of a Type I error is equal to α.

This seems to suggest that it would be wise to make α small.... But, unfortunately, it is not this simple—there are also errors of the second kind or *type II errors.*

A type II error consists of failing to reject a false null hypothesis. It is very difficult to determine the probability of a type II error, but we can get a general idea of how it is calculated if we return to our earlier example of coin tossing.[15]

The probability that type I and type II errors will be committed is inversely related. When the risk of making a type I error is minimized, the chance of making a type II error increases. The probability of committing a type II error is also inversely related to sample size. By increasing sample size, the researcher is able to minimize the risk of committing a type II error.[16]

STEPS OF HYPOTHESIS TESTING

We discussed hypotheses in Chapter 10, but at this time we consider the steps used in testing the hypothesis. There are seven steps to the testing process and these must be carried out in definite order. They are stated here briefly, since we do not intend to attempt to provide a statistics course within the discussion of research in nursing.

1. State the research hypothesis. The symbol used is H_1.
2. State the null hypothesis. The symbol is H_0. It is the null hypothesis that is actually being tested.
3. Select a statistical test. It should be appropriate for the level of scaling done and the kind of data on hand. The beginning student will, no doubt, need assistance in the selection of a statistical test.
4. Determine sample size (N) and level of significance (α).
5. Look up the sampling distribution of the statistical test under H_0. Usually, tables will be available.
6. Decide what the region of rejection will be. After looking at the hypothesis, decide whether a one-tailed or a two-tailed test is appropriate. Next, on the basis of α, select the outcomes that will be the cutoff for rejection of H_0.
7. Compute the statistics, and decide whether H_0 is to be accepted or rejected. If the result of the computation falls within the region of rejection, H_0 is rejected. If it falls outside the region, H_0 is accepted.

LIMITATIONS

In the *limitations,* the researcher discusses the weaknesses of the entire study, as the researcher perceives them. All weaknesses should be identified and reported. Researchers are expected to be their own most ardent critics. If an investigator does not recognize the flaws, the readers will pick them out and will criticize the investigator for not seeing the study's shortcomings. If the researcher observes some weaknesses, such as inadequate sample size or unclear definitions, early on in the study, every effort must be made to eliminate them before proceeding with the study. Revisions in the instrument should be

[15] Freeman, Linton C.: Elementary applied statistics: for students in behavioral science, New York, copyright © 1965, John Wiley & Sons, Inc., p. 154. By permission of John Wiley & Sons, Inc.
[16] *Ibid.,* p. 156.

PARAMETRIC—tests significance of interval & ratio data. Results are significant to generalize from a sample population.

	Purpose	Example	Use in Research
t TEST To test two means to differentiate at a selected probability value.	To compare observed differences with expected differences.	Are results significant at predetermined t value.	If results are significant we reject null hypothesis (accept working).
ANALYSIS OF VARIANCE (ANOVA) To test for significant differences of two or more means.	To find how much greater within group difference is than between group difference.	Compare differences between school A & B and within group differences on state board exams.	Are differences result of treatment or sampling error?
ANALYSIS OF COVARIANCE (ANCOVA) To match control groups on extraneous variables.	To control pretest differences in experimental designs.	Is post test difference due to experiment or another variable.	Increase power of statistical test by reducing within group variance.

NON PARAMETRIC—tests significance of nominal and ordinal data. Tests significances when nature of the population is not known.

	Purpose	Example	Use in Research
CHI SQUARE X^2 General test to measure strength of relationship between two variances.	Tests differences between observed and expected.	Do clients who receive intervention A recover faster than non intervention?	Measures strength of relationship between variables.
SPEARMANS RANK ORDER CORRELATION A test of the relationship between two ranked sets of data.	Measures correlation between ranked variables.	Compare correlation between nurses and doctors ranking of ten causes of coronary disease.	Useful for a precise measure of correlation from -1.0 to $+1.0$

FIGURE 23-23 Tests of significance.

	Purpose	Examples	Use in Research
REGRESSION	To find a linear equation of the relationship between two variances.	The relationship between health and exercise as they regress towards the mean.	To predict the strength of variable X with Y. Measures from +1.0 to −1.0 while 0 is no relationship.
META-ANALYSIS	To find a method of combining the ES (effect size) of several experimental control differences.	Twenty different studies report on nursing intervention plan Y. Both have control and experimental groups which report an effect size.	To summarize the results of a number of experiments of a similar nature into a single result.

FIGURE 23-24   Predicting and summarizing statistics.

made prior to the major study so that validity and reliability of the study will not be questioned.

In a research project there are two types of limitations the investigator should discuss—those that are recognized but are beyond the control of the researcher and those that are oversights and thus were unanticipated. It is this discussion of the limitations that is so valuable for future researchers when they review the literature. For example, a researcher would report that there was a major accident in the community on the day that she collected her data and many of the intended sample were unavailable to participate in her study. She planned for a sample of 50 staff nurses but only 25 were available, so sample size was an unexpected limitation. Another example of a limitation is, "The reliability of the instrument developed for the project was not systematically studied prior to its use, although the pilot study aided in refining the wording of many items."

Limitations refer to criticisms of the validity and reliability of the instrument, the content of the data, the evidence of subjective bias on the part of the investigator and the respondents, and the lack of data cross checking. An example of a limitation is, "The reliability of the instrument developed for the project was not systematically studied prior to its use, though the pilot study aided in refining the wording of many items."

SUMMARY

An important aim of the researcher is to be able to make generalizations from the results of a single study sample, which requires that the descriptive presentation of the data be systematic and objective.

Frequency distribution is one of the methods used to describe data. A frequency distribution is a systematic way to list a series of observations of a variable. This is done by listing the categories and then tabulating the frequency of each occurrence.

Three measures of central tendency are the mean, the median, and the mode. These measures are characteristic representatives of a group and are valuable for descriptions and comparisons.

The most frequently appearing value is the *mode.* It is quickly determined and is not affected by extreme scores; but it cannot be used for algebraic manipulation. The frequency distribution is bimodal when two modes appear in the clusters of observations or values.

, The *median* is a point in which half the number of values are above it and half are below it. It is easy to calculate and is a useful approximate measure of the average. The median is seldom affected by extreme scores; however, it cannot be handled algebraically.

The *mean* is computed by adding the scores and dividing the sum by the total number of scores. It is the most accurate and reliable of the three measures and is suitable for mathematical manipulation; however, it is influenced by extreme scores.

Distributions can often be described by their relationship to the normal curve, or normal distribution. The *normal curve* is the resulting symmetrical form of a frequency distribution. It begins and ends at a low point where there are few extreme scores and rises in the center where most scores cluster. In the normal curve, the mode, the median, and the mean all occur at the highest point of the distribution. These three measures of central tendency also divide the normal distribution into two equal parts, the left called the negative side and the right called the positive side. Theoretically, all populations, if large enough, approach the normal distribution. Frequency distributions with a cluster of units at one end are either negatively or positive skewed.

Standard deviation is a measure of dispersion and is an average of all deviation from the mean. The standard deviation, because it is algebraic, can be combined and used for a comparison of the data. It deserves its place as the master measure of variability.

Standard scores are units of the standard deviation. A standard score is the distance of any score or value from the mean of the distribution, expressed in standard deviation units. It is possible to compare standard scores or units. The standard score is expressed as a *z* score.

In rank-order *correlation,* two or more judges rank variables according to their order of frequency or strength. Statistics are applied and the resulting figure is the correlation between the judges' opinion of the rank of the variables.

Chi-square is a nonparametric test that shows the amount of difference between the frequencies observed and the frequencies expected. With the chi-square the researcher can tell if the findings are significant beyond chance. If so, he/she can attribute any difference between the observed and the expected frequencies to an independent variable.

A *t test* is a statistical formula used to determine if the differences between means are significant. *Analysis of variance* is a procedure to test the significant difference between three or more sets of data from three or more groups. *Regression* is the central tendency of a set of data represented by a line correlation of the mean values of the correlation between two variables plotted on a scatter diagram. *Meta-analysis* is a technique used to find the average increase of a number of research studies. The studies must have used control and experimental groups. The difference between groups after treatment is known as effect size. Meta-analysis combines effect sizes to summarize the result of several investigations concerning one particular theme.

DISCUSSION QUESTIONS

1 What do people usually mean when they say "average?"
2 Suggest three variables that would fall in approximately a normal curve.
3 Give an example of how standard deviation might be used in reporting an experience that you have had.
4 How could standard scores be used to make a comparison between a nurse and a social worker?
5 What is the purpose of statistics?
6 If we applied rank order correlation to some data and found a correlation of .88, what does it show?
7 Why are statistics preferable (if they are) to percentages?
8 Are statistics and percentages both desirable in a research study?
9 Give an example of how chi-square could be used.
10 Why do you think the mean, the median, and the mode all fall at the same point on a normal curve?

CLASS ACTIVITIES

Track I

1 Raw data on several topics are gathered from the students. The class mean, median, and mode are then computed for each variable.
2 Members of the class write their weight and sex on a slip of paper. These are collected and tallied. The mean and the standard deviation are figured according to sex and total class participants.

Track II (Steps in Research Project)

1 Each group or single researcher is to determine various descriptive measures using raw data collected in the study.
2 Apply descriptive and/or statistical analysis to data.
3 Make a table using number and percent for each item in the instrument, to be used in the appendix and for purposes of calculation.

SUGGESTED READINGS

Amos, J.R., Brown, F.L., and Mink, O.G.: Statistical concepts, a basic program, New York, 1965, Harper & Row Publishers.

Andrew, B.J.: Can professional competence be measured? In Loveland, E.H., guest editor: New directions for program evaluation, measuring hard-to-measure, no. 6, 1980.

Besag, F.P., and Besag, P.L.: Statistics for the helping professions, Beverly Hills, 1985, Sage Publications, Inc.

Boodo, G.M., and O'Sullivan, P.: Obtaining generalizability coefficients for clinical evaluations, Evaluation and the Health Professions 5(3):345–358, September 1982.

Burckhardt, C.S.: The measurement of change in nursing research, statistical considerations, Nurs. Res. 31:53, January–February 1982.

Campbell, D., and Elliott, J.F.: Utilizing nonparametric statistical techniques, evaluating management effectiveness of an alcoholic treatment center, Evaluation and the Health Professions 4(1):59–71, March 1981.

Cooper, H.M., and Rosenthal, R.: Statistical versus traditional procedures for summarizing research findings, Psychological Bulletin **87**:442–449, 1980.

Diers, D.: Research for nursing, ed. 3, New York, 1976, Appleton-Century-Crofts, Chapter 5.

Duncan, R.C. Knapp, R.G., and Miller, M.C., III: Introductory biostatistics for the health sciences, ed. 2, New York, 1983, John Wiley & Sons.

Feldman, M.J., and Ventura, M.R.: Evaluating change using noninterval data, Nurs. Res. **33**(3):182–184, May–June 1984.

Fox, D.J.: Fundamentals of research in nursing, ed. 4, Norwalk CT, 1982, Appleton-Century-Crofts.

Goodwin, L.D.: The use of power estimation in nursing research, Nurs. Res. **22**(2):118–120, March–April 1984.

Hartwig, F., with Dearing, B.E.: Exploratory data analysis, Series 07-016, Beverly Hills, 1979, Sage Publications, Inc.

Hays, W.: Statistics, ed. 3, New York, 1981, Holt, Rinehart & Winston, Chapter 2.

Henkel, R.E.: Tests of significance. In Uslaner, E.M., editor, Series: quantitative applications in the social sciences, no. 07-004, Beverly Hills, 1976, Sage Publications, Inc.

Iversen, G.R., and Norpoth, J.: Analysis of variance. In Uslaner, E.M., editor, Series: quantitative applications in the social sciences, no. 07-001, Beverly Hills, 1976, Sage Publications, Inc.

Jackson, N.E.: The statistically simple study: a guide for thesis advisers, Journal of Nursing Education **22**(8):351, October 1983.

Jacobsen, B.S.: A statistical tale of significance...to correlate audience and wakefulness at the conference sessions with...the program, Nurs. Res. **32**(6):376, November–December 1983. 1983.

Knapp, R.G.: Basic statistics for nurses, New York, 1978, John Wiley & Sons.

Kulik, C.C., Kulik, J.A., and Shwalb, B.J.: College programs for high-risk and disadvantaged students: a meta-analysis of findings, Review of Educational Research **53**(3):397–414, Fall 1983.

Kulik, J.A., Kulik, C.C., and Cohen, P.A.: Effectiveness of computer-based college teaching: a meta-analysis of findings, Review of Educational Research **50**(4):525–544, Winter 1980.

Kuzma, J.W.: Basic statistics for the health sciences, Palo Alto, CA, 1984, Mayfield Publishing Company.

Kviz, F.J. and Knafl, K.A.: Statistics for nurses, an introductory text, Boston, 1980, Little, Brown & Company.

Minium, E.W.: Statistical reasoning in psychology and education, ed. 2, New York, 1978, John Wiley & Sons.

Miller, P.McC., and Wilson, M.J.: A dictionary of social science methods, New York, 1983, John Wiley & Sons.

Nuttall, P.: The passionate statistician, International Nursing Review **31**(1):24–25, February, 1984.

Polit, D., and Hungler, B.: Nursing research: principles and methods, Philadelphia, 1978, J.B. Lippincott, Co., Chapter 24.

Reid, B.J.: Potential sources of type I error and possible solutions to avoid a "galloping" alpha rate, Nursing Research **32**(3):190, May–June 1983.

Reynolds, H.T.: Analysis of nominal data, In Uslaner, E.M., editor: Quantitative applications in the social sciences, no. 07-007, Beverly Hills, 1977, SAGE Publications, Inc.

Shelley, S.I.: Research methods in nursing and health, Boston, 1984, Little, Brown, & Company.

Waltz, C., and Bausell, R.B.: Nursing research: design, statistics, and computer analysis, Philadelphia, 1981, F.A. Davis Company.

Weiner, E.E.: Understanding the use of basic statistics in nursing research, American Journal of Nursing **83**(5):770, May 1983.

Williams, F.: Reasoning with statistics, ed. 2, New York, 1979, Holt, Rinehart & Winston.

CHAPTER 24

THE EVALUATION PROCESS

The term evaluation is used at least three ways in research: evaluation research, evaluation survey, and evaluation process.

Evaluation research developed and grew into a discipline as a result of the proliferation of human services programs that began during World War II. Questions of worth and merit demanded answers because public money was used to create these programs. Evaluation practice and evaluation research were initially influenced by such researchers as Campbell, Stanley, Scriven, and Donabedian. The development of terminology, concepts, and perspectives enhanced the evaluation approach to research. Most federal agencies now require an evaluation component in human services programs.[1]

Evaluation is the systematic appraisal of a phenomenon through the use of a set of procedures. Evaluation research is commonly conducted to rate the extent to which a program has attained its goals by considering such factors as cost, impact, activities, and results.

Evaluation of innovative programs is especially important because it adds to the knowledge base of a discipline. However, the measurement of changes in attitude, behavior, knowledge, and values resulting from public and educational programs is hindered by an inadequate number of valid and reliable tools and comparison experimental groups.

Evaluation survey, which was discussed in Chapter 12, is one type of descriptive research in which data are collected to provide a critical inspection or a comprehensive view of the situation. The evaluation survey determines and reports the findings as they currently exist.

The present chapter focuses on the evaluation process as it is related to a research project. After the data have been collected, the raw data must be prepared for analysis. Then the researcher interprets the meaning of the results as they are related to the phenomenon under study, to other individuals or groups, and to future research. Decisions concerning the phenomenon result from arbitrary evaluation by the researcher.

This chapter is concerned with evaluating the results of a research project. It is not concerned with the process of evaluating health and social programs, institutions, and policies. The researcher systematically uses techniques and methods in conducting evaluation research because it is a form of applied research.

---

[1]Kosecoff, J. and Fink, A.: Evaluation basics, Beverly Hills, 1982, Sage Publications, Inc.

The evaluation process begins after the data are analyzed. What insight has been gained? What new knowledge has come to light? These questions require further inquiry about generalizations and evaluations that can be extended from the data.

The term *generalization* has been mentioned before; but for the purpose of this book, generalization means extending the implications of the data at hand to a broader population. It is important that we make generalizations from the data to the population, since this is the very purpose for which the scientific method was established. If generalizations are important in the physical sciences, they are even more important in the health sciences. If we experiment with a new medicine, we must be certain that the data we have collected are so reliable that it is possible to generalize to the total population.

Suppose we reject our null hypothesis based on a 10% sample of the registered nurses currently licensed in our state. If we believe that the statistic test we used was appropriate and that the sample was truly representative of the remaining 90% of the registered nurses, then it is possible to extend (generalize) the conclusions based on our sample to the 90%. It would not be wise to generalize our findings to nurses in other states without replicating the study in several areas of the country first. If our findings were similar, then we could proceed to generalize.

HOW FAR CAN GENERALIZATIONS BE MADE?

Startling conclusions from factual evidence are necessary in some fields before changes will be made in traditional procedures. Inequalities that need to be erased have been found in the treatment of minorities. Human beings, human emotions, human responses, and humanity in general are all in need of change; however, it is necessary to have factual evidence before recommendations can be generalized to a whole group. It has been through small research studies that the public is now aware of the injustices done to minorities.

In research there is nearly as much interest in the process of obtaining data as in the results. This holds true in the generalization process. It is important to know the answers to certain questions, such as what was the sample like, was the sample large enough, and was the sample characteristic enough of the variable under study to permit the assumption that it was representative of the population in general?

One way to know how far to generalize is by means of statistical results or by the kind of correlation found in the evidence. In a sample, if the statistical probability is quite high, then the conclusions can be generalized to the population with some degree of confidence.

If, in the process of generalization, researchers begin to compare or to consider all the possible variables and begin to read in exceptions and contradictions to all the data, they will end up not being able to generalize at all. It is important, therefore, that at some point the researcher decides if it is better to learn a little about the general population or a lot of minute details about a great number of factors that do not fit together into the larger scheme. The fact that generalizations are based on accumulated evidence makes the scientific method productive. Broader generalizations that can be made to a larger population provide hypotheses and add possibilities and probabilities for future testing. At least other researchers inquiring into the general area will have stimulating ideas to test.

If, after a researcher has collected all the data and all the evidence, the conclusion is reached that generalization is beyond the study just completed, the study has been of little value. The researcher should explore the reasons for identified weaknesses and report possible solutions. If the researcher has the time and the interest, it may be profitable to repeat the study, making any necessary modifications.

Purposes of Generalizations

One use for generalizations lies in their powers to forecast the future from the past. Suppose we find that there is an upward trend in the number of people entering the health field. Can we assume that the trend is going to continue? If an increase was observed over a long period of time, we might have noticed several fluctuations. As it was, we chose a time to look at health field statistics when manpower was on the rise. If we were to generalize from the present to the future, we would certainly need to look at trends over a long period of time.

We suggest, however, that if predictions of future trends are necessary, past decades will provide better indications of long-term future trends, whereas the recent past is a relatively good indicator of the short-term future tendencies.

Generalizaitons contribute toward scientific conceptualization in that they can expand beyond a single study. Through careful analysis, the researcher may be able to conceptualize and develop further research investigations.

Generalizations are useful for determining the needs or requirements for fulfilling demands for decision making. Suppose it has been found that the inner city has different health needs than the suburbs. If, after replicating this study in a number of cities, the findings are similar, then city health planners can make decisions for inner cities in other areas.

A major use of generalizations is to reduce the cost and labor of researching a total population. If a sample can adequately portray the characteristics of the whole, why spend time and funds on the investigation of the total population?

There is always the possibility that the findings of any scientific research may be earthshaking. If the findings are true for the sample, then what?

Acceptance of Generalizations

The researcher may discover what appears to be valuable information for a discipline. He/she may, when writing up the report, generalize the findings to the population at large. The researcher's ideas and arguments may be widely distributed, but he/she cannot force anyone to accept the results of the study. If quality research has been done, the findings will stand on their own merit.

There are at least three steps a researcher can take to aid in the acceptance of his/her research by others. First, a research study should be well documented. Evidence of the researcher's inquiry into the general area, as well as into the particular area, must be shown. References to people, places, things, and occurrences must be accurately reported within the context of the report. Even then, of course, some individuals who learn of the research findings will not bother to change their routine way of thinking to incorporate the findings into their lifestyle or work habits.

Second, the researcher must explain his/her research study in exact detail to minimize misunderstanding. This does not mean that the study report must be lengthy or wordy, but a concise, full description must be given. Those persons prejudiced against a study are then less likely to reject or to question the results. As an illustration, application of research findings that permit one person to have power or control over others are not likely to be accepted by those who would lose power. It is best to anticipate and prepare for any criticism of study findings by including in the original report the answers to questions that might be raised later.

Third, distribution of the study findings should be as wide as feasible. If only a biased group learns about them, then, it can be anticipated that the study will not be well accepted. If the findings in nursing research are made known to those in related but interested disciplines, as well as nurses in various specialties, the findings are more likely to be accepted. What would have happened if Semmelweis' study of puerperal fever had received wider publicity?[2] Would someone in another country have repeated his research and confirmed his theory? We would like to think so.

For the sake of progress it is important that generalizations, based on positive evidence, be accepted by the population. Unfortunately, this does not always occur, and the researcher must be ready to continue his/her work, motivated by the awareness that truth is being discovered. It is hoped that the beginning researcher will have the satisfaction of reporting the project results to a receptive audience or instructor.

How far can the researcher generalize from any given sample? How far can the researcher stretch the conclusions from the sample findings to describe the total population? Let us use for an example a school of nursing that has an enrollment of 600 students. Suppose we study 100 of these individuals. Can we say that 100 students constitute a representative sample? Can we generalize and say that the attitudes and responses of the 100 students can be extended to include all 600? Will the 100 students under observation have the same general characteristics and attitudes as the other 500 who were not included in the study? Can we say that our findings can be extended to include all nursing students in the state? In the United States?

We can make one definite statement about how much to generalize from a study sample about total population by stating that the results are based on a given sample from a specified population, on such and such day, at a certain time, under specific conditions, using certain techniques and instruments. If we were to collect data from our school of 600 students using a sample of 100 students, we could say that for this time, with this sample, using the described methods, this is what was found.

If this study were repeated, using another group of students enrolled in a different school, and the findings were similar to those in the original investigation, we could report that similar findings were found in the second instance. If other researchers repeated the study in several regions of the United States, in a variety of situations and circumstances, and the same evidence was found, it would be permissible to generalize from our findings to the total population. There is a need in nursing for replication studies of this nature; repeated descriptive studies must be carried out until generalizations can be made. There must be continued replication on a much larger scale in the health professions and in the social sciences.

An example of a condition that has been found true so frequently that we can generalize about the total population is that women practice religion more than men.

---

[2]Thompson, Morton: The cry and the covenant, Garden City, N.Y., 1954, Doubleday & Co., Inc.

This study has been repeated so often that it is safe to say that women have a more strict religious behavior pattern (criterion: attend church more frequently) than men. Therefore, it can be generalized from repeated investigations that women do practice religion more than men.

A principle commonly followed in research is that generalizations can be made from findings if the data can be regarded as a reasonably fair sample of the population to which it is generalized. Care must be taken not to generalize beyond the group until there is certainty that the sample is truly representative.

Prediction is a special type of generalization that involves forecasting. This type of generalization is always difficult, because prediction involves moving from the known to the unknown. As an illustration, we can predict that health professionals will be required to spend more time learning to use complex health equipment in the future. This prediction is based on current trends and changes during the past 5 years. Predictions are not wild guesses; they stem from reports of observations, investigations, and extrapolations.

Of less certainty are predictions based on indefinite circumstances. It may or may not be safe to assume that population growth in the United States will not change drastically in the next 10 years or that the birth rate will not decrease in the next 10 years. It is important to note that the past circumstances or events are no guarantee of the future, and predictions should never be made totally on the basis of the past. For the sake of accuracy, it is much wiser to make predictions for the next 1 or 2 years based on the recent past than to predict future needs or circumstances for the next decade relying on history or events in the 1920s.

According to Jacox, empirical generalizations are established through inductive reasoning. By this process empirically observed events allow the researcher to argue from the particular to the general or from one event to other events.[3]

Generalizations and predictions are a form of inductive reasoning. In this case, researchers move from a known fact (based on data) to predicting the unknown (theoretical). They make the assumption that the unknown will be an extension of the known. Inductively, they take the findings of their research sample and extend the interpretations to include more than the sample. Through inductive reasoning they can develop hypotheses and theories for further testing.

Let us assume that we take a survey of health professionals to determine their need for continuing education. Our findings indicate that the majority of our sample of 50 persons from a total population of 324 wants to learn more about computer programming. The sample subjects complain that they do not have enough technical knowledge to use computers. From this information we could generalize that most of the health professionals in the population also feel that they have an inadequate understanding of computer use.

In contrast, using a deductive approach, it would be possible to test the hypothesis that consumer knowledge is always behind technology. We might want to test this hypothesis in other areas such as business, engineering, and so on to see if the same holds true.

The following steps demonstrate the use of the inductive reasoning process.

1. *Sample size (N = 50).* The total population of health care professionals at Hospital Y is 324. *Findings from sample:* Health care professionals do not think that they have enough knowledge to use computer-based machinery (the known).

[3]Jacox, Ada: Theory construction in nursing, Nurs. Res. **23**(1):7, 1975.

2. *Generalization:* The total population of Hospital Y feels the same way as the subjects in the sample (Fig. 24-1).
3. *Further generalizations, based on replication research in 3 other hospitals:* All health professionals from the 10 city hospitals in the area feel that they have inadequate knowledge of computer-based machinery.
4. Possibly, a theory could be developed that would predict that technology will always be ahead of the ability of the public to use it. This theory would be developed by extending the findings from the original sample of 50 health care professionals to the general population.
5. *Inductive reasoning:* Health care professionals need more instruction to utilize the capabilities of equipment linked to computers. Since this is true with the sample of health care professionals, it is probably true with all users of technology. Through logical and systematic study, we have taken the data from the sample of 50 subjects and extended the generalization to all users of technology.

Let us repeat, if we are sure that our sample is adequate, and that it is representative of the general or usual feelings of the study group, then we can generalize from our research findings. But if our sample is small and includes a number of exceptions, then we must be cautious about generalizing.

CONCLUSIONS

The conclusions are the ultimate findings of the research project. The evaluation process then determines the worth of the investigation based on the conclusions.

The following is an example of a conclusion. *RNs seem to base their choice of professional nursing on personal interests. Family members seem to play a relatively small role in such decision-making (Table X).*

The final section in a research report provides a discussion of the conclusions that can be drawn from the study findings. It is not enough for researchers to know the extent to which they can generalize the results; they also must synthesize and interpret the results. What do the findings really mean? Are they related to something that was observed or to something that was implicit in the study? Do statements that have been made hold for all of the respondents at all times or for only some of the respondents part of the time?

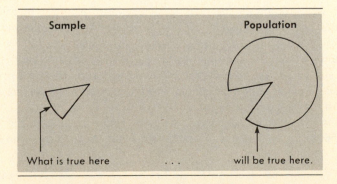

FIGURE 24-1   Generalization.

If we found that nurses were concerned people, the word *concerned* might have different connotations. Some people would probably interpret it as having a concern for health; others might assume it was a concern for emotional health; whereas still others might think it was a concern for people in general. In his/her conclusions the researcher should point out exactly what was learned from the study and should include an explicit explanation of the conclusions.

The present tense is used for stating general conclusions and no new material should be added; that is, no new facts should appear in the list of conclusions. The conclusions are for presenting the meaning of the data, not for presenting new findings. This section contains a review of outstanding facts and a comprehensive evaluation, generalization, and projection of new insights into what has already been presented. The section may begin by simply stating, "Six conclusions may be drawn from the findings." The major statement may be followed by a brief explanation and identification of a table(s) to clarify the conclusion.

Estimating the Value of Research

The value of a research project is seen most clearly at the time its conclusions are determined. Of course, researchers tend to have different reasons for beginning a research project in the first place. For some, it may have been an assignment, part of their job description; for others, it may have been for status or monetary gain. There are some researchers who do research for the pure joy and satisfaction that they get from it. These researchers think that the stimulation and pleasure received from investigating the unknown is reward enough. Still other motives for doing a research project are the hope and anticipation that the findings will contribute to the discipline's body of knowledge and that they will be relevant for a large segment of the population. The reason for being a researcher may be complex; many or all of these factors may be complex; many or all of these factors may contribute to a greater or lesser extent.

In the case of students, the completion of a research project may have been a requirement for a course, and the conclusions may not really hold great importance for them. Even though the research process may have been emphasized, a classroom assignment can contribute to the body of knowledge. It takes time to analyze findings and to draw conclusions, so sufficient time must be available for the researchers to ponder their findings.

Simon calls attention to another significant way of estimating the value of research. If the study tests an important theory, then the theory must seem worthy of being tested. Also, a study that tests a theory would, of itself, be important in contributing to the future of research.[4]

Another factor we can use in estimating the value of a research study is noting how unusual, how surprising, and how unexpected its results were. If, over a period of time, researchers and others have been assuming that the reverse of the present findings was true, then the study would be quite valuable.[5]

Suppose, for example, we found that women from a disadvantaged background seemed to be better nurses (however we measured better) than nurses who came from a

[4]Simon, J.L.: Basic research methods in social science, New York, 1969, Random House, Inc., p. 223.
[5]*Ibid.*, p. 224.

middle-class background; this discovery would be important information for the recruit-ment of students. Of course, further research on the why of the situation and on other questions arising from the findings would be needed, along with continued follow-up of the sample. The investigator could bring the findings to the attention of nursing educators and employers interested in hiring nurses.

When discussing the importance of generalization, the more universal the findings, the greater is the value of the study. As mentioned elsewhere in this book, the researcher is expected to suggest other studies that might be carried out as a result of the present findings. These may include repetitive investigations, as well as extensions from current research results. The number of studies that can be generated indicates, to a degree, the value of the present work. How many useful hypotheses or new theories does the study suggest? Research has been done to test the theories of such men as Max Weber, John Dewey, and Sigmund Freud. These men have suggested possibilities for further research, and investigators have since attempted to test the validity and reliability of these theorists' findings. Research based on these theories has provided possibilities for other investigators, making it clear that the second-generation research was valuable. Similarly, if the researcher can provide this quality of theory and this type of stimulus for future investigators, then such studies will be proven valuable.

Another estimate of the worth of a study is its importance to human beings. Since nursing is inextricably involved with human beings, all nursing research is ultimately aimed at improving health care. Every project in nursing research should be of value to the profession. An investigation that improves human living conditions would certainly have great importance. To know that more men then women travel by train may not be important; a new clinical procedure to make patients more comfortable is important.

The extent to which a study fits into a discipline or into other disciplines is an indicator of its value. If a study has implications that go beyond simple fact, if it builds toward a theory, or if it has implications for an additional discipline, its rating is increased among investigators. Quite often the real value of a research study cannot be tested or proved until many years later when the full impact of its extensiveness is realized.

The degree to which the findings of research are accepted by other members of the discipline or by the investigator's colleagues is a further indication of the study's worth. Researchers who are thorough, use systematic methodology, and design their research with understanding and insight gain the professional respect of their colleagues.

The type of criticism given a research project is important. If the study is published in a professional journal, it is interesting to note any criticism it may receive. Sometimes criticism cannot hide the worth of a truly valuable study. Freud has been greatly criticized for many years by some segments of the population; but in spite of the criticism, there are many who feel that his findings have real value.

Worthwhile research should suggest some uses for the findings. Why should research be done if it is not going to generate useful information? Research can be done for the pure joy of learning and because there is an interest in the topic; but it seems valuable, logical, and desirable to design a study that benefits people in general—a study that would go to the heart of some problem.

Researchers must consider the practicality of a study. Research on the scale of a grand theory, which is difficult to put to an empirical test, might not be as valuable as a study that is practical. Suppose, for example, that we were attempting to develop a new type of teaching technique for clinical nursing. The new technique would be more practical than a new nursing philosophy; yet a philosophy might prove more valuable in the long run. Certainly a new technique that resulted in improved clinical nursing would be more practical and could be put to immediate use. This is not to discount the possibility that philosophy could contribute to a practical effect.

IMPLICATIONS

Implications are concerned with the anticipated meaning or the value of the data. Through them, the researcher can explain the findings' potential influence on specific groups or populations. Helpful suggestions are given for using the new knowledge for making decisions.

Implications drawn from a research report are the offshoot of inductive and deductive reasoning. Data gathered during the collecting period must be interpreted. Although certain techniques can be carried out by mechanical means, nothing replaces the reasoning power and wisdom of the human mind. Researchers draw conclusions from their studies, but what do their project mean to the whole population? Would findings in their samples hold for the universe?

Researchers must have insight, vision, and creativity to discover the implications of the study for the discipline that it serves. By taking the bits of ingredients that made up the data, researchers formulate the questions: "What could result from the mixing and compiling of these bits and pieces?" "What could be the result of adding all the ingredients together?" Inductive reasoning makes possible the process of going from the specific to the whole.

On the other hand, if the effect, or the whole, was observed, what ingredients was it made of? What can be deduced or concluded from the whole? If the cause was studied as the whole, then what specific elements did the study reveal? The researcher will, of course, have to use inductive or deductive reasoning, depending on the approach to the problem or question under investigation. Skill in establishing possible implications from research is not developed overnight; but as the researcher continues to learn more about a discipline and its context, he/she will be better able to determine what benefits the study holds for his/her discipline, the community, and the population in general.

Implications are based on the researcher's conclusions and express specific suggestions for implementation. For example, high school counselors should be well informed about the various types of nursing programs as well as courses leading to RN licensure so that they may encourage students to make a discriminating choice of schools.

RECOMMENDATIONS FOR FURTHER STUDY

In the recommendations section, the researcher suggests two or three other studies that could be carried out as an extension of the present research project. He/she may recommend that most or all of the design be repeated on a larger scale or in another setting.

Recommendations are the consensus of agreement reached from implications, limitation, generalizations, and conclusions. The researcher bases his/her recommendations for similar studies or for other research on these statements. For example, the researcher might suggest: "A study of the reasons why more than 5 out of 10 students would advise a friend who wants to become a nurse to enroll in College Y rather than in College Z. A study could be conducted using students enrolled in both colleges in more than one selected year. In-depth responses could be obtained by using interviews."

Recommendations for further research may be presented as a list similar to that used for the conclusions. A brief description of the proposed methodology and a statement concerning the usefulness of such a study provides other researchers with ideas and encouragement to become involved in the present investigator's area of interest.

SUMMARY

The evaluation takes place after the data are analyzed and includes generalizations about the findings. Generalization is extending the results of the data at hand to a broader population. Generalizations move from the sample to the general world. Sample size is an important factor in determining how far we can generalize. The purposes of generalization are to predict and to control.

The extent to which the findings of research are accepted is another consideration in the evaluation process. There are three factors involved: (1) the study needs to be well documented; (2) the study must provide complete details; and (3) there must be wide distribution of the findings, if possible.

The final portion of the research report is a discussion of the conclusions and of the relationship of the findings to the real world. The conclusions should point out what was learned from the study.

The value of a study may be estimated by its relationship to an important theory, its new or unique results, its universality, its importance to human beings, its acceptance by other members of the discipline, and its publication.

DISCUSSION QUESTIONS

1 Why is it desirable to critique a research study?
2 Distinguish between generalizations made by the public and generalizations based on research findings.
3 Comment on the following statement, "The evaluation process is open to more personal bias than any other part of research."
4 Comment on the following statement, "If you can critique research studies, you will most likely be able to conduct good research." Defend your position.
5 Discuss the relationship between theory and evaluation research.
6 Why would it be possible for two researchers to arrive at different conclusions from the same piece of research? Or is it possible?
7 What is the difference between evaluation research and evaluating research?
8 What are the limitations of a generalization?
9 Why are the conclusions an important component of a research report?

10 What are the advantages of including the implications of the study with the study reports?
11 Of what benefit are the recommendations for further research?

CLASS ACTIVITIES

Track I

1 The instructor distributes research articles or reports to each group of three to five students. The groups are to critique the handouts.
2 The instructor distributes two research articles to each group of three or four students. Each group reads research articles A and B and then compares the quality of the articles as to their clarity, their completeness, and the quality of their research designs.

Track II (Steps in Research Project)

1 Each student is to determine the generalizations, conclusions, implications of their study findings and develop recommendations for further research.
2 Members of groups are to choose the best statements from each member for their research report.

SUGGESTED READINGS

Cooper, H.M., and Rosenthal, R.: Statistical versus traditional procedures for summarizing research findings, Psychological Bulletin **87**:442–449, 1980.

Fleming, J.W., and Hayter, J.: Reading research reports critically, Nurs. Outlook **22**(3):174–175, March 1974.

Gay, L.R.: Educational research: competencies for analysis and application, Ed. 2, Columbus, 1981, Charles E. Merrill Publishing Company.

Gulick, E.E.: Evaluating research requests: a model for the nursing director, J. Nurs. Admin. **11**(1):26–30, January 1981.

Issues in evaluation research, An invitational conference, Dec. 10–12, 1975. American Nurses' Association, ANA Publication Code No. G-124.

Kosecoff, J. and Fink, A.: Evaluation basics, Beverly Hills, 1982, Sage Publications, Inc.

Miles, M.B.: Qualitative data as an attractive nuisance: the problem of analysis. In Van Maanen, J., ed.: Qualitative methodology, Beverly Hills, 1983, Sage Publications, Inc.

Partridge, C.J.: The outcome of physiotherapy and its measurement, Physiotherapy **68**(11):362–363, November 1982.

Riddoch, J.: The future of research in physiotherapy, Physiotherapy **68**(11):358–360, November 1982.

Snow, R.E.: Representative and quasi-representative designs for research on teaching, Review of Educational Research **44**(3):270, Summer 1974.

Stetler, C.B., and Marram, G.: Evaluating research findings for applicability in practice, Nurs. Outlook **24**(9):559–563, September 1976.

Walberg, H.J.: Quantification reconsidered, in W. Gordon, ed.: Review of research in education, 11. Washington, D.C., 1984, American Educational Research Association.

Ward, M.J., and Fetler, M.E.: What guidelines should be followed in critically evaluating research reports? Nurs. Res. **28**(2):120–126, March–April 1979.

PART SIX

Presentation of Findings

Part Six, the concluding section of the book, contains three chapters that deal with the preparation of the research report, the publication process, and utilization of the research findings.

Chapter 25 contains a discussion of the format and process of writing up the report in an acceptable form for dissemination. This chapter also includes examples of visual aids that may be used within the text of the research report.

Chapter 26 contains information to assist the researcher in writing and preparing a manuscript for publication in periodicals, and books, as well as in monographs. The writing of abstracts and copyrighting details are included.

This section closes with a discussion, in Chapter 27, of the utilization of research by the practitioner, educator, and administrator.

CHAPTER 25

WRITING THE RESEARCH REPORT

Writing the research report is, of course, the pinnacle of the whole research process. Investigators have a moral obligation to share their research findings.

Beginning researchers will find good examples of content and format in professional journals. It is imperative that they be acquainted with the correct format and components of a research report so that their work will receive attention and approval.

The writing of the research findings, or for that matter any written report, is facilitated by use of a detailed outline. If a researcher needs a 10-page report that covers 5 important areas, that researcher should have perhaps 2 pages for each of the 5 areas. This outline should map out the logical sequence of the report, determine the length, and ensure complete coverage of the material. Such planning facilitates the writing process and establishes the format of the written report.

Even though the writing of the research report is the capstone of the process, it is often given the least amount of effort. Apparently, researchers, especially beginning investigators, spend so much time getting started that they rush the completion of the project and take shortcuts in writing the report. Original or first drafts are, without exception, unacceptable. More than one draft is required before a report is in polished form.

The format (discussed later) is usually the same regardless of the discipline. Some sections must be included in all research reports. The research report should follow the order of the original investigation. We cannot emphasize too often or too strongly that all details of the research process should be included. We have already stressed the need for replication studies; yet a good replication study can succeed only when the original researchers provide complete and thorough details of their research methods.

It is a well-known fact that many research studies have produced valuable information, were conceptually sound, were methodically researched, and presented new ideas and yet were not published because the authors were unable to communicate the results through the written word. Many authors do not use a straightforward style and language, perhaps because they do not know how important writing skills are in research reports. Two criticisms that can be made of many research reports are that they do not contain enough details and that they are not written in a concise, simple style.

Even in scholarly reports, it is often difficult to find the hypothesis. Beginning researchers especially seem unable to state their hypothesis in a single sentence. Perhaps

□For the writing of this chapter, we adapted classroom materials generously provided by Cyril J. Hoyt, University of Minnesota. Used with permission of Dr. Hoyt.

they do not take the time before the study to formulate a scientific hypothesis that is conceptually clear and empirically testable. A research report should state the hypothesis clearly: "The hypothesis is. . . . " If there are several hypotheses in a given study, it may be best to number them.

Writing a research report is similar to writing a good sermon. The pastor tells the people what he is going to say, then he tells them, and then he explains what he has told them. Jesus used examples as a means of clarification. Abstract ideas should be expressed as clearly, concisely, and simply as possible. Beyond that, an illustration may be given to reinforce or clarify ideas.

The study report need not be filled with large words to be scholarly, nor should the report be wordy. Part of the rewriting procedure involves striking out words like *these, that, those,* and *it* and substituting words that add clarity. The research findings should be readable and available to scholars and nonscholars alike. Most disciplines are criticized for having their own technical jargon. The use of nontechnical language in any research report increases the size of its audience. This is not to say that the writer cannot use literary techniques to enliven dull, flat prose.

The word *I* should be avoided in research reports. Substitute "it was found," "the research revealed," or some similar phrase. Avoid using such adjectives as *very* and *really*. Use terms that express definiteness, if possible. When the situation is not certain, words such as *probable, possibly,* and *seemingly* are appropriate substitutes.

Requirements for the well-written research report are conciseness, clarity, honesty, completeness, and accuracy.

Conciseness is the state of being brief, yet thorough. A concise report says a great deal in a few words. Concise writing is terse and succinct. A concise style saves the reader's time and requires fewer pages of reading material. It also forces the writer to rethink and refine his/her ideas.

Clarity is lucidity of expression. The thought or meaning is readily understandable. If a single reader does not understand a statement in the report, then the statement is not clear.

Honesty means free from fraud. It can mean admitting failure. Honesty is making clear the separation between opinions and facts, using accurate quotations and footnotes, admitting that the hypothesis was accepted or rejected, and not changing hypotheses for conscience's sake or capitalizing on serendipity as a substitute for insight.

Completeness requires that the researcher report all important details of the study. Writers must place themselves in the position of the naive, disinterested reader and include all the information needed for enlightenment. Often the researcher is afraid to reveal too many details about the sample or methods for fear of being criticized. We contend that the more a study can be criticized, the more completely (better) it has been written.

Accuracy is the quality of being precise and error free. It is difficult to be accurate because it is so tempting to estimate figures rather than to go to the trouble of rechecking; however, data should be exact. The researcher should avoid broad generalizations. Rounding off percentages to cover up "no response" answers is neither accurate nor honest. Such techniques as adding the pilot study data to the main project to enlarge the sample size are neither fair nor accurate. Accuracy often hurts one's pride but dishonesty may lower the reader's opinion of the investigator.

A researcher can expect to rewrite a report several times, so at least a week should be set aside for writing a 10- to 20-page research paper. How many themes, term papers, and research reports are written the night before they are due? Why minimize a good research project by placing it in a deficient package?

RESEARCH REPORT FORMAT

Whereas theses and dissertations are often divided into six chapters, research reports are divided into sections. These sections should follow the order in which the study is done. Professional research articles tend to follow this same basic format.

Just as the conceptual framework of a research study aids the researcher in designing the project, the format used in reporting the proceedings serves as the vehicle to transport the reader through the maze of information that makes up the formal report. In fact, the format of the research report provides the first notion about the quality of the contents just as the test for face validity carries an instant impression about an instrument.

The research paper may be divided into three parts: introduction; presentation and analysis of data; and summary, conclusions, and recommendations. Or it may have introductory pages (title, table of contents and lists of tables and figures); a main body (problem, purpose, definitions, review of literature, design of the study, descriptive techniques, presentation and analysis of data, summary, conclusions, implications and recommendations for future research); and a bibliography and appendix. Altschul urges researchers to report details of the beginning and the end of the research process.[1] To facilitate writing each section, the researcher must rethink the process that was involved in developing the design.

MECHANICS OF WRITING THE REPORT

The written report may use a combination of prose and visual presentations such as tables, charts, and graphs. Good visual aids assist the investigator in clarifying the meaning of the information, as well as improving the appearance and readability of the report. Poor visual aids undermine the quality of the research and confuse the reader. If the tables and graphs are slipshod and crowded, they can bring the accuracy of the entire paper into question. The researcher's basic objective in using the visual presentation is to arrange statistical material in a kind of order or classification so that its meaning and significance can be easily and quickly understood by the reader.

Illustrations

Any visual illustration other than a table is designated as a figure (Fig. or Figure). These include graphs, maps, blueprints, charts, photographs, and diagrams. Illustrations are numbered consecutively in each section or throughout the report. The figure number

[1] Altschul, Annie: "Beginning and End," *Nurs. Times* 70 (19): 718 (May 9, 1974), pp. 7, 8.

should be placed below the illustration along with a caption that explains the content of the figure.

A chart is a form designed to provide fluctuating information. It is often called a map or a graph. Distinguishing between charts, graphs, and maps can be difficult; some authors use the terms interchangeably.

A graph is a pictorial representation of a form of numerical data. It has connecting lines between a series of points and is most often drawn on ruled or lined paper. There are several types: line graphs, bar graphs, histograms, and pie graphs.

Graphs make use of lines to visually portray quantities or relationships of figures. They give an added dimension to tables by allowing for visual interpretation of the data. Pie graphs are often used to show proportions, such as how the nurse's work day is divided proportionally. Pie graphs show percentages, whereas bar graphs portray frequencies. A pie graph can be made by first drawing a circle and then using a protractor to divide the 360 degrees into sections similar to slices of pie. The sections represent portions of the whole. For example, in our illustration of the nurse's workday, the total number of hours would represent the whole, and each section of the pie would represent the amount of time spent doing each type of activity. If a nurse does one activity 20% of the time, it would be represented by 72 degrees of the circle. Pie graphs have a figure number, and in addition each section of the pie is identified by a label and by the corresponding percentage (Fig. 25-1).

A bar graph may be vertical or horizontal. Fig. 25-2 is an illustration of a bar graph. Fig. 23-12 is an example of a histogram. Note that the histogram is commonly built over the midpoint of each interval.

A diagram may take many forms. One of these, a sociogram, portrays the friendship patterns of a group of students (Fig. 25-3). Such a drawing could be used to visually present the data resulting from observations, interviews, and questionnaires.

An organization chart is another type of diagram (Fig. 25-4). Blueprints also may be called charts (Fig. 25-5). They provide the exact measurements and the design of a proposed physical facility. Another type of schematic drawing is a flow chart (see Fig. 1-1). It portrays a process or the steps in an activity.

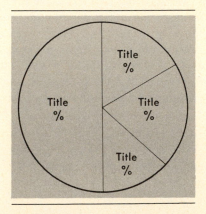

FIGURE 25-1   Pie graph.

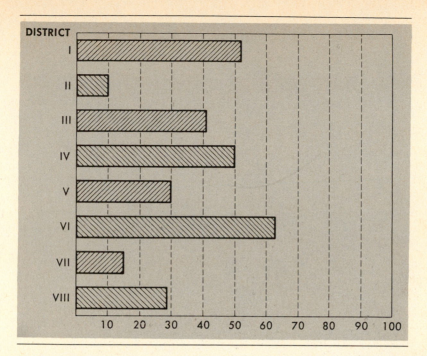

FIGURE 25-2 Bar graph: percent of members from each district who attended the state, convention (may be vertical or horizontal).

Hatwig and Dearing discuss the stem and leaf display.[2] The stem and leaf display is a type of visual interpretation of data which is a combination of frequency histogram or polygraph (see Fig. 25-6).

On the left side of the figure are the interval scores. The top line includes the range of scores from 31 to 40. On the right side of the figure, students earned scores of 35, 39, and 40. This type of display is similar to a histogram in a horizontal rather than a vertical position. It provides a useful visual display of data as well as a curve of frequencies. The stem leaf display has many possibilities for practical application to grading as well as to research.

The researcher should make creative use of any of these techniques to help the reader to understand the study results.

Arrangement of the Report

The report has a standard form similar to that of term papers, theses, and doctoral dissertations. The content may vary according to the type of research done, but the format remains basically the same. Research reports, whether done by a professional or by a beginning researcher, should follow a somewhat standardized form.

A standardized format meets some of the same demands as the standardizing of automobile parts. Three reasons for using a standardized form are as follows:

[2]Hartwig, F., with Dearing, B.E.: Exploratory Data Analysis, Series 07-016, Beverly Hills, 1979, Sage Publications, Inc.

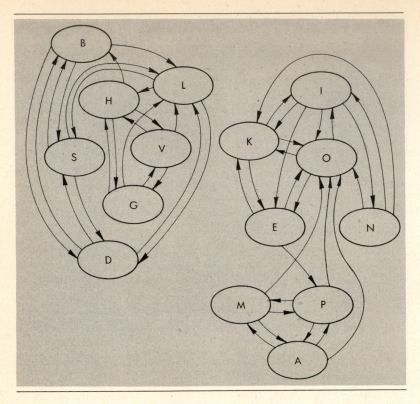

FIGURE 25-3   Sociogram.

1. Appearance. Arrangement in the prescribed format provides the most pleasing appearance.
2. Convenience. The traditional form was developed to meet the needs of those people who are constantly working in research. They have found that standardization makes for efficiency. They know where to look for the report title, author's name, bibliography, and so on, without having to search for them. Printers, readers, and workers in related fields can do their work more efficiently when there is standardization.
3. Guidelines. If there were no rules, researchers would find it difficult to write up the report of their findings. Organization of the report is easier when there are guidelines to follow.

The text of the research report follows several pages of introductory material beginning with the title page.

Title Page

The title page contains the name of the report, which may be typed in capital letters. If more than two lines are required for the title, these lines may be typed to form an inverted pyramid. The title should be worded in straightforward language so that the reader can have a clue as to the content of the report. These are so many different formats that no specific one can be recommended. The rule is, be consistent.

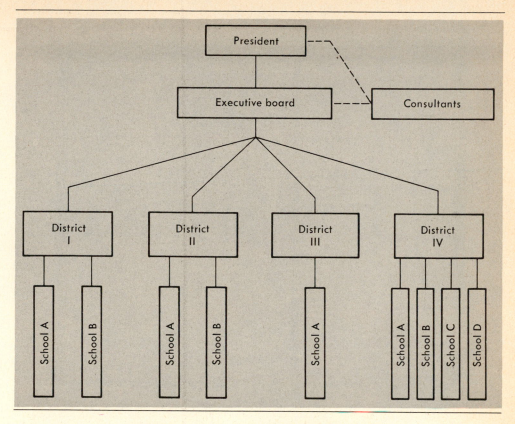

FIGURE 25-4   State nursing student organization plan.

The author's name may be typed near the center of the page or along one of the margins under the word "by." The center of the page is usually preferred. The name of the author may be capitalized and is spelled as it is normally written.

The purpose of the research project may be included at the bottom of the page under the title. The purpose of the project could be to fulfill an educational requirement for a course or a degree, or it could be to carry out a study for an organization, which has supplied funds for the project.

Acknowledgments

Acknowledgments may be made in the first section if they are deemed appropriate. The acknowledgment page may be titled in capital letters. It mentions those who contributed to the success of the research study and the preparation of the report.

Table of Contents

The table of contents may list each of the major headings and subheadings of the report along with their page numbers. No information in the report other than the headings and subheadings is provided in the table of contents. This means that there cannot be a table of contents if the headings have been omitted from the report. Every research report

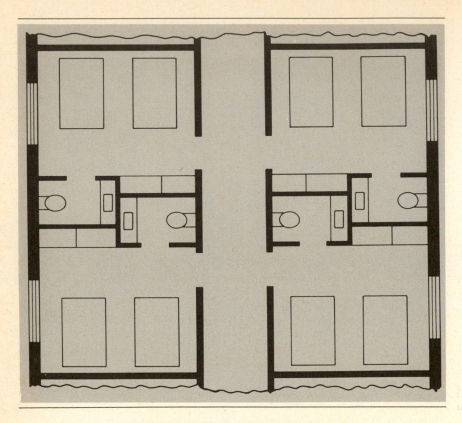

FIGURE 25-5 Blueprint of a hospital unit.

SCORES ON A HYPOTHETICAL EXAM	
31-40	5 9 0
41-50	4 6 8
51-60	3 3 7 8 9
61-70	4 5 7 8 9 9
71-80	1 2 2 4 6
81-90	1 6 8 9
91-100	2 3 3
interval	scores
(stem)	(leaves)

FIGURE 25-6 Stem and leaf display.

should have divisions that are identified in the text and are readily located in the table of contents.

If an outline is to be included in the research report, it may be placed after the table of contents.

List of Tables

Tables are listed in the order in which they are presented in the text of the report. The table number, full title, and page number should be included.

List of Figures

The list of figures follows the list of tables and is arranged in chronological order. It includes the figure number, the full title, and the page number.

Text

The body of the research report (text) follows the list of tables or figures if included. The title of the research project may be repeated at the top of the first page.

Headings show organization and assist the reader in determining the steps of the report, so they are a necessity. Major division headings are centered on the page and typed in all capitals. Subtopics are placed at the left margin, in regular type, and underlined. If an additional heading is needed in the text, several extra spaces may be used to set that heading off from the topic above and below.

Pages may be numbered at the upper righthand corner, except for the first page of each section where the number usually appears in the center bottom margin.

The text of the research report begins with the problem and purpose of the study. The hypotheses or study questions are cited, followed by the definition of terms, delimitations, and assumptions.

The literature review covers the pertinent studies that were related to the topic of interest and provides the reader with a background knowledge of similarities and differences between the present study and prior research. The sample and/or population and general collection procedures are described next. Revisions made as a result of the pilot study should be included. Findings compose the major part of the text; they need to be in visual and prose form. Results of each test of the hypotheses are reported. Reliability and validity of the instrument and the study are discussed along with the limitations. Any other pertinent findings are reported.

The conclusions, implications, and recommendations for further study make up the final section of the text. This is followed by the bibliography and appendices.

A research report can be dull reading. Including subjects' comments in the margins of questionnaires or asides made by interviewers adds flavor to the report.

Footnotes

Footnotes are an important part of a research report since they document the text. They may appear either at the bottom of the page or on a separate page at the end of the text. The footnotes, bibliography, and appendix complete the research report.

Credit is always given for any material quoted or paraphrased. Unique ideas or special wording also must be credited to the original author. In some cases it is difficult to know when to give credit.

A footnote should never refer to material contained in more than one paragraph unless it is a direct quotation of more than one paragraph. If there are complicated or extensive tables, lists, instruments, and so on, they may be placed in the Appendix along with a footnote stating that the reader may see the material (specified) in Appendix _____.

When material is quoted word for word, it must be enclosed in quotation marks or set apart as an indented paragraph if more than approximately 40 words in length. Suppose an hypothetical quotation is being considered for discussion. The basic quotation is cited in example 1. The quotation is placed correctly on the page and is footnoted, as it should be. Notice that the footnote number follows punctuation marks, except in the case of a dash.

Example 1: Quotation—Correct

Sociologists are often questioned concerning their interest in nursing as a research topic. Their interest is not limited to lack of opportunity in other disciplines but to the unique placement of the nursing profession within the emotion-laden sphere of critical personal involvement. Hour after hour, crucial decisions must be made. Death or life hangs in the balance. How long can the human machine stand the pressure of making commitments to preserve the health of society? Cases must eventually become only routine. "What happens," the sociologist asks, "when crisis becomes routine?"[1]

The rule is that if the paragraph is an entire or partial quotation, credit must be given to the source. It is correct for the writer to cite the name of the source along with a quotation, but the quotation must be in the originator's exact words. It would be incorrect if the student wrote the following statement, citing it as a part of the original quotation, when it is really just a poor paraphrase.

Example 2: Quotation—Incorrect

Smith has said, "Sociologists do not study nursing because it is unique, but rather because it is a discipline that accepts death and illness as a matter of routine."[1]

If Smith's original paragraph brings to mind something the writer already knew, there is no reason for him to give Smith credit. But if a writer quotes Smith directly or uses his exact terminology, then Smith must be given credit. In example 3 we find a statement that might be common knowledge to some people who have nursing experience. In this case, the statement need not be footnoted.

Example 3: Quotation—Correct

Sociologists are interested in studying the nursing field because in nursing life and death become routine matters.

Example 4 is incorrect because Smith's name is not included within the context of the quoted material and because many of the original words and phrases of the author were used. The correct method is given in example 5.

Example 4: Quotation—Incorrect

Sociologists are often asked why they study nursing. The answer seems to be the unique placement of the nursing profession in a position demanding crucial decisions. Death and life hang in the balance. Sociologists study nursing because nursing is a discipline that must face crisis on a routine basis.[1]

Example 5: Quotation—Correct

Smith remarks that sociologists are often asked why they study nursing.... [1]

Footnotes, either at the bottom of the page or at the end of the paper, have different contents from an alphabetically arranged bibliographical citation. The footnote furnishes the name of the author, title of the article or chapter, title of the book, editor's name (if there is one), and volume of the periodical or book. Date of publication and page number are included for both books and periodicals, whereas the place of publication and the publishing company also are included for book citations.

Some journals do not publish footnotes and bibliography separately. Rather, all references are given alphabetically (for the reader's convenience), with complete information. Each bibliographical citation is assigned a number in the text, and the footnote uses the corresponding bibliographical numbers. This system is difficult to handle, since the paper must be completely written before footnotes can be numbered.

A widely used procedure in professional journals is skipping footnotes entirely. References are simply noted by author's last name and year of publication (in parentheses) within the text of the report. To look up the source, the reader must refer to the bibliography. There are two major weaknesses in this method: (1) no page numbers are given to locate the bibliographic citation, and (2) the reader must turn to the bibliographical section to find the source. If the author happens to have written several books or articles, the reader is required to search through the titles until the correct one is found.

The most time-consuming method of footnoting for the writer but the most convenient for the reader is the placing of footnotes at the bottom of the page on which the quoted or paraphrased information appears.

The following examples of footnotes are fictitious. Note that the author's name is listed with given name first and that the format presented is only one of many that may be used.

Format for Book

Author's name, *Title of Book*, name of editor, translator, or compiler, edition (other than first) (place of publication, date of publication) volume in Roman numerals if more than one, page or pages referred to.

[1] Mary Smith, *Nursing in Utopia*, John Watson (ed.) (New York, 1980), pp. 16–18.
[2] Allen Foster, *The Male Nurse* (Chicago, 1982), p. 45.
[3] A.B. Lockhart and C.A. Banner, "The Second Child." In Margaret Reed, *The Family*, 2nd ed. (New York, 1981), I, 208.

Format for Periodicals

Author's name, "Title of Article," *Name of Periodical*, volume number in Roman numerals (date of periodical issue), page number.

[4] Pamela Waltman, "Care of the Handicapped Child," *Health Concepts*, XI (March, 1979), 403.
[5] Louann Richey, "The Future Nurse," *Journal of National Nursing*, X (April, 1980), 257.
[6] Don Michaels, et al., "Let's Write About Nursing," *Health Journal*, February 2, 1985, p. 14.

Abbreviations Used in Second Footnote References

We suggest that only the author's last name, volume number (for books) if there is more than one, and the pages be included in second references.

[6]Smith, p. 22.

[7]*Ibid.*, p. 22. (*Ibid.*, meaning "in the same place," is frequently used when the work referred to is the same as in the immediately preceding footnote.)

[8]Foster, *op. cit.,* p. 48. (*Op. cit.,* meaning "in work cited," is used when the work cited is not the one immediately preceding.)

[9]Richey, "The Future Nurse," p. 258. (When the author has written more than one work that is cited in the report, the title of the work should be included in the reference.)

[10]Richey, *loc. cit.* (*Loc. cit.,* meaning "in the place cited," is used when the page reference is the same as that cited the last time the work was referred to.)

Miscellaneous Abbreviations

Miscellaneous abbreviations

ca.	about, example: ca. 1941
cf.	compare, example: cf. (24)
comp.	compiled by, compiler
e.g.	for example
ed.	editor (pl. eds.), edition, edited
et al.	and others
f., ff.	and following pages
i.e.	that is
n.d.	no date, example: Los Angeles, n.d.
sec.	section
trans.	translated by, translator

Bibliography

The bibliography contains the list of authors cited alphabetically by last names. The bibliographical citation includes the author's name, name of article, and name of book or periodical (underlined). Inclusive pages of the periodical article and the book publisher's name also are included in the bibliography. It should be possible for a reader to look up one of the works cited on the basis of the information furnished in the bibliography.

When typing the bibliography, if more than one line is needed, note that the second line is usually indented five spaces. Footnotes and bibliographical citations are extremely important. If readers become interested in the content of a research report, they may look up a few of the references for themselves. However, unless sufficient information is provided, readers will not know where to look. The page number must be included in the footnotes to enable the readers to find the quotation or reference. A research report that uses careful footnoting indicates the author's honesty.

There is a growing confusion about the meaning of references and bibliography. A bibliography is a list of the sources used in the report, whereas a list of references sometimes includes other appropriate literature. References are usually citations of works that were referred to but may or may not have been quoted or paraphrased. If numbers are used in the text to identify citations, each citation may be numbered in order and listed at the end of the report as a reference. In this case, the first reference is listed first, and so on.

Illustrations of entries in a selected bibliography are as follows (fictitious).[3]

---

[3]The format for these bibliographical listings is one of many different formats that may be used.

Format for Books

Author (alphabetically). *Title*. City: publisher, year, pages.

Anderson, Betty (ed.). *Theories of Health Care*. Midwest, Ind.: Jackson & Company, 1980.

Olsen, Charles. "The Effects of Stress." in A.C. Collier (ed.). *Perceptions of Anxiety*. New York: Nelson Publishers, 1984, pp. 61–75.

Wilson, A.C., Jr. *The Management of Coronary Care Units*. New York: Nelson Publishers, 1985.

Format for Periodicals

Author (alphabetically). "Article." *Publication*, date, **volume**, pages.

Donaldson, James. "The Value of Hobbies." *State Health Systems*, 1986, **42**(3), 55–61. (NOTE: If each issue has independent pagination, the issue number follows the volume number, in parentheses.)

Field, Pamela. "Care of the Handicapped Child." *Health Concepts*, 1979, **42**, 400–405.

Michaels, Peter. "Why Nursing?" *Health Journal*, June 12, 1979, pp. 22–24.

Richey, Louann. "The Future Nurse." *Journal of National Nursing*, 1985, **10**, 250–260.

The major differences between the formats for footnotes and bibliographies are that in an alphabetically arranged bibliography the author's surname is listed first and periods are used to punctuate after the author's name, the title of the material, and the date. Commas and parentheses replace the periods in a footnote.[4]

Appendix

The appendix is placed at the end of the research report. It may include copies of the instrument, correspondence form letters, follow-up instrument, and detailed tables. It contains information that would be too extensive to be included in a footnote. When there is more than one type of inclusion (for example, copies of letters, charts, or tables), appendices should be titled and numbered or lettered consecutively (for example, Appendix 1, Appendix 2, etc., or Appendix A, Appendix B, etc). The pages of the appendix are numbered in consecutive order similar to the other sections of the report. If institutions participate in the research project, then they should be listed along with a description of their type, purpose, and so on, if this information is not part of the text. The appendix furnishes the reader with other materials that are either too bulky or too detailed to be included in the body of the paper. All information and data essential to the reader's understanding of the report should be included.

POSTER PRESENTATION

A new method of presenting a research study is known as a poster session. Traditionally research papers have been presented at conferences by researchers who read their report. Although scholarship is good and necessary, listening to 30 minutes of research findings presented in a monotone is not anticipated with enthusiasm. The answer to relief of boredom is a poster session. A poster session is a visual display of the basic information from a research study.

[4]A manual of style, ed. 12, Chicago, 1969, The University of Chicago Press, p. 340.

A large piece of poster board, approximately 18"×27", is used as a base to mount the 5 to 7 sections of a research report. Sometimes the report is printed or painted directly on the poster board. More often, pages are typed and pasted or stapled to the board. Posters should include the researcher's name, title of the research, hypothesis, research design, findings, data in tables, conclusions, a brief abstract, and a statement of accepting or rejecting the hypothesis and the level of significance.

The researcher often stands near the poster to interact with readers. Viewers can ask questions, make suggestions, discuss further research, and exchange addresses for future communication concerning additional research. On occasion, the researcher may provide a handout, have a slide presentation, overhead transparencies, or other visual aids.

Advantages

1. The presentation method is more interesting.
2. Viewers can observe several research studies in the time it would ordinarily take for the reading of one research report.
3. Viewers can select those projects they find most interesting.
4. Authors are available to answer questions, which may not be possible when one or two researchers present papers. Often, it seems that the first presenter takes most of the time allotted for presentation and each following presenter gets less and less.
5. The researcher is forced to condense the project to the essential information.

Disadvantages

1. The poster is difficult to transport and requires a stand or other support for display.
2. There may be 10 to 20 poster presentations in a room, all vying for attention. Potential viewers may be overwhelmed and not bother looking at any posters.
3. In a crowded room, it is often difficult to get close enough to read the details on typewritten pages.
4. After reading several poster projects, the novelty is gone and viewers lose interest. While attending a recent display of posters it was observed that many potential viewers looked in the display room but never entered.

One suggestion to improve poster sessions is for the researcher to vary his/her presentation by limiting a slide session to 6 to 10 slides shown over a 3- to 4-minute period of time.

SUMMARY

Writing the research report is the highlight of the research project. Most disciplines are criticized for their use of technical jargon. The number of readers can be increased by use of simple straightforward language. More than one revision is necessary to put the report in its final form.

The format for any written study is basically the same. A written report should follow the order of the original investigation and ought to include all the details of the research process. Good replication studies are possible only when the original researcher has given a thorough description of his study. Reports from beginning researchers frequently lack sufficient details and simple, concise language. Writers should avoid using words such as *these, that, those,* and *it.* Definite statements are preferred to vague generalities. The research report should be

1. Concise—not redundant. Conciseness saves the reader's time and forces the writer to refine his ideas.
2. Clear—lucidly expressed. Clarity helps the reader to understand the points being made.
3. Honesty—free from fraud. Honesty is necessary to maintain the respect of the reader and the integrity of the author.
4. Complete—fully detailed. Completeness helps the reader to evaluate the study.
5. Accurate—precise and error free. Accuracy is necessary to maintain the integrity of the author in the eyes of the reader.

The research report is generally divided into six sections that include (1) formulation of the problem, (2) review of the literature, (3) hypothesis, (4) design and conduct of the study, (5) analysis of data, and (6) conclusions. If one desires, the number of sections may be changed, but the content remains the same. The first section includes purpose, background, and assumptions.

The second section discusses the research findings of similar studies. The important literature can be summarized in a few pages. Often a broad approach to the review of literature is preferable to a narrow viewpoint that cites a few studies in detail.

The third section is usually reserved for a discussion of the hypothesis. The hypothesis should be explicit. It may be stated in either the null form or the scientific form. The null form does not suggest the end result, whereas the scientific or positive hypothesis predicts the anticipated findings.

The next section contains all details related to procedure. It describes the instrument, gives details of administration, considers tests of validity and reliability, and provides information concerning the sample.

The fifth section of the research report contains an analysis of the data. If space is available, the researcher should give a breakdown of responses to every item. Tables developed for those items judged relevant to the hypothesis are necessary. Discussion of the tables should precede their placement on a page. Tables, graphs, and charts are preferable to prose descriptions.

The final section provides a synthesis of the findings and relates the various aspects of the study to the discipline in general. The conclusion of the report is not a place for new material, but a place for comprehensive evaluation and generalizations. The limitations of the study are included in the final section. The purpose of citing the limitations is for the researcher to point out weaknesses and to criticize the research process. Limitations are especially valuable for readers who may attempt similar studies, because they can benefit from the shortcomings of the present research. Other topics of the final section are the implications and recommendations for further study.

The mechanics of a written report require a combination of skills in both verbal and visual presentation. Prose definitions can be assisted by visual aids in the form of graphs, charts, and tables.

The written report should have a consistent form and should include subheadings as well as major divisions. The standardized format is preferred because it is easy for printers and readers to follow, has a pleasing appearance, and provides suitable guidelines.

The major parts of the research report are the title page, acknowledgments, table of contents, list of tables, list of figures, text, footnotes, bibliography, and appendix. The honest writer must give full credit to other writers in the footnotes. Page numbers are valuable to the reader. There are different forms of footnoting. The method placing footnotes at the bottom of the page is the most difficult for the writer but the most convenient for the reader. The integrity of the writer is shown in his/her concern for accurate documentation.

Poster sessions are displays of the basic features of a research study. Hypotheses, study design, instrument, tables of data, and conclusions are presented in visual style on a large piece of poster board. Researchers stand beside their display to answer questions. Posters are more interesting than verbal presentations, but they are difficult to carry and display.

DISCUSSION QUESTIONS

1 What value is there for the researcher in writing the report?
2 What are the advantages and disadvantages of *not* writing the report?
3 Make a general statement about the contents of the research report.
4 Comment on the interplay between the prose discussion and the visual presentation in the research report.
5 Comment on the statement, "Tables should be able to stand alone."
6 Failure to document sources is a serious form of plagiarism. How and why has this developed?
7 What differences are there between writing a research report based on research conducted for a course and on research funded by a sponsor?
8 What type of information lends itself to visual presentation?
9 How many visual aids should be included in the text of a research report?
10 How does the information included in the appendix differ from that included in the text?

CLASS ACTIVITIES

Track I

1 Research reports are distributed by the instructor. Each student rewrites an assigned part of the report.
2 The instructor provides each student with a table of statistical data from newspapers or popular magazines. Each student analyzes the data and describes in prose what the table reveals.

Track II (Steps in Research Project)

1 Each student is to outline the format for writing the research report. One member of the group is selected to write the first draft. The first draft is then reviewed by the other group members.
2 Students are to draw illustrations and prepare the appendix.

SUGGESTED READINGS

Abdellah, Faye G., and Levine, Eugene: Better patient care through nursing research, ed. 2, New York, 1979, Macmillan, Inc.

Boehret, Alice C.: Without research we continue to reinvent the wheel, Am. J. Nurs. **74**(8):1408–1409, August 1974.

Boffey, Philip M.: Scientific data: 50 Pct. Unusable? Chronicle of Higher Education **10**(1):1, 6, February 24, 1975.

Brooks, Philip C.: Research in archives, the use of unpublished primary sources, Chicago, 1969, The University of Chicago Press.

Cheadle, J.: Presenting your research, Nurs. Mirror, pp. 26–28, May 4, 1978.

Daniels, L.B.: What is the language of the practical? Curriculum Theory Network 4(4):238–240, 1975, The Ontario Institute for Studies in Education, Toronto, Ontario, Canada.

Dunn, A.: How to write for publication: how to make the editor's life easier, Nurs. Times 74(40):1635–1636, October 1978.

Hall, E.T.: Why Americans can't write, Human Nature 1(8):74–79, August 1978.

Katz, S.B., and others: Resources for writing for publication in education, New York, 1980, Teachers College Press.

Knafl, K.A., and Howard, M.J.: Interpreting and reporting qualitative research, Research in Nursing and Health 7:17–24, 1984.

Kratz, C.: Preparing a research article, part 2, Nurs. Times 74:1634–1635, October 5, 1978.

Leedy, P.D.: Practical research planning and design, New York, 1980, Macmillan, Inc.

Mercer, Ramona T.: Eight stages of a doctoral dissertation, Nurs. Res. 23(5):435–436, 1974.

Myatt, W.: Stalking the wild semicolon, Santa Rosa, Calif., 1976, Thresh Publications.

O'Farrell, E.K.: Write for the reader, he may need to know what you have to say, Nurs. Educator 1(2):23–29, July–August 1976.

Powell, S.R., and others: Writing for publication: a group approach, Nurs. Outlook 27(11):729–732, November 1979.

Reproduction of copyrighted works by educators and librarians, Washington, D.C., 1978, Copyright Office, Library of Congress.

Strunk, W., and White, E.B.: The elements of style, ed. 3, New York, 1979, Macmillan, Inc.

University of Chicago. A manual of style, ed. 12, Chicago, 1969, University of Chicago Press.

Williams, Lillian B.: Evaluation of nursing care: a primary nursing project, Part I. Report of the controlled study, Supervisor Nurse 6(1):39, January 1975.

Zinsser, W.: On writing well, New York, 1976, Harper & Row Publishers.

CHAPTER 26

PUBLICATION OF THE RESEARCH REPORT

All research should be conducted with the publication of the findings in mind. Therefore the purpose of this chapter is to help beginning researchers share their findings with the public and their profession by offering them assistance in the preparation of their reports for publication. Regardless of how valuable the research findings are, unless they are made known, no one else can benefit from them.

A long research report may be from 300 to 500 pages in length, whereas a small study may be compressed into 10 pages. A long report, if suitable, could be published as a book or a monograph, and the findings and the description of a small study could be published as an article in a professional journal. One could also summarize the contents of a long report for publication in a periodical.

Although quantitative research methodology has been the major focus of this book, the authors have introduced qualitative research as another important type of research methodology. The publication of quantitative and qualitative research has some features in common and in other ways it differs. The general requirements for manuscripts, regulations for the use of quotations, the writing of abstracts, and copyrighting remain the same. What differs is the writing style and format. Qualitative research reporting will be especially welcomed by researchers who enjoy reading and writing the rich descriptive style that is the hallmark of qualitative research.

MANUSCRIPT FORMAT

The basic format for publication of quantitative research follows the order given in Chapter 25: formulation of the problem, review of the literature, hypotheses, design and conduct of the study, analysis of data, and conclusions. However, almost every publisher has a particular format that is unique to that organization. Therefore, the format will usually be outlined according to the editor's wishes. Many journals provide a brief description of the requirements for submitting a manuscript for publication and an address for further inquiry, which is usually found inside the front cover or with the table of contents.

General Requirements for Manuscripts

There are several general requirements for the preparation of manuscripts for publication. A manuscript should be typed, double-spaced, on quality paper with at least 1-inch margins. Wide margins provide space for the publisher to make comments and corrections. The size of the paper is the standard 8½ x 11 inches used in all research reports. Page numbers are usually placed in the upper righthand corner.

Other requirements concerning the length of the manuscript and the placement of footnotes, references, illustrations, and tables vary according to the publisher's preference. The usual manuscript length is from 1,000 to 2,000 words for articles in journals. Editors will specify the number of words in the prepared manuscript. They also will state the responsibilities the author has for preparing the manuscript and may set a deadline for submission.

The appearance of the manuscript should invite reading. Continuity, good grammar, correct punctuation, and appropriate headings and subheadings are expected. Visual material should be labeled for ease in understanding.

Periodicals

Before typing the manuscript for publication in a periodical, the researcher should investigate the current literature to find out which publishers usually accept such manuscripts. The librarian may be of assistance in suggesting additional periodicals with which the author is unfamiliar or which have only recently been established.

The researcher must consider four questions when selecting a publisher for the research report.

1. Is the article written in a style for the general reader or for professionals? Lay periodicals are designed for readers who may not have been educated in the profession but who have an interest in the findings. Sometimes the lay periodical contains material written by a professional that is free of the jargon peculiar to the discipline and is suitable for a lay reader. Professional periodicals are written for readers who have been educated in the discipline and who understand the technical vocabulary. News items pertinent to the profession, as well as job opportunities, may or may not be included.

2. What professional audience might be interested in the research results? Often, findings for a specific field also have implications for other disciplines. Many topics are of such a general nature that they may be of interest to more than one discipline. For example, findings in a nursing research study may be of great interest to anthropologists, sociologists, psychologists, and historians, as well as professionals in the health fields. It is true that the amount of literature published in any one discipline is so vast that professionals find it difficult to keep abreast of new research in their own area. Nevertheless, researchers will still find it worthwhile to consider publishing in the periodicals of other disciplines.

3. What type of publishing company publishes the kind of information contained in the article? A discipline may have a rather strict hierarchy of professional periodicals. The journal with the highest status, appropriate for more scholarly material, usually sets the highest standards for publication. This means that articles written by well-known writers and by those using technical language are given priority. Usually the prestigious periodical is interested in disseminating the findings of a large research project having a broad range of implications, a great deal of statistics, or a high level of theoretical abstraction. The

editor of the prestigious journal may be flooded with manuscripts, whereas the editor of smaller, lesser known journal may be in need of good manuscripts written by beginning researchers. Thus new authors should seek out a publisher and be satisfied to see their material published, no matter how small the distribution or the prestige of the publisher. The writer's commitment is to get the findings into print.

4. What type of articles does the journal usually publish? When a discipline is subdivided into a number of specialities, each may have one or more publications. Therefore, authors must determine which publications specialize in their type of manuscript. After having decided on one or two possible journals, the researcher should write the editor and either describe the article or enclose an abstract and ask if the editor is interested in reading the manuscript. If the editor is interested, he/she will inform the author of the next step to take. If the editor wishes to read the manuscript, he/she may request from one to three copies for review and enclose a list of guidelines for preparing the manuscript.

Monographs

Monographs, which are similar to books, deal with only one particular topic. Generally, the monograph is published in small book form and is based on a single study. Because it is longer than a journal article, it needs its own cover. If a research report is lengthy and its findings have implications for a wide distribution, book publishers known to publish monographs similar in nature to the research report should be contacted for permission to submit the report for consideration. A monograph may be valuable enough to be enlarged into a book, or the editor may suggest that the manuscript be shortened into a journal article.

Any rejected manuscript may be submitted to another publisher. The first editor may have rejected it for one of the following reasons: inappropriate for that particular journal, untimely subject material, or lacking content in a particular area. The manuscript also may have been rejected because of the idiosyncrasies of the publishing company; another publisher may be pleased with the manuscript and accept it for publication. Some editors may ask that the manuscript be revised or that additions or deletions be made before it is accepted. Frequently, if the necessary corrections are made the manuscript will be accepted. If writers do not want to take the time to make the suggested modifications or to change the meaning of a paragraph or a section, they can try another publisher.

Books

Authors of books should use the same submission procedure for their manuscripts as the authors of articles. Well-known writers may be approached by an editor to write a book or an article. Beginning writers must prove themselves, however, and may have some difficulty in getting their manuscripts accepted for publication.

Generally, periodical articles are written for prestige, and books are written for both prestige and profit. Often the publisher of a professional journal does not make a profit but is dedicated to publishing relevant information in the field. The author of a professional journal article is not reimbursed for a manuscript. Rather, writers bear all the expense of preparing the manuscript, and whether or not they receive printed copies of their article depends on the publisher. Some publishers may give them one or more copies of the entire journal containing the article; others may send several reprints.

Editors' reputations are based on quality manuscripts. They try to publish the best material available. A well-known writer has a wider market than an unknown writer, but there are always opportunities for beginning researchers who have something of value to share with their colleagues. Book publishers sell to a wide market, so they are looking for written material that is interesting, readable, thought provoking, controversial, original, or valuable to the discipline.

USE OF QUOTATIONS

To avoid plagiarism, special attention must be given to the sources of quotations. Quotations should be used only when they express an idea extremely well. Quotations also are included in a manuscript when specific remarks are directed toward something written by another author that agrees, disagrees, criticizes, or reinforces the ideas in the manuscript. Quotations should be used sparingly because the purpose of writing is to present an account of the author's own research study.

When material is published, permission to use the quotations must be obtained from the copyright holder. Extensive quoting requires considerable paperwork to obtain all the permissions. Requests may not be answered immediately or they may be refused, necessitating deletion of the quotation. In some cases publishers of journal articles may allow limited quotations without written permission if the article has not been previously copyrighted.

Quotations from individuals who participated in the study sample may be included in the manuscript if these people are not identified by name or description. Quotations are frequently used in published literature when the source of the statement is not revealed. They may be used to enliven the presentation or to illustrate a point.

WRITING ABSTRACTS

An abstract is a brief summary of the contents of the research report. Usually one or two sentences are written to describe each of the following steps: problem, purpose, hypothesis, sample, procedure, results, and conclusions. The abstract is used for two purposes. Researchers can mail a résumé of the study to editors who might be interested in publishing the article or the book, to participants, and to others who express interest in the project; or they can distribute a brief summary of their study to gain a wider dissemination of the results.

Researchers also can prepare a brief account to be published at the head of the article. This summary, or abstract, is printed, in this instance, in small type or italic lettering and enables the busy reader to glean the contents of the article. If the abstract interests readers, they may take time to read the entire report.

Abstracts vary in length depending on the purpose for which they are written. Some editors ask the writer for an abstract of a specific length. Usually the abstract appearing at the head of an article in a professional journal is about 200 words long, whereas abstracts of research articles sent to editors for possible publication tend to be from 300 to 500 words in length.

One of the marks of a profession is its research activity. The results of research studies must be disseminated to be useful to a profession. Abstract journals are established to disseminate research results, to categorize research topics, and to make all research reports that have appeared in current periodicals available for quick survey. Most disciplines or professions have their own abstracts or indexes or both. Abstracts of research results are needed for publication in each particular discipline's abstract journal. Some of the well-known abstract journals include *Psychology Abstracts, Religious and Theological Abstracts, Chemical Abstracts, Sociological Abstracts, Index Medicus, Nursing Abstracts,* and *Dissertation Abstracts.* Researchers need to investigate these sources when they are interested in locating articles dealing with specific subjects of concern. For example, reports of research projects done in the field of nursing appear frequently in *Sociological Abstracts.*

COPYRIGHT

Copyrighting is the process of securing the exclusive rights over printed material. The owner of the copyright is granted the right to print and publish, sell or distribute, transform or revise the work. A research report that the investigator wishes to have published should be coyrighted to protect the author's rights. When the work is published, the copyright is usually held by the publisher.

Unpublished works are eligible for either common law literary property protection or statutory copyright protection. The former arises automatically when the work is created and requires no action in the Copyright Office; it ends when the work is published or a copyright is secured.

Statutory copyright refers to federal protection granted under registration for material in unpublished form. Detailed information concerning copyright laws can be obtained by writing to:

Information and Publication Section
Copyright Office
Library of Congress
Washington, D.C. 20559
202-287-8700

The wise researcher-author will pay close attention to copyright laws.

Photocopying has become a major issue. The focus of attention is on the legality of reproducing material without reimbursing the author and publisher for their time and effort. Innumerable hours of labor on the part of these people go into the creation and production of scholarly works. Legal debate centers around the number of photocopies of copyrighted material that can be made by one individual.

RESEARCH-BASED ARTICLES

The researcher may decide to publish his/her report in its entirety or to include only certain sections, illustrations, and tables. Additional articles may be published, based on the research study, as long as they do not include a direct quotation from the published sections of the original copyrighted material. If the focus of the proposed articles lies in the unpublished portion of the report, it is often possible for the author to write one or more articles from the unpublished material. It is important to inform the copyright holder of any intention to publish such additional information before he/she begins preparing such an article for another publisher.

Editors of the large professional journals often select articles for publication through a system of readers or reviewers. In the blind method the author's name may be deleted from the manuscript and a team of readers independently decide if the article is appropriate for publication. Only after the readers have completed reviewing the manuscript is the name of the author revealed. The decision to publish an article is based on a majority vote and the author is informed of the acceptance or rejection of the article. The advantage of the blind method is that the little-known or unknown author has as great a chance to have an article published as the well-known professional.

In the writing and publishing field, nothing succeeds like success. Many articles are written and published at the request of editors. Often through a series of interlinking friendships or events, invitations are extended to authors to write articles based on their research findings. An informal conversation with someone associated with a publishing company or a question raised by a potential author at a convention may end with the publication of an article.

Every article has its own story of how it happened to get into print. By way of illustration, there was a case in which a university graduate student did a unique research study and was later asked by his professor to present the findings in the form of a paper at a convention. Someone at the convention happened to be a contributing editor to a professional periodical and asked that the revised research report be submitted for publication. The necessary modifications were made, and the paper was published some months later.

As another example, for a classroom assignment, an instructor compiled data collected from student's opinions concerning student involvement in patient selection. The data were originally compiled to be used to inform the clinical instructors of the students' attitudes; however, they had other professional implications. Further analysis of the data and development of the theme led to the publication of an article in a professional journal.

Frequently, well-known people inform editors and contributing editors of other friends and colleagues who are doing interesting research. The editor may, in turn, contact the researcher and ask for a manuscript. Assigned papers often provide students with opportunities for publication. The first publication is often a stepping stone for requests or motivation for a second article.

WRITING QUALITATIVE RESEARCH REPORTS

Meaning is the key consideration in qualitative research. Therefore the researcher should write in such a manner that the reader is led from the real world beyond mere storytelling to an interpretation of the domain he/she has systematically studied.

If the researcher has chosen to combine quantitative and qualitative techniques, the triangulation method may result in the inclusion of tables and various types of illustrations. Sensitivity to what is occurring at the time of data gathering should be set down in descriptive form so as to reveal what is really happening. A good qualitative study takes the commonalities from multiple sources of information and attempts to reveal or shed light on the type of behavior that is ordinarily displayed.

Specific examples will lend authenticity to the qualitative report. Clarity and conciseness combined with interpretative language carry the reader rapidly into the world being studied. Sufficient information about the conduct of the research study should be provided to permit readers to make adequate judgment of the conclusions. Because a qualitative research report is more inclusive than the descriptive report alone, the researcher shares his/her personal experiences in gaining permissions, relating with individual subjects and other activities that reveal social processes. The theory, concept, or proposition that explains the point of focus should be named. As with quantitative research, the reader should be informed about further research that should be conducted.

SUMMARY

Beginning researchers should have an outlet through which to share their research findings if the findings are to benefit the profession and the public. The printed page is the usual answer to the question, "How can I inform others of my research results?"

The research manuscript, when prepared for publication, may be from a few pages to several hundred pages in length. It should be typed on good quality $8\frac{1}{2}$ x 11 inch paper, double-spaced, with wide margins. Requirements for manuscript preparation vary from publisher to publisher, so the editor should be contacted before the manuscript is submitted for consideration. If the editor asks to see the manuscript, the author can be certain that the editor will give the manuscript his full attention.

There are at least four questions that must be considered in the selection of a publisher for a research report.
1. Is the article written for the lay reader or for the professional?
2. Does the article appeal to a specific group of readers, or does it have cross-disciplinary interest?
3. Is the article appropriate for the more prestigious and technical periodicals or for the lesser known journals?
4. Is the content of the article appropriate to one of the specialized journals of the profession?

Manuscripts may be submitted for possible publication as articles, monographs, or books, depending on the length of the manuscript or the purpose of the authors. After deciding on a possible periodical for publication, the author should write the editor to see if he/she is interested in the manuscript.

Quotations should be used sparingly and then only when they enhance the manuscript. Permission to quote published material must be obtained from the copyright holder. A copyright protects the holders' exclusive rights and allows the owners to print or publish and sell or distribute their work. The wise researcher-author will pay careful attention to copyright laws.

An abstract is a brief summary describing the purpose and the steps of the research study. Abstracts vary in length depending on their use. They are written chiefly for wide dissemination of the study results and for submission to publishers. The abstract also serves as a brief informative introduction at the head of an article in a professional journal.

Abstracts are printed in abstract journals for the purpose of dissemination of study results, categorization, and quick summary.

Publishers look for articles that are original, thought provoking, or interesting. Opportunities to publish articles come about through varied circumstances, perhaps by the request of an editor.

Good research is never complete until the findings appear in print.

The writing style of the qualitative research report differs from that of quantitative research in that it is less formal and rigid. Lacking an hypothesis to be tested, it does not contain all the steps of scientific quantitative research.

DISCUSSION QUESTIONS

1 Why is research almost worthless unless it is published?
2 We sometimes hear the statement, "I don't care how you footnote as long as you are consistent." why is consistency important?
3 Why is research easy and publishing difficult?
4 Would you approve or disapprove of being allowed only one photocopy of an article or a page from a book? Why?
5 If you had your choice, which of the following would you choose and why?
   a. Make a brilliant discovery through research but never receive credit.
   b. Make no really significant contribution to research but receive great acclaim for your work.
6 Why do you think the authors hope that students will place greater emphasis on intellectual curiosity than on monetary gain? Which do you think most researchers in the health professions place first?
7 How much time should pass between the completion of a research report and the publication of the findings?
8 Which is the most effective, publishing a research report in a new professional journal or presenting it as an oral report at the profession's state convention?
9 In what way is ethics involved in publishing the research report?

CLASS ACTIVITIES

Track II (Steps in Research Project)

1 Project groups and single researchers are to prepare the final draft of their report for typing. The format, grammar, and completeness of the report should be rechecked.
2 The members of each group are to determine how each researcher will participate in the oral presentation of their group research report.

SUGGESTED READINGS

Altschul, Annie: Beginning and end, Nurs. Times 70(19):719, May 9, 1974.
Brosnan, J., and Kovalesky, A.: Perishing while publishing, Nurs. Outlook 28(11):688–690, November 1980.
Carnegie, M. Elizabeth: A serious omission, Nurs. Res. 24(2):83, March–April 1975.
Evans, N.: Authors and publishers: the mutual selection process, Am. J. Nurs. 81(2):350–352, February 1981.

Fuller, E.O.: Preparing an abstract of a nursing study, Nursing Research 32(5):316, September–October 1983.

Gortner, Susan R.: Scientific accountability in nursing, Nurs. Outlook 22(12):766, December 1974.

King, D., and others: Disseminating the results of nursing research, Nurs. Outlook 29(3):164–169, March 1981.

Knafl, K.A., and Howard, M.J.: Interpreting and reporting qualitative research, Research in Nursing and Health 7:17–24, 1984.

Lewis, Edith P.: Editorial, What bugs editors, Nurs. Outlook 23(8):491, August 1975.

Lindeman, C.A.: Dissemination of nursing research, Image Vol. XVI(2):57–58, Spring 1984.

McCloskey, J.C. and Swanson, E.: Publishing opportunities for nurses: a comparison of 100 journals, Image Vol. XIV(2):50–56, June 1982.

Need for information on current nursing research, Nurs. Res. 23(1):63–64, 1974.

Powell, S.R., and others: Writing for publication: a group approach, Nurs. Outlook 27(11):729–732, November 1979.

Stuart, G.W., and others, Nurs. Outlook 25(5):316–318, May 1977.

Swanson, E. and McCloskey, J.C.: The manuscript review process of nursing journals, Image Vol. XIV(3):72–76, October 1982.

Van Dyne, L.: "Spreading chaos" seen in scholarly publishing, Chronicle of Higher Education 10(17):11, July 7, 1975.

Van Til, W.: Writing for professional publication, Rockleigh, NJ, 1981, Allyn & Bacon, Inc.

Winkler, K.J.: Revisions in the U.S. copyright law, Chronicle of Higher Education 10(18):6, July 21, 1975.

CHAPTER 27

THE CRITICAL CONSUMER

Educational research takes place in classrooms where teachers and students interact. Administrative research is interested in leadership, management, budgets, staffing, and training. Clinical research is conducted in the health care area where nurses come into contact with patients and clients. It occurs from the time patients enter health care facilities until they are well. Clinical research can take place within the hospital, clinic, community, or home.

Clinical researchers propose that investigations are conducted for the purpose of improving patient health through better nursing care. Nursing research can refer to clinical research or to nurses and nursing in general. The study of nursing as a profession would be considered research in nursing; however, nursing research is the study of the problems which occur in nursing practice. Most research conducted by nurses is clinical research. Loomis found that 78.4% of dissertations were related to clinical nursing and 21.6% concerned social issues in nursing.[1] It is quite apparent that clinical research is the most common type of investigation. Clinical research may include prevention of disease and infection, promoting recovery, interaction of client and nurse, health teaching, and nursing intervention plans, to name but a few pertinent topics.

Broad categories of clinical research encompass the following terms (the word *nursing* could be added to each):

occupational health nursing	mental health
specialties in nursing practice	health care management
critical care nursing	hospice
emergency nursing	long term care
neurosurgical nursing	allied health
gerontological nursing	nursing home
midwives	practitioners
maternal-child	health assessment
nephrology	family process
cancer	psychiatric
oncology	perinatal
rehabilitation	prenatal
geriatric	pediatric

The methods used in clinical research are the same methods and techniques utilized in any other research.

[1]Loomis, M.E.: Emerging content in nursing: an analysis of dissertations abstracts and titles 1975 to 1982, Nursing Research **34**(2):113–118, March–April 1985.

BORROWING METHODS AND FINDINGS

There is no reason why some of the methods of one discipline cannot be used in another. As an illustration, content analysis was first used in World War II as a means of finding out what was happening in Germany. Copies of German newspapers were available in many large cities and they contained train schedules, deaths of soldiers, factory openings, and other valuable information. Over a period of time, fluctuations and changes were recorded and meaningful relationships became apparent to persons knowledgeable about war conditions and preparations.

Content analysis has often been used in nursing research. Elmes, et al have noted that Freud's id, ego, and superego are analogous to a hydraulic valve. The flow of the id is controlled by the valve-like ego and superego.[2]

Some of the Campbell and Stanley quasi-experimental designs—the time-series experiment, for example—could easily be adopted for evaluating patient-teaching and other treatment interventions.[3]

Findings in one discipline also can be used in another discipline. Research in social psychology has found that liking and interaction have a positive correlation and this knowledge is useful for nursing. A nurse-patient relationship should grow more positive over time. Therefore, if possible, the same nurse should be assigned to a client as long as he/she is under a nursing care plan.

Formal organization theory contains a considerable amount of knowledge related to leadership qualities. Organizational research has revealed that democratic styles of leadership are more satisfying and effective than authoritarian styles. The use of this information in nursing could extend to such areas as nursing administration, employees under a nurse manager, patients under the care of a professional nurse, health training in a factory by an occupational health nurse, or teaching a pregnant woman about prenatal care.

The field of sociology has spent considerable time studying conformity. Some of the information about conformity could be applied to the problem of convincing clients that they should take their medication and follow the guidance of the nurse's care plan. The use of findings and methods employed by one discipline and applied to another (nursing) allows for greater flexibility of approaches and an expanded scope of understanding of the interrelationship of ideas and research findings.

DEVELOPMENT AND IMPLEMENTATION OF NURSING RESEARCH

Nursing research techniques can be utilized by many levels of the health team. Dr. Virginia Mermel believes that staff nurses holding B.S.N. degrees are in an ideal position to implement research.[4] Some of the reasons why staff nurses can be in the forefront in research are:

[2]Elmes, D.G., Kantowitz, G.H., and Roediger, H.L. III: Research methods in psychology, 2nd ed., St. Paul, 1985, West Publishing Co., p. 41.
[3]Campbell, D.T., and Stanley, J.C.: Experimental and quasi-experimental designs for research, Chicago, 1963, Rand McNally & Company, p. 37.
[4]Dr. Virginia Mermel was instrumental in suggesting many of the issues during her address to the Beta Kappa Chapter, Sigma Theta Tau, University of Virginia, April 20, 1985.

1. Staff nurses are at the heart of the action when the patient/client is most in need of care.
2. Staff nurses are able to note the discrepancies between what should be and what is. The wise researcher will seek the advice of staff nurses at every phase of the investigation.
3. Staff nurses can help to select the correct wording for the instrument or questionnaire since they are in constant contact with the health care environment.
4. Validity in the real world is assured when real-world people such as staff nurses are involved.
5. Nurses are trained to be good at interviewing and observing. These are important skills in research.
6. Research needs subjects, and who could be more knowledgeable than the staff nurses about appropriate subjects?
7. When the time comes in the research process to carry out experiments, and the researcher wants to test nursing intervention plans, it is necessary to have the assistance of the nursing staff.
8. Evaluating the results of the research requires the expertise of staff nurses. They are especially well qualified if they have been involved in the study.
9. Staff nurses are enthusiastic about the research process when they can be involved.
10. Research brings a fresh experience to the nursing profession and encourages the staff to think in new ways. Both the staff nurse and the research project benefit from this combination.

Implementing Findings

In addition to developing the research, the staff nurse is also the implementer of the findings. As such, she is the *consumer* and responsible, as any consumer, for critically evaluating any research outcome she may implement. Implementing the findings means utilization of the results of research. If a new intervention plan to improve patient care has been effective, it should be incorporated in the nursing care plan. The following reasons are suggested for involving staff nurses in implementation of research results.

1. If staff nurses do not implement research results, who will?
2. Staff nurses are the most logical and qualified persons to test new health care techniques.
3. If staff nurses are involved in the process of developing research, they should be the most knowledgeable in implementing research.
4. Staff nurses are on the front line of patient/client care and are in the most advantageous position to use research findings.

WHAT IS GOOD RESEARCH?

An often-asked question concerns how good research can be identified. The answer is both obvious and evasive. Obvious, because how is anything measured as "good"? Often books, food, cars, and clothes are labeled good. What real criteria is used to define anything as "good"? Evasive, because "good" is a very subjective measure. Chapter 4 contains a long list of criteria and variables which should be considered when critiquing research. The following ideas should at least be considered in evaluating the quality of research:

1. Were the findings significant? At what level? If the experimental group difference is only slightly larger than the control, the result may be caused by chance.

2. What worthwhile value does the research have? A study of the SAT scores of freshmen students does not seem as valuable as some new treatment to reduce the pain suffered by burn victims.

3. Does the research produce results in real-life situations as effectively as in the laboratory? Obviously, the research which resulted in polio vaccine was "good" research. When someone finds the cause of or cure for cancer, it will be considered "good" research.

4. In the academic world, the test of an hypothesis or a theory is considered on a par with the findings. It bears repeating that "how" an hypothesis is tested is as important as what is found.

5. Research that produces a cheaper method or a better product is "good." Research that developes a faster, more effective method of treatment is "good." Research results that please clients, promote wellness, and reduce pain are "good."

6. Unexpected findings, especially if they are the opposite of what was anticipated, are often labeled "good."

7. The person who declares that a certain piece of research is "good" frequently provides the standard of judgment. Publishing of the research results in a professional journal, a positive evaluation by a panel of experts, or reference to the research by other writers are all measures of worth.

8. If well-known authors, researchers, or public figures label a piece of research "good," then public acceptance is almost assured.

9. Readers or users are free to place their personal stamp of "good" on a study.

10. In the end, history may contribute the final analysis. Semmelweis made a great contribution to health with a very convincing piece of research. His peers were not impressed, but time, the ultimate judge, has labeled his product "good research." Florence Nightingale has weathered the critics and withstood the bards. Today she stands on a pinnacle alone. Her research methods and dedication have won her accolades as a "good researcher."

SUMMARY

Clinical research is developed and implemented for the purpose of improving the health of clients and patients. Nursing research can refer to clinical research or to the broader aspects of the profession.

Research in nursing is the study of nursing as a profession. Seventy-eight percent of the research conducted by nurses is in the clinical area. Research in all the nursing speciality areas is considered clinical research.

Staff nurses are the logical persons to be involved in developing research since they are most often involved with patients. The staff nurse is a valuable consultant for developing questionnaires, assuring validity, interviewing and observing, conducting research, and evaluating results.

Clinical research can borrow from the findings and theories of other disciplines to improve patient care and the quality of nursing practice. All disciplines have developed and tested theories which are applicable to nursing including education, sociology, psychology, business, and the physical sciences.

Staff nurses are, again, the logical implementers or consumers of clinical research findings. They are the most qualified, and in the best position to evaluate the results and use of new knowledge.

An evaluation of what is good research is both obvious and evasive. Everyone has some ideas of what is "good," but to define the term "good" is more difficult. Some criteria for evaluating research are the same as those for critiquing a research study. Value for patients, level of significance, results, methods used to collect data, kinds of findings, opinions of experts, published results, and historical acceptance are all measures of "good research."

CLASS ACTIVITIES

Tracks I and II

1 Each student is to write a letter to the editor of a journal in which he or she would like to have a research article published.
2 The students are to write a 500-word abstract of a scientific investigation for a professional journal. Either the instructor or the students may select the research article.

SUGGESTED READINGS

Bergman, R.: Omissions in nursing research, Int. Nurs. Rev. **31**(2):55–56, 1984.
Butts, P.A.: Dissemination of nursing research findings, Image Vol. **XIV**(2):62–64, June 1982.
Fawcett, J.: Utilization of nursing research findings, Image Vol. **XIV**(2):57–59, June 1982.
Hockey, L.: Bridge-building, Nurs. Times **79**(22):64, June 1, 1983.
Kratz, C.R.: Research—how can we challenge nursing practice? Nursing Times **78**(44):128, November 3–9, 1982. Occasional papers.
Morse, J.M.: Putting research into practice, Canadian Nurse **8**:40, September–October 1982.
White, J.H.: The relationship of clinical practice and research, J. Adv. Nurs. **9**(2):181–187, March 1984.

EPILOGUE

Research in any discipline can be a monetary affair based on research grants, or it can be a matter of desire and a means of satisfying intellectual curiosity. We sincerely hope that you encounter the latter before the former.

A research study is an extension of you—treat it well. Added to the systematic investigations of others, it may contribute more to the improvement of human health than you can ever dream.

GLOSSARY

abscissa— the horizontal line on a scattergram which represents increasing values from left to right. The ordinate represents frequencies on the vertical line.

accidental sample— a group of subjects obtained by convenience.

ad hoc explanation— an explanation for a specific case or purpose.

aggregate— a group of subjects with similar characteristics.

alpha error— in statistics, a type I error; that is, rejecting the null hypothesis when it is true.

alternate-forms reliability— a state in which the same results are obtained using a parallel form of the instrument.

alternate hypothesis— another explanation for the relationship between two variables.

analysis— the process of carefully scrutinizing data by placing it in categories, calculating the mean, and applying statistical procedures.

analysis of covariance— a statistical test similar to analysis of variance, which analyzes the effects of experimental treatment on a dependent variable.

analysis of variance— a statistical procedure that compares within-group differences with between-group differences in experimental research.

applied research— research which is conducted to solve an everyday problem or question.

a priori method— before the fact; a method of logic which is characterized by reason alone or by deduction.

archival research— the process of using historical records as a source of data.

area sampling— a procedure in which specific geographic areas of the population are sampled.

array (matrix)— the arrangement of data in rows and/or columns for purposes of analysis.

assumptions— ideas or beliefs which are strongly considered to be true.

attitude scale— an instrument or tool which measures the subject's mood or feeling.

balanced Latin square— the process of assigning experimental groups of subjects to conditions which allow each group to precede or follow every other group; valuable for assessing pretest-posttest effects.

baseline— the peak average or maximum used as a measure against which the treatment is introduced in an experiment. The baseline is the pretest norm.

basic research— scientific study aimed at testing theory or satisfying curiosity as opposed to applied research.

Bayesian statistics— a method of analyzing data using known distribution (prior data) and new data to predict probable outcomes.

before-after design— an experimental design using a before test and an after test to determine the effect of treatment.

between group variance— a measure of the spread of scores between groups; usually found in experimental research.

bimodal distribution— spread of data in which there are two points where most scores or values occur.

biserial coefficient— use of the normal distribution to estimate the correlation between two variables.

bivariate— a term for referring to two variables as opposed to one variable (univariate).

blind experiment— an experiment in which the subjects are unaware of whether they are in the experimental or the control group.

block randomization— the assigning of groups into experimental groups by chance. Often used in the Latin-square design.

carryover effect— the result which occurs when subjects retain (carryover) knowledge from pretest to posttest.

case study— an in-depth research study of a single individual, single unit, or single organization.

categorization— the process of placing data into categories (groups) according to some plan or order.

causal modeling— developing a model (replication of something real) to create an imaginary possible vehicle for studying cause-effect relationship.

cause— the phenomena that determines the dependent variable. The dependent variable is caused by the independent variable.

central-limit theorem— the belief that if the sample size is large enough, it approximates the normal curve in spite of the distribution.

central tendency— measures or averages which are often referred to as the mean, median, and mode.

chi-square (X^2)— a statistical formula which compares observed frequencies with expected frequencies to test for significance.

class interval— the scores within a given unit or the range of scores in an interval.

closed question— an item in a questionnaire which is limited to the answers provided, as opposed to open questions which allow the respondent freedom to provide the response.

cluster analysis— a process used to arrange or sort scores or values into groups.

cluster sample— a part of the population selected from a particular segment of the population on the basis of some characteristic(s).

cohort— a group of people in the same age span, same socioeconomic condition, or similar stage in their life cycle.

concept— a term or idea which has a specific meaning within the context of a general field of study; a notion that substitutes for a definition of several words.

conceptual framework— a structure showing the basic design of a research process as it relates to the relationship among variables.

conceptual replication— the repetition of a former research study using a new operational definition of the original hypothesis.

concept validity— the adequacy of an operational definition to reflect the meaning of a construct or concept.

concomitant variable— the name for a variable that interacts with another variable, usually has an effect on the dependent variable, and occurs concurrently.

concurrent validity— a means to affirm the truth (validity) of a measure or instrument by correlation with a known valid measure.

confidence interval— statistical assurance that a value is within the level of confidence chosen by the researcher.

confidence level— assurance that the degree of significance is not due to chance; confidence in the validity of findings.

confidentiality— the pledge that research information will not reveal the identity of the subject.

confounding variables— those qualities or quantities that vary and which may have an effect upon the variables under observation; variables which may influence the cause-effect relationship.

consensual validation— the process of determining validity by using experts or judges.

construct validity— the state in which the test or instrument is valid as related to other concepts (constructs).

content analysis— the reviewing of the content of some form of communication for consistent use of word or idea.

content validity— the extent to which the elements of an instrument represent the meaning of the concept under study. The instrument has content validity when judged so by a panel of experts.

contingency analysis— a form of cross-tabulation of one variable with any other variables in a study to find correlation.

contingency table— a table which shows the occurrence of two variables or two dimensions.

control group— in an experimental design, the experimental group receives a treatment (experiment) while the control group is left unchanged. A test is given to the two groups to determine the difference in response.

control variable— a group or object held constant for comparison with the experimental group.

correlation— a relationship between two variables.

correlation coefficient— a measure of the relationship between two variables as indicated by correlation coefficients from -1.0 to +1.0.

counterbalancing— varying the order of pre- and posttests to determine the effects of the tests. Used in experimental research to avoid carryover from pretest to posttest.

covariance— the statistical measure of the relationship (covariance) between two variables.

criterion validity— a type of validity established by comparing one criterion with another quality which has high validity.

cronbach's alpha— the name for a statistical procedure to measure reliability through an internal consistency.

cross-cultural research— collecting data from two or more nationalities or countries (cultures). Because cultural variables are often different, cross-cultural validity is stronger than single-culture validity.

cross-sectional studies— a sample of many subjects to ascertain change at a given point in time. Longitudinal studies, on the other hand, sample one group over a long period of time.

cross-sectional survey— a survey in which data are gathered from a variety of subjects at one point in time as opposed to a longitudinal study of the same group over a long period of time.

cumulative distribution— an arrangement of scores in which values are continually totaled (accumulated) as the number of frequencies goes higher.

curvilinear regression— a line of values (averages) which follows a curve rather than a straight line.

data— the information gathered in a research study.

debriefing— a session in which the researcher tells the subjects what he/she wanted to learn and counsels them if necessary.

deception— the process of tricking subjects in order to conduct an experiment.

deduction— the process of reasoning from the world to an individual; from general to specific.

degrees of freedom— the number of units or variables which influences statistical significance.

delimitations— the limits placed on the sample and research design by the investigator.

Delphi technique— a process in which a questionnaire administered three times to a cross-disciplinary group of experts who then see a summary of each administration for the purpose of forecasting the future.

demand characteristics— the elements or conditions which enable a subject to second guess the researcher in an experiment. Subjects are aware of what the researcher wants and will answer is expected.

dependent variable— the variable (quantity or quality) that is the result (effect) of the independent variable.

descriptive research— a study in which the data are collected to define or describe some group or phenomena.

descriptive statistics— the process of defining (describing) data utilizing the mean, normal curve, and other statistics.

design— in research, the plan or strategy for conducting the study.

discriminant analysis— a procedure to determine the degree or power of an item or test to discriminate or differentiate between high and low.

discrimination power— the ability or power to discriminate; to differentiate between items with very high to very low values.

dispersion— the spread of scores or values from most to least; similar to range.

distribution— the arrangement of scores or values in groups, by frequencies, from low to high.

domal sampling— a type of area sampling which specifies every n^{th} subject.

double blind— an experimental approach in which neither the subjects nor the researcher is aware of who is in the experimental and control groups.

empirical— a verifiable method of finding data and facts based on objective techniques which can be measured or observed.

empirical evidence— data which is capable of being measured by mechanical or mathematical means.

empirical validity— the quality exhibited by a study that tests what it proposes to test and can be verified by objective measures.

endogenous variable— characterized as internal as opposed to an exogenous (external) variable.

equal-appearing intervals— the same distance between items on an altitude scale; as items move along a scale from low to high they are an equal distance apart.

error of measurement— the degree to which a value deviates from its true value due to inaccuracy.

error, random— the amount of mismeasurement which occurs while measuring a value or score.

experiment— usually refers to a comparison of an experimental group and a control group. The experimental group receives a treatment and the control does not.

experimental control— the process of controlling (manipulating) variables to reduce their effect on the dependent variable.

experimental design— the plan or strategy which is developed to conduct experimental research and test relationships between two variables.

experimental research— a scientific process whereby data are gathered to test the cause-effect relationship between two or more variables.

exploratory study— a preliminary research project to ascertain some problem or possibility for future research.

ex post facto— after the fact. The results are confirmed after the experiment or from the analysis of some data.

ex post facto explanation— a statement to explain something after the fact of after the occurrence.

external criticism— the process used to confirm the validity or truthfulness of data by applying tests from other sources.

external validity— a term concerned with generalization beyond the study; related to the use of findings.

extraneous variable— a quantity or quality (variable) which may have an effect on research results that are outside or beyond the control of the researcher.

face validity— a type of validity in which an instrument is valid (tests what it proposes to test) because it appears valid.

factor analysis— a process of analysis which entails finding the relationship of several variables (factors) on any single variable through a sophisticated technique.

factor loading— part of the process of factor analysis. Factors or variables are considered one-by-one in relationship to several other variables.

field experiment— research conducted in a real-world setting as opposed to a laboratory. May be similar to a lab experiment except in a natural setting.

field research— data gathering in the real world when subjects are unaware of being observed as opposed to a laboratory situation.

forced-choice method— a technique that usually refers to a questionnaire in which items are limited to the choices listed.

F ratio— a statistical procedure which compares within-group difference to between-group difference.

frequency— the number of times an event or value occurs.

frequency distribution— the spread of scores, values, or data from a research study; usually displayed in visual form or points on a scale where variables intersect.

frequency polygon— a visual distribution of scores or values on a line from high to low.

generalizability— the assurance with which the researcher can predict (project) findings from the sample to the population.

goodness-of-fit test— a statistical test to determine how close a group or distribution of a score approaches or conforms to the expected or normal.

grouped distribution— the process of placing scores or values into categories or intervals with no overlap.

H_0— a symbol used in statistics to represent the null hypothesis (a statement of no difference between two variables).

H_1— a symbol used in statistics to represent the working hypothesis.

H_2— a symbol used to represent the alternate hypothesis.

hawthorne effect— the result which occurs when subjects change their behavior because they are aware of being observed. The name was derived from the Hawthorne plant study.

histogram— a graph in which vertical bars indicate the number of units or subjects that received each score or value.

historical research— data collected from records and artifacts which have special contemporary meaning.

homoscedasticity— the condition which occurs when two variables change at the same time in the same direction.

hypothesis— the statement of the relationship between two variables.

hypothesis testing— the attempt to accept or reject a hypothesis through research and or statistics.

hypothetical construct— a mental image of a concept or variable which may explain the existence of an event or relationship.

impressionistic analysis— the process of analyzing or describing some visual observation. Used in research when an observer describes something currently under observation.

independent variable— the cause variable. An hypothesis states the relationship between the independent (cause) variable and a dependent (effect) variable.

induction— the process of reasoning or moving from a particular instance to a larger group; generalizing from the specific to the population.

inductive theory— a theory developed from research or specific data as opposed to a broader or more general source.

inference— the process of applying characteristics of the sample to the population.

inferential statistics— a kind of data analysis which allows the researcher to infer or make generalizations based on the strength of the findings.

inferential validity— the kind of validity which exists when a true relationship found in the laboratory also exists in real life.

informed consent— a condition that exists when the subject agrees to take part in a research project after being told about the details and potential results.

interaction-process analysis— a method of observing and recording group interaction with a 12-category checkoff list. Robert Bales is the author of such a method.

internal criticism— a process of testing or asserting validity using within-criteria.

internal validity— truth which is evident from within the data or results of research. If the independent variable is the cause of the dependent variable, it has a measure of internal validity.

interval data— information that is scaled in equal units. The difference between units has the same value.

intervening variable— a factor which has an effect on the independent or the dependent variable.

interview— the process of asking questions of subjects verbally in order to collect data.

invalid— not valid; does not test what it proposed to test.

inverted U-shaped relationship— a curved line similar to the normal curve; shaped like an upside-down U.

jackknife— to close; a statistical analysis of small sections of data as compared with the whole in order to find a confidence level.

Kendall's tau coefficient— a statistic which compares a series of two ranked sets of variables in order to find a correlation.

Kuder-Richardson Formula 20— a statistical formula used to measure internal reliability by comparing dichotomous items.

kurtosis— the degree of flatness used to describe a frequency distribution in relation to the normal curve.

latin square— an experimental design in which groups are randomly assigned to various treatment or control groups in order to reduce interactive effects.

law— a statement which is true under all situations.

least-squares regression— a technique which is utilized along with other measures to ascertain distance from the mean.

leptokurtic— the degree of height used to describe a frequency distribution that is more pointed than the normal curve.

level of significance— a statistical number indicating the possibility that such results could have occurred by chance; related to degrees of freedom.

likert scale— a rating of opinions or attitudes on a scale from 1 to 5, ranging from strongly agree to strongly disagree.

limitations— weaknesses of the study which should be reported by the researcher.

linear— a term that refers to a line in statistics; a linear relationship refers to a scattergram in which a change in one value corresponds to a similar change in another value.

longitudinal survey— a study in which data are collected from the same subjects over a long period of time.

main effect— the chief or most apparent reason for the dependent variable, often used in analysis of variance.

manipulation— refers to changing one variable to learn how it will affect another variable.

Mann-Whitney U test— a nonparametric test to find significant differences between two samples.

matched groups design— a method of assigning subjects to groups that allows a particular variable or variables to be present in every group.

matched sample— a process in which two groups with similar characteristics are selected for comparison purposes.

matching— a process of assuming that each group has similar (matched) subjects.

mathematical modeling— the process of using mathematics to simulate a replica of a real-life interaction in order to find or test a relationship.

maturation— from the word mature, growing older or changing; in research, a confounding variable in which social and historical change may influence results.

mean— the arithmetic average of a group of scores. To determine the mean, all scores are added, then divided by the total number of scores.

mean deviation— the degree a value deviates (moves away) from the mean (average).

mean square— a process used in analysis of variance; an average of the squared measures. To determine the mean square, the sum of squares is divided by the degrees of freedom.

measurement— the use of an instrument to ascertain the dimensions of a variable.

measurement error— the mistakes (errors) in ascertaining and observing variables which may invalidate the results.

measurement, standard error of— a measurement of the difference between a series of observed scores and the actual or true scores.

measures of central tendency— statements of averages expressed as either mean, median, or mode.

median— that point or score which is half above and half below the other scores.

MEDLARS (Medical Literature Analysis and Retrieval System)— a system for retrieval of literature through a computer search of medical research, including nursing.

MEDLINE— a MEDLARS online data retrieval of Index Medicus citations.

method of least squares— a technique used to obtain an average or mean (regression line) of the values of two variables on a scattergram. The line passes through or near the average of the scores that are most frequent.

methodology— the study of the manner of collecting research data.

mode— a measure of central tendency (average); the most frequently appearing score.

monotonic relationship— the name for the relationship that exists when one variable continuously moves with another.

multidimensional scaling— a statistical method of assigning items to units for analysis; many as opposed to one unit.

multiple-regression analysis— the method used to analyze and measure the relationship between several variables.

multivariate— a term that usually refers to analyzing several variables, as opposed to univariate (one), or bivariate (two).

naive subject— a participant in research, usually experimental, who is unaware of being a subject and who therefore reacts naturally.

nominal data— data which fits in only one category or unit. For example, subjects are male or female.

nominal scale— a value or variable which can be classified in only one way, according to a rule.

nomothetic— a method of research and gathering data by quantifying and observing a number of subjects for the purpose of discovering universal behavior. Idiographic is a single-case approach.

nonequivalent control group— a second control (nontreatment) group which serves as a comparison. It is often a group that is simply convenient, not exactly equivalent.

normal curve— a graph whose line extends from almost zero to a peak in the center, and approaches almost to infinity at the extreme end. The normal distribution is unimodal in which the mean, median, and mode are at the exact center.

normal distribution— a group (distribution) of scores or subjects that is average (normal) as compared with the normal curve.

null hypothesis (H_o)— a statement of no difference used in testing the relationship between two variables.

nursing research— scientific study conducted by nurses concerning nursing practice, the profession, and its interests.

observation— a technique that utilizes visual measures to collect data.

one-shot case study— a research technique involving a single group of individuals studied in depth.

one-tailed test— a technique which considers one end of the normal curve or distribution.

open-ended question— a type of item in an instrument which allows subjects great freedom in their responses.

operational definition— a phrase derived by converting hypotheses into an empirically testable statement.

opinionnaire— a type of questionnaire in which subjects are asked their beliefs about a topic.

ordinal data— quantities and qualities which can be placed in order from high to low.

ordinate— the vertical dimension on a graph or plot.

organismic variable(s)— a term that refers to physical, physiological, or psychological variables (anything that changes).

p— probability; the symbol used for probability. This symbol refers to the probability that such results could occur by chance. ($P < .01$)

panel study— a research study in which the investigator interviews his/her subjects several times during a period of months or years in order to observe change.

paradigm— a kind of model or framework for explaining or describing a theory.

parsimony— the simplest explanation is the best explanation.

partial correlation— a statistical approach allowing the researcher to measure the relationship between some variables or partials while ruling out other variables.

participant observations— a type of research in which the research observer joins a group under the guise of a member in order to collect data about the group.

path analysis— a statistical technique which charts a path of the relationship of one variable, with another variable and the strength of that relationship.

Pearson product-moment correlation— a statistical procedure to measure from -1.0 to +1.0 correlation between two variables.

Pearson r— a symbol which refers to Pearson product movement correlation coefficient; a statistical procedure used to find the correlation between two variables from -1.0 to +1.0.

percentile— a term that refers to dividing a distribution into units from 1 to 100. For example, a person ranking at the 25th percentile means 24% were below and 75% were above.

pilot study— a ministudy conducted before the major study in order to make revisions and find flaws in the methodology. It should include every step expected in the major study.

placebo effect— the condition that exists among subjects who believe the treatment is real when it is only a noneffective substitute. Subjects often react in the same manner as those in the treatment group.

plausible-rival hypothesis— an alternative reason or guess which may be as likely as the original hypothesis.

population— the total number of units from which a sample is selected.

positive correlation (positive relationship)— the relationship between two variables in which a change in one induces the same change in the other.

postexperimental interview— an interview (face-to-face conversation) with subjects in an experiment after it is completed. Often, the subject has some insight into the experiment.

posttest— a test given after the experiment to determine the change caused by the treatment.

power (of a statistical test)— a term that refers to the ability of the statistical test to provide a reliable, valid test of the probability that the results were caused by chance.

predictive validity— the condition that exists when the results of a test or research are deemed valid (true) because they predict or forecast accurately.

predictor— anything that forecasts. Usually, a variable has predictive ability if it explains or predicts another variable. For example, a good memory is a predictor of intelligence.

pretest-posttest design— the strategy used in experimental research in which a group is given a pretest to measure a variable, followed by treatment and a posttest. Results of the pretest are compared with those of the posttest to determine the degree of change.

primary source— data gathered by the researcher as original information.

projection— the act of extending beliefs, thoughts, and attitudes to another person.

projective techniques— a method of interpreting statements, drawings, and pictures produced by subjects that imply their true personalities.

Q— the symbol for interquartile; the range between scores or values divided into four parts of 25% each.

Q-sort— a technique in which the subjects arrange statements into stacks from high to low as those statements apply to their beliefs.

quantitative data— information gathered from a sample in the form of numerical quantities.

quasi-experiment— an experiment in which the researcher does not use all four aspects of a true experimental design: before and after tests, and experimental and control groups.

questionnaire— a written question-and-answer sheet which provides data about a subject's attitudes, beliefs, habits, and socioeconomic background.

quota sample— a sample in which a specified number of units is collected, often in a convenient manner rather than at random.

random— selection by some form of chance which allows any unit equal opportunity to be chosen.

random error— a mistake that can occur by chance or a fluctuation that can unintentionally alter the results of research.

random sample— a selection of subjects which allows every unit in the total population equal opportunity to be included in the sample.

range— the extent of the spread of scores from highest to lowest in a variable or value.

rank— the term used to describe an order of values from high to low. For example, the runners were ranked in order of finishing the race.

rank-order correlation— a statistical technique which finds a correlation (relationship) between two sets of data in a high to low continuum (rank order). Two persons or groups are asked to rank the variables in descending order. +1.0 is perfect positive correlation.

rapport— a condition that occurs when the researcher and subject are able to communicate with ease.

rating scale— an instrument for assigning numerical values to data.

raw scores— data or values from research which have not been placed in order, in units, or in categories.

real limits— the range between two points or intervals. On a scale of ages from 40 to 50, the real limits would be 39.5 to 50.49.

regression— a statistical procedure for fitting a line to a group of data describing the relationship between two variables. A regression line provides the best visible summary of the data in a scattergram.

regression to the mean— the phenomena of all variables to return (regress) toward the mean when measured often enough.

relevant variable— a variable which has an effect. A relevant variable produces a change in another variable; a nonrelevant variable would not cause a change.

reliability— a characteristic which occurs time after time. A test is reliable when the results are consistent.

repeated-measures design— an experimental treatment which is repeated with varying amounts of the treatment each time.

replication— the process of repeating a study using the identical methods as in the original study.

representative sample— a sample (part of whole) which is similar to (representative of) the population.

research— a process of utilizing quantitative and qualitative methods to collect and analyze data for the purpose of prediction and explanation.

sample— a part of the whole. In research, the sample is selected in such a manner that it is representative of the population.

sample bias— a part of the whole (sample) which does not represent the population because of a nonrandom procedure. An error (bias) results if the study becomes inaccurate.

sample, cluster— a sample selected because it represents a natural group of people within the population.

sample, matched— see matched sample.

sampling— the process of selecting a representative part of the whole (population).

sampling error— a mistake (error) in selecting a part (sample) of the population. For example, the research erred in sampling by failing to include part-time nurses in the sample of employed nurses.

scale— an instrument or device used to assign some measure or value to a variable.

scatter diagram— a table with vertical and horizontal values. For example, a point representing education on one axis and income on the other should show a correlation between the two.

scattergram— see scatter diagram.

scientific method— a step-by-step, systematic process to predict and explain. The process includes problem, hypothesis, conceptual design, gathering of data, analysis of data, and conclusions.

score— a number or quantity which is representative of a value. For example, a student received a score of 95 out of 100 points.

secondary source— data obtained from records and other nonprimary sources.

sensory impression— a measure of some value ascertained by the senses: eye, ear, touch.

serendipity— the acquisition of valuable information as the result of researching something else; an unplanned find.

set— a manner or condition which develops into a habit; a (set) way of reacting.

significance, statistical— a measure determined by statistics (mathematical calculation) which indicates if such results could have occurred by chance.

sign test— a statistic used to ascertain if one variable occurred more significantly often than another.

skewness— a word used to define the slant of scores or values which are either more frequent on the left or right of the curve. A higher frequency on the left is negative, on the right positive.

slope— the incline or decline of a line on a graph.

small-n-design— a technique in which a small number of (few) students is used in a research study.

sociogram— the chart of friendship choices in a group when subjects are asked to list X number of friends with whom they want to associate.

Solomon four-groups design— a very controlled assignment of experimental and control groups with or without pre- and/or posttests.

Spearman-Brown Prophecy Formula— a statistic used to determine the reliability of a split-half test. The means of the two halves are compared for reliability.

Spearman rank difference method— a statistical technique to find the correlation between two ranked sets of data.

split-half reliability— a comparison of one-half of a test (odd versus even numbered items) to see if the total scores of each half are similar; done at the time of scoring.

spurious correlations— a false relationship which exists when two variables occur at the same time.

standard deviation— a statistical calculation to indicate how far each score in a distribution is from the mean.

standard error— see measurement, standard error.

standard error of the mean— the error (or difference) between the means of the sample and the population means.

standardized test— a test which is often used because it has been tested for validity and reliability.

standard score— scores (values) which are determined by the distance of any score from the mean of the distribution expressed in standard deviation units; may be used to compare the scores of two distributions that are scaled differently.

statistical hypothesis— see hypothesis

statistical inference— a type of statistics which facilitates predicting or explaining from the data to a larger population.

statistical significance— the possibility that such results could have occurred by chance; expressed numerically.

statistical test— a mathematical calculation for determining the significance of research data and the probability of chance.

statistics— a mathematical discipline which analyzes research findings for significance.

stratified random sample— samples taken from two or more levels or strata which are used to make inferences about the population.

structured interview— the obtaining of verbal responses in a carefully planned, face-to-face exchange between researcher and subject.

student's test— a statistical technique to determine if the difference between two means is significant or if it could have occurred by chance.

subject attrition— those subjects (persons) in a research study who leave, die, or drop out of the study.

sum of squares (SS)— a part of analysis of variance which measures differences between and within groups.

survey research— collecting data from a group, usually by questionnaire or interview, to learn some of the subjects' characteristics.

symbols— signs used in place of words; used most often in statistics.

synergism— a term which refers to the interaction of variables; often noticed in replication research when results differ between the two studies.

target population— the subjects which will be sampled from the total group of interest to the researcher.

test— a measure of quality or ability as related to some variable; may be an instrument or tool to assess.

test-retest reliability— a method of determining if a test or instrument is faithful over time by administering the same test twice to see if results are the same.

test of significance— a statistical procedure to determine if the results of research are so significant as to be greater than chance.

theoretical framework— a structure showing the basic design of a research process using a theory for developing an hypothesis or testing other theories.

theory— an hypothesis which has been tested and accepted numerous times and has been promoted to the status of theory.

Thurstone's method of equal-appearing intervals— a technique to find items in a questionnaire which differentiate equally along a continuum.

trace measures— evidence based on the result of physical activity.

t test— a statistical procedure to determine the difference between two means by standard deviation; usually considered the same as a T test.

two-by-two factorial design (2 X 2)— a technique in which two levels of the independent variables are placed in a two-by-two table to allow for a comparison.

two-tailed test— a statistical procedure which involves using both ends of the normal curve in considering the rejection of the hypothesis.

Type I error— see alpha error.

Type II error— in statistics, a beta error; that is, accepting the null hypothesis when it is false.

ultimate causation— the real cause or actual final cause of any variable.

uncontrolled variable— a variable which the researcher cannot control for reasons of ability, knowledge, or authority.

universe— all the subjects in the population of interest.

unobtrusive measure— a method to obtain data from subjects who are unaware of being observed.

unstructured interview— an open-ended verbal exchange between subject and researcher in which the researcher is free to explore as motivated by the subject's responses.

validity— the state in which a test has validity when it tests what it proposes to test.

variable— something which varies. A variable is capable of having a variety of characteristics from one extreme to another.

variability— the ability of a unit or person to change; involves degree or range of change.

AUTHOR INDEX

SUBJECT INDEX

Systematic sampling, 218
Systems analysis, 350–351
   advantages of, 351
   ambiguity of, 351
   disadvantages of, 351
   relationships, 350
   theoretical, 351

T

T-scores, 243
T test, 437–438, 439, 448
Table of contents, 473, 474
Tables, 42, 60, 378, 385–395, 414
   clarity of, 385–386
   construction of, 390–393
   description of, 390
   format of, 392
   labelling, 392
   list of, 475
   parts of, 388–390
   for pilot studies, 393–395
   proportions, 390
   types of, 386–390
   vertical lines in, 390
TALENT project, 355–356
Tally marks, 417
Type recorder, use of 237–238, 312, 345
Taxonomy, 79
TDB (Toxicology Data Bank), 101
Techniques, research;
   see Research techniques
Telephone, use of, 313
Teletype, 411, 412
Terman, study of gifted children, 179
Tests, development of, 259–261
   discriminating, 259–260
   and experiments, 243
   standardized, 244
Test-retest, 257, 258
Testing, 241, 254
Text, 475
Thematic Apperception Test, 370
Theoretical approach, different from problem-solving, 75
Theoretical perspectives, 75–76
Theoretical reviews, 99
Theories, 75, 80, 85
   classified by use, 77
   comparisons of, 99
   empirical testing of, 77

   logical deduction of, 81
   parallel, 84
   summaries of, 99
Theoria, 74
Theoros, 74
Theory, 47, 48, 52, 66, 74–75, 80, 145, 146, 263, 378, 380, 459
   accepted or rejected, 76
   and approach, 48
   building of, 50, 77–79, 83
   and comparison, 81
   and data, 82
   development of, 75
   and observation, 73
   vs. speculation, 74
   empirical routes in, 74
   evaluation of, 83
   grounded, 81
   guiding research, 72
   and health sciences, 79–80
   and hypotheses, 47–50
   kinds of, 77
   and knowledge, 76–77, 84
   from library search, 79
   and metaphor, 78
   and method, 72–88
   by miniaturizing, 78
   from models, 79
   partial, 78
   and reality, 75
   and research, 73–74, 81, 84–86
   and schematic drawing, 78
   and serendipity, 81
   testing of, 80
   through taxonomy, 79
   effectiveness of, 77
   inductive construction, 77
Theory borrowing, 78
Theory extension, 78
Theory integration, 78
Theory reworking, 78
Thermometers, 39, 256
Theses, 469, 471
Third-person, 468
3 × 5 card, 94, 95, 96, 102, 109
Thurston scale, 352, 361
Time element, confounds research, 186
Time-series analysis, 180, 203
Time-series experiment, 194
Time sharing, 413

World Health Organization (WHO), 13
WHO, 30, 105, 321
WHO Export Committee on Nursing, 19
Writers, 26
Writing, 489–90
   mechanics of, 469–479
   scholarly, 93

Writing style, 109
Written records, 325

Z

Z scores, 243, 432–433